the portable internist

the portable internist

Anthony J. Zollo, Jr., MD
Assistant Professor of Clinical Medicine
Department of Medicine
Baylor College of Medicine
Houston, Texas
Chief Medical Officer
Department of Veteran's Affairs Outpatient Clinic
Lufkin, Texas

HANLEY & BELFUS, INC./ Philadelphia
MOSBY/ St. Louis • Baltimore • Boston • Chicago
London • Philadelphia • Sydney • Toronto

Publisher   HANLEY & BELFUS, INC.
              210 South 13th Street
              Philadelphia, PA 19107
              (215) 546-7293
              Fax (215) 790-9330

North American and Worldwide sales and distribution:

              MOSBY
              11830 Westline Industrial Drive
              St. Louis, MO 63146

In Canada: Times Mirror Professional Publishing Ltd.
              130 Flaska Drive
              Markham, Ontario L6G 1B8
              Canada

Library of Congress Cataloging-in-Publication Data

Zollo, Anthony J., 1954–
     The portable internist / Anthony J. Zollo, Jr.
        p.   cm.
     Includes bibliographical references and index.
     ISBN 1-56053-066-9
     1. Internal medicine—Handbooks, manuals, etc.   I. Title.
     (DNLM: 1. Internal Medicine—handbooks. WB 39 Z86p 1994)
RC55.Z65 1994
616—dc 20
DNLM/DLC
for Library of Congress   94-29734
                                                              CIP

The Portable Internist   ISBN 1-56053-066-9

Library of Congress catalog card number 94-29734

Last digit is the print number: 9 8 7 6 5 4 3 2 1

CONTENTS

CONTRIBUTORS

Ridha Arem, M.D.
Associate Professor, Division of Endocrinology and Metabolism, Department of Medicine, Baylor College of Medicine, Houston; Chief, Endocrinology Service, Harris County Hospital District; and Medical Director, Endocrine Laboratory, The Methodist Hospital, Houston, Texas

Carol M. Ashton, M.D., M.P.H.
Assistant Professor, Department of Medicine, Baylor College of Medicine, Houston; Staff Physician, General Medicine Section, Veteran's Affairs Medical Center, Houston, Texas

Mary Anne Doherty, M.D.
Associate Chief of Staff for Ambulatory Care, Edith Nourse Rogers Memorial Veteran's Hospital, Bedford, Massachusetts

Sheila Goodnight-White, M.D.
Assistant Professor, Department of Medicine, Baylor College of Medicine, Houston; Director, Ambulatory Care Education and Pulmonary Ambulatory Care Clinics, Medical Service, Veteran's Affairs Medical Center, Houston, Texas

Gabriel B. Habib, M.D., FACC
Director, Coronary Care Unit, and Assistant Chief, Section of Cardiology, Veteran's Affairs Medical Center, Houston, Texas

Richard J. Hamill, M.D.
Assistant Professor, Departments of Medicine and Microbiology/Immunology, Baylor College of Medicine, Houston; Associate Chief, Medical Service, Veteran's Affairs Medical Center, Houston, Texas

Mary P. Harward, M.D.
Assistant Professor, Department of Internal Medicine, University of Florida Health Sciences Center, Gainesville, Florida

Teresa G. Hayes, M.D.
Assistant Professor, Department of Medicine, Baylor College of Medicine, Houston; Staff Physician, Veteran's Affairs Medical Center, Houston, Texas

Sondra L. Khalil, M.D.
Staff Physician, Internal Medicine, Department of Veteran's Affairs Outpatient Clinic, Lufkin, Texas

Christopher J. Lahart, M.D.
Assistant Professor, Department of Medicine, Baylor College of Medicine, Houston; Chief, AIDS Unit, Veteran's Affairs Medical Center, Houston, Texas

Edward C. Lynch, M.D.
Professor and Associate Chairman, Department of Medicine, Baylor College of Medicine, Houston, Texas

Sharma S. Prabhakar, M.D.
Staff Nephrologist and Chief of Dialysis, Bronx Veteran's Affairs Medical Center, Bronx, New York

Loren A. Rolak, M.D.
Department of Neurosciences, The Marshfield Clinic, Marshfield, Wisconsin

Richard Alan Rubin, M.D.
Clinical Instructor, Division of Rheumatology, Department of Medicine, Baylor College of Medicine, Houston, Texas

Gary Trey, M.D.
Assistant Professor, Division of Gastroenterology, Department of Medicine, Baylor College of Medicine, Houston; Attending Physician, The Methodist Hospital, Houston, Texas

Mark M. Udden, M.D.
Associate Professor of Clinical Medicine, Department of Medicine, Baylor College of Medicine, Houston, Texas

Karen Woods, M.D.
Assistant Professor, Department of Medicine, Baylor College of Medicine, Houston; Chief, Therapeutic Endoscopy, Harris County Hospital District and The Methodist Hospital, Houston, Texas

Nelda P. Wray, M.D., M.P.H.
Associate Professor of Clinical Medicine, Department of Medicine, Baylor College of Medicine, Houston; Chief, General Medicine Section, Veteran's Affairs Medical Center, Houston, Texas

Anthony J. Zollo, Jr., M.D.
Assistant Professor of Clinical Medicine, Department of Medicine, Baylor College of Medicine, Houston; Chief Medical Officer, Department of Veteran's Affairs Outpatient Clinic, Lufkin, Texas

PREFACE

This book represents a distillation of the broad field of internal medicine. The goal was to cover a mix of important topics and to offer the reader a synthesis of the vast amount of information available. Obviously, this book is not intended to replace one of the "standard" textbooks of internal medicine, but rather it is meant to be a truly portable volume that the busy clinician, house officer, or student can consult throughout the day. It is intended to be carried on rounds, to the clinic, and all other areas as a ready source of key information. For further reading on any topic, we have provided references to key articles or textbooks. In the absence of such listing, the reader is referred to one of the standard textbooks.

This book, in keeping with The Portable Series, is arranged in alphabetical order to facilitate the rapid location of information. Because abbreviations are both ubiquitous and efficient, we have used them whenever practical. To avoid confusion, a glossary of abbreviations is included at the end of the book.

I wish to thank all of the contributors for their hard work and expertise. I would also like to thank Linda Belfus, our publisher, for her confidence and assistance. Finally, I would like to thank my wife, Mary B. Zollo, for reading and re-reading the manuscript during the editing process.

Anthony J. Zollo, M.D.
Houston, Texas

DEDICATION

To the memory of W. A. "Jim" Crow, III, M.D.

Our friend and colleague

A

ABDOMINAL AORTIC ANEURYSM

Abdominal aortic aneurysm (AAA) is defined as an aortic diameter greater than 3 cm below the renal arteries. About 95% of AAAs are infrarenal, but aneurysmal dilation of the abdominal aorta above the takeoff of the renal arteries is not that uncommon. The prevalence is 2% in those older than age 65, but 10% in those with HTN or CAD aged 60–75. AAAs are the tenth leading cause of death for men over 65.

Most AAAs are asymptomatic. They are often discovered by physical exam (abdominal exam is 50% sensitive, but with decreased sensitivity in the obese) or by abdominal ultrasound, x-ray, or CT performed for another indication. Rupture of an AAA produces symptoms of groin, back, or abdominal pain and shock. The mortality of rupture is greater than 50% with or without emergency surgery. The operative mortality rate in elective aneurysmectomy is less than 5% but doubles in patients older than age 75. Perioperative complications are those of coexistent CAD and cerebrovascular disease. The preoperative evaluation should focus on these areas.

The size of the AAA measured by ultrasound determines treatment:

- **If 3–4.4 cm in diameter:** Surveillance with abdominal ultrasound every 6 months.
- **If 4.5–6 cm in diameter:** Elective repair if life expectancy is greater than 10 years or surveillance with ultrasound every 6 months. If the diameter increases more than 0.5 cm/year or pain develops, then repair.
- **If greater than 6 cm:** Surgical repair is recommended because the risk of rupture is very high (up to 80%).

Recent Mayo Clinic experience demonstrated that with AAAs greater than 5 cm, the risk of rupture within 5 years was 25%; however, only 3% of AAAs less than 5 cm ruptured within 10 years. During the surveillance period, 25% were found to be "rapid expanders" (> 0.4 cm/yr) while the remaining 75% were found to be "slow expanders" (< 0.2 cm/yr).

References: Reuler JB, et al: Abdominal aortic aneurysms. J Gen Intern Med 6:360–366, 1991.

Nevitt MP, et al: Prognosis in abdominal aortic aneurysms. A population based study. N Engl J Med 321:1009–1014, 1989.

ABDOMINAL PAIN

Abdominal pain is a nebulous and perplexing symptom. The first and most basic principle is an accurate description of the pain, prompted by appropriate questions. The precipitating and ameliorating factors, character of the pain, level of acuity, and chronological progression all must be included in the depiction in order to give an accurate diagnosis. Lack of accurate characterization by either the physician or the patient is probably the most common cause of errors. Once the pain is characterized, it is usually fairly easy to classify it into several main areas and further narrow the diagnosis.

Pain with a short history may be infectious or vascular in origin, whereas pain of longer duration may be cancer or one of the inflammatory bowel diseases. Precipitating factors include food, toxins, allergens, and drugs. Pain of peritoneal inflammation is exacerbated by pressure or change in tension of the peritoneum. Pain from obstruction of hollow viscera is intermittent or colicky. Pain associated with occlusion of vascular structures of the abdomen may be sudden and diffuse, as with embolism, thrombosis, or rupture of an aneurysm, but may also be mild and continuous for several days prior to vascular collapse or peritoneal inflammation. Pain in the abdominal wall is usually constant and aching and aggravated by movement, while referred pain takes on the characteristics of its primary site. Referred pain from compression of nerve roots in the spine is exacerbated by coughing, sneezing, or straining, as well as by hyperesthesia over the involved dermatomes. Abdominal pain can also be referred from intrathoracic processes such as myocardial or pulmonary infarction, pneumonia, pericarditis, or esophageal disease. Physical exam in these situations will reveal a totally benign abdomen. Psychogenic pain usually shows no correlation between signs and symptoms and fits poorly into any diagnostic category.

The following table is useful to categorize abdominal pain:

Important Causes of Abdominal Pain

I. Pain originating in the abdomen
  A. Parietal peritoneal inflammation
    1. Bacterial contamination: perforated appendix, pelvic inflammatory disease.
    2. Chemical irritation: perforated ulcer, pancreatitis, mittelschmerz.
  B. Mechanical obstruction of hollow viscera: small or large intestine, biliary tree, ureter.
  C. Vascular disturbances: embolism, thrombosis, vascular rupture, pressure or torsional occlusions, sickle-cell anemia.
  D. Abdominal wall: distortion or traction of mesentery, trauma, infection of abdominal wall muscles.
II. Pain referred from extra-abdominal sources
  A. Thorax: pneumonia, referred pain from coronary occlusion.
  B. Spine: radiculitis from arthritis.
  C. Genitalia: torsion of the testes.
III. Metabolic causes
  A. Exogenous: black widow spider bite, lead and other poisonings.
  B. Endogenous: uremia, diabetic ketoacidosis, porphyria, allergic factors (C′1 esterase inhibitor deficiency).
IV. Neurogenic causes
  A. Organic: tabes dorsalis, herpes zoster, causalgia, others.
  B. Functional

Modified from Silen W: Abdominal pain. In Wilson JD, et al (eds): Harrison's Principles of Internal Medicine, 12th ed. New York, McGraw-Hill, 1991, p 105.

The physical exam will usually confirm the initial diagnostic impression. Absence of bowel sounds occurs with severe chemical peritonitis of sudden onset. Contrary to usual teachings, bowel sounds may be weak or normal in the presence of obstruction. Direct tenderness without rebound minimizes the possibility of peritoneal inflammation, while rebound tenderness increases that possibility. A rectal and, in females, a pelvic exam must be done in all patients with abdominal pain. When the exam is normal, attention should be paid to intrathoracic or genital disease.

Laboratory tests should include hematocrit and urinalysis to assist in determining the state of hydration of the patient and the presence of blood loss. Leukocytosis is often present, but a normal white count does not rule out intra-abdominal pathology. Plain and upright films of the abdomen are helpful in the diagnosis of obstruction. Air-fluid levels are seen with obstruction, and pneumoperitoneum may be seen with a perforated viscus. In chronic pain, CT or MRI scan of the abdomen may be helpful, although it must be cautioned that these imaging procedures are expensive and should not be used in place of the careful completion of a thorough history and physical exam.

ACETAMINOPHEN TOXICITY

Large doses of acetaminophen result in severe hepatotoxicity and ultimate death from acute liver failure. Ingestion of 15 grams or more is usually necessary to cause a severe or fatal reaction, but lower doses have been shown to be severely hepatotoxic in certain patients. To be effective, treatment to prevent hepatotoxicity must be initiated early in the course of the injury. It is important to attempt to learn the timing and dose of the ingestion. Since the dose ingested may not be reliably obtained from the suicidal or psychotic patient, determination of acetaminophen blood levels has been employed with some success and can be used to predict those patients in whom serious liver injury is likely to occur. The following graph can be used to determine the likelihood of hepatic toxicity based on the patient's acetaminophen plasma level and the time since ingestion:

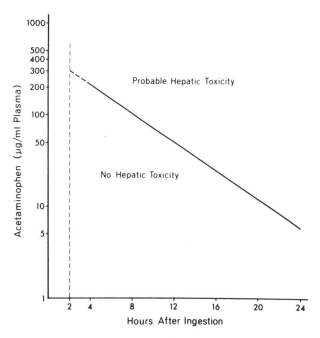

Plasma acetaminophen levels vs. time. (From Rumack BH, Matthew H: Acetaminophen poisoning and toxicity. Pediatrics 55:871, 1975, with permission.)

N-acetylcysteine (Mucomyst) is the drug of choice for treatment of acetaminophen overdose. It may be administered orally but has been shown to be effective only if treatment is initiated within the first 10–12 hours after ingestion. There are two clinical settings when the drug should be used:

1. When the patient's parameters, fitted to the above graph, indicate the patient is at risk, or
2. When blood acetaminophen levels are not rapidly available but there is good reason to believe that a significant overdose has occurred.

The initial dose is 140 mg/kg orally followed by maintenance doses of 70 mg/kg every 4 hours for a total of 72 hours. In addition, gastric contents should be lavaged free of any remaining pill fragments and the patient should be monitored closely hemodynamically. Over 90% of patients may be expected to recover completely if treated in the early phases after ingestion.

Reference: Bass NM, Ockner RK: Drug-induced liver disease. In Zakim D, Boyer T (eds): Hepatology. A Textbook of Liver Disease, 2nd ed. Philadelphia, W.B. Saunders, 1990, pp 754–791.

ACID-BASE DISORDERS

Metabolic Alkalosis

Metabolic alkalosis is an acid-base disturbance characterized by a primary increase in the plasma HCO_3^- level and an increase in the pH of the blood. It is a common acid-base disorder, which, when severe (pH >7.55), can be fatal. This is particularly true in surgical patients with multisystem failure.

Metabolic alkalosis is usually the result of loss of acid from the extracellular fluid (ECF) space, such as loss of H^+ from the stomach, from the kidneys, or internally into the cells. The secretion of HCl into the stomach leaves behind a cation and HCO_3^- in the ECF. Loss of HCl from the stomach leads to a proportionate rise in plasma HCO_3^-. In addition, the kidney secretes H^+, thus generating a HCO_3^- into the ECF, and when the latter exceeds the net acid production in the body, the HCO_3^- concentration in the plasma increases. In severe K^+ deficiency, the intracellular K^+ may shift into extracellular space to maintain a near normal ratio of K^+ in the ECF and intracellular fluid (ICF) compartments. The intracellular K^+ is then replaced by H^+ derived from carbonic acid in the ECF, which yields a HCO_3^- in the ECF, resulting in transient alkalosis. Sometimes metabolic alkalosis is due to the addition of HCO_3^- or its precursors, such as citrate, lactate, or acetate, at a rate greater than the net acid generation. In the presence of normal kidneys, most of such added alkali is excreted so that only mild alkalosis occurs.

The systemic adaptations of metabolic alkalosis are three-fold: First, there is buffering of systemic alkalemia in the body fluids by H^+ derived from intracellular phosphates and proteins. About one-third of excess HCO_3^- is thereby titrated. Second, there is respiratory adaptation in the form of hypoventilation resulting in secondary hypercapnia and hypoxia. The degree of respiratory adaptation is limited by the requirement for oxygen, since P_aO_2 will be reduced by hypoventilation, and therefore the P_aCO_2 rarely exceeds 55 mm Hg. Thus, if P_aCO_2 is normal or subnormal in metabolic alkalosis, a superimposed respiratory alkalosis is likely to be present. Third, renal compensation includes rapid excretion of excess HCO_3^- in the urine, resulting in normalization of plasma HCO_3^- concentration. The factors that impair this renal excretion of HCO_3^- in the urine, thereby perpetuating metabolic alkalosis, include severe ECF volume depletion, hyperaldosteronism, Cl^- depletion, K^+ depletion, and hypoventilation. Depending on the urinary Cl^- concentration and on the response to administration of Cl^- salts, metabolic alkalosis can be classified into two types: Cl^- responsive and Cl^- resistant.

Clinical manifestations of metabolic alkalosis include muscle cramps, weakness, and hyperreflexia. Alveolar hypoventilation can lead to signs of hypoxia. Severe metabolic alkalosis (pH > 7.6) is associated with cardiac arrhythmias, especially in those with a diseased heart.

Laboratory evaluation reveals increased plasma pH and HCO_3^-. Respiratory compensation will increase the P_aCO_2. Hypokalemia and hypochloremia are invari-

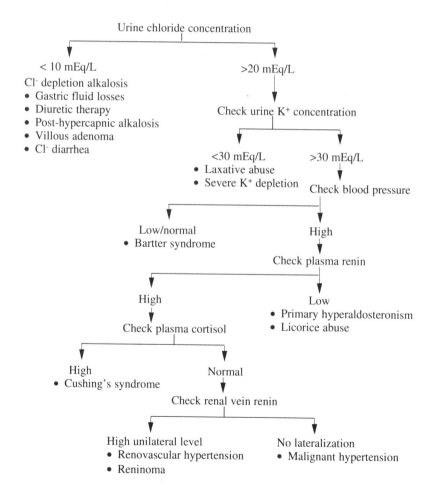

Diagnostic algorithm for metabolic alkalosis.

able accompaniments. Hypokalemia is usually due to renal K^+ losses as a result of enhanced distal K^+ secretion, which persists as long as metabolic alkalosis persists. Blood urea nitrogen and serum creatinine may be elevated if there is associated volume contraction. Urinary Cl^- concentration can be used as a marker to distinguish between Cl^--responsive and Cl^--resistant types of metabolic alkalosis. A spot urine Cl^- concentration of more than 20 mEq/L indicates that volume depletion is not a critical factor in the maintenance of alkalosis except when diuretics have been taken in the preceding 12 hours. The urine Na^+ concentration is often not helpful, since it may be increased during periods of bicarbonaturia despite volume contraction. Bicarbonaturia also increases renal K^+ loss.

Management depends on the etiology and the type of metabolic alkalosis. In all instances, the underlying disease process should be treated, but unlike the situation in metabolic acidosis, this alone would not ameliorate the acid-base disorder. For Cl^--sensitive alkalosis, treatment usually involves administration of NaCl solutions and K^+ to correct K^+ deficits. Patients with Cl^--resistant alkalosis and severe K^+ depletion may require large amounts of KCl before NaCl can be effective in correcting alkalosis. In addition, treatment of an excess mineralocorticoid state may require removal or ablation of secretory tumors or blockade of mineralocorticoid effects with spironolactone.

Additional forms of therapy may be needed in special situations. Gastric H_2 blockers like cimetidine or ranitidine are useful in preventing or treating metabolic alkalosis in patients with excessive nasogastric suction or Zollinger-Ellison syndrome. The carbonic anhydrase inhibitor acetazolamide is useful in patients with metabolic alkalosis and volume expansion (as seen in congestive heart failure). However, one should note that adequate K^+ supplementation may be needed with acetazolamide. Hemodialysis has been employed to correct metabolic alkalosis in patients with renal failure by using dialysate containing low HCO_3^- concentration. Occasionally, dilute HCl or NH_4Cl has been used to correct serious metabolic alkalosis rapidly in instances when NaCl administration would be too slow in correcting the disorder.

Reference: Galla JH, et al: Pathophysiology of metabolic alkalosis. Hosp Pract 22:95, 1987.

Mixed Disorders

A mixed acid-base disorder is said to exist when there is more than one primary acid-base disturbance. It could be a combination of one respiratory and one or two metabolic disorders or one metabolic and one or two respiratory disorders. Mixed acid-base disorders are suspected on the basis of clinical situation (e.g., a patient with cor pulmonale on diuretics or a uremic patient with vomiting), and the diagnosis is confirmed by some laboratory clues. If a given set of acid-base lab values falls out of range for an expected compensation of a given acid-base disorder, then a mixed disorder is suspected. A nomogram for interpreting acid-base values follows. A point falling outside the indicated predictive bands suggests a mixed acid-base disturbance.

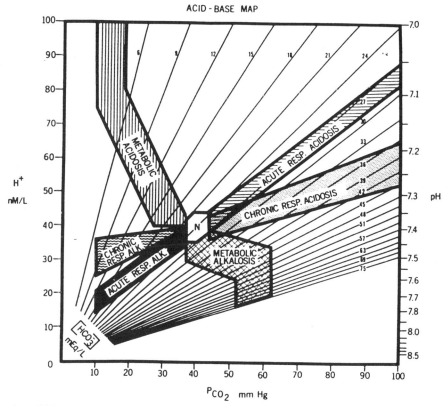

An acid-base nomogram with shaded areas representing the confidence limits after full compensation. (From Goldberg M, et al: Computer-based instruction and diagnosis of acid-base disorders. JAMA 223:269–275, 1973, with permission.)

Expected Compensation in Acid-Base Disorders

DISORDER	H^+	pH	(HCO_3^-)	P_aCO_2	COMPENSATION
Metabolic acidosis	↑	↓	↓↓	↓	P_aCO_2 ↓ 11–15 mm Hg per 10 mEq/L ↓ in HCO_3^-
Metabolic alkalosis	↓	↑	↑↑	↑	P_aCO_2 ↑ 6–7 mm Hg per 10 mEq/L ↑ in HCO_3^-
Respiratory acidosis	↑	↓	↑	↑↑	Acute: 1 mEq/L ↑ in HCO_3^- per 10 mm Hg ↑ P_aCO_2 Chronic: 3.5 mEq/L ↑ in HCO_3^- per 10 mm Hg ↑ P_aCO_2
Respiratory alkalosis	↓	↑	↓	↓↓	Acute: 2.5 mEq/L ↓ in HCO_3^- per 10 mm Hg ↑ P_aCO_2 Chronic: 5 mEq/L ↓ in HCO_3^- per 10 mm Hg ↓ P_aCO_2

Mixed Acid-Base Disorders

DISORDERS	ADAPTATION	pH
Inadequate response		
1. Metabolic acidosis and respiratory acidosis	P_aCO_2 too high and HCO_3^- too low for simple disorders	↓↓
2. Metabolic alkalosis and respiratory alkalosis	P_aCO_2 too low and HCO_3^- high for simple disorders	↑↑
Excessive response		
1. Metabolic acidosis and respiratory alkalosis	P_aCO_2 too low and HCO_3^- too low for simple disorders	Normal or slightly ↑ or ↓
2. Metabolic alkalosis and respiratory acidosis	P_aCO_2 too high and HCO_3^- too high for simple disorders	Normal or slightly ↑ or ↓
Triple disorders		
1. Metabolic alkalosis, metabolic acidosis, and either respiratory acidosis or alkalosis	P_aCO_2 and HCO_3^- not appropriate for simple disorders and anion gap >20 mEq/L	Variable

1. **Respiratory alkalosis and metabolic acidosis:** This combination is often seen in patients with septicemia, salicylate intoxication, hepatic failure with lactic acidosis, and hyperventilation with renal acidosis. Respiratory alkalosis lowers the P_aCO_2 below the range of respiratory compensation for the given degree of metabolic acidosis. The pH may be normal or near normal, and hence the disorder itself does not need treatment.

2. **Respiratory alkalosis and metabolic alkalosis:** This is probably the most common mixed acid-base disorder. Examples are seen in patients with hepatic failure who hyperventilate and/or use diuretics. The pH is markedly elevated while the plasma HCO_3^- is normal or elevated and the P_aCO_2 is variable. Treatment of the metabolic alkalosis with Na^+ or K^+ chloride solutions and correction of underlying respiratory disorder are necessary.

3. **Respiratory acidosis and metabolic alkalosis:** This situation is seen in patients with respiratory failure who retain CO_2 and develop congestive heart failure. When diuretics are given in such patients, the plasma HCO_3^- is elevated more than warranted for the degree of respiratory acidosis. The pH may be normal or slightly higher. Quite often, if the clinical information is not forthcoming, this combination could be falsely interpreted as a single primary acid-base disorder. The presence of a large A-a gradient (>15 mm Hg) often gives a clue to the underlying respiratory disorder.

4. **Respiratory acidosis and metabolic acidosis:** This is seen in patients with cardiorespiratory arrest and in patients with chronic lung disease who develop septic shock. The P_aCO_2 is high for the degree of metabolic acidosis, as the respiratory acidosis prevents the compensatory fall in P_aCO_2. Similarly, the elevation of HCO_3^- in response to respiratory acidosis is prevented by the presence of concomitant metabolic acidosis. The actual levels of P_aCO_2 and HCO_3^- are determined by the predominant acid-base disorder. The pH is, however, very low. Treatment should be directed against both of the disorders.

5. **Metabolic acidosis and metabolic alkalosis:** This is seen in patients with profound vomiting who develop volume depletion, shock, and lactic acidosis. The disorder is suspected in a patient with metabolic acidosis with inappropriately high anion gap.

· 6. **Triple acid-base disorders:** These are said to exist when a respiratory disorder supervenes in a patient with metabolic acidosis and alkalosis. As mentioned previously, the combined metabolic disorders generate a large anion gap while the superimposition of respiratory alkalosis in such a patient would decrease the P_aCO_2 below the level warranted for simple metabolic acidosis.

Renal Tubular Acidosis

Renal tubular acidosis (RTA) refers to those conditions in which metabolic acidosis results from decreased net tubular H^+ secretion despite normal or adequate renal function. In contrast, the acidosis in renal failure is characterized by normal or sometimes supranormal H^+ secretion per residual nephron or for a given GFR.

There are at least two major forms of RTA depending on the site of defect: the proximal (type II) and the distal. Distal RTA is divided into hypokalemic (type I) and hyperkalemic (type IV) varieties. Hyperkalemic RTA is due to a specific tubular defect or hypoaldosteronism.

Causes of Renal Tubular Acidosis

DISTAL	PROXIMAL (TYPE II)
Hypokalemic or normokalemic (type I)	Primary
Primary	Outdated tetracycline
Nephrocalcinosis	Cystinosis
Multiple myeloma	Wilson's disease
Hepatic cirrhosis	Lead toxicity
Lupus erythematosus	Cadmium toxicity
Amphotericin B	Amyloidosis
Lithium	Multiple myeloma
Toluene	Nephrotic syndrome
Renal transplant rejection	Early renal transplant injury
Medullary sponge kidney	Medullary cystic disease
Hyperkalemic (type IV)	
Hypoaldosteronism	
Obstructive nephropathy	
Sickle-cell nephropathy	
Lupus erythematosus	
Cyclosporine nephrotoxicity	

Pathophysiology

Proximal RTA results from decreased HCO_3^- reabsorption in the proximal tubule. Normally about 85% of HCO_3^- is reabsorbed in the proximal tubule and the remaining 15% is reabsorbed in the distal tubule. The HCO_3^- level falls due to increased fractional excretion of HCO_3^-. Eventually the plasma HCO_3^- falls to a level at which all the filtered HCO_3^- that is presented to the distal tubule is entirely reabsorbed. This causes the urine pH to fall below 5.5; the systemic acidosis remains mild (HCO_3^- approx. 15 mEq/L) and stable.

Distal RTA can result from several mechanisms. Decreased ammonium excretion plays a major role in the hyperkalemic RTA of hypoaldosteronism. Urine ammonium is measured by urine anion gap:

$$\text{Anion gap} = \text{Urine Cl}^- - (\text{Urine Na}^+ + \text{Urine K}^+)$$

Damage to the H^+ pump in the collecting tubule is responsible for RTA in urinary obstruction and medullary sponge kidney, while amphotericin causes back-leak of H^+ or H_2CO_3. There are incomplete forms of RTA in which acidosis is mild.

Clinical Features

Distal RTA (type I) clinically presents as musculoskeletal weakness or pain, recurrent renal stones, and nephrocalcinosis. In children, complete forms can present with severe acidosis and hypokalemia (often presenting as periodic paralysis). Proximal RTA presents in children with growth retardation, rickets, vomiting, volume depletion, and lethargy. Hyperkalemic RTA (type IV) is characterized by mild to moderate metabolic acidosis and hyperkalemia disproportionate to the degree of renal failure. Most patients have diabetes mellitus or interstitial nephritis, a creatinine clearance of less than 45 ml/min, and a serum K^+ of greater than 5.5 mEq/L. Other features are shown in the following table:

Laboratory and Clinical Features of RTA

	DISTAL			PROXIMAL
	Hypokalemic	Hyperkalemic		
		Tubular Defect	Hypoaldosteronism	
Low serum HCO_3^-	Common	Common	Common	Always
Serum K^+	Decreased	Increased	Increased	Decreased
Renal stones and nephrocalcinosis	Common	Rare	Very rare	Rare
Bone disease	Common	Rare	Very rare	Common
UpH after NH_4Cl	>5.4	>5.4	<5.5	<5.5
UP_aCO_2 after $NaHCO_3$	<60	<60	>70	>70
FE HCO_3^-	<5%	<5%	<5%	>15%

UpH = urinary pH, UP_aCO_2 = urinary P_aCO_2, FE HCO_3^- = fractional excretion of HCO_3^-.

Therapy

Distal RTA (type I) requires oral HCO_3^- supplementation of 1–2 mEq/kg/day to correct the acidosis. Potassium citrate is often needed to treat hypokalemia. Proximal RTA requires much higher doses (10–15 mEq/kg/day) to correct the defect. As the FE HCO_3^- increases, it promotes kalliuresis and causes severe hypokalemia. Rickets is corrected by vitamin D and sodium phosphate. Hyperkalemic RTA often can be managed by a combination of dietary restriction of K^+, use of diuretics, and small doses of HCO_3^- as in type I RTA. Only in some cases is replacement of mineralocorticoids (fludrocortisone) needed.

References: Rocher LL, et al: The clinical spectrum of renal tubular acidosis. Annu Rev Med 39:319, 1986.

Battle DC, et al: The use of urinary anion gap in the diagnosis of hyperchloremic metabolic acidosis. N Engl J Med 318:594, 1988.

Respiratory Acidosis

Respiratory acidosis is an acid-base disturbance characterized by a primary increase in P_aCO_2 and an increase in the plasma pH and carbonic acid concentration. The increase in P_aCO_2 is primarily because of decreased elimination rather than increased production.

Pathophysiology

The increased carbonic acid concentration as a result of retained CO_2 is buffered primarily by hemoglobin and phosphates. This results in a small increase in plasma HCO_3^-. The renal response to respiratory acidosis consists of increased H^+ secretion, regenerating HCO_3^- in the plasma, and increased Cl^- excretion. Thus, the compensatory result is an elevation of plasma HCO_3^- along with a reduction of plasma Cl^- concentration. The anion gap is unaffected. The acidosis causes a shift of serum Na^+ and H^+ into the cells while the K^+ moves out of the cells. This causes an elevation of serum K^+.

Causes of Respiratory Acidosis

ACUTE	CHRONIC
Neuromuscular abnormalities	Neuromuscular abnormalities
Brain stem injury	Chronic narcotic or sedative ingestion
High cord injury	Primary hypoventilation
Guillain-Barré syndrome	Pickwickian syndrome
Myasthenia gravis	Poliomyelitis
Botulism	Diaphragmatic paralysis
Narcotic, sedative, or tranquilizer over-dose	Thoracic-pulmonary disorders
Airway obstruction	Chronic obstructive pulmonary disease
Foreign body	Kyphoscoliosis
Aspiration of vomitus	End-stage interstitial pulmonary disease
Laryngeal edema	
Severe bronchospasm	
Thoracic-pulmonary disorders	
Flail chest	
Pneumothorax	
Severe pneumonia	
Smoke inhalation	
Severe pulmonary edema	
Vascular disease	
Massive pulmonary embolism	
Respirator-controlled ventilation	
Inadequate frequency, tidal volume settings	
Large dead space	
Total parenteral nutrition (increased CO_2 production)	

Clinical and Systemic Effects

In acute respiratory acidosis, hypoxemia—which often accompanies the hypercapnia—predominates the picture. Patients usually have tachypnea, restlessness, and altered mental status. They may become comatose. In chronic respiratory acidosis there are few signs of CO_2 retention. Most often papilledema and findings of the underlying pulmonary disease predominate.

Laboratory Features

In acute respiratory acidosis there is elevation of P_aCO_2 and plasma HCO_3^- and a low pH. P_aO_2 is often decreased, while plasma Na^+, K^+, and Cl^- are often normal. In chronic respiratory acidosis, arterial pH is never less than 7.25, despite severe CO_2 retention. The anion gap is normal and the plasma electrolytes are normal except for a slightly decreased plasma Cl^-.

Therapy

Restoration of adequate ventilation is the mainstay of treatment. The acidosis is usually managed with moderate amounts of $NaHCO_3^-$ until definitive therapy is effective. Since HCO_3^- equilibrates across the blood-brain barrier more slowly than CO_2 does, there may be initial intracerebral acidosis. Chronic respiratory acidosis is often impossible to reverse completely due to the nature of underlying pulmonary pathology. Supportive measures such as pulmonary toilet and the treatment of respiratory infections or CHF can alleviate the symptoms significantly. The acidosis per se is quite often inconsequential except when it causes venous constriction and cardiac decompensation following fluid administration. The prognosis is that of the underlying chronic pulmonary disease.

Reference: Malony D, et al: Respiratory acid-base disorders. In Kokko JP, et al (eds): Fluid and Electrolytes, 2nd ed. Philadelphia, W.B. Saunders, 1990.

Respiratory Alkalosis

Respiratory alkalosis is an acid-base disturbance characterized by a primary decrease in P_aCO_2 and a rise in pH of the blood. This often results from alveolar hyperventilation, which could be due to central or peripheral neural stimulation, increased ventilation from mechanical ventilators, or increased conscious effort.

Causes of Respiratory Alkalosis

Increased CNS drive for respiration
    Anxiety—hyperventilation
    CNS infection/infarction/trauma/tumor
    Drugs—salicylates/nicotine/aminophylline
    Fever/sepsis—especially gram-negative sepsis
    Pregnancy/progesterone
    Liver disease
    Pain
Increased stimulation of chemoreceptors
    Anemia, asthma
    Carbon monoxide toxicity
    Pulmonary edema/pneumonia
    Pulmonary emboli
    Interstitial lung disease
    Reduced, inspired O_2 tension—high altitude
Increased mechanical ventilation—iatrogenic
    Multiple mechanisms
    Hepatic insufficiency
    Gram-negative sepsis

Pathophysiology

The acute response to respiratory alkalosis consists of buffering by intracellular proteins. The plasma HCO_3^- must be decreased to normalize the pH in the face of decreased P_aCO_2 by the following net reaction:

$$H^+ + HCO_3^- \longrightarrow CO_2 + H_2O$$

The H^+ is released from the intracellular buffers. Buffering is completed in a few minutes and persists for a few hours. The renal adaptation constitutes the chronic response to respiratory alkalosis. This is accomplished by decreased HCO_3^- reabsorption leading to bicarbonaturia or decreased NH_4^+ and titratable acid excretion, resulting in diminished net acid excretion. The decreased NH_4^+ excretion is compensated by the excretion of Na^+ and K^+ ions. The renal compensation starts in a few hours and is completed in 1–2 days, after which the excretion of these electrolytes returns to normal and a new steady state is established. A general rule of thumb is that the decrease in plasma HCO_3^- in acute respiratory alkalosis is 1–3 mEq/L for each 10 mm Hg decrease in P_aCO_2, and in chronic respiratory alkalosis, 2–5 mEq/L for each 10-mm Hg decrement below a normal P_aCO_2 of 40 mm Hg.

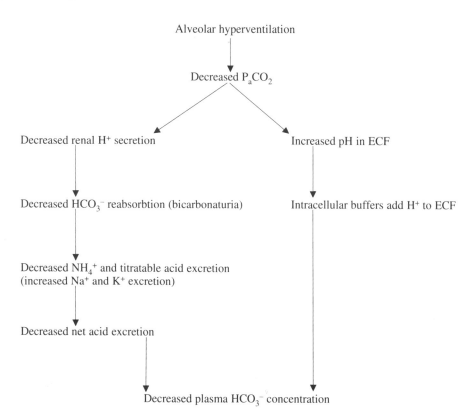

Clinical Features

Clinically, neuromuscular stimulation and irritability result from respiratory alkalosis, manifesting as paresthesia, cramps, hyperreflexia, tetany, and seizures. Chvostek's and Trousseau's signs can also be elicited. Atrial and ventricular tachyarrhythmias are seen with severe alkalosis.

Laboratory Features

Respiratory alkalosis is characterized by elevation of pH and decreased P_aCO_2 and HCO_3^-. There is a slight increase in plasma Cl^- and a slight reduction in plasma K^+ and phosphate concentration. Urine pH may be alkaline in the acute hypocapnic stage. There may also be an increase in the plasma lactate concentration.

Therapy

The mainstay is to treat the underlying disorder. Correction of hypoxemia often ameliorates the symptoms. In patients with hyperventilation syndrome, breathing into a large paper bag held over the nose and mouth may cause disappearance of signs and symptoms. In cases when alkalosis is secondary to mechanical hyperventilation, decreasing the minute ventilation, increasing the dead space, or use of an inhaled gas mixture containing 3% CO_2 is helpful for short periods of time. It is necessary that the P_aCO_2 be restored to normal rather slowly so that the compensatory metabolic acidosis does not result in a dangerously low pH.

ACLS PRINCIPLES

Cardiac Arrest

Principal factors influencing chances for successful resuscitation

1. Quick application of defibrillation for ventricular fibrillation (VF) or pulseless ventricular tachycardia (VT).
2. Institution of effective CPR with establishment of a secure airway (preferably endotracheal intubation) and administration of 100% oxygen.
3. Use of epinephrine in dosages sufficient to maintain coronary and cerebral perfusion.
4. Prognosis with cardiac asystole is poor.

Principles for managing cardiac arrest

1. Initiate CPR and call for help.
2. With arrival of resuscitation team and equipment:
   a. Place patient on cardiac board.
   b. Insert oral airway and ventilate mouth-to-mask or bag-to-mask with 100% oxygen.
   c. Continue chest compression.

3. Assess patient, get history of events leading to cardiac arrest, assign tasks to helpers (team members).
4. Apply quick-look paddles as soon as available to determine cardiac rhythm.
5. If the rhythm is VF or pulseless VT, proceed to immediate electrical defibrillation using ACLS algorithm. In this algorithm, three sequential attempts are made to defibrillate using 200 joules, then 200–300 joules and 360 joules. If unsuccessful, one proceeds with other measures sequentially with 0.5–1.0 mg epinephrine (1:10,000) IV, intubation, further attempts at electrical defibrillation, lidocaine 1 mg/kg IV, more defibrillation, and then bretylium followed by defibrillation.
6. Establish venous access with antecubital or preferably a central vein.
7. Endotracheal intubation: check tube position, hyperventilate, and oxygenate. Do not interrupt CPR more than 30 seconds to intubate.
8. Administration of drugs for the cardiac rhythm problem: VF or VT resistant to defibrillation, cardiac asystole, bradycardia.
9. Frequent reassessment of:
   a. Pulse generated by CPR.
   b. Appearance of spontaneous pulse after intervention.
   c. Adequacy of ventilation.
   d. Development of spontaneous breathing after return of pulse.
   e. Blood pressure if spontaneous pulse is present.
10. Draw blood specimens for: arterial blood gases, BUN, serum creatinine, electrolytes, other blood studies as needed.
11. Keep accurate records of entire resuscitation effort.
12. Control the crowd at bedside.

Reference: American Heart Association: Chapter 16. Putting It All Together: Resuscitation of the Patient. In Textbook of Advanced Cardiac Life Support, 2nd ed. Dallas, American Heart Association, 1990.

ACNE

Acne vulgaris presents as open comedones (called "blackheads" because of the black keratin plug at the lesion's center), closed comedones, and inflammatory papules and cysts. Papules are less than 1 cm in diameter and cysts are greater than 1 cm in diameter. Acne commonly occurs on the face, neck, shoulders, upper arms, and back. It is most common in adolescence but can continue until the age of 40. Acne flares may occur just before menses in menstruating women but improve during pregnancy. The lesions usually resolve within 7–10 days but sometimes leave scars and color changes.

Therapy for mild to moderate acne (comedones and small pustules) includes daily skin cleansing. Women should avoid oil-based cosmetics. Keratin plugs can be removed through peeling agents such as 5% benzoyl peroxide that are available over the counter. Benzoyl peroxide should be applied nightly after skin cleansing. If 5% benzoyl peroxide is ineffective after a week of use, it can be applied twice daily, or a 10% strength can be used. Mild erythema and chapping predictably occur, and patients need to be advised about these side effects.

For patients who do not respond to benzoyl peroxide, retinoic acid may help. A 0.025% gel of retinoic acid is available by prescription (Retin-A). It is usually applied nightly, but the strength and application frequency can be increased as needed. Combination therapy with daily benzoyl peroxide and nightly retinoic acid may help severe cases.

Patients with pustules require antibiotics. Men can take 1,000 mg erythromycin daily, although tetracycline and its derivatives such as doxycycline and minocycline can also be used. Patients using tetracyclinelike agents should be warned about the possibility of phototoxic reactions. Women frequently develop vaginal candidiasis with use of daily oral antibiotics. Topical antibiotics such as 1.5–2% erythromycin or 1% clindamycin used twice daily can be prescribed for female patients. Some prescription preparations combine benzoyl peroxide and an antibiotic in one topically applied agent. Other therapies available for the most severe cases of acne include birth control therapy for women and 13-*cis*-retinoic acid (Accutane). These agents should be used under the guidance of a dermatologist.

ACROMEGALY

Acromegaly is a condition resulting from excess secretion of growth hormone from the anterior pituitary, where somatotrophs constitute more than 50% of the cell population. Release of growth hormone from the pituitary is controlled by two hypothalamic factors: growth hormone-releasing hormone (GHRH), which stimulates its release, and somatostatin, which inhibits its release. Linear growth depends on the action of growth hormone to stimulate the production of somatomedins such as somatomedin C (insulinlike growth factor), which is produced primarily in the liver. If growth hormone hypersecretion occurs prior to puberty, gigantism results. If it occurs after puberty, acromegaly results.

Most cases of acromegaly are caused by pituitary macroadenomas. The condition is uncommon, with a reported prevalence of 40 cases per million. Less than 1% of cases are GHRH induced. These are sometimes associated with bronchial carcinoids and pancreatic islet cell tumors and rarely hypothalamic gangliocytomas. Symptoms are as follows:

Manifestations of Acromegaly

LOCATION	SYMPTOMS	SIGNS
General	Fatigue Increased sweating Heat intolerance Weight gain	—
Skin and subcutaneous tissue	Enlarging hands and feet Coarsening facial features Oily skin Hypertrichosis	Moist, warm, doughy hand-shake Skin tags Acanthosis nigricans Increased heel pad
Head	Headaches	Parotid enlargement, frontal bossing
Eyes	Decreased vision	Visual field defects
Ears	—	Otoscope speculum cannot be inserted
Nose-throat-paranasal sinuses	Sinus congestion Increased tongue size Malocclusion Voice change	Enlarged furrowed tongue Tooth marks on tongue Widely spaced teeth Prognathism

Table continued on next page.

Manifestations of Acromegaly (Cont.)

LOCATION	SYMPTOMS	SIGNS
Neck	—	Goiter
		Obstructive sleep apnea
		Enlarged sinuses
Cardiorespiratory system	CHF	Hypertension
		Cardiomegaly
		Left ventricular hypertrophy
GU system	Decreased libido	—
	Impotence	
	Oligomenorrhea	
	Infertility	
	Kidney stones	
Neurologic system	Paresthesias	Carpal tunnel syndrome
	Hypersomnolence	
Muscles	Weakness	Proximal myopathy
Skeletal system	Joint pains (shoulders, back, and knees)	Osteoarthritis

From Daniels GH, et al: Neuroendocrine regulation and diseases of the anterior pituitary and hypothalamus. In Wilson JD, et al (eds): Harrison's Principles of Internal Medicine, 12th ed. New York, McGraw-Hill, 1991, p 1662, with permission.

The best screening test involves measuring serum growth hormone levels 60–120 minutes after the ingestion of 100 gm of glucose (a normal level is < 2 µg/L). Random growth hormone testing is unreliable, since the hormone level may be elevated in normal individuals. Conventional skull or sella turcica views usually detect the responsible pituitary tumor, but CT or MRI is necessary to delineate tumor size prior to institution of therapy. Additional testing for hypopituitarism, possible MEN type 1 syndrome (hyperparathyroidism and pancreatic islet cell tumors), and elevated prolactin levels should also be performed. Acromegaly has been reported in association with pheochromocytomas or hyperaldosteronism.

Successful therapy aims at lowering the growth hormone level below 2 µg/L while maintaining normal pituitary function. Transsphenoidal surgery can realize these goals rapidly, especially for patients with preoperative growth hormone values less than 40 µg/L. Radiation therapy works more slowly and may lead to the development of hypopituitarism in up to 50% of patients so treated. Bromocriptine used alone is infrequently successful in lowering growth hormone levels below 5 µg/L but may help relieve clinical symptoms when used as adjunctive therapy. Octreotide is a long-acting analogue of somatostatin that may find usefulness as either primary or adjunctive therapy, but it has the drawback of requiring subcutaneous injections every 6–8 hours.

ADDISONIAN CRISIS

Addisonian crisis should be considered when hypotension and peripheral vasoconstriction occur in a patient who has either a history of chronic adrenal insufficiency or one of the known causes of adrenal insufficiency. In most patients, the stigmata of chronic adrenal insufficiency are present and the crisis has been precipitated by either the failure to take the glucocorticoid replacement or an intercurrent illness (e.g., infection or major stress). Clinical features include weakness and abdominal pain, nausea, diarrhea, hypotension, fever, clouded sensorium, and dehydration. Shock can occur in severe cases. The prostration is often out of proportion to the severity of the intercurrent illness.

Acute adrenal crisis occurs rarely in a patient without the stigmata of chronic adrenal insufficiency. Addisonian crisis may also occur in patients with pituitary or hypothalamic disease (e.g., pituitary apoplexy) or in patients receiving chronic glucocorticoid therapy who have not had the dose adjusted to cover an intercurrent illness.

Common laboratory findings include hypoglycemia, electrolyte imbalance (e.g., hyponatremia, hyperkalemia), hypercalcemia, metabolic acidosis, and prerenal azotemia.

The diagnosis is often one of suspicion. If an acute Addisonian crisis is suspected on clinical grounds, immediate tests such as BUN, electrolytes, blood glucose, CBC, and plasma cortisol should be drawn and glucocorticoid therapy initiated. A cortisol level of less than 25 µg/dl during stress is of little diagnostic value, and further dynamic testing should be carried out to definitely exclude the diagnosis. In the meantime, steroid replacement should be continued using dexamethasone, which does not measure in cortisol assays. Further investigation should also be carried out to determine the etiology of the crisis and other possible associated endocrine abnormalities.

The treatment of acute adrenal insufficiency should include high doses of IV glucocorticoids (200–300 mg/24 hr, hydrocortisone or equivalent), and an IV infusion of saline. Mineralocorticoids may also be necessary. Clinical improvement should be noticed within 3 hours after initiation of therapy. As the patient's condition improves, the dose of steroids is gradually tapered down to maintenance requirements.

ADENOPATHY

Differential Diagnosis and Evaluation

A normal lymph node is less than 1 cm in diameter, freely mobile within a restricted area, and nontender and firm without being hard. Thus, in the normal state, lymph nodes are barely, if at all, palpable. Enlargement of lymph nodes may occur either due to proliferation of cells normally present within the node or due to infiltration by other cells (e.g., malignant). Nodal enlargement can be a presenting sign in a wide variety of medical conditions. Enlargement of lymph nodes in a particular area is often a sign of a local, or regional, process involving the area drained by those nodes. More generalized adenopathy, involving nodes at two or more sites not serving the same area of the body, is a sign of a systemic, or generalized, process.

Localized adenopathy should prompt an evaluation of the structures that drain into the involved nodes. Some nodes are classically described in certain conditions, such as Virchow's node (a left supraclavicular node indicating a possible intraabdominal malignancy). Proper evaluation requires a working knowledge of the anatomic drainage patterns. Most frequently, the etiology is discerned after a directed history and physical examination. Local axillary node enlargement is often explained by trauma to the upper extremities such as minor abrasions, insect bites, and localized cellulitis. Similar etiologies exist for the inguinal nodes and the lower extremities, but sexually transmitted diseases are included in the list. At times the involved nodes may not be palpable but may be picked up by radiographic studies. In these cases, the adenopathy may actually assist in forming a better differential diagnosis. For example, a patient with pneumonia seen on a chest x-ray may have a pulmonary infiltrate without characteristics that aid the clinician in determining whether the cause is viral, bacterial, or mycobacterial. The presence of hilar adenopathy, however, may be more suggestive of a mycobacterial etiology. This distinction can be even more helpful in a patient infected with HIV, when hilar adenopathy would be unusual for PCP but may be the only clue toward TB.

Generalized adenopathy can be more difficult to evaluate, since one is not afforded the luxury of focusing on a particular body site. Causes of generalized adenopathy can be listed under three main categories: infectious, neoplastic, and others. Although these categories also pertain to localized adenopathy, the conditions within the categories are dramatically different, as shown in the table that follows. A close examination of the causes reveals many of these conditions to be readily diagnosed with a thorough history and physical exam accompanied by basic laboratory studies often including serologic tests. Several of the more common disorders are also of a self-limited nature, highlighting the need for careful history taking and patience in the requesting of invasive testing. Only in the minority of cases is a lymph node biopsy necessary.

Causes of Generalized Lymphadenopathy*

Infections†

Bacterial
  Scarlet fever
  Syphilis
  Brucellosis
  Leptospirosis
  Tuberculosis
  Atypical mycobacterial infection
  (Melioidosis)
  (Glanders)
Parasitic
  Toxoplasmosis
  (Kala-azar)
  (Chagas' disease)
  (African trypanosomiasis)
  (Filariasis)
Fungal
  Histoplasmosis

Viral
  EBV and CMV
    Infectious mononucleosis syndrome
  Hepatitis B
  Measles
  Rubella
  HIV
    AIDS-related complex
    AIDS
  (Dengue fever)
  (West Nile fever)
  (Epidemic hemorrhagic fevers)
  (Lassa fever)
Rickettsial
  (Scrub typhus)

Miscellaneous
  Sarcoidosis
  Other chronic granulomatous diseases
  SLE
  RA
  Hyperthyroidism
  Lipid storage diseases
  Generalized dermatitis
  Serum sickness
  Phenytoin administration

Neoplasms
  Lymphoma
  Acute lymphocytic leukemia
  Chronic lymphocytic leukemia
  Other chronic lymphoproliferative
    disorders
  Immunoblastic lymphadenopathy
  Reticuloendothelioses

*Parentheses indicate infections that are uncommon or not reported in the united States.

†Other infections that characteristically produce regional lymphadenopathy (e.g., tularemia, Lyme disease, lymphogranuloma venereum) may rarely cause generalized lymphadenopathy.

From Libman H: Generalized lymphadenopathy. J Gen Intern Med 2:48–58, 1987, with permission.

ADRENAL INSUFFICIENCY

Signs, Symptoms, and Laboratory Evaluation

The two most common causes of adrenal insufficiency are autoimmune adrenalitis and tuberculosis (TB). In developing countries, TB may be more prevalent than autoimmune adrenalitis. Autoimmune Addison's disease is often part of the polyendocrine deficiency syndrome type I and type II. Type I is an illness of childhood characterized by adrenal insufficiency, hypoparathyroidism, and mucocutaneous candidiasis and may include hypogonadism, pernicious anemia, chronic active hepatitis, and alopecia. Type II is a disorder of young adults. It is characterized by the presence of adrenal insufficiency, autoimmune thyroid disease, and insulin-dependent diabetes mellitus.

Causes of Adrenal Insufficiency

ETIOLOGY (OCCURRENCE, %)

I. Primary adrenal insufficiency
 A. Autoimmune (70%)
 B. Tuberculosis (20%)
 C. Others (10%)
  1. AIDS
   syndrome
  2. Fungal infections
  3. Adrenal hemorrhage
  4. Amyloidosis
  5. Sarcoidosis
  6. Congenital adrenal hyperplasia
  7. Hemochromatosis
  8. Adrenoleukodystrophy
  9. Adrenomyeloneuropathy
  10. Metastatic neoplasia
  11. Congenital unresponsiveness to ACTH
II. Secondary adrenal insufficiency
 A. Adrenal suppression from exogenous glucocorticoids or ACTH
 B. Following cure of Cushing's syndrome (removal of endogenous glucocorticoid excess)
 C. Hypothalamic and pituitary lesions

The clinical features of chronic adrenal insufficiency are often vague. The most characteristic manifestation is increased pigmentation, which is present in more than 90% of the cases. It is more readily seen in areas exposed to light or pressure, such as the face, the back of the hands, elbows and knees, buccal mucosa, conjunctiva, nails, and skin creases. Other manifestations include:

- Weakness
- Anorexia
- Vague abdominal pain
- Postural hypotension (dizziness, fainting)
- Hypoglycemia
- Weight loss
- Nausea
- Diarrhea or constipation
- Impaired ability to recover from physical and surgical stress
- Salt craving

The most widely used initial diagnostic tests for primary adrenal insufficiency are the measurement of early morning plasma cortisol and plasma ACTH levels, the short ACTH stimulation test (250 µg of IV cosyntropin), and measurement of cortisol at 0, 45, and 60 minutes postinjection. An inappropriately elevated plasma ACTH level is often indicative of primary adrenal insufficiency. The lack of cortisol response to ACTH stimulation does not distinguish primary from secondary insufficiency. A normal response of cortisol to ACTH is defined by an increment of at least 7 µg/dl and an absolute cortisol value exceeding 18 µg/dl.

The diagnosis of primary adrenal insufficiency is confirmed by a prolonged ACTH stimulation test (infusion of 800 µg ACTH/day for 2 days) and measurement of 24-hour urine 17-hydroxy steroids and 17-ketosteroids, prior to and after ACTH stimulation. Plasma cortisol levels increase after several hours of prolonged ACTH stimulation in secondary adrenal insufficiency and remain low in primary adrenal insufficiency. Patients who received glucocorticoids for more than 4 weeks within the past year should have an ACTH stimulation test to determine if they will require glucocorticoid treatment during stress or surgery. Other laboratory features are:

- Normocytic normochromic anemia
- Eosinophilia and relative lymphocytosis
- Hypercalcemia
- Hyponatremia
- Prerenal azotemia
- Fasting hypoglycemia

CT scan or ultrasound of the adrenal glands may be helpful in establishing the cause of adrenal insufficiency. The finding of large adrenal glands suggests a primary adrenal insufficiency (autoimmune, amyloidosis, granulomatous, and metastatic disease). The presence of adrenal calcifications usually suggests TB. Atrophic glands suggest idiopathic and autoimmune causes.

ADRENAL TUMORS AND MASSES

Adrenal masses and tumors are very common, occurring in 2–8% of the adult population in autopsy series. Adrenal masses in the adult may be:

- Cortical adenomas
- Pheochromocytomas
- Cysts
- Adenolipomas
- Cortical carcinomas
- Ganglioneuromas
- Myelolipomas
- Metastases from other tumors

CT scan is the preferred method for imaging of the adrenals. It can detect 99% of normal left adrenal glands and 95% of normal right adrenals. The current resolution ability of CT scan allows visualization of masses as small as 1 cm in diameter. The attenuation coefficient of the mass may also provide an indication as to the nature of the mass.

MRI is slightly less reliable than CT scan at defining normal adrenal glands. However, the ability of MRI to recognize adrenal abnormalities is comparable to that of CT scan. MRI may become the procedure of choice for initial localization of pheochromocytoma. It also may be useful in the differential diagnosis of adrenal masses, because it can distinguish benign adenomas from morphologically identical metastatic disease, adrenal carcinomas, and pheochromocytomas.

The third technique used for imaging is a **venogram,** which can be combined with selected adrenal venous sampling and is very useful in functioning adrenal masses (e.g., an aldosteronoma, or an adrenal tumor producing glucocorticoids). However, adrenal venography can cause the rupture of the adrenal vein and infarction of the gland in 2–10% of the cases.

Because of the frequent use of abdominal CT scan, unsuspected adrenal tumors are detected in approximately 1% of all the scans performed. Less than 10% of asymptomatic adrenal masses are functional. An adrenal carcinoma is seldom less than 3 cm in diameter, whereas an adrenal adenoma is seldom greater than 6 cm. About 30–50% of carcinomas are nonfunctional.

If a mass was originally discovered on CT scan, an MRI may be helpful in providing information concerning the presence or absence of a malignant lesion. Even though most adrenal masses discovered on CT scan are nonfunctioning, evaluation of function is required.

The extent of the endocrine evaluation is controversial. Measurement of DHEA-S; an overnight dexamethasone suppression test; 24-hour-urine measurement of cortisol, catecholamines, and metanephrines; and dynamic tests for hyperaldosteronism are recommended, although a more limited testing battery may be sufficient. If endocrine evaluation is negative, a conservative approach is usually taken when the tumor is less than 4 cm. A repeat CT scan 3–6 months later should be performed and surgery is indicated if there is evidence of growth. If the size remains unchanged, another CT scan is done one year later. If the mass is greater than 6 cm, surgery is indicated because of the high incidence of carcinoma in large adrenal tumors. No additional therapeutic or diagnostic intervention is recommended if the radiologic procedure is diagnostic of an adrenal myelolipoma or cyst or if the patient is known to have metastatic disease from a known primary.

Fine-needle aspiration has a limited value. In cystic lesions, clear fluid is usually associated with a benign lesion; bloody fluid may be due to either a benign or a malignant lesion.

Reference: Copeland PM: The incidentally discovered adrenal mass. Ann Intern Med 98:940–945, 1983.

ADULT RESPIRATORY DISTRESS SYNDROME

The term *ARDS* applies to acute, life-threatening lung injury of diverse etiology, in which there is an initial noxious event followed by an interval of normal lung function and then progressive hypoxemia and pulmonary infiltrates. This noncardiogenic pulmonary edema is the result of increased interstitial and alveolar water due to an increase in capillary permeability.

Clinical Characteristics

1. Arterial hypoxemia
2. Reduced thoracic compliance
3. Normal pulmonary capillary wedge pressure
4. Diffuse pulmonary infiltrates

Causes

Disorders Retrospectively Associated with ARDS

Shock
  Septic (including toxic shock syndrome)
  Hemorrhagic
  Cardiogenic
  Anaphylactic
Trauma*
  Direct pulmonary contusion/concussion
  Nonpulmonary, multisystem
  Multiple major fractures
Fat embolism syndrome
Severe head injury/intracranial bleeding
Surface burns
Aspiration of gastric contents (especially
  low pH)*
Near-drowning*
Lung infection*
  Viral pneumonia
  Bacterial pneumonia (staphylococcal,
    streptococcal, *Klebsiella,*
    pneumococcal, enterococcal,
    Pseudomonas)
  Miliary TB
  Legionnaires' pneumonia
  Pneumocystis carinii
  Blastomycosis
  Coccidioidomycosis
  Cytomegalovirus
  Mycoplasma
Malaria
Rocky Mountain spotted fever
Sepsis* (gram-negative rods most common,
  but also other gram-negative and positive
  organisms, including clostridial and gono-
  coccal septicemia)
Pancreatitis

Multiple (massive) transfusions
DIC
Bowel infarction
Irritant gas or chemical inhalation (NO_2, Cl_2,
  SO_2, NH_3, H_2SO_4, phosgene, mercury,
  cadmium, perchlorethylene, organo-
  phosphates)
Smoke inhalation
O_2 toxicity
Drug overdoses
  Heroin, methadone
  Ethchlorvynol, aspirin, proproxyphene
  Tricyclic antidepressants
Drug idiosyncratic reaction (colchicine, hy-
  drochlorothiazide, ampicillin)
Thrombotic thrombocytopenic purpura
Leukemia, AIDS
Venous air embolism
Bone marrow transplantation
Cardiopulmonary bypass/hemodialysis
Toxic ingestions (ethylene glycol, paraquat,
  kerosene)
Radiation
Lymphangiography
Chemotherapy
High altitude
Hanging
Re-expansion of collapsed lung
Uremia
Liver failure
Heatstroke
Transfusion reaction
Postpartum complications
Amniotic fluid emboli
Diabetic ketoacidosis

*Common risk of ARDS.

From Pepe PE: The clinical entity of adult respiratory distress syndrome: Definition, prediction, and prognosis. Crit Care Clin 2:377–403, 1986, with permission.

Severity (Lung Injury Score)

The lung injury score was developed to characterize the presence and extent of the clinical manifestations of acute pulmonary damage. The lung injury score attempts to quantify the presence, severity, and evolution of acute and chronic pulmonary damage. Four parameters are measured:

1. CXR: presence and extent of disease
2. Gas exchange: P_aO_2/F_IO_2 ratio
3. Level of positive end-expiratory pressure (PEEP) required to maintain adequate oxygenation
4. Lung compliance

Components and Individual Values of the Lung Injury Score

		VALUE
1. CXR score		
No alveolar consolidation		0
Alveolar consolidation confined to 1 quadrant		1
Alveolar consolidation confined to 2 quadrants		2
Alveolar consolidation confined to 3 quadrants		3
Alveolar consolidation in all 4 quadrants		4
2. Hypoxemia score		
PaO_2/F_IO_2	≥300	0
PaO_2/F_IO_2	225–299	1
PaO_2/F_IO_2	175–224	2
PaO_2/F_IO_2	100–174	3
PaO_2/F_IO_2	<100	4
3. PEEP score (when ventilated)		
PEEP	≤5 cm H_2O	0
PEEP	6–8 cm H_2O	1
PEEP	9–11 cm H_2O	2
PEEP	12–14 cm H_2O	3
PEEP	≥15 cm H_2O	4
4. Respiratory system compliance score (when available)		
Compliance	≥80 ml/cm H_2O	0
Compliance	60–79 ml/cm H_2O	1
Compliance	40–59 ml/cm H_2O	2
Compliance	20–39 ml/cm H_2O	3
Compliance	≤19 ml/cm H_2O	4

5. The final value is obtained by dividing the aggregate sum by the number of components that were used.

	Score
No lung injury	0
Mild-to-moderate lung injury	0.1–2.5
Severe lung injury (ARDS)	>2.5

From Murray JF, et al: An expanded definition of the adult respiratory distress syndrome. Am Rev Respir Dis 138:720–723, 1988, with permission.

Clinical Management

Despite increased understanding of the pathophysiology of ARDS, mortality remains high (greater than 50%). No specific pharmacologic therapy for ARDS is available, and management is limited to supportive measures:

1. Treat the underlying precipitating condition.
2. Establish adequate oxygenation.
3. Maintain euvolemia.
4. Support hemodynamics.
5. Support nutritional status.
6. Recognize and prevent clinical complications.

Complications Associated with ARDS

I. Pulmonary	III. Renal
A. Pulmonary emboli	A. Renal failure
B. Pulmonary barotrauma	B. Fluid retention
C. Pulmonary fibrosis	IV. Cardiac
D. Pulmonary complications of ventilatory	A. Arrhythmia
and monitoring procedures	B. Hypotension
1. Mechanical ventilation	C. Low cardiac output
a. Right mainstem intubation	V. Infection
b. Alveolar hypoventilation	A. Sepsis
2. Swan-Ganz catheter	B. Nosocomial pneumonia
a. Pulmonary infarction	VI. Hematologic
b. Pulmonary hemorrhage	A. Anemia
3. Tracheal intubation	B. Thrombocytopenia
a. Laryngeal injury	C. DIC
b. Tracheal stenosis	VII. Other
II. Gastrointestinal	A. Hepatic
A. Gastrointestinal hemorrhage	B. Endocrine
B. Ileus	C. Neurologic
C. Gastric distension	D. Psychiatric
D. Pneumoperitoneum	

From Pingleton SK: Complications associated with the adult respiratory distress syndrome. Clin Chest Med 3:143–155, 1982, Table 1, p 144, with permission.

References: Bone RC: Adult respiratory distress syndrome (symposium). Clin Chest Med 3:1–215, 1982.

Suchyta MR, et al: The adult respiratory distress syndrome: A report of survival and modifying factors. Chest 101:1074–1079, 1992.

ALCOHOL WITHDRAWAL SYNDROME

Alcohol withdrawal syndromes may be categorized as minor or major. Minor withdrawal is uncomfortable for the patient but not life threatening. Major withdrawal syndromes, including alcoholic hallucinosis, seizures, and delirium tremens, can be life threatening.

Minor withdrawal symptoms can occur as early as 6–8 hours after the cessation of drinking. Symptoms are those of autonomic hyperactivity and include inability to concentrate; irritability; a coarse, generalized intention tremor; sweating; sleeplessness; and bad dreams. Anorexia is present and, at times, nausea and vomiting. The minor withdrawal state is of relatively short duration; symptoms are most intense on days 1 and 2, resolving by day 4 or 5.

The therapeutic intent in minor withdrawal is to provide symptomatic relief during the period the manifestations are their most troublesome. Except for alcohol ingestion, there is no way to prevent minor withdrawal symptoms, so there is no reason to institute therapy until the symptoms become manifest. One common method of outpatient treatment is a 4-day decreasing regimen of oral chlordiazepoxide: 50 mg QID on day 1, 50 mg TID day 2, 50 mg BID day 3, 50 mg in morning of day 4. This dosage schedule capitalizes on the fact that chlordiazepoxide is a benzodiazepine with five active metabolites, some of which have a half-life of up to 96 hours in normals. Other practitioners prefer to use a benzodiazepine with a short half-life, such as oxazepam. Beta-blockers can control autonomic signs and reduce the craving for alcohol but may need to be supplemented with sedatives. Clonidine may be an effective alternative to benzodiazepines.

Major withdrawal syndromes pose some degree of threat to life, and so the therapeutic intent is to both relieve symptoms and prevent death. Alcoholic hallucinosis is a very uncommon syndrome in which the patient has a clear sensorium but has auditory hallucinations. The content of the hallucinations is threatening, and the patient's emotional response is appropriate to the content. Suicides have been reported. The syndrome resolves over a 2-week period of abstinence. Psychiatric consultation should be obtained, as such a patient needs psychotropic drugs and may need a psychiatric hospital stay.

Alcohol withdrawal seizures are tonic-clonic, generalized seizures. The peak period of seizure activity is 8–24 hours after the last drink. Withdrawal seizures can be precipitated by a drop in the blood alcohol level and may occur while alcohol is detectable in the blood. Withdrawal seizures can occur singly or in bursts of two to six. Status epilepticus is rare. Withdrawal seizures are never focal, and therefore, an alcoholic who presents with a focal seizure must be presumed to have an intracranial lesion. The use of phenytoin to prevent seizures is controversial. Many physicians administer prophylactic phenytoin to newly abstinent alcoholics who have a history of withdrawal seizures.

About 30% of patients who have a withdrawal seizure will go on to develop delirium tremens (DTs), a distinct withdrawal syndrome (the term should not be used as a wastebasket for all alcohol withdrawal). DTs is associated with a significant mortality rate (up to 5%). The usual onset is 3–5 days after the cessation of drinking, though it can occur up to 12 days afterward. DTs is a state of profound confusion, delusions, vivid visual and tactile hallucinations (delirium), severe agitation, tremor (tremens), and sleeplessness. There is massive overactivity of the autonomic nervous system, with fever as high as 104°F, hypertension, tachycardia, profuse diaphoresis, and dilated pupils. Fluid and electrolyte requirements are extensive. Management difficulties are compounded by the ever-present need to rule out infectious explanations for the fever and structural CNS lesions. Moreover, liver insufficiency and comorbid conditions such as COPD are often present.

Once DTs have been recognized, treatment should be instituted aggressively. Because of its unpredictable absorption after oral ingestion and its long half-life, oral chlordiazepoxide is not the treatment of choice in DTs. (Chlordiazepoxide is not a good parenteral agent; absorption after intramuscular injection is unpredictable and intravenous use often causes hypotension.) A reasonable approach is to institute treatment immediately after diagnosis, using diazepam 5 mg intravenously every 5 minutes until the patient is sedated. A peak blood level is achieved rapidly, and the half-life is long enough that few (if any) repeated intravenous doses are necessary over the ensuing hours and days. About 80% of patients with DTs regain normal mental status by 3 days or less.

There is no clear evidence that administering benzodiazepines can prevent the development of DTs. In fact, attempts to prevent DTs often lead to both inadvertent overdosage of benzodiazepines and the attendant dangers of altered mental status and stupor. Treatment should not begin until the diagnosis is made. (See also Ethanol Abuse.)

References: Turner RC, et al: Alcohol withdrawal syndromes: A review of pathophysiology, clinical presentation, and treatment. J Gen Intern Med 4:432–444, 1989.
Sellers EM, et al: Alcohol intoxication and withdrawal. N Engl J Med 294:757–762, 1976.

ALDOSTERONE: PRIMARY HYPERALDOSTERONISM

Primary hyperaldosteronism is responsible for less than 1% of all cases of HTN. The three main causes are an adrenal tumor (70% of cases), bilateral hyperplasia of the zona glomerulosa (30%), and glucocorticoid suppressible hyperaldosteronism (familial, rare). The single most important screening test for primary hyperaldosteronism is the measurement of serum K^+ levels. K^+ levels may be normal as a result of a low-salt diet or the use of an ACE inhibitor. In such patients, overt hypokalemia is revealed with the use of a thiazide diuretic. Hypokalemia is usually more profound in adenoma than in hyperplasia.

The clinical features are HTN and manifestations of K^+ depletion, including fatigue, weakness, muscle cramps, and polyuria. Some patients may have an impaired glucose tolerance, hypomagnesemia, mild hypernatremia, and alkalosis. Some patients may have intermittent hypokalemia.

Differential Diagnosis of Primary Hyperaldosteronism

1. Defect of the cortisol-cortisone interconversion
2. Licorice ingestion
3. Tumor secreting excess deoxycorticosterone
4. Secondary hyperaldosteronism (high renin)

Diagnosis

The diagnosis of primary hyperaldosteronism is confirmed by a salt-loading test. Two liters of intravenous saline are infused over a 4-hour period, and plasma aldosterone is measured in the supine position along with plasma cortisol and

K+ level. A high, nonsuppressed aldosterone level is consistent with primary hyperaldosteronism.

Several clues and tests are used to differentiate between the three mains causes of primary hyperaldosteronism:

1. Hyperplasia is associated with lower aldosterone levels and less marked hypokalemia than adenomas.
2. An increase in aldosterone levels following a change from the supine to the upright position is seen in hyperplasia but not in adenoma (associated with a fall).
3. 18-Hydroxycorticosterone (a precursor of aldosterone) is much higher in adenoma than in hyperplasia. A supine, fasting 18-hydroxycorticosterone higher than 100 ng/dl suggests an adenoma.
4. Adrenal imaging techniques such as CT allow visualization of the adenoma. However, some patients with bilateral hyperplasia may develop a nodule, and many adenomas that may be smaller than 1 cm are not seen on CT scan.
5. Glucocorticoid-suppressible hyperaldosteronism can be suspected in young patients. A 2-day course of dexamethasone causes a reduction of aldosterone to the normal range.
6. Simultaneous venous sampling from adrenal veins and measurement of aldosterone and cortisol can be carried out. A diagnosis of adenoma is established when aldosterone concentrations are higher than 1,000 ng/dl from one side and the concentration in the other side is similar to that in the inferior vena cava. It has 95–100% accuracy when the radiologist is well experienced.
7. Iodocholesterol scan has a lower diagnostic yield than adrenal vein sampling.

Treatment

The treatment of primary hyperaldosteronism due to an adenoma consists of surgical removal of the tumor. Hypokalemia and hyperplasia are managed with spironolactone. Males may not tolerate the antiandrogen effect of spironolactone and can be alternatively treated with amiloride or other potassium-sparing diuretics.

ALOPECIA

Current understanding of the alopecias (hair loss) is incomplete. Morphologically, the alopecias are divided into cicatricial (scarring) and noncicatricial (normal scalp). Cicatricial alopecias occur because of damage to the hair follicle such that hair can no longer be produced. Noncicatricial alopecia results from transformation of the hair follicle either into a "resting" telogen phase or into a vellus follicle that produces insignificant, short, fine, nonpigmented hair. Observations that may prove helpful include whether the hair loss is patchy or diffuse, the appearance of the scalp, and the duration of hair loss.

It has been estimated that up to 20% of the hair can be lost before the patient notices and 50% before others notice thinning; therefore, the patient's assessment of loss is more critical than the physician's assessment.

Causes of Alopecia

PATCHY		DIFFUSE
SCARRING	NONSCARRING	DIFFUSE
Tinea capitis with bacterial infection	Alopecia areata	Male-pattern baldness
Discoid lupus erythematosus	Tinea capitis infections	High fever
Third-degree burns	Secondary syphilis	Pregnancy
Trauma	Hair-pulling	Chemotherapy
Herpes infections		Radiation therapy
Neoplasms		Exfoliative dermatitis
Lichen planus		Systemic lupus erythematosus
Scleroderma		Dermatomyositis
		Hypothyroidism
		Cushing's syndrome
		Hypopituitarism
		Anticoagulants
		Oral contraceptives

From Haynes H, et al: Dermatology in primary care. In Branch WT Jr (ed): Office Practice of Medicine, 2nd ed. Philadelphia, W.B. Saunders, 1987, with permission.

Classification of Cicatricial Alopecias

Developmental defects and hereditary disorders:
   Aplasia cutis congenita
   Recessive X-linked ichthyosis
   Epidermal nevi
   Facial hemiatrophy (Romberg's syndrome)
   Generalized follicular hamartoma
   Incontinentia pigmenti
   Porokeratosis of Mibelli
   Scarring follicular keratosis
   Darier's disease
   Epidermolysis bullosa (recessive dystrophic type)
   Polyostotic fibrous dysplasia
   Conradi's syndrome
Infection:
   Bacterial
   Fungal
   Protozoan
   Viral
Neoplasms:
   Basal cell carcinoma
   Squamous cell carcinoma
   Metastatic tumors
   Lymphomas
   Adnexal tumors

Physical/chemical agents:
   Mechanical trauma (including factitial)
   Burns
   Radiation
   Caustic agents
   Other chemicals/drugs
Dermatoses of uncertain origin and clinical syndromes:
   Lupus erythematosus
   Sarcoidosis
   Scleroderma/morphea
   Lichen sclerosus et atrophicus
   Necrobiosis lipoidica diabeticorum
   Dermatomyositis
   Cicatricial pemphigoid
   Graham-Little syndrome
   Follicular mucinosis
   Acne keloidalis/sycosis nuchae
   Erosive pustular dermatosis
   Pseudopelade of Brocq
   Folliculitis decalvans
   Alopecia parvimacularis
   Dissecting perifolliculitis of the scalp (perifolliculitis capitis abscedens et suffodiens)
   Lipedematous alopecia
   Amyloidosis

From Fitzpatrick TB, et al (eds): Dermatology in General Medicine, 3rd ed. New York, McGraw-Hill, 1987, Tables 65–3 & 65–4, pp 632–635, with permission.

Classification of Noncicatricial Alopecias (Cont.)

Androgenetic alopecia
Hereditary syndromes with noncicatricial alopecia
Alopecia areata
Noncicatricial alopecia associated with systemic diseases or processes:
    Telogen effluvium
    Deficiency states (nutritional/metabolic)
    Endocrine disease
    Drugs and chemical agents
    Syphilis
Traumatic noncicatricial alopecia:
    Trichotillomania
    Traction alopecia
    Other causes

From Fitzpatrick TB, et al (eds): Dermatology in General Medicine, 3rd ed. New York, McGraw-Hill, 1987, Tables 65–3 & 65–4, pp 632–635, with permission.

ALPHA-FETOPROTEIN

Alpha-fetoprotein (αFP) is an oncofetal protein found in the serum of normal fetuses and adults with certain types of cancer. In the fetus, αFP serves many of the same functions that albumin does in the adult. In pregnant women, serum αFP elevation is used to screen for the presence of fetal neural tube defects. Nonneoplastic αFP elevation in adults is also seen in conditions with regenerating liver cells such as viral hepatitis, postnecrotic cirrhosis, alcoholic cirrhosis, and primary biliary cirrhosis. Elevated levels of αFP are found in many types of cancer including hepatocellular carcinoma; testicular carcinoma; adenocarcinomas of the pancreas, stomach, and colon; lung cancer; and metastases to the liver from various tumor types.

Most benign liver diseases are associated with αFP values under 500 ng/ml. The highest levels (>1,000 ng/ml) are associated with germ cell tumors and hepatomas. Levels higher than 3,000 ng/ml are thought to be specific for hepatoma.

In testicular carcinomas, only embryonal cells and yolk sac cells stain for αFP. Pure seminomas do not cause elevation of serum αFP. In a patient with a diagnosis of pure seminoma, elevation of serum αFP indicates the presence of undetected embryonal cells. Such tumors should be treated as mixed germ cell tumors. (See also Cancer: Tumor Markers)

Reference: Bartlett NL, Freiha FS, Torti FM: Serum markers in germ cell neoplasms. Hematol Oncol Clin North Am 5:1245–1260, 1991.

ALZHEIMER'S DISEASE

Alzheimer's disease is by far the most common cause of dementia, accounting for well over 50% of all cases. Most elderly patients who were once termed "senile" probably had Alzheimer's disease, which is now felt to be a specific, distinct disease rather than the mere loss of intellectual functions with normal aging.

The diagnosis of Alzheimer's disease requires finding a loss of several cognitive functions (not just memory), which is progressive over time and for which there is no other identifiable cause. Because there is no biological marker short of a brain biopsy (showing neurofibrillary tangles, amyloid plaques, and granular vacuolar degeneration), the diagnosis depends on clinical criteria as follows.

Clinical Diagnosis of Alzheimer's Disease

1. Proof of dementia by formal neuropsychological testing
2. Deficits in two or more areas of cognition (i.e., not just memory loss)
3. Progressive worsening
4. No disturbance of consciousness
5. Onset between ages 40 and 90 (usually after age 65)
6. Absence of other causes of dementia (To a large degree, the diagnosis of Alzheimer's disease is one of exclusion.)

Therefore, the diagnostic evaluation in a patient suspected of having Alzheimer's disease consists of measures to exclude other causes of dementia. These include imaging of the brain, EEG, and laboratory studies for endocrine, hematologic, and metabolic imbalances. Patients with Alzheimer's disease generally have normal brain imaging. There may be some atrophy, but the correlation between atrophy and cognitive function is very loose, at best. Sometimes, the MRI will show increased signal in the white matter—a nonspecific finding in a large segment of the elderly population. The EEG is often moderately slow, but there are no abnormalities in the spinal fluid or blood tests.

Two conditions that are not true dementing illnesses but are often mistaken for Alzheimer's disease are depression and Parkinson's disease.

The cause of Alzheimer's disease remains elusive. The neurotransmitter acetylcholine seems to be important for memory, and there are deficits in the acetylcholine systems of the brain in Alzheimer's disease. However, it is not clear that these are specific changes or fundamental to the cause of the illness. Approximately 10% of cases are familial and the gene has been located on chromosome 21, closely linked to the genes for apo-protein and for beta amyloid, which are present in increased concentrations in Alzheimer brains.

There is no therapy for Alzheimer's disease, though most research has focused on enhancing the acetylcholine system. Recently, the cholinesterase-inhibiting drug tacrine was found to have some influence on Alzheimer's disease, but not sufficient to endorse it strongly as a treatment.

References: McKhann G, et al: Clinical diagnosis of Alzheimer's disease: Report of the NINCDS-ADRDA Work Group. Neurology 34:939–944, 1984.

Mayeux R: Therapeutic strategies in Alzheimer's disease. Neurology 40:175–180, 1990.

AMENORRHEA, PRIMARY

Primary amenorrhea refers to the absence of menarche by the age of 16 years. In **secondary amenorrhea,** a woman has previously had menses but currently has had no menstruation for at least three months. In an evaluation for primary amenorrhea, attention must be given on physical examination to development of the breasts, uterus, and cervix. Breast development means exposure to estrogens. The presence of pubic and axillary hair results from androgenic stimulation. If the uterus and cervix are present and do not have primary disease, amenorrhea is indicative of a disorder of the hypothalamic-pituitary-ovarian axis. The more common causes of primary amenorrhea are:

Chromosomal abnormalities
  1. Turner's syndrome: Affected patients usually have:
     Gonadal dysgenesis, with undifferentiated streak gonads
     45,X chromosomal karyotype
     Female phenotype
     Sexual infantilism
     Short stature
     Physical abnormalities such as webbed neck, low-set ears, and cardiovascular abnormalities such as coarctation of the aorta or aortic stenosis
  2. Pure gonadal dysgenesis: Affected patients have:
     Streak gonads
     Karyotype of 46,XX or 46,XY
     Female phenotype
     Normal stature
     Absence of the physical abnormalities of Turner's syndrome

Distal genital tract obstruction
  1. Congenital malformations of the malarian duct are associated with:
     Primary amenorrhea, with certain anomalies such as aplasia of all müllerian derivatives, vaginal aplasia, and imperforate hymen
     Normal hormonal levels
     Normal pubertal development

Physiologic delay of puberty

Anorexia nervosa (functional hypothalamic anovulation)

Hormonal abnormalities
  1. Kallmann's syndrome: Characteristics are:
     A familial syndrome of hypogonadotropic hypogonadism
     Anosmia
     Color blindness (rare in women)
     Cleft lip and palate (sometimes)
     Sexual infantilism
     Inherited by women as an X-linked recessive trait
     Low FSH and LH
     Other normal pituitary hormones
  2. Hypopituitarism: Principal causes are:
     Primary pituitary tumors
     Craniopharyngioma
     Hyperprolactinemia, due to tumor or other causes
     Histiocytosis X

3. Adrenal hyperplasia
   Cushing's syndrome
   Congenital adrenal hyperplasia
   21-hydroxylase deficiency
   11-hydroxylase deficiency
4. Primary hypothyroidism

Evaluation of Primary Amenorrhea

Physical examination
Breasts
Cervix
Uterus
Vagina
Signs of virilization
FSH level; if elevated, obtain karyotype
Prolactin level
T_4, TSH
17-Hydroxyprogesterone level for diagnosis
of 21-hydroxylase deficiency
Testosterone level
Radiographic evaluation of sella turcica

AMYLOIDOSIS

Amyloid is an amorphous, homogenous protein that is deposited in tissues in a wide variety of illnesses. Amyloid is eosinophilic in histologic sections stained with hematoxylin and eosin, and it shows a unique apple green birefringence under polarized microscopy after staining a tissue section with Congo red. There are many different types of amyloid, reflecting differences in the biochemical characteristics of the amyloid protein. Classification of amyloidosis proceeds according to the type of precursor protein:

Classification of Amyloidosis

CLINICAL DISORDER	AMYLOID PROTEIN PRECURSOR	AMYLOID PROTEIN
Primary systemic amyloidosis	Immunoglobulin light chain	AL
Amyloidosis with multiple myeloma	Immunoglobulin light chain	AL
Secondary (reactive) amyloidosis	Serum amyloid A protein	AA
Familial Mediterranean fever	Serum amyloid A protein	AA
Familial nephropathy	Serum amyloid A protein	AA
Familial amyloid polyneuropathy	Transthyretin (prealbumin)	ATTR
Systemic senile amyloidosis	Transthyretin (prealbumin)	ATTR
Amyloid of chronic dialysis	Beta-2 microglobulin	AB_2M
Alzheimer's disease	Amyloid beta protein precursor	ABP
Down's syndrome	Amyloid beta protein precursor	ABP
Jakob-Creutzfeldt disease	Scrapie protein	AScr
Medullary carcinoma of thyroid	Procalcitonin	ACal
Atrial amyloidosis	Atrial natriuretic factor	AANF
Type II diabetes mellitus	Islet amyloid polypeptide	AIAPP
Insulinoma	Islet amyloid polypeptide	AIAPP

In primary systemic amyloidosis or the amyloidosis associated with multiple myeloma or macroglobulinemia, the amyloid protein (AL) contains portions of kappa or lambda light chains. Serum amyloid A protein is a circulating precursor of the AA protein of secondary amyloidosis, familial Mediterranean fever, and the familial nephropathy associated with urticaria and deafness. In the United States, the principal disorders associated with secondary amyloidosis are rheumatoid arthritis, Crohn's disease, tuberculosis, and osteomyelitis. There are a large number of rare familial syndromes in which amyloidosis occurs related to the precursor protein transthyretin (i.e., prealbumin). Most of these syndromes are characterized by neuropathy or cardiomyopathy or both, sometimes with vitreous opacities. In patients maintained on chronic dialysis, the carpal tunnel syndrome may occur due to amyloid deposits containing beta-2 microglobulin. The plaques of Alzheimer's disease contain amyloid, caused by a new protein termed amyloid beta protein (ABP). This protein is also part of the amyloid deposits in Down's syndrome and in hereditary cerebral amyloidosis. The amyloid plaques of Jakob-Creutzfeldt disease and the animal disease scrapie contain prion protein. In medullary carcinoma of the thyroid, amyloid, containing calcitonin, is deposited locally. In senile cardiac amyloidosis, amyloid deposits in the heart contain prealbumin. Atrial natriuretic factor has been found in isolated atrial deposits of amyloid. The hyaline material in the pancreatic islets of Langerhans in type II diabetes mellitus is amyloid, containing a new protein—islet amyloid peptide.

Reference: Cohen AS: Amyloidosis. Bull Rheum Dis 40(2):1–12, 1991.

AMYOTROPHIC LATERAL SCLEROSIS

ALS, also known as Lou Gehrig's disease, is an idiopathic degenerative disease usually appearing insidiously in middle to later age and progressing to death within 3–5 years. It is best thought of as motor neuron disease since it has signs of both upper and lower motor neuron disease.

UPPER MOTOR NEURON DISEASE	LOWER MOTOR NEURON DISEASE
Weakness	Weakness
Spasticity	Flaccidity
Hyperreflexia	Hyporeflexia
Clonus	Atrophy
Babinski signs	Fasciculation

In ALS, only the motor neurons are damaged. Patients experience weakness, with atrophy, fasciculation, and at least some muscle groups showing spasticity and hyperreflexia, but there will be no dementia, sensory loss, bowel or bladder changes, ataxia, or other neurologic symptoms.

The differential diagnosis of a patient with isolated upper and lower motor neuron findings is, however, surprisingly short, and most of the conditions are rare.

Differential Diagnosis of ALS

1. Cervical spondylosis
2. Lead intoxication
3. Hyperparathyroidism
4. Paraneoplastic syndromes
5. Inflammatory myopathies

The evaluation of a suspected case of ALS generally includes:

1. Electromyography and nerve conduction velocity studies. These show denervation of the muscle without significant nerve slowing.
2. Cervical spine imaging. MRI is useful to exclude spondylosis.
3. Muscle biopsy to show denervation and exclude other conditions.
4. Blood studies, including lead levels, serum protein electrophoresis, Ca^{++}, PO_4^{--} and CPK.

Because progressive swallowing and breathing impairment leads to death within a few years, physicians must verify the diagnosis before discussions with the patient and family. There is no treatment for ALS. Management focuses on chronic care of the debilitated patient and ethical issues of prolonged life support.

Note: Lou Gehrig, who hit behind Babe Ruth in the Yankee lineup, played every game from June 2, 1925, until May 2, 1939, setting a record of 2,130 consecutive games, which still stands. He was the first modern player to hit four consecutive home runs in one game and holds the lifetime record for most grand slams, at 23. Knowing he was dying, he told his fans at his farewell tribute at Yankee Stadium on July 4, 1939, that because of their support and friendship, "Today I consider myself the luckiest man on the face of the earth." ALS was probably named after him because his lifetime batting average of .340 was much higher than that of Jean-Martin Charcot, the French neurologist who had described the disease 100 years earlier.

Reference: Mitsumoto H, et al: Amyotrophic lateral sclerosis. Recent advances in pathogenesis and therapeutic trials. Arch Neurol 45:189–202, 1988.

ANALGESICS, NARCOTIC

The narcotic analgesics are extremely useful in the treatment of pain. As they also are highly addictive, their use in therapy of nonmalignant pain is generally limited to short courses for specific indications (e.g., postoperative pain). In cancer pain, narcotic analgesics are one of the mainstays of therapy. Although physical dependence and tolerance occur in the cancer patient, psychologic addiction is rare in the presence of severe pain. If the source of pain is removed, it is usually possible to rapidly taper and discontinue the narcotic.

All of the opiate derivatives have a similar spectrum of side effects, including constipation and the potential for nausea, somnolence, and mental confusion. Stool softeners and bowel stimulants should be given concurrently with narcotic therapy. Among the narcotics, codeine is the most frequent cause of allergic reactions, which usually manifest as pruritus or a pruritic rash. Patients allergic to codeine can usually be switched to a different narcotic without recurrence of the rash.

For mild to moderate pain, the following opiate derivatives are equivalent in analgesia to 650 mg of aspirin or 650 mg of acetaminophen when taken orally:

MEDICATION	EQUI-ANALGESIC DOSE (mg)	DURATION (hr)	PLASMA HALF-LIFE (hr)	COMMENTS
Propoxyphene (Darvon)	65	4–6	12	Biotransformed to potentially toxic metabolite; used in combination with acetaminophen (Darvocet)
Codeine	32	4–6	3	Biotransformed to morphine; often used in combination with acetaminophen (Tylenol #3, Tylenol #4)
Meperidine (Demerol)	50	4–6	3–4	Not suitable for chronic use because of buildup of toxic metabolite normeperidine

For severe pain, the following narcotic analgesics are equivalent in analgesia to 10 mg of morphine sulfate IM:

MEDICATION	EQUI-ANALGESIC DOSE (mg)	DURATION (hr)	PLASMA HALF-LIFE (hr)	COMMENTS
Morphine, IM	10	4–6	2–3.5	Can also be given SC, IV, sublingually, or by low- or high-potency elixirs. Slow-release tablets (MS Contin, Roxanol SR) can be administered orally or rectally
Morphine, oral	60	4–7		
Hydrocodone, oral (Hycodan)	5–10	4–8	4	Used as antitussive; also combined with acetaminophen (Vicodin)
Codeine, IM	130	4–6	3	Biotransformed to morphine; useful as initial narcotic analgesic; often combined with acetaminophen
Codeine, oral	200	4–6	3	
Oxycodone, IM	15	3–5	–	Available as 5-mg dose in combination with aspirin (Percodan) or acetaminophen (Percocet, Tylox)
Oxycodone, oral	30			
Hydromorphone, IM	1.5	4–5	2–3	Available as rectal suppository and in high-potency form (10 mg/ml) for cachectic patients; significant street abuse potential
Hydromorphone, oral (Dilaudid)	7.5	4–6		
Meperidine, IM	75	4–5	3–4	Contraindicated in patients with renal disease; accumulation of toxic metabolite normeperidine produces CNS excitation and seizures
Meperidine, oral (Demerol)	300	4–6	12–16	
Methadone, IM	10	—	15–30	Good oral potency; requires careful titration of the initial dose to avoid drug accumulation
Methadone, oral (Dolophine)	20			
Fentanyl, transdermal (Duragesic)	2.5	72	13–22	For long-term control of chronic pain; avoids peaks and valleys of pain control compared to drugs with shorter half-life

Modified from Foley KM: The treatment of cancer pain. N Engl J Med 313:84–95, 1985.

ANEMIA

Anemia is a symptom, not a disease. It therefore merits a disciplined and standardized approach to the evaluation of its causes. Anemia is present when the hemoglobin is less than 2 SD below the mean of a normal population. (A diagnosis of anemia can just as well be made on the basis of hematocrit or RBC count). In adult males living at sea level, the lower level of the reference range is 13.5 g/dl; in females, 12.0 g/dl. In men older than age 70, the normal curve is shifted to the left, and the lower bound of the reference range falls by 1–2 g/dl, but elderly women do not exhibit a similar decline. Therefore, adults older than age 70 with a hemoglobin under 12.0 g/dl meet the criterion for anemia.

A careful Hx & PE starts the clinician's exploration of the potential etiologies found in the differential diagnosis of anemia. This, together with six initial tests, leads to a firm diagnosis of the cause of anemia in more than 75% of patients. The low hemoglobin (or hematocrit) starts the diagnostic cascade: it is supplemented by an examination of the peripheral blood smear, reticulocyte count, MCV, WBC count and differential, platelet count, and serum ferritin level. The result of each test needs to be interpreted in the clinical context and in light of results from the other tests.

Though many anemias are multifactorial, in general anemias can be categorized as **marrow-failure anemias, hemolytic anemias,** and **blood-loss anemias.** In the latter two, the bone marrow is responding normally to an abnormal stimulus: there is a higher-than-average production of RBCs but the rate of loss is greater than the rate of production. Therefore the key diagnostic clue that directs the work-up to or away from marrow failure is the reticulocyte count. It is high in hemolytic anemia and blood-loss anemia and low in marrow-failure anemia.

Most anemias seen in clinical practice are marrow-failure anemias. These can be subcategorized as normocytic (MCV 80–100), microcytic (MCV <80), and macrocytic (MCV >100). The causes of normocytic anemia are iron deficiency (in the early phase of iron deficiency, hematocrit drops before the MCV), anemia of chronic disease, renal failure, liver disease, endocrine disorders such as hypothyroidism, and a rarer set of disorders termed primary marrow disorders, including such conditions as myelodysplasia and myelofibrosis.

The serum ferritin distinguishes iron deficiency anemia from the other marrow-failure anemias. The serum ferritin reflects marrow iron stores accurately but may be falsely elevated in patients with inflammatory diseases or liver or kidney disease. However, a low serum ferritin is always interpretable, even if inflammatory disease or liver or kidney disease is present. Microcytic anemia due to marrow failure is due either to iron deficiency or to anemia of chronic disease. Again, the serum ferritin helps to distinguish the two. Macrocytic anemias due to marrow failure include cobalamin deficiency, folate deficiency, alcoholism, some drugs, and some of the primary marrow disorders. Radioisotopic assays of serum cobalamin and RBC folate are helpful.

Autoimmune Hemolytic Anemia

Autoimmune hemolytic anemia (AIHA) is an important hemolytic disorder caused by the presence of autoantibodies against components of the RBC membrane. Warm AIHA is caused by IgG antibodies that react at 37°C with the Rh antigens present on the RBCs of all individuals except those rare individuals who are Rh_{null} (lacking Rh factors). Cold agglutinin disease is caused by an IgM that reacts with either I or i on RBCs and also fixes complement. Cold agglutinins typically react at

4°C, although some individuals are blessed with IgM antibodies that have a high thermal amplitude and react at temperatures up to 20°C.

Clinical Manifestations

Patients may have symptoms of anemia: fatigue, pallor, weakness, or dyspnea on exertion. Jaundice with fever and splenomegaly may be present. Spherocytosis is found upon examination of the peripheral blood film. Reticulocytosis in the face of anemia confirms hemolysis.

The Coombs test or direct antiglobulin test is the most important. In warm AIHA there are relatively small numbers of antibodies on the RBCs. These are not capable of directly agglutinating the RBCs. The addition of a rabbit or other antihuman Ig antibody in the direct Coombs test will agglutinate RBCs if an autoantibody is present. The initial Coombs test used is polyspecific (it will detect antibody and complement). More specific Coombs reagent for complement or IgG may be used to fully characterize the types of antibodies present on the RBCs. The indirect Coombs test detects antibodies in the plasma by incubating the patient's plasma with a panel of donor cells representing a variety of antigen types.

After incubation of the serum with the panel of test cells, the Coombs reagent is added. Agglutination indicates the presence of antibodies in the serum, reactive with the RBCs. The pattern of agglutination is informative: a specific pattern indicates the presence of an alloantibody, whereas pan-agglutination indicates the presence of an autoantibody reactive with Rh. Alloantibodies arise after sensitizing events such as pregnancy or transfusion. These antibodies recognize specific antigens related to blood groups such as Kid, Kell, or Duffy that are not present on the RBCs of the patient. Thus the direct Coombs test is not positive.

| | COOMBS TEST | |
	Direct	Indirect
Autoimmune hemolytic anemia	+	+/–
Alloimmunization	–	+

Differential Diagnosis

- *Causes of spherocytosis:* Hemolytic transfusion reaction, Rh isoimmune disease, hereditary spherocytosis, oxidant hemolysis, fragmentation hemolysis, burns, microangiopathic hemolytic anemia.
- *Causes of warm AIHA:* Idiopathic, collagen vascular disease (SLE, RA, autoimmune thyroiditis, autoimmune hepatitis, Evans' syndrome [ITP + AIHA]), chronic lymphocytic leukemia, non-Hodgkin's lymphoma, Hodgkin's disease, drug-induced, HIV infection, brown recluse spider bite.
- *Causes of cold agglutinin disease:* Chronic cold agglutinin disease, mycoplasma (specificity for I), mononucleosis (specificity for i), lymphoma, Waldenström's disease, paroxysmal cold hemoglobinuria.

Management

Folate replacement is advised just as it is for any chronic hemolytic process. Corticosteroids are often effective in the initial management. Splenectomy is sometimes effective in AIHA, but not nearly as successful as it is in the management of ITP. Danazol has been effective in some patients, providing good enough control of the disease to avoid splenectomy in high-risk patients. Concurrent use of danazol sometimes allows patients to be managed on low doses of prednisone. In some patients, immunosuppressive therapy with cyclophosphamide or other immunosuppressive agents has been required.

IV gamma globulin has also been employed successfully in patients with AIHA. The mechanism of action is not entirely clear, but blockade of the RES by small aggregates of the globulin may be responsible for the transient benefits.

For severe anemia, transfusions may be lifesaving. Although it may be a difficult cross match, patients do no worse with transfusions than with their own blood. In the selection of units for transfusion, some attempt to characterize the autoantibody should be made, as rare cases exist in which the autoantibody has a restricted antigenic activity. It is also important to look for alloantibodies in patients who could have been sensitized by pregnancy or prior blood transfusions. This may be done by stripping the patient's RBCs of their autoantibody and then using the stripped cells to absorb their own serum. The antibody remaining in the serum after absorption is most likely to be an alloantibody. Thus the patients usually receive type-specific units that do not have the specific antigen recognized by a concurrent alloantibody. There is also anecdotal experience showing that patients with AIHA are more prone to venous thrombotic disease.

Reference: Engelfriet CP, et al: Autoimmune hemolytic anemia. Semin Hematol 29(1):3–12, 1992.

Hypochromic, Microcytic Anemias

Causes of Hypochromic, Microcytic Anemias

1. Thalassemia
   Alpha thalassemia
     Alpha thalassemia minor
     Hemoglobin H disease
     Hydrops fetalis
2. Anemia of chronic disease
3. Iron deficiency
4. Sideroblastic anemia
   Hereditary
   Myelodysplastic syndrome

   Beta thalassemia
     Beta thalassemia minor
     Beta thalassemia major
   Thalassemia intermedia

   Drug, toxin induced

Laboratory Differentiation of Hypochromic, Microcytic Anemias

	SERUM IRON	TIBC	% SATURATION	FERRITIN	BONE MARROW
Iron deficiency	↓	↑	↓ (<10%)	↓	Absence of iron
Iron overload	↑	→	↑	↑	Adequate iron
Anemia of chronic disease (inflammation)	↓	↓	Variable	↑	Adequate iron
Beta thalassemia	→	→	→	→	Adequate or ↑ iron
Sideroblastic anemia	↑	→	↑	↑	Ringed sideroblasts

TIBC = total iron-binding capacity

Thalassemia

Alpha thalassemia minor and beta thalassemia minor are both associated with mild anemia and microcytosis. Clues to their presence include subtle punctate polychromasia on the peripheral blood film and a narrow RBC size distribution or red cell distribution width index coexisting with microcytosis. Thalassemia patients require genetic counseling.

Alpha thalassemias are present in Asian, Mediterranean, and black populations. These disorders result from deletion of one or both genes on chromosome 16. In an individual with normal alpha hemoglobin synthesis, there are four functioning genes. Deletions of one or multiple genes results in the alpha thalassemic syndromes depicted in the table above. In blacks, a chromosome with a single deletion is the general rule so that the typical alpha thalassemia detected is only thalassemia minor. In Asians, chromosomes with one deletion or a chromosome with both genes deleted is prevalent. Thus in Asians, births of individuals with three or four gene deletions result in Hb H disease or hydrops fetalis, respectively. Hb H disease results in a mild hemolytic anemia, whereas hydrops fetalis results in fetal demise.

The α-Thalassemia Syndromes

SYNDROME	GENOTYPE	HEMATOLOGIC ABNORMALITIES	HEMOGLOBIN VARIANTS At birth	Later
Normal	αα/αα	None	None	None
Silent carrier state (α-thal-2)	–α/αα	None	Hb Bart's (0–2%)	None
α-thal-minor				
α-thal-1 (heterozygous)	––/αα	Mild anemia, thalassemic morphology	Hb Bart's (2–10%)	None
α-thal-2 (homozygous)	–α/–α	Mild anemia, thalassemic morphology	Hb Bart's (2–10%)	None
Hb H disease	––/–α	Chronic hemolytic anemia	Hb Bart's (10–40%)	Hb H (5–30%) Hb Bart's (trace)
	––/XX			
	––/αCS			
Hydrops fetalis	––/––	Fatal anemia in utero	Hb Bart's (> 80%) (also Hb H and Hb Portland)	—

X = nondeletional gene of α locus; CS = gene for Hb Constant Spring). (From Jandl JH: Blood: Pathophysiology. Cambridge, MA, Blackwell Scientific Publications, 1991, p 139, with permission.)

Beta thalassemia minor results from the inheritance of one of multiple mutations in the beta globin locus on chromosome 11. In beta thalassemia, the typical mutation results in defective mRNA synthesis or processing. Patients with beta thalassemia minor may have a palpable spleen tip or a family history of microcytic anemia. Thalassemia is often recognized in patients who have failed to completely respond to a trial of iron therapy. Hemoglobin electrophoresis in beta thalassemia minor discloses an increased Hb A$_2$ and sometimes an increased Hb F level. It is usually prudent that the clinician show that iron stores are normal before ordering an electrophoresis, as concurrent iron deficiency will depress the usually elevated Hb A$_2$ found in beta thalassemia minor.

Beta thalassemia in both parents may result in thalassemia major in the offspring. Prenatal diagnosis, through the use of specific probes to identify DNA haplotypes, is possible and enables couples to avoid the birth of a severely affected child. Thalassemia major results in a tremendous expansion of the bone marrow because of (1) the inability of cells to complete hemoglobin synthesis and (2) the toxicity of the alpha tetramer to the RBC membrane. Treatment involves transfusions coupled with iron chelation to avoid iron overload. Recent experience from Italy suggests that bone marrow transplantation when carried out in young individuals without liver disease is a reasonable approach to therapy for those children with suitable HLA-identical donors.

Anemia of Chronic Disease

ACD may be associated with microcytosis or a normal RBC size. It is the most common cause of anemia in hospitalized patients. However, the criteria for diagnosis are not well established. The anemia is usually mild and accompanied by typical underlying diseases. Most commonly these are related to infections, chronic inflammation, or tumor. The anemia is mild and associated with reticulocytopenia and a characteristic pattern of iron studies. Typically there is a reduced serum iron, a reduced TIBC (transferrin), and a reduced percent saturation of the TIBC. Last, there is usually an increased serum ferritin or increased storage iron in bone marrow histiocytes with scanty incorporation into developing RBCs. A recent study demonstrated that ACD was remarkably prevalent in a hospitalized population when defined by iron studies alone. ACD may also be found in patients who do not have a typical infectious, inflammatory, or neoplastic disease. In certain disorders such as RA, iron deficiency may coexist with ACD, but this is not likely when the serum ferritin is above 50–60 ng/ml.

Iron Deficiency Anemia

IDA is a very common disorder. Unfortunately, the normal person is unable to acquire much more than 1 mg Fe/day from the diet. In normal men, this amount approximates the daily iron loss, but in women with menstrual losses and the need for additional iron to support pregnancy and delivery, iron intake may be insufficient unless supplemented at critical times. In postmenopausal or older women, as well as in men, the discovery of IDA should lead to an investigation for GI bleeding. IDA may accompany blood loss from peptic ulcers, gastritis, and varices, as well as angiodysplasia, polyps, or cancer of the colon. Sometimes iron loss may occur as a result of hemoglobinuria associated with valve hemolysis or paroxysmal nocturnal hemoglobinuria. IDA may be found in infants and in some adults with malabsorption due to achlorhydria, gastric resection, or sprue. In less developed countries, hookworm infestation is a common cause.

In addition to anemia and microcytosis, iron deficiency may be accompanied by a smooth atrophic tongue; brittle, spoon-shaped nails (koilonychia); and esophageal webs. A very common finding is pica. If the iron-deficient patient is questioned carefully and with sensitivity, a patient physician is often rewarded with a history of eating ice, dirt, clay, starch, paper, or other strange substances. Ice eating is so common that it has its own term: pagophagia. Emotional lability and lagging intellectual development may occur in iron-deficient children. However, it is possible that such problems may be due to the effects of inappropriately high levels of lead, which may accompany the pica associated with iron deficiency.

The diagnosis of IDA relies on characteristic iron studies: low serum iron, increased TIBC, reduced percent saturation of the TIBC, and reduced ferritin. When there is a concurrent disorder that may result in ACD, then the ferritin level may need to be interpreted with caution. In straightforward IDA, the serum ferritin is usually very low (<12 ng/ml). Because of concurrent ACD, IDA may be present when the ferritin is in the range of 12–50 ng/ml. Treatment with ferrous sulfate 325 mg/day is usually successful. Reticulocytosis should occur in 7–10 days. Once the anemia has been corrected, the ferritin should be checked to determine that iron stores are present. In individuals who also have thalassemia, the anemia and microcytosis may not correct entirely, and ferritin must be checked to avoid iron overload.

Sideroblastic Anemia

In this disorder there is a failure of iron to leave the mitochondria. In the bone marrow stained with Prussian blue, there are increased iron storage and the presence of pathological erythroid cells containing large chunks of iron distributed around the nucleus: the ringed sideroblast. Iron studies of the peripheral blood disclose an increased serum iron and an increased percent saturation of the TIBC. The serum ferritin is also increased.

Sideroblastic anemia may occur uncommonly as a hereditary disorder or as a result of certain drugs or toxins. Lead poisoning or plumbism is an important cause of sideroblastic anemia and should be suspected when coarse basophilic stippling is observed on the peripheral blood film. Alcohol is another frequent culprit. Drugs used for the chemotherapy of TB such as rifampin and pyrazinamide are also causes of sideroblastic anemia. Acquired sideroblastic anemia is also one of the myelodysplastic syndromes.

Reference: Cash JM, et al: The anemia of chronic disease: Spectrum of associated disease in a series of unselected hospitalized patients. Am J Med 87: 638, 1989.

Megaloblastic Anemia

Causes of Megaloblastic Anemia

I. Folate deficiency
   A. Dietary
   B. Alcoholism
   C. Malabsorption: sprue, other malabsorption syndromes, inhibition of intestinal conjugase (phenytoin, oral contraceptives)
   D. Relative deficiency due to increased requirements: pregnancy, hemolysis (sickle-cell anemia, hereditary spherocytosis)
   E. Inhibition by drugs (methotrexate, trimethoprim, pyrimethamine)
II. B_{12} deficiency
   A. Dietary (strict vegetarians, breast-fed infants of vegetarians)
   B. Malabsorption due to ileal disease (Crohn's disease, malignancy, resection, sprue, Whipple's disease)
   C. Malabsorption due to unavailability of B_{12} (pernicious anemia, overgrowth of intestinal bacteria, fish tapeworm [*Diphyllobothrium latum*], chronic pancreatitis, gastric resection)

Megaloblastic anemia most often results from folate or B_{12} deficiency and has characteristic morphologic features in the peripheral blood and bone marrow. In peripheral blood there are marked macroovalocytosis and hypersegmented granulocytes. Eosinophils may also show an increased number of lobes so that three or four lobed eosinophils are commonly seen. The bone marrow is often hypercellular, with increased numbers of large, aberrant, erythroid precursor cells that display asynchrony of nuclear and cytoplasmic maturation. The nuclear maturation lags behind that of the cytoplasm and is associated with a more delicate chromatin pattern or nuclear fragmentation. Giant metamyelocytes are also present.

Megaloblastic maturation is sometimes recognized in other tissues such as the epithelial cells identified in a Pap smear or in an intestinal biopsy. Megaloblastic anemia is also encountered as part of the myelodysplastic syndrome, congenital dysplastic anemias, congenital abnormalities in the synthesis of folate and B_{12}, acute leukemia, thiamine-dependent megaloblastic anemia, and pyridoxine-responsive anemia. Megaloblastic anemia and neuropathy is associated with chronic exposure to nitrous oxide. Early recognition of congenital abnormalities in folate and B_{12} metabolism is important as initiation of appropriate replacement therapy may prevent the mental developmental abnormalities associated with these disorders.

Laboratory findings also include anemia with an increased MCV. Neutropenia and thrombocytopenia may also be present. Occasionally, Howell-Jolly bodies and megaloblastic nucleated RBCs may be identified in the peripheral blood film. Other laboratory findings are consistent with ineffective erythropoiesis. These include increased serum iron and ferritin; increased serum unconjugated bilirubin and LDH; and a decreased haptoglobin. Occasionally, these findings and the presence of marked anisocytosis and poikilocytosis lead to the erroneous impression of a hemolytic process. In megaloblastic anemia there may be some shortening of the RBC survival, but the absence of reticulocytosis indicates that ineffective erythropoiesis is the mechanism of the anemia.

The diagnosis depends on the demonstration of a low serum B_{12} level or a low RBC folate level. Often, patients have a low serum folate level in the absence of megaloblastic anemia, making the serum level an invalid index of deficiency. Folate and B_{12} levels are usually obtained together because the RBC requires B_{12} to accumulate folate. Serum B_{12} reflects tissue levels and is a good index of deficiency.

Folate and B_{12} Levels in Deficiency States

	SERUM B_{12}	SERUM FOLATE	RBC FOLATE
B_{12} deficiency	↓	→ or ↑	↓
Folate deficiency	→	↓	↓

Folate deficiency is most often dietary in origin. Teenagers on a steady diet of junk food, unrelieved by green leafy vegetables, as well as aged individuals on a skimpy diet of tea and toast may be folate deficient. Alcohol use is associated with anemia for a number of reasons, including dietary insufficiency of folate and the antifolate effect of alcohol. Patients with malabsorption syndromes are also likely candidates for folate deficiency, as are patients receiving phenytoin or oral contraceptives. A relative deficiency may develop in those who require more than the usual folate intake. Thus, patients who are pregnant, who have hemolytic anemia, or who are on dialysis (folate is dialyzable) may benefit from folate supplementation. Of special interest is the possible association between folate and risk for neural tube defects (including spina bifida) in addition to the recent recommendation by the CDC that all pregnant women receive folate supplementation to reduce this risk. Antifols are frequently used in the treatment of AIDS-related infections such as toxoplasmosis and PCP. These drugs may precipitate folate deficiency and may require coadministration of folinic acid.

B_{12} deficiency is most often due to malabsorption. Dietary inadequacy is uncommon and occurs in strict vegetarians who eat no meat, eggs, or milk products. A common cause is pernicious anemia (PA), which is due to atrophic gastritis with absence of intrinsic factor. Intrinsic factor is necessary for the absorption of B_{12} in the distal ileum, and its absence in PA is associated with other features of autoimmunity. PA is marked by a progressive, severe, but surprisingly well-tolerated anemia. Glossitis, anorexia, and diarrhea are also common. Neurologic abnormalities are sometimes a striking feature and include dorsal column disease and cerebral dysfunction, peripheral neuropathy, weakness, and spasticity. Recently it has become clear that neurologic disease may be present in B_{12} deficiency without anemia. In some centers, testing for the increased methylmalonic acid or homocysteine associated with B_{12} deficiency is possible and may help to clarify the etiology of the neurologic problems.

The diagnosis of PA rests on establishing a low B_{12} level and a demonstration of atrophic gastritis or B_{12} malabsorption corrected by intrinsic factor (Shilling test). Some experts believe that the malabsorption of B_{12} is often subtle, so that the typical laboratory evaluation of B_{12} absorption may be normal. They have developed a test based on the absorption of B_{12} from a specially prepared meal.

Therapy for B_{12} deficiency is straightforward, but replacement of B_{12} in some anemic individuals may be complicated by hypokalemia. The anemia of B_{12} deficiency may be corrected by administration of pharmacologic doses of folate. However, neurologic disease is often exacerbated by folate administration.

Reference: Lindenbaum J, et al: Neuropsychiatric disorders caused by cobalamin deficiency in the absence of anemia or macrocytosis. N Engl J Med 318:1720–1728, 1988.

Microangiopathic Hemolytic Anemia

The microangiopathic hemolytic anemias are characterized by intravascular hemolysis and thrombocytopenia due to disorders of small blood vessels. Examination of a peripheral blood film discloses erythrocyte fragmentation with schistocytes (schizocytes), helmet cells, and spherocytes. Intravascular hemolysis results in elevations in the values of the plasma hemoglobin, serum LDH, and SGOT. In addition, hemoglobinuria and/or hemosiderinuria and ferritinuria are found. Thrombocytopenia occurs because of incorporation of platelets in microthrombi or destruction of platelets in the microcirculation.

Causes of Microangiopathic Hemolytic Anemia

Thrombotic thrombocytopenic purpura (TTP)
Hemolytic uremic syndrome: infantile form, adult form, related to chemotherapeutic agents
Pregnancy: preeclampsia, eclampsia, HELPP syndrome
Malignant hypertension
Primary renal disease: acute glomerulonephritis
Connective tissue disorders: SLE, polyarteritis nodosa, systemic vasculitis, progressive
   systemic sclerosis
Renal allograft rejection
Disseminated malignancy
Vascular malformations: Hemangioendothelioma of liver or spleen, Kasabach-Merritt syndrome
Disseminated intravascular coagulation (DIC)

The classic triad of TTP is hemolytic anemia with RBC fragmentation, thrombocytopenia, and fluctuating neurological deficits. The addition of fever and renal abnormalities makes a pentad. Hemolytic uremic syndrome is similar to TTP but is characterized by more severe renal manifestations and absence of direct CNS involvement. It generally occurs in children below the age of 2 years and in association with an infectious disease, particularly a diarrheal illness such as those due to *E. coli* or *Shigella*. The principal chemotherapeutic agents associated with hemolytic uremic syndrome are mitomycin C and cisplatin.

The acronym HELPP refers to a syndrome in pregnant women characterized by hemolysis, elevated liver enzymes, and low platelet count. Affected women have HTN and a preeclamptic state. Control of HTN is essential in patients with HELLP, preeclampsia, or malignant HTN in order to alleviate the hematologic abnormalities.

Primary glomerular disorders, usually of an immune causation, are occasional causes of microangiopathic hemolytic anemia. SLE with microangiopathic hemolytic anemia is uncommon but when present closely resembles TTP clinically. Disseminated malignancy may result in microangiopathic hemolytic anemia by reason of either widespread intravascular tumor or DIC. DIC of any etiology may lead to RBC fragmentation, usually mild in degree.

Sideroblastic Anemia

In patients with sideroblastic anemia, the mechanism of the anemia is ineffective erythropoiesis. There are abundant erythroid precursors in the bone marrow, but production of new erythrocytes is decreased. In the peripheral blood there is a subpopulation of hypochromic microcytic erythrocytes along with normochromic normocytic RBCs, giving the classical dimorphic appearance. With the recognition of macrocytes in some affected patients, the RBC population may actually be trimorphic. The reticulocyte count is low, reflecting impaired erythropoiesis. Dysplastic changes in erythroid precursors are common, particularly in acquired primary sideroblastic anemia. The unique feature of sideroblastic anemia is that many erythroblasts are ringed sideroblasts, that is, RBC precursors with a ring of Prussian blue-staining iron in mitochondria surrounding the nucleus.

Classification of Sideroblastic Anemias

Hereditary
Acquired
    Myelodysplastic syndrome (MDS): primary sideroblastic anemia, other forms of MDS, secondary MDS
    Secondary sideroblastic anemia: alcohol, drugs, lead poisoning, malignancies

---

Hereditary sideroblastic anemia is rare and may be inherited as an X-chromosome-linked disorder or as an autosomal recessive disease. The anemia is hypochromic and microcytic. Some patients' anemia responds to pharmacologic doses of pyridoxine.

Acquired primary (or refractory) sideroblastic anemia is now generally regarded as one form of the primary myelodysplastic syndrome. In primary sideroblastic anemia, 15% or greater of the erythroblasts in the marrow are ringed sideroblasts. Lesser numbers of ringed sideroblasts may be found in other categories of the myelodysplastic syndrome such as refractory anemia with excess blasts (RAEB) and chronic myelomonocytic leukemia (CMML). Alkylating agent chemotherapy and excessive exposure to benzene or irradiation may lead to the myelodysplastic syndrome, sometimes with sideroblastic erythropoiesis. In approximately 15% of patients with primary sideroblastic anemia, the illness terminates as acute myeloblastic leukemia (AML). Termination in AML is more frequent in patients with RAEB or CMML.

Alcoholism is a major cause of secondary sideroblastic anemia. Affected patients are also commonly deficient in folic acid. Drugs that may be responsible for sideroblastic anemia are isoniazid, pyrazinamide, cycloserine, and chloramphenicol. Patients with lead poisoning may have a mild hypochromic microcytic anemia with identifiable ringed sideroblasts in the bone marrow. Although anemia with ringed sideroblasts has been observed in patients with solid neoplasms and chronic inflammatory conditions, it is unclear whether this relationship is causal.

ANGINA PECTORIS

Medical vs. Surgical Therapy of Stable Angina

Three major clinical trials published in the early 1980s have contributed a great deal to our present therapeutic approach in patients with stable exertional angina. These clinical trials—the Coronary Artery Surgery Study (CASS),[1] the European Collaborative Study (ECS),[2] and the Veterans Administration Cooperative Study of Coronary Bypass Surgery (VACS)[3]—were randomized, prospective trials that evaluated the following common hypothesis: Does CABG decrease total and cardiovascular mortality compared to medical antianginal therapy in patients with stable exertional angina? The follow-up in these trials ranged from 5 to 11 years.

Based on the results of these three clinical trials, some general recommendations can be made about indications for CABG in patients with stable angina pectoris.

1. *Three-vessel CAD with depressed LV function:* Patients with at least 70% narrowing involving all three coronary vessels (left anterior descending [LAD], left circumflex [LCX], and right coronary artery [RCA]) as well as an LVEF of 35–50% have a significantly improved survival with CABG compared to medical therapy. Patients with three-vessel CAD and an LVEF less than 35% are at an increased operative risk and would benefit from CABG if the latter is expected to have an operative mortality less than 8%.

2. *Two- or three-vessel disease with involvement of the proximal LAD artery:* In the ECS, patients with two- or three-vessel CAD, one of which involves the proximal portion of the LAD (defined as the portion of the vessel proximal to the first septal perforator), have been shown to have an improved survival with CABG. Interestingly, all patients in the ECS had a normal LVEF. Thus, these patients as defined previously would benefit from CABG despite a normal LVEF.

3. *Left main CAD:* In the VA cooperative trials published in the 1960s, it was clearly demonstrated that the natural history of left main disease (defined as >50% narrowing of the left main coronary artery) is very poor and that CABG has a beneficial effect on survival in these patients, decreasing mortality to that usually found in patients with one-vessel CAD.

4. *Three-vessel CAD with a positive exercise test:* Both the VACS and the ECS revealed that patients with three-vessel CAD and a positive treadmill exercise test have an improved survival with CABG.

References: 1. CASS Principal Investigators and Their Associates: Coronary artery surgery study (CASS): A randomized trial of coronary artery bypass surgery. Survival data. Circulation 68:939–950, 1983.

2. European Coronary Surgery Study Group: Long-term results of a prospective randomized study of coronary artery bypass in stable angina pectoris. Lancet 2:1173–1180, 1982.

3. The Veterans Administration Coronary Artery Bypass Surgery Cooperative Study Group: Eleven-year survival in the Veterans Administration randomized trial of coronary bypass surgery for stable angina. N Engl J Med 311:1333–1339, 1984.

Medical vs. Surgical Care of Unstable Angina

The natural history of unstable angina is significantly worse than that of stable exertional angina. Unstable angina is a potentially life-threatening cardiac condition and can result in sudden cardiac death, fatal or nonfatal MI, serious cardiac arrhythmias, or CHF exacerbations. Thus, patients with unstable angina should be admitted to the hospital for close observation and ECG monitoring. The early clinical recognition of unstable angina is very crucial to its optimal management.

In addition to the absence of clear-cut ECG and cardiac enzyme changes diagnostic of acute MI, the definition of unstable angina depends on the presence of one or more of three historical features: (1) crescendo angina, defined as more severe, prolonged, or frequent angina; (2) angina at rest as well as on minimal exertion; (3) angina pectoris of new onset (usually within one month). Clinical management consists of the following:

1. **Bed rest:** Patients with unstable angina should generally be hospitalized in a monitored cardiac unit, placed on bed rest to minimize myocardial oxygen consumption, and monitored for worsening anginal symptoms, cardiac arrhythmias, and infarct evolution.

2. **Nitrates:** IV nitrates offer the following advantages: (a) more consistent control of ischemic episodes during 24 hours, (b) optimal titration of drug therapy, (c) reduction of symptomatic episodes of ischemia, and (d) reduction of the need for sublingual nitroglycerin use. The nitroglycerin regimen should be titrated to control symptoms of angina and to lower mean arterial BP by about 10%. Excessive doses of nitrates may result in hypotension and can thus be counterproductive, because hypotension may worsen myocardial ischemia by reducing coronary artery blood supply.

3. **Beta-blockers:** The main advantage of the addition of beta-blockers to intravenous nitrates in patients with unstable angina is the reduction of myocardial oxygen consumption mediated by a reduction of heart rate and myocardial contractility. The dose of the beta-blocker can be titrated to achieve a resting heart rate of 45–55 beats per minute without causing symptomatic hypotension or bradycardia. Beta-blockers should be used cautiously in patients with moderate LV systolic dysfunction (defined as an LVEF of 30–40%) and only rarely in patients with severe LV systolic dysfunction (defined as an LVEF of <30%).

4. **Calcium antagonists:** When used in combination with nitrates, calcium antagonists are about as effective as beta-blockers in relieving anginal

symptoms in patients with unstable angina. Selection of a calcium antagonist over a beta-blocker may be desirable in patients with angina at rest accompanied by transient ST-segment elevations consistent with a vasospastic etiology. The use of a dihydropyridine calcium antagonist with minimal negative inotropic effects, such as nifedipine, is recommended in patients with unstable angina and moderate or severe LV systolic dysfunction who remain symptomatic on nitrates, heparin, and aspirin and who do not tolerate a heart-rate-lowering calcium antagonist such as diltiazem.

Three clinical situations typify a worse clinical prognosis for unstable angina. The first involves patients with chest pain refractory to intensive medical therapy within 48 hours of therapy. The second involves patients who have either persistent ECG changes with angina or documented episodes of silent ischemia detected by continuous ECG monitoring. The third involves the subset of patients with post-MI angina. Patients recovering from acute MI who have recurrent angina during initiation of ambulation in the early hospitalization period have a poor prognosis if revascularization is not performed. In these patients, early coronary angiography is recommended during the initial hospitalization. If such patients have either angina refractory to medical therapy or angina at rest or angina at a low exercise threshold, then the possibility of revascularization with either percutaneous transluminal coronary angioplasty (PTCA) or CABG should be seriously considered. The selection of PTCA versus CABG depends on both the extent of CAD (single-vessel disease, unlike multivessel disease, favors PTCA over CABG) and the technical suitability of the obstructive coronary disease to PTCA (proximal, noncomplex, noncalcified lesions shorter than 1 cm are usually amenable to PTCA).

Whether to manage the patient with unstable angina by means of a medical regimen or with revascularization is often a difficult decision that should be tailored to the particular clinical situation and the needs of the patient. Clinical trials have been conducted in patients with unstable angina to provide the clinician with more rational scientific grounds for these difficult decisions. One should always remember, however, that the results of clinical trials can provide for the clinician only general guidelines rather than strict rules.

In a recent prospective, randomized, and controlled clinical trial—a Veterans Administration Cooperative Study—CABG was compared to medical antianginal treatment in 468 patients with unstable angina and critical coronary artery lesions as defined by a ≥75% luminal narrowing. CABG was shown to be superior to medical therapy in prolonging survival in patients with unstable angina and depressed LV function (defined as an LVEF of 30–59%). However, surgery was as effective as medical therapy in prolonging survival in patients with unstable angina, particularly those with normal LV systolic function.

Reference: Luchi RJ, et al: Comparison of medical and surgical treatment for unstable angina pectoris. Results of a Veterans Administration Cooperative Study. N Engl J Med 316:977–984, 1987.

ANKLE SPRAIN

Ankle sprains result from inversion or eversion foot injuries and frequently occur in sports or with a misstep such as occurs when stepping off a curb or step. Sprains range from first degree (stretched ligament) to second degree (torn ligament without disruption) to third degree (disrupted lateral ligament). Most minor sprains involve the lateral ligaments; third-degree sprains usually involve the anterior talofibular ligament. Medial or anterior symptoms suggest severe injury and should be referred to an orthopedist.

Characteristics of Ankle Sprains

TYPE (DEGREE)	SIGNS AND SYMPTOMS	EXAMINATION	X-RAY	TREATMENT
First	Swelling	Limited swelling and pain; no ecchymosis or joint laxity	Negative	RICE (rest, ice, compression, elevation)
Second	Tearing sensation	Diffuse swelling and pain; ecchymosis; slight joint laxity	Negative	RICE, immobilization (use crutches)
Third	Tearing sensation	Diffuse swelling, tenderness, and ecchymosis; joint laxity	Negative or small bone chip	RICE, no weight bearing, walking cast when swelling decreases

Reference: Birnbaum JS: The Musculoskeletal Manual, 2nd ed. New York, Academic Press, 1986.

ANKYLOSING SPONDYLITIS

Ankylosing spondylitis, only recently differentiated from RA, was initially called rheumatoid spondylitis and was believed to be a unique manifestation of RA. Currently, we think of ankylosing spondylitis as the prototypical spondyloarthropathy. It is a chronic axial arthropathy with a male predominance of 3:1. The overall prevalence in the population is 0.1–0.2% in white Americans and less in African-Americans and Asian-Americans. Haida and Pima Indians may have the highest prevalence (10% and 20% of their adult male populations, respectively). Onset is usually between puberty and 35 years, peaking in the mid-20s. Although diagnostic criteria exist, these are most useful for broad population surveys rather than individual diagnosis.

The pathogenesis remains unknown. The dramatic association with the class I MHC protein HLA B27 has been shown with epidemiologic studies. In addition, the placement of the HLA B27 gene in rodents (transgenic mice) has resulted in the development of a characteristic spondyloarthropathy.

Patients present with pain and stiffness in the lower back, which worsens with inactivity and lessens with exercise. This is an obvious distinction from mechanical or degenerative back pain, which usually worsens with exercise and lessens with rest. In patients younger than age 35 who present with back pain, ankylosing spondylitis is suggested by pain that awakens the patient from sleep as well as morning stiffness of greater than 30 minutes' duration. The disease may be heralded by a peripheral arthritis. As many as 50% of patients may eventually develop a symmetric peripheral arthropathy involving large joints such as the hip and knee.

Physical examination is often normal in early disease, but one can elicit tenderness over the sacroiliac or lumbar regions. There is distinct loss of lumbar flexion and extension, as well as lateral bending. The hips and shoulders may show some limitation of motion, and the peripheral joints can be involved.

Plain x-rays show sacroiliitis, and in general, this is required for the diagnosis. Early lesions include sclerosis of bone adjacent to the sacroiliac joint with frank bony fusion (ankylosis) occurring later. Although CT scan may help with early diagnosis, it offers no advantage as the disease progresses. The primary site of inflammation is the enthesis (site of insertion of the tendon to bone). On x-rays, this appears as spurring or squaring of the vertebra. Progression can lead to fusion of the apophyseal joints. Ligamentous ossification produces the classic bridging syndesmophytes, leading to the well-described bamboo spine.

Extra-articular manifestations are most common with advanced or long-standing disease but may rarely predate pain. About 13% of young men who require pacemakers for idiopathic rhythm disturbances have HLA B27 phenotype. More severely, aortic regurgitation can be seen in 5% of patients. Patients with ankylosing spondylitis may have anterior uveitis. Neurologic complications can occur on the basis of fragility of the fused spine. Thus, in these patients, neck pain after an automobile accident must be worked up aggressively. Pulmonary fibrosis has been noted in about 1% of patients with long-standing disease.

The prognosis is generally good. The course for the first 10 years is often a good predictor of subsequent disease. More severe disease usually occurs early. The presence of aggressive peripheral arthropathy and early onset of extra-articular features are poor prognostic findings. The disease increases mortality, and cervical fractures, cardiac disease, and amyloidosis are contributing factors.

Treatment should begin with supportive measures such as physical therapy. Goals should include maintenance of functional capacity and prevention of deformity. NSAIDs, particularly indomethacin, remain useful. Injection with glucocorticoid and local anesthetic into peripheral joints is helpful when such joints are involved. Glucocorticoids are not generally used systemically. In refractory cases, sulfasalazine may add benefit.

Reference: Khan MW, at al: Ankylosing spondylitis and other spondyloarthropathies. Rheum Dis Clin North Am 16:551–579, 1990.

ANOREXIA IN CANCER

Anorexia is one of the most common complications of cancer and, after pain, is the problem that most often afflicts patients and families. However, its pathophysiology is poorly understood and its remedies are few and unsatisfactory. It may result in the loss of only a few pounds at the onset of disease, or it may be a terminal event with cachexia as its result. It is well-known that weight loss correlates with survival. About two-thirds of patients with cancer experience anorexia, and slightly less than that report weight loss. The amount of weight loss varies with disease site. The most common association with weight loss occurs with gastric cancer, although pancreatic cancer can be associated with the most rapid and severe losses. The cause of death in cancer patients has been attributed to cachexia, but it is not clear if this is cause or effect. (See also Weight Loss in Cancer.)

The constellation of symptoms associated with anorexia has been termed the **cancer anorexia-cachexia syndrome**. It is associated with abnormalities of glucose, fat, and protein metabolism. Increased gluconeogenesis and Cori cycle activity create an energy-losing cycle between tumor and host. Because body glycogen mass is decreased, body glucose consumption is increased. Varying degrees of insulin resistance have been found to be present. Enhanced lipid mobilization, decreased lipogenesis, decreased lipoprotein lipase activity, elevated TG, decreased HDL, increased venous glycerol, and deceased glycerol clearance from the plasma have been reported. Abnormal activity of lipoprotein lipase appears to be the central derangement of lipid metabolism.

Since the pathophysiology of anorexia in cancer is unclear, treatment is difficult, but a few things are known. The causes may be simple and obvious, such as physical invasion by the tumor itself into the GI tract at the level of the mouth, esophagus, or stomach. Iatrogenic causes such as radiotherapy or chemotherapy can contribute to the anorexia. Pain, depression, and emotional causes all take their toll. However, severe anorexia may occur in the absence of, or out of proportion to, other factors, and it is clear that a humoral mechanism enters into the cycle in most cases. Such "humors" have been called anorexins. Appetite is controlled by thermostatic, glucostatic, hormonal, digestive, and cerebral neurotransmitters, but cessation of eating due to loss of appetite alone does not account for the weight loss seen in these patients. The basal metabolic rate, rather than decreasing in response to starvation, is normal or increased. Patients often complain of changes in taste sensation, early satiety, or even aversion to food, especially red meat. It has been shown that the extent of these abnormalities relates directly to the degree of tumor burden. Hormonal changes have been described in some patients, with findings of increased serum cortisol, reduced serum testosterone, and reduced serum triiodothyronine. But the relationship of these abnormalities to the development of anorexia is not clear. Cytokines have also been studied in this setting. IL-1, TNF-alpha, and IL-6 are all endogenous pyrogens and anorectic agents. The first two may exert their effect on the hypothalamus and GI tract. They probably also increase resting energy expenditure and promote skeletal muscle wasting.

Treatment of anorexia of cancer is simple, but unfortunately it is rarely useful. Patients should be scrupulous about mouth care and should avoid foods they have found to cause aversion. Some patients tolerate best a high-carbohydrate, low-protein diet, often avoiding heated foods; the American Cancer Society publishes written material containing suggestions in this area. Enteral supplements are useful in some patients. TPN is of limited benefit, with a relatively high risk/benefit ratio. Many oncologists reserve TPN for those patients who are undergoing treatment that affects the appetite or oral intake but who have a reasonable expectation of recovery if properly supported through this period. Many drugs have been tried with limited success. The most commonly used are megestrol acetate in high doses, corticosteroids, cyproheptadine, dextroamphetamine, and delta-9-THC.

In some cases, identification and treatment of related problems may help alleviate anorexia. In this context, treating gastroparesis with metoclopramide, pain with analgesics, depression with psychotropics, nausea with antiemetics, hypersecretion with H_2-blockers, and vitamin deficiencies with vitamin supplements can be helpful.

Reference: Nelson K, et al: Management of the anorexia cachexia syndrome. Cancer Bull 43(5):403–406, 1991.

ANTIBIOTICS

Adverse Effects

Aminoglycosides

Ototoxicity
1. Vestibular (streptomycin)
2. Cochlear (neomycin, kanamycin, amikacin)
3. Both (tobramycin, gentamicin)

Nondepolarizing neuromuscular blockade
Nephrotoxicity

Cephalosporins

Hypoprothrombinemia
Coombs-positive hemolytic anemia
Interstitial nephritis

Disulfiram-like reaction (cefamandole, cefoperazone, moxalactam)

Chloramphenicol

Bone marrow suppression
1. Dose-related, manifested by reversible anemia, leukopenia, or thrombocytopenia
2. Aplastic anemia, probably idiosyncratic "Gray" syndrome in neonates, manifested by abdominal distention, vomiting, cyanosis, hypothermia, irregular respirations, and vasomotor collapse due to accumulation of drug because of infant's inability to conjugate

Diarrhea
Glossitis
Nervous system disorder (digital paresthesias, peripheral neuritis, encephalopathy, optic neuropathy)

Clindamycin

Nausea, vomiting, epigastric distress

Antibiotic-associated pseudomembranous colitis

Erythromycin

Epigastric distress, nausea
Hearing loss (IV)
Phlebitis with infusions

Diarrhea
Cholestatic hepatitis (estolate)

Imipenem/Cilastatin

Seizures (esp. in patients with renal insufficiency)

Antibiotic-associated pseudomembranous colitis

Metronidazole

Metallic oral taste
Furring of tongue, glossitis and stomatitis
Sensory polyneuropathy, convulsions, encephalopathy

Nausea and vomiting
Neutropenia
Disulfiram-like reaction

Nitrofurantoin

Nausea and vomiting
Acute pulmonary reaction (fever, cough, dyspnea, eosinophilia, and infiltrates)
Interstitial pulmonary fibrosis
Hepatocellular and cholestatic liver injury
Headache, dizziness, nystagmus, drowsiness
Hemolysis (in G6PD–deficient individuals)

Hypersensitivity reactions: rash, urticaria, and pruritus; eosinophilia; drug fever

Drug-induced lupus syndrome
Ascending sensorimotor peripheral neuropathy
Granulocytopenia, leukopenia

Penicillins

Gastric distress and diarrhea
Neurotoxicity (confusion, agitation, myoclonus, seizures)
Hemolysis
Hypokalemia (carbenicillin, ticarcillin)
Platelet dysfunction
Interstitial nephritis (methicillin)

Antibiotic-associated pseudomembranous colitis
Hypersensitivity reactions, rash
1. Immediate
2. Urticarial eruptions
3. Drug fever
4. Thrombocytopenia

Quinolones

Nausea and vomiting
Headaches and dizziness

Rash

Rifampin

Staining of excretions and soft contact lenses
Gastrointestinal complaints
Light-chain proteinuria
Increased serum bile acids
Eosinophilia, tubulointerstitial nephritis, thrombocytopenia

Rash
Liver enzyme elevations, hepatitis
Flulike syndrome with fever, chills, and myalgias (worse with intermittent administration)

Sulfonamides

Hypersensitivity reactions: rash; eosinophila; drug fever; erythema multiforme
Crystalluria
Jaundice
Kernicterus (in newborns)
Megaloblastosis

Nausea, vomiting, diarrhea
Serum sickness (fever, joint pain, urticaria)
Drug-induced lupus syndrome
Hemolytic anemia (in G6PD–deficient individuals)
Granulocytopenia, thrombocytopenia

Tetracyclines

Thrombophlebitis (IV only)
Diarrhea
Antibiotic-associated pseudomembranous colitis
Suppression of long-bone growth in premature children
Benign intracranial HTN

Epigastric distress, nausea, vomiting
Superinfection (e.g., yeast vaginitis)
Teeth discoloration (children)
Photosensitivity, manifested by abnormal sunburn reactions or skin paresthesias
Dizziness, vertigo, ataxia (minocycline)

Vancomycin

Urticaria, flushing, tachycardia and hypotension with rapid infusion
Rash
Leukopenia, thrombocytopenia (rare)

Phlebitis at infusion site
Ototoxicity (high frequencies)
? Nephrotoxicity

Reference: Conte JR Jr, et al (eds): Manual of Antibiotics and Infectious Diseases, 6th ed. Philadelphia, Lea & Febiger, 1988.

Dose Adjustments for Renal Insufficiency

Most antibiotics require some degree of dosage adjustments for renal impairment. Several different nomograms and sets of guidelines are available. In order to calculate the appropriate dose, several steps are required:

1. Calculation of lean body weight (LBW):
   Males = 50 kg + 2.3 kg/inch over 5 feet
   Females = 45.5 kg + 2.3 kg/inch over 5 feet
   a. In obese patients whose actual body weight (ABW) is greater than 30% above the LBW, the dosing weight is calculated as follows:
   Dosing weight = [(ABW − LBW) × 0.4] + LBW

2. Calculation of creatinine clearance (C_{Cr}):
   Males: $C_{Cr} = \dfrac{(140 - \text{age}) \times (\text{Dosing weight in kg})}{72 \times \text{serum creatinine}}$
   Females: $C_{Cr} = 0.85$ of male value

3. Find fraction of antibiotic dose to be administered: Look up the particular antibiotic in the table that follows, and determine which line it falls on. Then find the calculated (or measured) creatinine clearance along the horizontal axis of the graph that follows, follow it up to the appropriate line, and read the dose fraction on the vertical axis.

Dosing Lines for Various Antibiotics for Use in Patients with Impaired Renal Function

Amikacin..A	Cephalothin..A	Nafcillin..D
Ampicillin..B	Cephapirin..C	Netilmicin..A
Azithromycin..H	Cephradine..A	Nitrofurantoin..D
Azlocillin..C	Chloramphenicol..G	Ofloxacin..B
Aztreonam..D	Ciprofloxacin..F	Oxacillin..F
Carbenicillin..B	Clarithromycin..D	Oxytetracycline..C
Cefaclor..D	Clindamycin..G	Penicillin G..B
Cefamandole..B	Cloxacillin..F	Piperacillin..D
Cefazolin..A	Dicloxacillin..D	Rifampin..H
Cefonicid..B	Doxycycline..H	Spectinomycin..B
Ceforanide..B	Erythromycin..D	Streptomycin..A
Cefoperazone..G	Gentamicin..A	Sulfamethoxazole..G
Cefotaxime..E	Imipenem..D	Tetracycline..B
Cefotetan..C	Kanamycin..A	Ticarcillin..B
Cefoxitin..A	Lincomycin..E	Tobramycin..A
Ceftazidime..B	Lomefloxacin..F	Trimethoprim..F
Ceftizoxime..A	Methicillin..B	Trimethoprim-sulfa-
Ceftriaxone..B	Metronidazole..H	methoxazole..F
Cefuroxime..B	Mezlocillin..D	Vancomycin..A
Cephalexin..A	Moxalactam..B	

Figure on page 55 modified from Brody M, et al: Antimicrobial induced renal failure: Choice of antimicrobials in renal insufficiency and/or urinary tract infection. In Rieselbach RE, et al (eds): Cancer and the Kidney. Philadelphia, Lea & Febiger, 1982, pp 824–854, with permission.

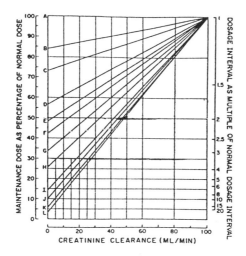

Mechanisms of Action

Mechanism of Action of Antimicrobial Agents

AGENT	SITE OF ACTION	EFFECT	CIDAL	STATIC
Penicillins, cephalosporins	Cell wall	Inhibit cross-linking of peptido-glycan resulting in spheroplast formation	+	Occ
Vancomycin	Cell wall	Block transfer of pentapeptide from cytoplasm to cell membrane	+	Occ
Polymyxin B, colistin	Cytoplasmic membrane	Bind phospholipid and disrupt membrane	+	
Aminoglyco-sides	Ribosome	Bind to 30S ribosomal subunit, thereby inhibiting attachment of mRNA; also affect tRNA	+	
Tetracyclines	Ribosome	Bind to 30S subunit and inhibit binding of tRNA		+
Chloramphenicol	Ribosome	Bind to 50S subunit and inhibit mRNA translation	Occ	+
Erythromycin, clindamycin	Ribosome	Inhibit mRNA translation	Occ	+
Rifampin	Nucleic acid synthesis	Impaired RNA formation by in-hibiting DNA-dependent RNA formation by inhibiting DNA-dependent RNA-polymerase	+	Occ
Metronidazole	Nucleic acid synthesis	Damages nucleic acid structure	+	
Quinolones	Nucleic acid synthesis	Inhibit DNA gyrase	+	
Sulfonamides	Nucleic acid synthesis	Competitive inhibition of *para*-amino benzoic acid, thereby blocking formation of thymi-dine and purines		+

Occ = occasionally. Modified from Young LS: Antimicrobial therapy. In Wyngaarden JB, et al (eds): Cecil Textbook of Medicine, 18th ed. Philadelphia, W.B. Saunders, 1988, p 113, with permission.

Drug Interactions

Important Antibiotic Drug Interactions

ANTIMICROBIAL AGENT	INTERACTING DRUG	RESULT
Amphotericin B	Curariform drugs	Increased curarelike effect
Aminoglycosides	Neuromuscular blockers (e.g., tubocurarine, pancuronium)	Additive blockade
	Diuretics: ethacrynic acid, furosemide	Increased ototoxicity
	Antibiotics: amphotericin B	Increased nephrotoxicity
	Carbenicillin/ticarcillin (other penicillins)	Inactivation, resulting in reduced activity
Ampicillin/amoxicillin	Allopurinol	Rash
Azithromycin	Antacids	Decreased maximal azithromycin serum concentration
Cephalosporins (cefamandole, cefoperazone, moxalactam, cefotetan, cefmetazole)	Alcohol	Disulfiram reaction
Chloramphenicol	Warfarin	Decreased warfarin metabolism and inhibition of vitamin-K-producing gut bacteria, thus increasing prothrombin time
	Phenytoin	Decreased phenytoin metabolism
	Oral hypoglycemics	Increased hypoglycemia
	Phenobarbital	Decreased phenobarbital levels
Clarithromycin	Carbamazepine	Increased carbamazepine levels
	Theophylline	Increased theophylline levels
	Zidovudine	Decreased maximal zidovudine concentration
Erythromycin	Theophylline	Increased theophylline levels
	Digoxin	Increased digoxin levels
	Carbamazepine	Increased carbamazepine levels
	Cyclosporine	Increased cyclosporine levels
	Methylprednisolone	Reduced steroid clearance
	Warfarin	Increased prothrombin time
Fluconazole	Warfarin	Increased prothrombin time
	Phenytoin	Increased phenytoin levels
	Sulfonylureas	Increased sulfonylurea levels
	Rifampin	Decreased fluconazole levels
	Cyclosporine	Possible renal impairment due to increased cyclosporine levels
Isoniazid	Warfarin, phenytoin	Increased risk of toxicity by decreased drug metabolism
	Disulfiram	Psychosis
	Rifampin, PAS	Additive hepatotoxicity
	Oral contraceptives	Decreased contraceptive effect

Table continued on next page.

Important Antibiotic Drug Interactions (Cont.)

Isoniazid (*cont.*)	Alcohol	Increased isoniazid metabolism
	Al-containing antacids	Decreased isoniazid absorption
Itraconazole	Antacids, H_2-antagonists	Decreased itraconazole absorption
	Warfarin	Increased prothrombin time
	Terfenadine, astemizole	Increased antihistamine levels; ventricular arrhythmias
	Rifampin	Decreased itraconazole levels
	Cyclosporine	Renal impairment due to increased cyclosporine levels
	Oral hypoglycemics	Hypoglycemia due to increased levels
	Digoxin	Digoxin toxicity due to decreased metabolism
	Phenytoin	Reduced itraconazole levels
Ketoconazole	Antacids, H_2-antagonists	Decreased ketoconazole absorption
	Cyclosporine	Renal impairment due to increased cyclosporine levels
	Warfarin, phenytoin	Decreased warfarin and phenytoin metabolism
	Isoniazid	Increased isoniazid levels
Metronidazole	Alcohol	Disulfiram-like reaction (nausea)
	Disulfiram	Psychosis
	Warfarin	Increased PT
Nalidixic acid	Warfarin	Increased PT
Polymyxins	Curariform drugs	Increased curarelike effect
Quinolones	Theophylline, caffeine	Decreased clearance of xanthines
	Al^{++}- and Mg^{++}-containing antacids, multivalent cations	Decreased quinolone absorption
	NSAIDs	Decreased quinolone absorption
	Probenecid	Decreased quinolone clearance
Rifampin	Warfarin, phenytoin	Decreased warfarin, phenytoin effect
	Isoniazid	Additive hepatotoxicity
	Methadone	Withdrawal symptoms
	Oral contraceptives	Decreased contraceptive effect
	Steroids	Decreased steroid effect
	Digitalis derivatives	Decreased digitalis levels
	Azole antifungals	Decreased azole levels
	Quinidine	Decreased quinidine levels
	Cyclosporine	Decreased cyclosporine levels
Sulfonamides	Procaine	Decreased sulfonamide effect
	Hypoglycemics	Hypoglycemia
	Warfarin, phenytoin	Displace drugs from protein-binding sites, causing increased warfarin and phenytoin effects
Tetracyclines	Antacids, oral iron, calcium	Decreased tetracycline absorption

ANTICOAGULANTS

Heparin

Heparin is a glycosaminoglycan consisting of chains of D-glucosamine alternating with gluconic or iduronic acid. Commercial, standard heparin is a heterogenous mixture of polysaccharides with molecular weights ranging from 5,000 to 30,000 daltons. Heparin blocks the action of thrombin, as well as the activated factors of X, XII, XI, and IX. These effects require the participation of anti-thrombin III. The binding of heparin results in a conformational change in antithrombin III so that it is capable of inactivating thrombin, Xa, and IXa. The results of heparin administration are complex and reflect binding of heparin to many plasma proteins, and endothelial cells as well as uptake by phagocytic cells. One consequence of this complexity is the disproportionate effect of heparin as the administered dose increases. Thus the administration of heparin to obtain a therapeutic goal is sometimes difficult, as an increase in the rate of heparin administration may suddenly have greater than the desired effect.

Clinical Uses of Heparin

CONDITION	EFFECTIVE HEPARIN REGIMEN
Venous thromboembolism	
Prophylaxis of DVT and PE	5000 U SC Q 8 or 12 hrs, or adjusted low-dose heparin*
Treatment of DVT	IV bolus of 5000 U, followed by 30,000–35,000 U/24 hrs by IV infusion or 35,000–40,000 U/24 hrs SC, adjusted to maintain APTT at 1.5–2.5 times control value†
Coronary heart disease	
Unstable angina	IV bolus of 5000 U, followed by 24,000 U/24 hrs by IV infusion, adjusted to maintain APTT at 1.5–2.5 times control value†
Acute MI	
Prevention of mural thrombosis	12,500 U, SC BID (fixed dose)
Prevention of death and reinfarction	IV bolus of 2000 U, 12,500 U SC BID (fixed dose)
After thrombolytic therapy	
Patency‡	IV bolus of 5000, followed by 24,000 U/24 hrs, adjusted to maintain APTT at 1.25–2.5 times control value†
Mortality§	IV bolus of 2000 U, 12,500 U SC BID (fixed dose)

*3500 U of heparin SC every 8 hours, adjusted to an APTT in the upper normal range.

†Equivalent to a heparin level of 0.2–0.4 U/ml by protamine titration or 0.35–0.7 U/ml according to the level of inhibition of factor Xa.

‡After treatment with tissue plasminogen activator (tPA).

§After treatment with streptokinase.

Adapted from Hirsch J: Recommendation for the use of heparin. N Engl J Med 324:1565–1574, 1991, with permission.

The clinical uses of heparin are summarized in the table above. Heparin is frequently used to maintain patency of venous and arterial lines, during angiography, and sometimes in the treatment of DIC associated with thrombosis (i.e., Trousseau's syndrome). For prophylaxis of DVT, 5,000 U Q 8–12 hours is administered. Treatment of DVT or PE requires a bolus of 5,000 U, followed by 30,000–35,000 U during 24 hours or a suitable rate of administration to maintain the activated PTT 1.5 and 2.5 times the control value. A brief duration (5 days) of treatment may be possible for DVT, whereas PE may require longer initial treatment (10 days).

Recently, a new class of low-MW heparins (LMWH) have been produced with MW between 4,000 and 6,500. Also in clinical trials are the heparinoids, which are a mixture of heparan sulfate and dermatan and chondroitin sulfates. LMWH and heparinoids may have a number of advantages over commercial heparin. The LMWH are more potent inhibitors of factor Xa and less potent inhibitors of thrombin, are not inactivated by platelet factor 4, have a longer half-life, and, at lower doses, have an increased plasma recovery compared to similar amounts of standard heparin. Recent clinical trials have shown LMWH to be safe and effective anticoagulants. Because of the favorable pharmacokinetics and the absence of effects on the PTT, LMWH are given once daily and without frequent PTT monitoring.

Complications of Heparin Therapy

Hemorrhage
Thrombocytopenia
   Alone
   With thrombosis (venous and/or arterial)
Osteoporosis
Skin necrosis
Alopecia
Hypoaldosteronism

The risk for bleeding while receiving heparin is increased with increasing dose and with concurrent aspirin use. Some patients have experienced hypersensitivity reactions and hypoaldosteronism. Osteoporosis is seen with long-term heparin administration.

Perhaps the most significant hazard associated with heparin use is heparin-induced thrombocytopenia. Prolonged administration or repetitive administration of heparin may induce the production of antibodies that are platelet reactive in the presence of heparin. Thus, after 10–14 days of heparin administration there is a precipitous drop in the platelet count. This event may be associated with recurrent arterial thrombi, DVT, or PE. The unsuspecting internist or cardiovascular surgeon may mistakenly continue or increase the rate of administration of heparin. It is extremely important to monitor the platelet count when heparin is given and to discontinue heparin administration immediately when the platelet count takes a significant tumble. The loss of a limb due to thrombotic occlusion by "white thrombi"; fatal strokes; saddle emboli; and acute MI have occurred as a result of heparin-induced thrombocytopenia. In patients who have previously received heparin, this disorder may occur after relatively brief periods of heparin administration. Low-dose heparin for prophylaxis or to maintain line patency has also been implicated in thrombocytopenia. Once thrombocytopenia has been recognized, elimination of heparin from all lines is mandatory.

Warfarin

Warfarin continues to be the mainstay of oral anticoagulation in patients with high risk for thrombosis. A summary of indications is shown in the table.

Warfarin management has undergone a revolution sparked by recognition that the coagulation test used to monitor therapy—the PT test—is variable and that lower dosage regimens are effective for most indications. The variability depends on the source of the thromboplastin used in the test. There may also be substantial differences in the PT measured even when kits from the same manufacturer are used. For example, it was recognized that average warfarin doses administered in England

Effectiveness of Oral Anticoagulant Therapy with Warfarin

CONDITION	INTERNATIONAL NORMALIZED RATIO (INR)*	
	Minimal Effective	Recommended
Deep-venous thrombosis		
Prevention	1.5–2.5	2.0–3.0‡
Treatment	2.0–2.3	2.0–3.0
Acute MI		
Prevention of stroke	2.0	2.0–3.0
Prevention of recurrence	2.7–4.5	3.0–4.5‡
Reduction of mortality	2.7–4.5	3.0–4.5‡
Peripheral arterial disease—prevention of death	2.6–4.5	—
AF—prevention of systemic embolism	1.5–2.5§	2.0–3.0‡
Cardiac-valve replacement		
Tissue valves	2.0–2.3	2.0–3.0
Mechanical valves	1.9–3.6	3.0–4.5‡
Cerebral embolism	Not evaluated	—
Native valvular heart disease	Not evaluated	—

*For thromboplastin with an ISI of 2.3, the INRs and the corresponding prothrombin time (PT) ratios are as follows:

INR	1.5	2.0	2.5	3.0	3.5	4.0	4.5	5.0
PT ratio	1.20	1.35	1.49	1.61	1.72	1.83	1.92	2.01

‡A lower range might be effective.

§Based on ISI of 2.3.

Adapted from Hirsh J: Oral anticoagulant drugs. N Engl J Med 324:1865–1875, 1991, with permission.

were lower than those prescribed in the United States. In England, brain thromboplastins are used and the PT is more sensitive to anticoagulation, which results in the apparent need for smaller doses with equal efficacy against thrombosis, but with a lower incidence of bleeding complications.

In order to standardize warfarin anticoagulation, an international standard was developed. Now, an International Sensitivity Index (ISI) is provided for each thromboplastin. This allows for the adjustment of the PT by converting the ratio of the patient's PT to the normal PT, to an international normalized ratio (INR). This is done using the formula $INR = (PT \ ratio)^{ISI}$. For example, if a patient's PT is 18 seconds using a PT kit with a normal of 12 seconds and a thromboplastin with an ISI of 2.4, the PT ratio is 18/12, or 1.5. The INR is the PT ratio raised to the power of the ISI, or $(1.5)^{2.4} = 2.65$. The desirable range for the INR for most indications is 2–3. The example shows that the warfarin dosage for the hypothetical patient described is appropriate. Until manufacturers are able to solve the problems in making a uniform thromboplastin, it will be necessary for physicians to make this calculation or have it provided for them by the clinical laboratory.

The pharmacology of warfarin is complex. Warfarin reduces the activity of vitamin K, which is essential for the γ-carboxylation of the anticoagulant proteins C and S and the procoagulant proteins (factors II, VII, IX, and X). It is readily absorbed from the gut, bound extensively to albumen, and metabolized by the liver. Inactive metabolites are excreted in the urine. Warfarin's potency is sensitive to changes in vitamin K production by gut flora, absorption of warfarin, warfarin's binding to albumen, and hepatic function. There is little need to adjust warfarin dosage for renal insufficiency.

Initiation of warfarin therapy should not be aggressive. Large loading doses may be associated with a disproportionate effect on the anticoagulant proteins C and S. In patients receiving high doses of warfarin without concomitant heparinization, skin necrosis has been observed, usually involving thrombosis of small vessels in fatty tissues of the breast, thigh, or ear lobe. Warfarin necrosis may occur in patients with protein C deficiency as a cause of their thrombosis. Thus it is desirable to initiate warfarin therapy when patients are on heparin, or very slowly when they are not.

Maintenance dosage should be kept as simple as possible, using multiples of a single tablet. When it is necessary to vary the daily dose, the schedule should be based on days of the week rather than calendar or odd/even days. Changes in diet or administration of antibiotics may alter vitamin K availability and prolong the PT. Certain drugs reduce the hepatic metabolism of warfarin. As shown in the table that follows, there are numerous drug interactions to consider. Patients should be encouraged to consult their physician before taking any drug (over-the-counter or prescription). Aspirin may potentiate bleeding during warfarin therapy by inactivating platelets. In recent studies, the duration of warfarin anticoagulation after DVT need be for only three months.

The most important complication of warfarin therapy is bleeding. Bleeding in the face of a normal INR suggests the possibility of an underlying lesion. Warfarin produces a characteristic embryopathy in women who receive the drug early in pregnancy. Warfarin must be avoided in the first trimester, and it should probably also be avoided in the second and third trimesters. Heparin is now the preferred treatment for the pregnant woman who is at risk for DVT or needs prophylaxis for an artificial heart valve.

*Drugs That Alter Prothrombin Time by Interacting with Warfarin,
According to Type of Interaction*

PHARMACOKINETIC (DRUGS THAT CHANGE WARFARIN LEVELS)	PHARMACODYNAMIC (DRUGS THAT DO NOT CHANGE WARFARIN LEVELS)	MECHANISM UNKNOWN (DRUGS WHOSE EFFECT ON WARFARIN LEVELS IS UNKNOWN)
Prolongs prothrombin time	**Prolongs prothrombin time**	**Prolongs prothrombin time**
Stereoselective inhibition of clearance of *S* isomer:	Inhibits cyclic interconversion of vitamin K:	Evidence for interaction convincing:
Phenylbutazone	2nd- and 3rd-generation cephalosporins	Erythromycin
Metronidazole	Other mechanisms:	Anabolic steroids
Sulfinpyrazone	Clofibrate	Evidence for interaction less convincing:
TMP-SMX	Inhibits blood coagulation:	Ketoconazole
Disulfiram	Heparin	Fluconazole
Stereoselective inhibition of clearance of *R* isomer:	Increases metabolism of coagulation factors:	Isoniazid
Cimetidine*	Thyroxine	Piroxicam
Omeprazole*		Tamoxifen
Nonstereoselective inhibitions of clearance of *R* and *S* isomers:		Quinidine
Amiodarone		Vitamin E (megadose)
		Phenytoin
Reduces prothrombin time	**Inhibits platelet function**	**Reduces prothrombin time**
Reduces absorption:	Aspirin	Penicillins
Cholestyramine	Other NSAIDs	Griseofulvin†
Increases metabolic clearance:	Ticlopidine	
Barbiturates	Moxalactam	
Rifampin	Carbenicillin and high doses of other penicillins	
Griseofulvin		
Carbamazepine		

*Causes minimal prolongation of the prothrombin time.
†Has been proposed to cause increased metabolic clearance.
From Hirsh J: Oral anticoagulant drugs. N Engl J Med 324:1865–1875, 1991, with permission.

ANTIPHOSPHOLIPID ANTIBODY SYNDROME

Understanding of the role of circulating antibodies to phospholipids (aPL) has expanded dramatically in recent years. An association between aPL and rheumatic diseases began in the 1940s, when patients with SLE were found to have a high incidence of biologic false-positive tests for syphilis. The antigen, initially called reagin, was found to be the phospholipid cardiolipin. A second association came with the detection of the so-called lupus anticoagulant (LAC), now also known to be an aPL. In 1988, the association between a definable clinical syndrome (venous and arterial thromboses, recurrent miscarriages, and thrombocytopenia) and the presence of circulating aPL was documented. These features are associated with the presence of aPL whether the antibodies represent the only manifestation of autoimmunity (primary antiphospholipid antibody syndrome) or whether there is also another associated rheumatic disease present.

The aPL recognize the negatively charged phosphodiester group in anionic phospholipids. There is strong evidence that the LAC is also an antibody to negatively charged phospholipids. More recent data also suggest the importance of a cofactor in aPL binding.

The mechanism by which aPL are associated with hypercoagulability is unknown, although a number of hypotheses have been advanced. Because phospholipids are required throughout the clotting and fibrinolytic cascade, it has been suggested that by interfering with phospholipid availability, aPL could lead to clotting. Binding of endothelial cells by an aPL could disrupt the normal anticoagulant function (reduction in prostacyclin has been suggested) and promote thrombosis.

The prevalence of aPL in the general population ranges from 2 to 5%, although data suggest an increase with age. In SLE the frequency ranges from 7 to 58%. In women with a history of recurrent fetal loss it is 13–40%. About 46% of young stroke patients were found to have either the LAC or aPL in circulation. Levine et al. suggest that aPL may be an important factor in roughly 10% of all strokes.

The primary clinical manifestations of the aPL syndrome revolve around clotting. Levine et al. carefully cataloged the presence of both strokes and transient ischemic attacks in young people without other predisposing risk factors. This phenomenon may help explain pathologic studies of CNS disease in SLE that show infarcts without active inflammation. Other arterial lesions have been associated, including renal and retinal arterial thromboses, distal gangrene, MI, and mitral valve lesions. Venous lesions are also seen and range from livedo reticularis to DVT and PE. Budd-Chiari syndrome has also been associated with the presence of circulating aPL.

Another associated clinical feature of aPL is recurrent fetal loss, at any time in pregnancy, often with evidence of placental infarction. Second- and third-trimester losses are most strongly associated with high levels of aPL in circulation. Migraine headaches are also well-known clinical manifestations of aPL. The last common manifestation is thrombocytopenia, which is usually mild and does not require intervention.

No single test adequately evaluates for the presence of aPL. The presence of anticardiolipin can be detected with an ELISA or a positive VDRL. The LAC is classically detected by an elevated PTT. Either the dilute Russell's viper venom time or the kaolin clotting time is useful.

Treatment remains controversial, and published regimens range from 80 mg of aspirin daily to high-dose glucocorticoids with plasmapheresis and cytotoxic agents. Prophylaxis is generally not required if no previous clinically associated events have occurred. If other risk factors for clotting are present, or titers of aPL are high, some have suggested aspirin or SC heparin. Oral anticoagulation (in nonpregnant patients) can be accomplished with warfarin and titrated by following the PT. Occasionally this is not successful, and a more aggressive regimen is required. In women with multiple miscarriages, high-dose prednisone has been successful. Recently, low-dose heparin has been shown to be as effective as 40 mg of prednisone and with fewer maternal complications.

References: Asherson RA, et al: The "primary antiphospholipid syndrome": Major clinical and serologic features. Medicine 68:366–374, 1989.

Levine SR, et al: Cerebrovascular ischemia associated with lupus anticoagulant. Stroke 18:257–263, 1987.

Cowchock FS, et al: Repeated fetal losses associated with antiphospholipid antibodies: A collaborative randomized trial comparing prednisone with low-dose heparin treatment. Am J Obstet Gynecol 166(5):1318–1323, 1992.

AORTIC INSUFFICIENCY

Physical Findings

1. **Apical impulse:** The precordial apical impulse will be accentuated because of the accompanying LVH.
2. **Austin-Flint murmur:** A soft, low-pitched, rumbling mid-diastolic murmur produced by anterior displacement of the mitral valve by the aortic regurgitant stream.
3. **Corrigan pulse (water-hammer pulse):** The high pulse pressure results in a very sharp upstroke of the pulse wave and a precipitous fall in the downstroke.
4. **Duroziez's sign:** While listening with the stethoscope, the clinician applies gradual pressure over the femoral artery with the stethoscope bell, producing a to-and-fro sounding murmur.
5. **Head bobbing:** The patient may be noted to bob the head slightly with each systolic pulse.
6. **Mayne's sign:** Moderate or mild degrees of aortic regurgitation may be detected by demonstration of a diminution of more than 15 mm Hg in the diastolic BP in an arm when it is elevated over the head compared with values taken when the arm is at heart level.
7. **Murmur:** The murmur of aortic insufficiency is a high-pitched blowing, decrescendo murmur heard best in the second right or third left intercostal space. The murmur may be elicited better when the patient is sitting up and leaning forward. Isometric maneuvers accentuate the murmur.
8. **Pistol-shot sound:** When the stethoscope bell is placed lightly over the femoral artery, a sharp sound like a gunshot can be heard.
9. **Pulse pressure:** The pulse pressure, or the difference between the systolic and diastolic BP, is normally 30–40 mm Hg. Widening of the pulse pressure occurs regularly in aortic insufficiency with both elevation of the systolic component and lowering of the diastolic component.
10. **Quincke's pulse:** An alternating flushing and paling of the skin at the root of the nail when pressure is applied gently to the tip of the nail.

APHASIA

Aphasia is an acquired disturbance of language function. It is not synonymous with a disturbance of speech, which is merely spoken language and which is referred to as dysarthria or mutism. Instead, aphasia implies a disturbance in all or most spheres of language, including not only speech but also writing, reading, comprehension, naming, and repetition. Evaluation of a patient with suspected aphasia is not sufficient if it checks only verbal speech. The patient must be made to write as well, because writing is also a language function. A patient who cannot speak, or who has very disordered verbal language but who is able to write normally, almost certainly does not have aphasia (or a left hemisphere cortical lesion).

Language function resides primarily in groups of neurons around the sylvian fissure in the left cerebral cortex. Although language function is often conceptualized in terms of dominant handedness, most left-handed people nevertheless also have language function in their left cerebral cortex.

Manipulation of languages is an extremely complex neural process, but for practical purposes, clinically, aphasias can be divided into two types: fluent (Wernicke's aphasia) and nonfluent (Broca's aphasia).

Wernicke's aphasia results from damage to the posterior part of the temporal lobe. Synonyms include fluent, posterior, receptive, and sensory aphasia. Patients with Wernicke's aphasia can speak fluently and uninterruptedly, but the content of their language is distorted. They make many paraphasic errors, substituting nonsense sounds (e.g., "swelt" for "belt") or entire words (e.g., "nothkit," "fwembley"). Comprehension is usually severely affected, so that such patients are unable to appreciate the garbled nature of their own speech, nor comprehend what others tell (or write to) them. The ability to name and repeat is similarly impaired. In fact, although speech is fluent, all other aspects of language show abnormalities.

A clinical pearl: Because Wernicke's area is located away from the motor, sensory, and visual areas, damage there, such as from a stroke, may produce no findings whatsoever except for the aphasia. Clinically, this would present as the sudden onset of fluent nonsensical speech (i.e., patients "talk out of their head," and, because comprehension is impaired, they do not understand what they are told). Therefore, a high percentage of patients with Wernicke's aphasia are admitted to a psychiatric unit initially.

The other important type of aphasia—Broca's aphasia—is caused by damage just in front of the face of the homunculus in the motor strip, in the left frontal lobe. Synonyms include nonfluent, anterior, expressive, and motor aphasia. Patients are nonfluent and cannot generate even as much as 15 words of spontaneous speech per minute. They have a hesitant, choppy, telegraphic, frustrated speech and often grope for words. Comprehension is relatively spared, leaving them the ability to appreciate their inadequate speech, thus enhancing their frustration. The ability to name and repeat is impaired, as might be expected in patients who have difficulty generating spontaneous speech. Because Broca's area lies so close to the motor strip, damage there almost always produces a right hemiparesis or at the very least, some weakness on the right side of the face.

Aphasia: Broca's vs. Wernicke's

TYPE	FLUENT	NAMES	REPEATS	COMPREHENDS
Broca's	No	No	No	Yes
Wernicke's	Yes	No	No	No

Ischemic strokes cause almost all cases of aphasia, and embolic strokes are particularly likely to produce these cortical deficits. Both Broca's and Wernicke's areas lie in the distribution of the middle cerebral artery, although Broca's is in its most anterior reach and Wernicke's is in its most posterior.

Treatment for aphasia is frustrating. Because they are unable to comprehend well, patients with Wernicke's aphasia make very little progress in speech therapy. Patients with Broca's aphasia may fare better, but the exact role, timing, and techniques of speech therapy remain debated.

Reference: Albert M, et al: Diagnosis and treatment of aphasia. JAMA 259:1043–1047, 1205–1210, 1988.

APHTHOUS ULCERS

Aphthous ulcers are painful lesions occurring on the buccal mucosa and the floor of the mouth. They have a central crater filled with a white coagulum and a surrounding violaceous rim. Lesions may be single or multiple and usually remain for 7–10 days. The occurrence of aphthous ulcers rarely indicates systemic disease or an immune disorder but can be associated with Behçet's syndrome, ulcerative colitis, or Crohn's disease.

Treatment is purely symptomatic and includes oral analgesics such as viscous lidocaine or oral antibiotic suspensions such as tetracycline. The solutions are swirled in the mouth, then expectorated. Topical steroids, such as triamcinolone in 0.5% hydrocortisone acetate oral paste (Kenalog in Orabase) or 0.05% fluocinonide (Lidex) gel can also be applied to individual lesions.

ARRHYTHMIAS

Diagnosis

Cardiac arrhythmias result from disordered impulse formation and/or conduction. Impulse generation in myocardial tissue results from the property of automaticity (i.e., the ability of certain cardiac cells to generate an action potential that is propagated to adjacent cells). This property is observed in the sinus node, certain other atrial cells, and His-Purkinje tissues. Of these, the sinus node normally discharges most rapidly and serves as the normal pacemaker. Disorders of impulse formation result when either the normal pacemaker discharges at an abnormal rate or an ectopic pacemaker takes over control. Disordered impulse conduction often causes bradyarrhythmias that allow reentry mechanisms to develop with sustained tissue reactivation and subsequent tachyarrhythmias.

Symptoms that may indicate arrhythmias include palpitations, syncope or near-syncope, dizziness, dyspnea, and progressive edema. Patients who complain of palpitations should be questioned as to the speed and rhythm of the beats, whether or not the palpitations come and go suddenly or gradually, what maneuvers slow the beats, and their use of alcohol, caffeine, nonprescription medications, or illegal drugs.

Laboratory evaluation should include electrolyte measurements, thyroid function testing, and serum levels of possible associated medications (e.g., theophylline, digoxin, and antiarrhythmic medications). Careful review of the ECG may not only define the specific arrhythmia but also suggest the presence of associated CAD, LVH, or accessory pathways. Holter monitoring is often helpful, as is treadmill stress testing. Invasive electrophysiologic testing may have both diagnostic and therapeutic applications in difficult cases.

Characteristics of Major Arrhythmias

MAJOR ARRHYTHMIAS	CHARACTERISTICS	ASSOCIATED CONDITIONS	TRACING
Sinus node dysfunction (includes sick sinus syndrome and tachy-brady syndrome)	Atrial rate <50 bpm Prolonged sinus pauses sometimes associated with paroxysmal atrial arrhythmias	Older age, hypothyroidism, hypothermia, hypoxia, acidosis, liver disease	A
Premature atrial complexes (PACs)	P waves with morphology different from sinus P waves	Myocardial ischemia, infection, stimulants, COPD	B
Paroxysmal supraventricular tachycardia (SVT)	Regular rate 150–230 bpm, QRS <100 msec, abrupt onset and termination	AV nodal reentry, AV reentry via accessory pathway	C
Atrial flutter	Sawtooth baseline, atrial rate 250–350 bpm	Heart disease, hyperthyroidism, alcohol, pericarditis	D
Atrial fibrillation (AF)	Absent P waves, irregular atrial rate of 350–600 bpm, fibrillatory waves	Cardiomyopathy, pericarditis, rheumatic heart disease, hyperthyroidism, ischemic heart disease, PE	E

Table continued on next page

Characteristics of Major Arrhythmias (Cont.)

MAJOR ARRHYTHMIAS	CHARACTERISTICS	ASSOCIATED CONDITIONS	TRACING
Nonparoxysmal junctional tachycardia	Regular junctional rhythm, rate 70–130 bpm	Inferior wall MI, digitalis toxicity	F
Preexcitation syndromes	PR interval <0.12 sec, QRS >0.12 sec, initial slurring of QRS	WPW syndrome (accessory AV pathway)	G
First-degree AV block	PR interval ≥0.20 sec	Cardiomyopathy, beta- and calcium channel blockers, viral and rheumatic myocarditis, digitalis toxicity	H
Second-degree AV block:			
Type I (Wenckebach)	Progressive prolongation of PR interval until P wave finally fails to conduct	Inferior wall MI, digitalis toxicity, beta- and calcium-channel blocker toxicity	I
Type II	Failure of P wave to conduct without preceding PR prolongation	Anteroseptal MI, primary or secondary degenerative diseases of the heart	J
Third-degree AV block	Nonconduction of any atrial impulses	Endocarditis, electrolyte disorders, cardiomyopathy, hypothyroidism, ischemic heart disease, digitalis or beta- or calcium-channel blocker toxicity	K
Premature ventricular complex (unifocal, multifocal, couplets) (PVC)	No preceding P waves, wide QRS with unusual morphology, usually followed by full compensatory pause	Infection, ischemic heart disease, stimulants, anesthesia, mental stress	L
Ventricular tachycardia (VT)	3 or more sequential PVCs, rate >100 bpm, unsustained (lasting <30 sec) or sustained	Ischemic or valvular heart disease, cardiomyopathy	M
Torsade de pointes	VT with constantly changing QRS morphology, prolonged QT interval	Congenital, antiarrhythmic drugs, tricyclic antidepressants	N
Accelerated idioventricular rhythm	3 or more ventricular beats in a row at a regular rate of 60–100 bpm	Acute MI, digitalis toxicity	O
Ventricular flutter	Sine wave baseline 150–300 bpm	Acute MI, antiarrhythmic drugs, hypoxia	P
Ventricular fibrillation (VF)	Absence of distinct QRS complexes with varying electrical waveform	Acute MI, antiarrhythmic drugs, hypoxia	Q

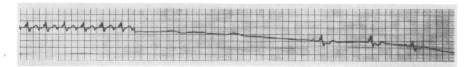

A, Tachycardia-bradycardia syndrome. Rhythm strip of ECG lead II showing spontaneous cessation of SVT followed by a 5.6-sec pause prior to resumption of sinus activity. The patient was asymptomatic during SVT, but the sinus pause caused severe light-headedness.

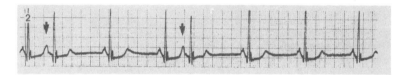

B, Atrial premature complexes (arrows) in sinus rhythm on ECG lead II. Note the difference in P-wave configuration between sinus and the premature atrial complexes. In addition, note that the PR interval of the premature complexes is prolonged, due to slowed conduction of the premature impulse through the AV conduction system.

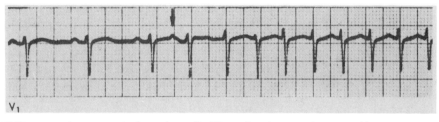

C, Paroxysmal supraventricular tachycardia. Three sinus beats are interrupted by a premature atrial systole (arrow), which conducts with P-R prolongation and initiates the SVT. The most common mechanisms of this arrhythmia are AV nodal reentry and AV reentry using an accessory pathway as the retrograde limb.

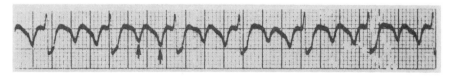

D, Atrial flutter. Flutter waves are indicated by arrows. The conduction ratio is 3:1 (i.e., three flutter waves to one QRS complex) and is a less common conduction ratio.

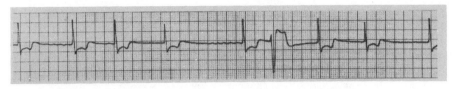

E, Atrial fibrillation. Atrial activity is present as the undulating wavy base line seen in the midportion of the ECG strip. The premature ventricular complex must be differentiated from aberrant supraventricular conduction.

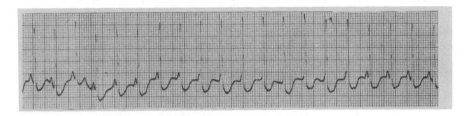

F, Nonparoxysmal junctional tachycardia with AV dissociation.

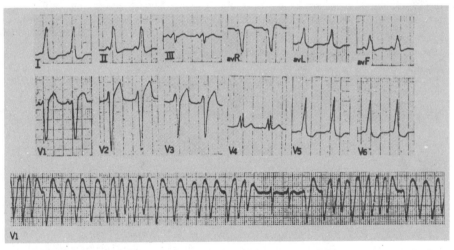

G, Preexcitation syndrome in 12-lead ECG (short PR interval, wide QRS, delta wave). During atrial fibrillation the ventricular rate is extremely rapid, at times approaching 350 bpm. The gross irregularity of the cycle lengths, wide QRS complexes interspersed with normal QRS complexes, and very rapid rate should suggest the diagnosis of AF and an AV bypass tract.

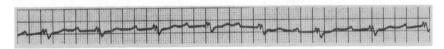

H, First-degree AV block. The PR interval is prolonged.

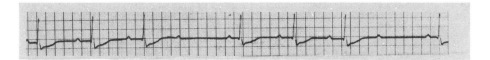

I, Second-degree AV block, type I (Wenckebach), characterized by progressive PR prolongation preceding the nonconducted P wave. In the setting of a normal QRS complex, Wenckebach almost always occurs at the level of the AV node.

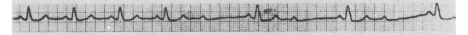

J, Second-degree AV block, type II. LBBB is present in this recording of lead I. Sudden failure of AV conduction results, without antecedent PR prolongation.

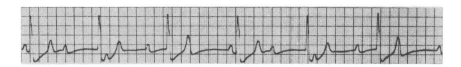

K, Acquired third-degree (complete) AV block. Complete AV dissociation is present owing to complete AV heart block. Atria and ventricles are under control of separate pacemakers.

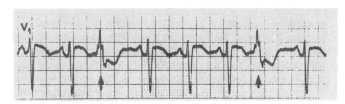

L, Premature ventricular complex (single ventricular ectopy). During sinus rhythm PVCs (arrows) occur. Note that the QRS configuration is bizarre, different from that during sinus rhythm. The presence of ventricular complexes are not preceded by P waves. The QRS width of the premature complexes is approximately 160 msec. The pause surrounding the premature complexes is fully compensatory, so that the next sinus beat occurs on time.

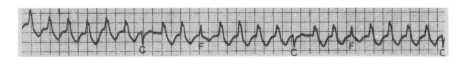

M, Ventricular tachycardia. A regular wide complex tachycardia is present. Atrial activity is not readily apparent. The complexes marked C and F most likely represent capture and fusion complexes that confirm the ventricular origin of the arrhythmia.

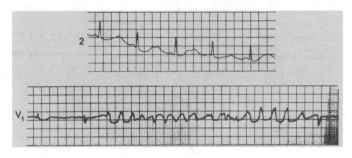

N, Torsade de pointes. During sinus rhythm (lead II) a markedly prolonged QT interval is present. Lead V₁ shows polymorphic VT.

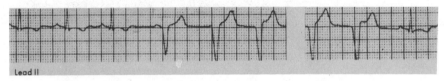

O, Accelerated idioventricular rhythm. The sinus rate slows slightly and allows the escape of an idioventricular rhythm. A fusion beat with a short PR interval results. Subsequently the sinus node once again regains control of the ventricular rhythm.

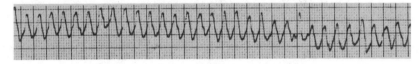

P, Ventricular flutter. Ventricular depolarization and repolarization appear as a sine wave with regular oscillations. The QRS complex cannot be distinguished from the ST segment or T wave.

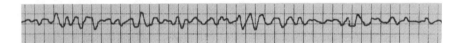

Q, Ventricular fibrillation. The baseline is irregular and undulating without any electrical evidence of organized ventricular activity.

Tracings from:

Josephson ME, et al: The bradyarrhythmias and the tachyarrhythmias. In Wilson JD, et al (eds): Harrison's Principles of Internal Medicine, 12th ed. New York, McGraw-Hill, 1991, pp 904, 909, 910, and 919, with permission.

Andreoli TE, et al: Cecil Essentials of Medicine, 2nd ed. Philadelphia, W.B. Saunders, 1990, pp 94, 97, 99, and 101, with permission.

A difficult diagnostic challenge lies in assessing the origin of a wide QRS complex tachycardia (whether it is a ventricular arrhythmia or a supraventricular arrhythmia with aberrant conduction). The distinction is critical, because treatment of VT with IV verapamil may result in hypotension and hemodynamic collapse. ECG findings diagnostic of VT in this setting include:

Absence of RS in precordial leads
Longest RS interval >100 msec
AV dissociation (fusions, captures)
Concordant morphology pattern in both V1 and V6

Reference: Andries EW, et al: An algorithm for diagnosing wide QRS complex tachycardia. Prim Cardiol 18:29–46, 1992.

Wide-Complex Tachycardias

Often, the emergency physician and general internist are faced with the diagnostic challenge of a patient presenting with a wide-complex tachycardia. A correct diagnosis is important in order to plan the therapeutic approach for these patients. An incorrect diagnosis can be fatal in some patients. For example, the administration of verapamil to a patient with V tach may lead to sudden cardiac death or severe hypotension. Despite some controversy about the most reliable methods of differentiating V tach from SVT in the ED setting, the following ECG features have been shown to favor a ventricular origin for a wide-complex tachycardia:

1. **AV dissociation,** one of the most reliable indicators of V tach, refers to the absence of any relation between the atrial and ventricular rhythms.
2. **Fusion beats and capture beats** are often present if long ECG rhythm strips are obtained. A capture beat is a normally conducted sinus beat with a normal QRS duration in the midst of a wide-complex tachycardia. A fusion beat is a beat with a QRS complex that is intermediate in morphology and duration between a normal QRS complex of a sinus-conducted beat and a wide QRS complex of V tach.
3. **Northwest QRS axis,** that is, a QRS axis between −90 and ±180°, is extremely uncommon in patients with an SVT, and it almost always implies a ventricular origin for the tachycardia.
4. **RBBB with a QRS complex duration >140 msec.**
5. **LBBB with a QRS complex duration >160 msec.**
6. **LBBB with a leftward QRS axis.**
7. **Positive QRS concordance:** QRS complexes that are predominantly positive in all precordial ECG leads.

In addition to these ECG characteristics, it is important to remember that any wide-complex tachycardia in a patient with a known history of a prior MI should be suspected to be V tach until proven otherwise. The large majority of wide-complex tachycardias in patients with prior MI are V tach. If a recent ECG can be obtained, a drastic change in the QRS morphology between a recent ECG and the current ECG would also favor V tach. It is also important to recognize that neither the presence of hypotension or chest pain nor the rate of the tachycardia is a particularly helpful clue.

The treatment of choice in a patient with a wide-complex tachycardia complicated by ``hemodynamic compromise'' evidenced by the presence of hypotension (systolic BP <90 mm Hg), acute MI, acute ischemic chest pain, acute pulmonary edema, and signs or symptoms of cerebral hypoperfusion is *electrical cardioversion,* regardless of whether it is SVT or V tach! It is extremely important to avoid verapamil in patients with wide-complex tachycardia and in patients complicated by hypotension, acute or chronic CHF, or a previous history of preexcitation syndrome (such as Wolff-Parkinson-White). (See also Supraventricular Tachycardia.)

ARTHRITIS

Monarticular vs. Polyarticular

Differential Diagnosis of Monarticular Arthritis

USUALLY MONARTICULAR	OFTEN POLYARTICULAR
Septic arthritis (bacterial, TB, fungal, Lyme disease)	Rheumatoid arthritis
Gout	Osteoarthritis
Internal derangement	Psoriatic arthritis
Ischemic necrosis	Reiter's syndrome
Hemarthrosis (coagulopathy, warfarin)	Calcium pyrophosphate deposition disease
Trauma and overuse	Chronic articular hemorrhage
Pauciarticular JRA	Most JRA and juvenile spondylitis
Neuropathic	Erythema nodosum/sarcoid
Congenital hip dysplasia	Serum sickness (acute hepatitis B, rubella)
Osteochondritis dissecans	Henoch-Schönlein purpura
Reflex sympathetic dystrophy	Systemic lupus erythematosus
Hydroxyapatite deposition	Lyme disease
Hemoglobinopathies	Parvovirus
Loose body	Dialysis arthropathy
Palindromic rheumatism	
Paget's disease involving joint	
Stress fracture	
Osteomyelitis	
Osteogenic sarcoma	
Metastatic tumor	
Synovial osteochondromatosis	

Modified from McCune WJ: Monarticular arthritis. In Kelley WN, et al (eds): Textbook of Rheumatology. Philadelphia, W.B. Saunders, 1989, pp 442–454.

Differential Diagnosis of Polyarticular Arthritis

A. Inflammatory
  1. Peripheral with axial involvement
     a. Ankylosing spondylitis
     b. Reiter's syndrome
     c. Enteropathic arthritis
     d. Psoriatic arthritis
  2. Peripheral pauciarticular
     a. Psoriatic arthritis
     b. Reiter's syndrome
     c. Rheumatic fever
     d. Polyarticular gout
     e. Enteropathic arthritis (ulcerative colitis, regional enteritis, bypass enteritis, Whipple's disease)
     f. Peripheral polyarticular
     g. AIDS arthropathy
     h. Relapsing polychrondritis
     i. Sarcoidosis
     j. Lyme arthritis
     k. Amyloid arthropathy
  3. Peripheral polyarticular
     a. Rheumatoid arthritis
     b. Systemic lupus erythematosus
     c. Subacute bacterial endocarditis
     d. Scleroderma

Table continued on next page.

Differential Diagnosis of Polyarticular Arthritis (Cont.)

B. Noninflammatory Osteoarthritis (OA)
1. Hereditary OA
   a. OA of the hands
2. Traumatic OA
   a. OA following local injury
   b. OA in obese and elderly persons
3. Metabolic diseases
   a. Hemochromatosis
   b. Ochronosis

b. Primary generalized OA

c. Chondromalacia following aggressive exercise programs
d. Charcot's arthropathy

c. Acromegaly
d. Hypothyroidism

Modified from Sergent JS: Polyarticular arthritis. In Kelly WN, et al (eds): Textbook of Rheumatology. Philadelphia, W.B. Saunders, 1993, pp 381–388, with permission.

ASCITES

Classification and Evaluation

Ascites is the accumulation of fluid in the peritoneal cavity. The patient usually presents complaining of weight gain, peripheral edema, abdominal distension, or malaise. Ascitic fluid accumulation of greater than 2 liters can be detected on physical examination by signs of shifting dullness or a fluid wave. The diagnosis of ascites can be confirmed by ultrasonography or CT scan. Once the diagnosis is made, paracentesis should be performed and fluid tested for albumin, protein, WBC with differential count, and, in some cases, TG, amylase, and LDH.

Exudative ascites usually demonstrates the following:

1. Protein content of the fluid >3 g/dl
2. A ratio of ascitic fluid to serum protein >0.5
3. An ascitic fluid LDH concentration >200 U/L
4. A ratio of ascitic fluid to serum LDH >0.6
5. An albumin gradient >1.1

The serum/ascitic fluid albumin gradient (serum albumin minus ascitic fluid albumin) reflects the oncotic pressure gradient between the vascular bed and the ascitic fluid. It is elevated in association with increased portal pressure and decreased with other causes. The various etiologies of ascites can be separated using this gradient.

Serum–Ascites Albumin Gradient

TRANSUDATIVE FLUID	EXUDATIVE FLUID
Wide gradient (>1.1 g/dl)	Narrow gradient (<1.1 g/dl)
Chronic liver disease, cirrhosis	Peritoneal carcinomatosis
Massive hepatic metastases	Peritoneal inflammation
Veno-occlusive disease	TB and fungal infections
Budd-Chiari syndrome	Serositis
Cardiac (RV failure)	Hollow organ leak
Myxedematous	Pancreatic
Hemodialysis with fluid overload	Bilious
Nephrotic syndrome	Chylous
Hypoalbuminemia	Ureteric
	Oncotic
	Nephrotic syndrome
	Protein-losing enteropathy
	Chronic disease
	Idiopathic

Patients with narrow-gradient ascites should have imaging studies (ultrasound or CT) done, and the fluid should be sent for cytology and fungal culture. Patients with high-gradient ascites should have a Doppler ultrasound performed to look for hepatic tumors and hepatic vessel potency. Fluid should be collected in blood culture bottles for culture and sensitivity. The final diagnosis of narrow-gradient ascites may require laparoscopy.

Treatment

The development of ascites in patients with cirrhosis is a sign of moderate to severe disease. However, ascites per se is a relatively benign condition and, apart from causing discomfort, is not life threatening. In contrast, the management of ascites may be dangerous. Some 10% of patients are estimated to die from iatrogenic complications of treatment of their ascites. Ascites formation is a reflection of Na^+ retention, so treatment must be aimed at creating a negative balance between Na^+ intake and excretion. Only 500–1,000 ml of ascites fluid can be reabsorbed into the vascular compartment in a 24-hour period. Thus, any additional loss in nonedematous patients results in depletion of intravascular volume and may result in shock, encephalopathy, and further renal impairment. In the management of ascites, a careful history is needed to exclude precipitating events: alcoholic binges, excessive salt intake or use of NSAIDs, or a recent bleed or infection. Target losses in patients without peripheral edema should be 0.5 kg per day.

Patients with cirrhosis often excrete exceedingly small amounts of Na^+ in their urine. A 24-hour urine Na^+ is helpful in the management of ascites. Patients who excrete less than 10 mEq of Na^+ in 24 hours require strong diuretics and might be resistent to diuretic treatments; those who excrete between 10 and 25 mEq of Na^+ in 24 hours are easily controlled with diuretics; and those who excrete more than 25 mEq of Na^+ should be controllable on a 2-gm Na^+ diet. One kilogram of weight loss equals 130 mEq of Na^+, and therefore, the goal in treatment is for patients to excrete 65 mEq more of Na^+ than they take in. One gram of salt contains 44 mEq of Na^+. There are four methods of treating ascites: diet, diuretics, repeat paracentesis, and peritoneal venous shunt. All patients should be placed on a 2-gm Na^+ diet.

If this course does not result in weight loss, patients should be started on a combination of a loop and distal-acting diuretics. Because cirrhotic patients have high levels of aldosterone, the loop diuretics, such as furosemide, should not be used alone except in patients with renal impairment. Doing so leads to rapid K^+ depletion. Treatment should start with 50 mg of spironolactone BID together with furosemide 40 mg every day. Alternatively, amiloride 20 mg can be used in place of the spironolactone. The aim is for the patient to lose 1 kg every 48 hours. If after 3 days on this therapy the patient is not losing weight, the dose can slowly be increased.

During the initial phase, electrolytes should be checked every second day. After a stable dose is found, electrolytes can be followed every couple of weeks. Some patients are resistent to diuretics, which means that they have either a very poor response to high doses of diuretics or unacceptable side effects, namely renal impairment or hepatic encephalopathy. Such patients are usually treated with both continued diuretics at a low dose and repeated paracenteses. Patients are reassessed from once weekly to once monthly, depending on the amount and rapidity of their ascitic fluid accumulation, and on each visit for paracentesis, their ascites is tapped dry. They are usually given 5 gm of albumin for each liter of ascites fluid taken out. The other possible treatment for refractory patients is peritoneal venous shunt;

however, these shunts have had complications of infection and DIC, and therefore paracentesis is the preferred method. The transjugular intrahepatic portosystemic shunt (TIPS) is an effective treatment for refractory ascites but has a high rate of occlusion, necessitating repeat procedures.

Steps in Management of Ascites

- Check 24-hour urine Na$^+$: if <10 mEq, patient will need diuretics; if >10 mEq, try low-Na$^+$ diet.
- If low-Na$^+$ diet does not result in loss of 0.5 kg per day, try diuretics. Starting dose is 100 mg of spironolactone and 40 mg of furosemide. If after 3 days on this dose the desired diuresis has not been obtained, double both doses while adjusting the dose of spironolactone and furosemide in order to ensure adequate potassium level and a ratio of BUN:creatinine less than 20:1.
- It is imperative that patients do not lose more than 750 gm per day in weight.
- Patients who are resistent to diuretics or in whom unacceptable complications ensue should be treated with intermittent paracentesis.

ASPERGILLOSIS

Allergic Bronchopulmonary Aspergillosis

Only recently recognized (first case in England in 1952, first U.S. case in 1968), allergic bronchopulmonary aspergillosis is related to the development of tissue hypersensitivity to antigens of the *Aspergillus* species. The organism actually grows in the airways. Immediate (type I), immune complex (type III), and perhaps cell-mediated (type IV) secondary allergic responses to the antigens of the organism lead to lung damage.

The clinical syndrome is one of moderately severe asthma, fever, and cough productive of brown or blood-streaked sputum. Weight loss and peripheral eosinophilia are common. Five clinical stages have been suggested:

Stage 1: acute disease
Stage 2: remission
Stage 3: exacerbation, as manifested by otherwise unexplained new infiltrates on CXR and at least a twofold rise in total serum IgE levels over baseline
Stage 4: corticosteroid-dependent asthma
Stage 5: chronic lung fibrosis, as manifested by irreversible obstructive and restrictive patterns on PFTs and fibrosis on CXR

The CXR findings seen during acute episodes are transient and are thought to represent immune complex reactions occurring in the lung parenchyma. They are homogeneous densities ranging from patchy infiltrates to lobar consolidation, and the borders are often ill defined. CXRs sometimes look worse than the patient does. In stage 5 disease, CXRs reveal interstitial fibrosis and bronchiectasis.

In most patients, aspergillosis is diagnosed between the ages of 30 and 60, but it often goes unrecognized for years because physicians fail to keep it in the differential diagnosis. The diagnostic criteria proposed by Greenberger and Patterson help resolve uncertainty:

(1) asthma
(2) infiltrate on CXR
(3) immediate cutaneous reactivity to *A. fumigatus*
(4) elevated total serum IgE
(5) serum precipitins to *Aspergillus* sp.
(6) peripheral eosinophilia
(7) elevated specific serum IgE and IgG antibodies to *A. fumigatus* antigens
(8) central bronchiectasis.

Prednisone is the treatment of choice. The goal is to control acute exacerbations and prevent the development of fibrosis. Systemic antifungal therapy is not effective.

Reference: Greenberger PA, et al: Diagnosis and management of allergic bronchopulmonary aspergillosis. Ann Allergy 56:405–414, 1986.

ASTHMA

Diagnosis and Management

Asthma affects an estimated 10 million people in the United States and has a significant impact on public health and health care. Asthma is a lung disease with the following characteristics: airway obstruction that is reversible either spontaneously or with treatment (although it may not be completely reversible in some patients), airway inflammation, and increased airway responsiveness to a variety of stimuli.

The diagnosis of asthma is based on the medical history and physical exam, as well as laboratory test results. Symptoms include cough, wheezing (see differential diagnosis below), chest tightness, and minimal sputum production. Effort should be made to determine other conditions associated with asthma (nasal polyposis, rhinitis, sinusitis, and atopic dermatitis), precipitating factors, and symptom pattern.

Differential Diagnosis of Asthma

Causes of Wheezing in Infants and Children

Foreign body	Laryngotracheomalacia
Vascular rings	Tumor/enlarged lymph nodes
Laryngeal webs	Tracheostenosis/bronchostenosis
Viral bronchiolitis	Cystic fibrosis
Aspiration	Bronchopulmonary dysplasia

(For differential diagnosis of asthma in adults, see Wheezing.)

Pathophysiologic Changes in Acute Bronchial Asthma

Expiratory airflow obstruction (FEV_1 and expiratory airflow are reduced)
Breathing at high lung volumes to prevent airway closure at resting lung volumes (vital capacity is reduced)
Pulmonary HTN (P pulmonale and RV strain on ECG)
Large fluctuations in pleural pressure with respiration (pulsus paradoxus)
V/Q mismatch

Objective Evaluation of Acute Asthma

Vital signs: tachycardia and pulsus paradoxus
Physical examination: use of accessory muscles of respiration with sternocleidomastoid
contractions
Spirometry: initially reduced FEV_1 with an increase in FEV_1 after administration of
bronchodilators
CXR: hyperinflation
ECG: acute cor pulmonale
ABGs: low P_aO_2, low or high P_aCO_2
Sputum smear and culture: eosinophils or evidence of infection

From Bleecker ER, et al: Obstructive airways disease. In Barke LR, et al: Principles of Ambulatory Medicine, 3rd ed. Baltimore, Williams & Wilkins, 1991, p. 612, with permission.

Overview of the Management of Asthma: Goals of Therapy

1. Maintain normal activity levels.
2. Maintain normal or near normal pulmonary function.
3. Prevent symptoms.
4. Prevent recurrent exacerbations.
5. Avoid adverse effects from asthma medications.

MANAGEMENT OF ASTHMA
Overview of Therapy

SEVERITY	THERAPY	OUTCOME
Mild/episodic	Inhaled beta2-agonist PRN	Controlled symptoms
Moderate	Additional therapy / Daily medication	Reduced PEFR variability
		Normalized tests of pulmonary function
	Anti-inflammatory agents + Bronchodilators / • Cromolyn • Inhaled beta2-agonist / • Inhaled • Oral theophylline / corticosteroids • Oral beta2-agonist	Prevention of acute exacerbations
Severe	Addition of oral corticosteroids	Maintenance of normal activity levels

From Guidelines for the Diagnosis and Management of Asthma. National Asthma Education Program Expert Panel Report, NIH Publication No. 91–3042, August 1991, Chap. 7: Management of Asthma, p.73.

Oral steroid therapy ''bursts'' may be indicated for some patients with acute exacerbation of asthma. Only in a minority of patients is chronic steroid therapy indicated, and it should be given in the lowest possible effective dose for the shortest time possible. Both patients and physicians should be aware and alert to complications of steroid therapy, for the cornerstone of asthma management lies in patient education.

Medical Complications and Indications for Hospitalization

Medical Complications of Asthma

1. Respiratory failure
2. Spontaneous pneumothorax/pneumomediastinum
3. Development of irreversible airway obstruction
4. Mucoid impaction
5. Allergic bronchopulmonary aspergillosis
6. Bronchiectasis
7. Complications of steroid therapy
8. Complications of bronchodilator therapy (paradoxical fall in arterial oxygenation, paradoxical bronchospasm, cardiac arrhythmias)
9. Pulmonary infections (bronchitis, pneumonia)
10. Atelectasis

Indications for admission: Patients with a *good response* to therapy (asymptomatic, no wheezing, and PEFR or $FEV_1 \geq 70\%$ predicted) for an acute exacerbation of asthma can be discharged after observation of 30–60 minutes postbronchodilator therapy. Patients with a *poor response* (symptomatic, wheezing, or PEFR or $FEV_1 \leq 40\%$ predicted) need to be admitted for continued observation and intensive treatment. Patients with *complications* (pneumonia, significant atelectasis, pneumothorax, vomiting, etc.) need to be admitted. Patients with an *incomplete response* (persistence of some symptoms, some wheezing, PEFR or $FEV_1 > 40$ but $< 70\%$ predicted) following therapy need to be considered for admission.

Factors Favoring Admission in Asthma

1. Borderline PEFR or FEV_1 values
2. Recent prior ED visit or hospitalization for asthma
3. Multiple ED visits or hospitalizations for asthma within 1 year
4. Past history of respiratory failure
5. Prolonged asthma symptoms (≥ 1 week) prior to presentation
6. Exacerbation despite multiple antiasthma medications
7. Exacerbation despite use of systemic corticosteroids
8. Infants
9. Inadequate follow-up care at home
10. Depression, psychosis, or serious psychiatric disorder

Adapted from Guidelines for the Diagnosis and Management of Asthma. National Asthma Education Program Expert Panel Report, NIH Publication No. 91–3042, August 1991.

Status Asthmaticus

The term "status asthmaticus" refers to refractory asthma that is unresponsive to traditional therapy. Such a refractory event implies that inflammatory changes have occurred that are not easily reversed with standard bronchodilator therapy. This represents severe life-threatening bronchospasm.

Staging of Asthma Based on Arterial Blood Gases

	P_aCO_2	P_aO_2
Stage 1	Normal	Normal
Stage 2	Decreased	Normal
Stage 3	Decreased	Decreased
Stage 4	Normal	Decreased
Stage 5	Increased	Decreased

Stage 1 is characterized by normal ABGs. Stage 2 is characterized by an increased A-a oxygen gradient ($P_{(A-a)}O_2$), with normalization of the P_aO_2 because of hyperventilation. In stage 3, hyperventilation is no longer able to compensate for the progressive widening of the $P_{(A-a)}O_2$. In stage 4, inspiratory fatigue is occurring and the P_aCO_2 begins to rise to normal levels. Stage 5 indicates impending respiratory failure. A normal P_aCO_2 should alert the physician to respiratory fatigue and the danger of respiratory arrest.

Indicators of Significant Respiratory Failure

1. PEFR 20% below predicted
2. FEV_1 less than 50% of predicted
3. Minimal response to bronchodilators in 1 hr
4. Respiratory rate greater than 30/min
5. Pulsus paradoxus
6. Use of accessory muscles
7. Marked decreased breath sounds without wheezing
8. Paradoxical breathing
9. Increasing P_aCO_2

Indications for Intubation

Apnea or near-apnea
Central cyanosis
Altered mental status
Significantly elevated P_aCO_2 with acidemia
Marked increased work of breathing despite initial therapy

ATAXIA

Ataxia refers to the clumsy, off-balanced, wide-based gait characteristic of cerebellar disease. The word "stagger" is an excellent one for expressing this symptom to laypersons. Patients with ataxia almost always describe it to their physician in terms of drunkenness, probably because alcohol use is one of the commonest causes of ataxia and certainly the one most familiar to patients. Other cerebellar signs may accompany ataxia: tremor, nystagmus, dysarthria, and hypotonia.

Almost all causes of ataxia relate to cerebellar disease:

1. Structural lesion
   A. Ischemic stroke
   B. Hemorrhage
   C. Tumor, almost always metastatic in adults
   D. Multiple sclerosis
2. Degenerative
   A. Friedreich's ataxia
   B. Other spinocerebellar degenerations, which are often sporadic in adults
3. Drugs
   A. Alcohol
   B. Phenytoin
   C. Fluorouracil
4. Hyperthyroidism

Evaluation of a patient with ataxia depends heavily on the imaging of the cerebellum with CT scanning or MRI so as to exclude stroke, hemorrhage, or tumor and to show any atrophy or degeneration. Of special diagnostic significance is atrophy of the anterior part of the cerebellum, called the vermis, which is characteristic of alcoholic cerebellar degeneration.

The commonest cause of ataxia is alcoholism. Alcohol is a cerebellar toxin that causes a staggering, ataxic gait. The patient may have some deficits on heel-to-shin cerebellar testing in the legs and possibly on finger-to-nose testing in the arms, but the usual pattern of alcoholic disease is that the gait is affected more than the legs, which are affected more than the arms.

The most dangerous cause of ataxia is a cerebellar hemorrhage. This is a life-threatening medical emergency because any mass or swelling in the cerebellum can compress the adjacent brain stem, with fatal consequences. The abrupt onset of ataxia thus mandates a CT scan or MRI. If a hemorrhage is found, it can be surgically evacuated and disaster averted. Occasionally, swelling occurs after an ischemic stroke as well, so this, too, must be considered a serious condition.

Sensory ataxia refers to the clumsiness and incoordination that results from loss of proprioception and position sense. Patients who do not know where their feet are will stagger when they walk. The commonest cause of sensory ataxia is a peripheral neuropathy that impairs perception, such as tabes, DM, or alcohol (again). Sensory ataxia is usually indistinguishable from cerebellar ataxia and can often be differentiated only by finding the sensory loss in the limbs. The old adage that sensory ataxia worsens in the dark whereas cerebellar ataxia doesn't is very unreliable.

Ataxia is among the hardest of symptoms to treat in all of neurology. Physical therapy is sometimes useful, with exercises to enhance balance and even the use of weights on the wrists and ankles to increase stability. A few drugs have modest effects on cerebellar function, including isoniazid, clonazepam, primidone, and propranolol, but none consistently produce good results.

References: Amarenco, P: The spectrum of cerebellar infarctions. Neurology 41:973–979, 1991.

Charness ME, et al: Ethanol and the nervous system. N Engl J Med 321:442–454, 1989.

ATRIAL ENLARGEMENT

Differential Diagnosis

By far, the most reliable ECG lead in the differentiation between left and right atrial enlargement is standard (or limb) lead II. The ECG characteristics of **left atrial enlargement** (LAE) are:

1. **Widened P wave:** >120 msec, in lead II.
2. **Bifid P wave:** A P wave characterized by two positive deflections, in leads II or III. In contrast, a biphasic P wave is a P wave with both a positive and a negative deflection. A biphasic P wave in lead II is not indicative of LAE. A bifid P wave in lead II is the most specific finding for LAE.
3. **Biphasic P wave:** In precordial lead V1, with a P-terminal force >40 msec-mV, biphasic P wave is a sensitive but nonspecific finding for LAE. The P-terminal force is defined as the product of the duration (expressed in msec) and depth (expressed in mV) of the terminal negative portion of the P wave in V1. If the duration of the terminal negative portion of the P wave exceeds 40 msec and if the depth of the terminal negative portion of the P wave in V1 exceeds 1 mV, then the P-terminal force will exceed 40 msec-mV.

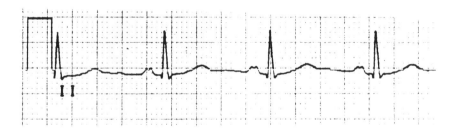

The characteristic features of LAE: a widened bifid P wave in standard lead II.

The ECG characteristics of **right atrial enlargement** (RAE) are:

1. **Tall P wave:** >2.5 mV in amplitude, in standard (or limb) lead II.
2. **Narrow P wave** in standard lead II.

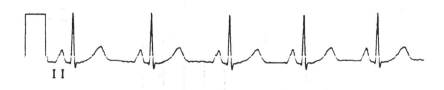

The characteristic features of RAE: a tall, narrow P wave in standard lead II.

Because the largest left atria are found at autopsy in patients with mitral valve disease, particularly in patients with mitral regurgitation, LAE by ECG is often referred to as *P-mitrale*. In patients with pulmonary parenchymal disease, such as COPD, secondary pulmonary HTN results in RV hypertrophy and RAE. Thus, RAE is commonly found in patients with pulmonary disease. RAE by ECG is thus commonly referred to as *P-pulmonale.*

ATRIAL FIBRILLATION

AF is defined as rapid, uncoordinated generation of electrical impulses by the atria at a rate of 300–500 per minute. The diagnosis is made by finding an irregularly irregular pulse and the absence of an "A" wave in the jugular venous pulse. The S_4 is absent and the S_1 is of variable intensity. The ECG demonstrates low-amplitude baseline undulations at a rate of 300–600 complexes per minute, with an irregularly irregular ventricular response.

Causes of Atrial Fibrillation

Cardiovascular

Hypertension	Acute myocardial infarction
Rheumatic and nonrheumatic valvular heart disease	Pericarditis
	Postcardiotomy
Cardiomyopathy	Sinus node dysfunction
Dilated (ischemic and nonischemic)	Tumors
Hypertrophic	Wolff-Parkinson-White syndrome
Infiltrative	

Noncardiovascular

Hyperthyroidism	Pulmonary hypertension
Pulmonary embolism	Chronic lung disease
Alcohol (acute or chronic intoxication)	Electrocution
Physical or emotional stress	Stimulant drugs (e.g., cocaine, amphetamines, caffeine, nicotine)

Modified from DeAntonio HG, et al: Atrial fibrillation: Current therapeutic approaches. Am Fam Physician 45:2557, 1990.

Thromboembolic Events

In the Framingham Heart Study, A fib is an important risk factor for thromboembolic events. The most devastating and unfortunately the commonest thromboembolic event in patients with A fib is a stroke. All patients with A fib are at increased risk of stroke, although it is greater in patients with valvular heart disease complicated by A fib as opposed to patients with A fib in the absence of valvular heart disease (also called nonrheumatic A fib). It is estimated that the risk of stroke in patients with nonrheumatic A fib is five times greater than that in patients in sinus rhythm.

It is thought that stasis of blood in the atria (particularly the left atrium) is the major pathogenetic factor explaining the propensity of patients with A fib to develop thromboembolism. It is thus conceivable that anticoagulation would reduce thrombus formation in the left atrium and thus reduce the risk of thromboembolism. Several clinical trials have evaluated the prophylactic role of oral anticoagulation with warfarin in patients with nonrheumatic A fib. These clinical trials have consistently shown a benefit of anticoagulation in lowering the risk for stroke. A recent clinical trial reported a *79% reduction in cerebral infarction,* from 4.3% to 0.9% per year in 525 patients with no previous history of a cerebral infarction. In the subset of 228 patients older than age 70 years, warfarin reduced the stroke risk from 4.8% to 0.9%.

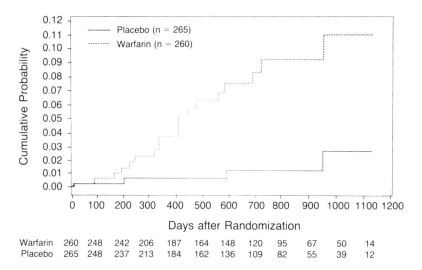

| Warfarin | 260 | 248 | 242 | 206 | 187 | 164 | 148 | 120 | 95 | 67 | 50 | 14 |
| Placebo | 265 | 248 | 237 | 213 | 184 | 162 | 136 | 109 | 82 | 55 | 39 | 12 |

Cumulative probability of cerebral infarction. The numbers below the figure are the numbers of patients at risk for a cerebral infarction at each point. There was a significant reduction in risk in the warfarin group as compared with the placebo group (risk reduction, 0.79; $p = 0.001$). From Ezekowitz MD, et al: Warfarin in the prevention of stroke associated with non-rheumatic atrial fibrillation. N Engl J Med 327:1406–1412, 1992, with permission.

AUTOIMMUNE LIVER DISEASE

Autoimmune chronic active hepatitis usually affects women in their early teens or middle age. The patient generally presents with malaise and jaundice and appears to be having a typical attack of acute viral hepatitis. On examination, patients usually have spider nevi, acne, and mild hirsutism. In the early stages, they have hepatomegaly. Recurrent episodes of acute liver disease ending in cirrhosis are the usual clinical course without treatment. Hepatic biochemistries usually show high SGPT/ SGOT (ALT/AST) and serum gamma globulins. With normal serum albumin being maintained until the latest stages of the disease, specific antibodies such as ANA are present in 80% of patients. Smooth-muscle antibody is detectable in 70% of patients. Anti-liver-kidney-microsomal antibody is present in 50% of patients. The etiology of this disease is unknown but obviously has an immune component. On hepatic histology, cellular infiltrates consisting largely of lymphocytes and plasma cells are seen in zone 1 and are infiltrating between the liver cells.

Treatment of the condition is gratifying. The initial treatment is 30 mg of prednisone for 1 week, reduced to a maintenance dose of 10–15 mg daily after 1 month. Within this 2-month period, patients usually become asymptomatic and their transaminases revert to normal. As a way to decrease the prednisone to 10 mg daily, patients are often started on 6 mercaptopurine or azathioprine at a dose of 50–100 mg daily. Patients are maintained on this medication for at least 2 years prior to attempts at withdrawal. However, most patients require maintainance with immunosuppression for life, and 75% will experience a relapse. All patients presenting with acute hepatitis who do not have a positive viral serology should be tested for autoimmune hepatitis with an ESR, serum protein electrophoresis, ANA, and anti-smooth-muscle antibody. If there is any chance that a patient may have autoimmune hepatitis, a month's course of steroids should be given.

B

BEHÇET'S SYNDROME

Behçet's syndrome is a systemic inflammatory condition that presents with oral, nasal, and genital ulcers. Other manifestations have been recognized, and the expanded diagnostic criteria are shown in the table. Behçet's is more frequent and severe in Japan and Mediterranean countries than in the United States. Men may be more commonly affected, and onset usually begins in the thirties. Multiple genetic associations have been hypothesized, including an increased frequency of HLA B51 among Asians with the complete form of the disease. Circulating immune complexes and neutrophilic vasculopathy suggest an autoimmune pathogenesis.

O'Duffy and Goldstein Criteria for the Diagnosis of Behçet's Disease

Criteria
  Aphthous stomatitis, genital aphthae, uveitis, cutaneous vasculitis, synovitis, meningo-encephalitis
Diagnosis
  Complete form: At least three criteria present, including oral aphthosis
  Incomplete form: Two criteria present, including oral aphthosis
Exclusions
  Inflammatory bowel disease, SLE, Reiter's syndrome, orogenital herpesvirus infection

From McCalmont TH, et al: Behçet's disease. In Churg A, et al (eds): Systemic Vasculitides. New York, Igaku-Shoin, 1991, p. 222, with permission.

The primary manifestation is mucocutaneous ulceration. By definition, aphthous stomatitis occurs in 100% of patients, producing clusters of small, sharp-bordered, painful ulcers that often last up to 2 weeks. Genital lesions look like the oral lesions and can occur on the scrotum, vulva, bladder, cervix, or glans penis. Whereas penile lesions are uniformly painful, vulvar lesions can occasionally be asymptomatic and should be routinely sought if suspicion is high. There are no clinical features to distinguish Behçet's syndrome ulceration from the common aphthous stomatitis, although biopsy may show vasculitis. Other cutaneous manifestations include erythema nodosum and pathergy (cutaneous hypersensitivity to development of sterile pustules after needle puncture).

Ocular involvement is the manifestation of most concern. Uveitis can occur in the anterior or posterior chamber. Anterior uveitis with hypopyon (pus in the anterior chamber) is the classically described ocular lesion of Behçet's syndrome. Other ocular lesions include iridocyclitis, retinal detachments, and chorioretinitis. Behçet's syndrome is one of the most common causes of acquired blindness in Japan.

Half of affected patients have some degree of peripheral arthropathy. Although early investigators suggested an increased frequency of the HLA B27 seronegative spondyloarthropathies in Behçet's syndrome, the association has not been confirmed.

Neurologic manifestations occur in 10–25% of patients. Although headache is the most common symptom, more severe CNS involvement can occur with meningoencephalitis. Vasculitic infarction can occur in the brain stem and cerebellum, resulting in ataxia and quadriparesis.

Deep venous occlusion (in up to a third of patients) and both larger and small arterial occlusions are well documented. Gangrene of the fingertips and avascular necrosis of bone have also been described. Rupture of an aneurysm secondary to inflammatory vasculopathy remains the most common cause of death in this disease. GI manifestations commonly include pain, diarrhea, and malabsorption. Endoscopic or pathologic review of tissue can show erosions and ulcerations. Occasionally, cardiomyopathy, pulmonary vasculopathy, and renal involvement may occur.

There is no specific diagnostic test; thus a strong clinical suspicion is important. Circulating immune complexes have been documented in up to 50% of patients. A polyclonal gammopathy is usually present, and the ESR and C-reactive protein are generally elevated during a flare. ANA and RF are generally not detected. The presence of anticardiolipin antibodies and cryoglobulins have been documented, although no correlation seems to exist between the presence or the titers and thrombosis. Histologically there is lymphocytic infiltration of tissue.

Treatment is difficult and no single agent is uniformly favored. Glucocorticoids are helpful symptomatically but do not prevent the catastrophic complications of vasculitis. Colchicine is used based on its antichemotactic properties. Treatment should be aggressive when there is a question of active CNS or ocular involvement. Azathioprine and methotrexate have both been used, but alkylating agents are generally the most efficacious, with chlorambucil (0.1 mg/kg/day) having documented efficacy. Cyclosporine has been used in patients not tolerating chlorambucil.

Reference: O'Duffy, JD: Vasculitis in Behçet's disease. Rheum Dis Clin North Am 16:423–432, 1990.

BIRTH CONTROL

Birth Control Methods

METHOD	FAILURE RATE (%)*	SIDE EFFECTS	COMMENTS
None	85–85	None	—
Spermicide	22–26	Increased risk of vaginal infection, vaginal irritation	May reduce risk of STD; should be used 10–30 min before intercourse
Periodic abstinence	14–20	None	Most likely to fail in women with irregular menses
Withdrawal	14–28	None	—
Diaphragm	13–40	Increased risk of vaginal and urinary infections, toxic shock syndrome if left in place >8 hrs	Must remain in place 6–8 hrs after coitus
Cervical cap	13–40	Increased risk of vaginal and urinary infections	May be difficult to fit
Condom	10–19	Allergic reactions	May reduce risk of STD; latex rubber condoms with spermicide are most protective; do not use with lotions or lubricants

Table continued on next page.

Birth Control Methods (Cont.)

METHOD	FAILURE RATE (%)*	SIDE EFFECTS	COMMENTS
Oral contraceptives	4–9	Thromboembolism, stroke, MI, HTN, hypertension	Progestin-only pills have fewer side effects but higher failure rate
Medroxyprogesterone acetate	<1–<1	Irregular menses, headaches, weight gain	Long-term safety not yet established; requires local anesthesia
Male sterilization	0.1	—	—
Female sterilization	0.4	—	—

*Average accidental pregnancy during first year of use. "Low" and "high" rates refer to rates among U.S. women likely to use the method correctly.

Adapted from Hatcher RA, et al: Contraceptive Technology, 15th ed. 1990–1992. New York, Irvington, 1990, p 134; and Choice of contraceptives. Med Lett 34:111–114, 1992.

BRAIN TUMORS

Brain tumors of the primary type occur in approximately 5 per 100,000 persons per year and are found in 1–2% of autopsy exams. Unlike other tumors, brain tumors rarely metastasize, and small ones become symptomatic early due to the anatomic confines of the skull. Symptoms usually progress gradually. Presenting symptoms include:

1. Focal neurologic defects
2. Headache
3. Vomiting
4. Papilledema
5. Seizures
6. Hemiparesis
7. Visual field defects
8. Speech difficulties
9. Altered mental status

The differential diagnosis includes congenital lesions, trauma, vascular disorders (e.g., strokes), infections (e.g., meningitis, abscess, or encephalitis), toxic-metabolic disorders (e.g., drug overdose, uncontrolled DM, exogenous toxins), and pseudotumor cerebri. Metastatic tumors to the brain represent about 50% of all intracranial neoplasms. Metastases from lung and breast cancers are the most common. Primary lymphomas of the brain are seen mainly in immunocompromised patients, such as transplant recipients or AIDS patients.

Types of Brain Tumors

TYPE	% CASES
Glioma	60%
Glioblastoma	
Astrocytoma	
Ependymoma	
Oligodendroglioma	
Medulloblastoma	
Meningioma	20%
Pituitary adenoma	6%
Craniopharyngioma	6%
Neurinoma	6%
Miscellaneous	1–2%

The diagnosis is made by CT or MRI of the brain and subsequent biopsy for tissue type. Typical configurations on these tests often give diagnostic clues to the cell type. If surgery is to be utilized in treatment, then angiography is often performed to delineate blood supply and help direct that surgery.

Treatment of primary brain tumors is surgical. Steroids are almost universally used to control concomitant edema. Unfortunately, characteristically the tumor extends, with projections far beyond the easily visible nidus, so complete resection is usually not possible. However, debulking is an important maneuver that often allows return to active life for up to 12 months. It also allows time for the patient to respond to other modalities such as radiotherapy and chemotherapy. Radiotherapy has been shown to increase survival and decrease morbidity in these patients. Doses of 6,000 rads or more are necessary for maximum control. The Brain Tumor Study Group has reported increased survival with a combination of radiation and carmustine (BCNU) following resection. Median survival of patients with glioblastoma multiforme was 8.5 months; for those with astrocytoma, 29 months. Intra-arterial cisplatin has also been reported to increase survival when used in conjunction with carmustine and radiotherapy postoperatively. Conjugated monoclonal antibodies, IFN, IL-1 and -2, TNF, LAK cells, and tumor-infiltrating lymphocytes for use in biologic therapy are all currently undergoing study both in vitro and in vivo to determine their effectiveness in this disease.

BREAST CANCER

Breast cancer incidence has been increasing dramatically in the United States since 1982. However, at least some of the rise may be due to an increase in the use of screening mammography for early detection. This is suggested by the fact that incidence rates for localized and in situ cancers rose while rates for regional and distant cancer stayed flat. In addition, among women found to have localized cancers, the proportion with tumors less than 3 cm in size increased while the proportion with tumors more than 3 cm did not.

Breast cancer is a complex disease. For the general internist, the most important decisions are when to biopsy and what to do when malignancy is found. However, the internist's role should focus on early detection as well as treatment. More breast cancers are detected by women who feel a mass in the breast than by screening mammography (by definition, "screening" mammography is mammography performed on a woman who has no clinical evidence of breast cancer). The diagnosis is often delayed because physicians fail to fully evaluate a benign-feeling mass or a palpable mass that does not appear on the mammogram. Up to 20% of women with pathologically documented breast cancer have normal mammograms.

Nipple retraction, bloody discharge from the nipple, dimpling of the skin, and fixation of the mass to underlying tissue suggest malignancy. Benign masses are mobile and well demarcated. It is important to note, however, that physical examination comes up with the correct distinction between a benign and malignant breast mass in only 60–85% of women. It is therefore necessary to systematically evaluate all breast masses. Donegan has recently offered a sensible algorithm for the evaluation of a palpable breast mass, as reproduced in the accompanying figure.

If cancer is found, consideration for treatment includes lumpectomy, quadrantectomy, and modified or radical mastectomy. The last is rarely used today, having been replaced by the others. For minimal surgery, the optimal lesions are less than 2–4 cm, with no palpable axillary nodes; there are no other lesions on exam or mammography, there is an infiltrating ductal pathology, and breasts are of a size that

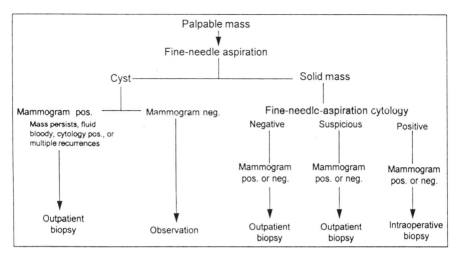

Suggested management of palpable breast masses in women. Mammography is not used to evaluate adolescents, and subareolar masses are not removed from the developing breasts of pubertal girls. Whether observation is an appropriate alternative in the management of a palpable mass that is benign according to physical examination, mammography, and cytologic examination is controversial. Pos. denotes positive, and neg. negative. (From Donegan WL: Evaluation of a palpable breast mass. N Engl J Med 327:937–942, 1992, with permission.)

will give an adequate cosmetic result. Concurrent with the surgery, patients should be staged so that appropriate treatment can be planned. Other tests may be done in order to make accurate prognostic estimates, such as flow cytometry, mitotic index, and hormone receptors.

Recurrent breast cancer is rarely controlled, so efforts must be directed toward early detection, diagnosis, and treatment. Adjuvant therapy of early tumors has been developed during the past several decades to effect a decrease in the recurrence rates of breast cancer. Patient age, number of positive nodes, and estrogen and progesterone receptor status of the primary tumor are all important prognostic factors. Long-term retrospective studies suggest that more than 50% of patients with node-negative breast cancer are cured of their cancer with local therapy alone. National Surgical Adjuvant Breast Project (NSABP) trials have shown that for both estrogen-receptor-positive and -negative patients treated with adjuvant therapy, 80% or more are free of disease after 4 years. However, although certain subsets of patients benefit from adjuvant therapy, other subgroups have unfortunately shown only marginal gains, and a large portion of breast cancer patients still die of their disease. Overall, the reduction in 5-year mortality of patients receiving adjuvant therapy through the NSABP trials has ranged from 20% to 25%.

Recurrent or advanced disease requires systemic therapy, and several agents in combination are most frequently used. Hormonal therapy can also be used in selected patients who have tumors that are hormone receptor positive, have a limited extent of metastasis, have a good performance status, and have no life-threatening metastases. Radiation therapy is usually used for treatment of bony metastases, although it has a place in selected patients in an adjuvant setting, particularly following segmentectomy.

Reference: Miller BA, et al: Recent incidence trends for breast cancer in women and the relevance of early detection: An update. CA 43:27–41, 1993.

BRONCHIECTASIS

Bronchiectasis is the result of destruction of the elastic and muscular wall of the bronchi leading to the irreversible dilation of the bronchi. Such dilation and destruction lead to increased sputum production, recurrent respiratory infections, cough, and hemoptysis. Blood-streaked sputum is common, but severe and life-threatening hemoptysis, usually from the systemic bronchial circulation, can occur. The incidence has declined with the use of antibiotics, and now most cases arise from congenital abnormalities.

Causes of Bronchiectasis

Congenital abnormalities
  Cystic fibrosis
  Kartagener's syndrome
  Young's syndrome (sinopulmonary infections and obstructive azoospermia)
  Congenital hypogammaglobulinemia
  Tracheobronchomegaly (Mounier-Kuhn syndrome)
  Bronchial cartilage deficiency (Williams-Campbell syndrome)
  Yellow nail syndrome (yellow nails, lymphedema, and, occasionally, bronchiectasis)
  Possibly alpha$_1$-antitrypsin deficiency
Inflammatory/infectious
  Complication of measles, pertussis, and lower respiratory influenza
  Postnecrotizing pneumonia
  Post-TB
  Postfungal (histoplasmosis, coccidioidomycosis)
  Aspiration
  Allergic bronchopulmonary aspergillosis
Associated with proximal airway obstruction
  Endobronchial tumor or foreign body
  Bronchostenosis
  Extrabronchial obstruction
Idiopathic

Symptoms of Bronchiectasis

  Cough
  Recurrent respiratory infections
  Airflow obstruction
  Sputum production
  Hemoptysis

Extrathoracic Manifestations of Bronchiectasis

  Clubbing
  Amyloidosis
  Brain abscesses

Diagnosis: The diagnosis is suggested by the symptom complex and an abnormal CXR in 90% of cases. Further measures are often required to identify affected segments. These include bronchography (considered the gold standard) and, more recently, CT scanning.

Treatment: Supportive treatment includes antibiotic therapy for exacerbations. Surgical management is reserved for localized lesions, absence of an underlying abnormality likely to recur, or significant/recurrent hemoptysis.

Reference: Chang S-W, et al: Hemoptysis with a normal chest roentgenogram. In Schwarz MI (ed): Pulmonary Grand Rounds. Toronto, B.C. Decker, 1990.

BUNDLE BRANCH BLOCK

Differentiation Between Left and Right

We are commonly faced with a widened QRS complex (defined as a QRS complex duration >120 msec) and with the differentiation between LBBB and RBBB. The first bundle branch to be depolarized is the left bundle branch followed by the right bundle branch. Thus, LBBB affects the entire QRS complex, whereas RBBB affects only the terminal portion of the QRS complex.

The characteristic ECG findings of RBBB are:

1. Wide terminal S wave in standard lead I
2. QRS with RSR′ configuration in V1 or V2: An RSR′ configuration refers to a QRS configuration characterized by an initial positive deflection (the R wave), followed by a negative deflection (the S wave), then by a second positive deflection (the R′ wave). That RSR′ configuration is also referred to as the M-shaped QRS pattern.
3. QRS complex duration >120 msec

Both the terminal wide S wave in standard lead I and the terminal wide R′ wave in V1 are indicative of delayed conduction in the terminal phase of the QRS complex due to block in conduction in the right bundle branch.

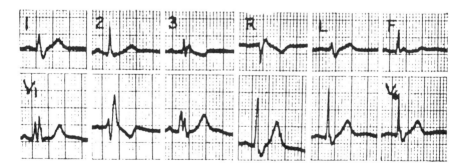

Characteristic changes of RBBB in a 12-lead ECG of an asymptomatic subject: a terminal wide negative deflection (called S wave) in standard lead I and precordial lead V6 and an RSR′ QRS pattern in precordial lead V1.

The characteristic ECG findings of LBBB are:

1. Wide monophasic R wave in standard lead I
2. Wide and deep S wave in V1 or V2
3. QRS complex duration >120 msec

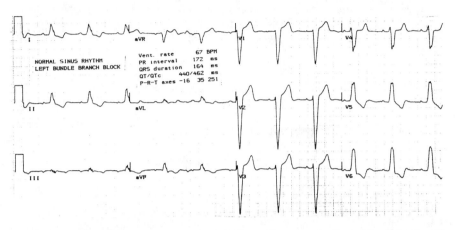

Characteristic changes of LBBB in a 12-lead ECG: a wide, monophasic positive deflection (R wave) in standard lead I and precordial lead V6 and a deep and wide negative deflection (S wave) in precordial lead V1.

Neither LBBB nor RBBB requires the presence of any specific QRS axis. However, the combination of LBBB with right axis deviation is extremely uncommon.

The presence of RBBB in an asymptomatic subject does not require any diagnostic workup. Unlike RBBB, which is commonly present in the absence of structural cardiac disease, LBBB is very rarely present in structurally normal hearts. The presence of LBBB in an asymptomatic subject should warrant further diagnostic workup to exclude subclinical ischemic heart disease.

CANCER

Adjuvant Therapy

Adjuvant therapy refers to treatment given after complete surgical resection of a cancer. Typically, radiotherapy to the tumor bed or chemotherapy is given in order to eradicate any undetected residual microscopic disease. Adjuvant therapy can increase the chance of long-term survival by up to 30% in certain types of malignancies.

Cancers in Which Adjuvant Treatment Has Been Shown to be Beneficial

TYPE AND STAGE OF CANCER	ADJUVANT THERAPY
Breast cancer, stage I and II	
Estrogen receptor negative	Chemotherapy
Estrogen receptor positive	Chemotherapy ± tamoxifen
Colon cancer, Dukes C	5-Fluorouracil and levamisole for 1 year after surgery
Rectal carcinoma, Dukes B or C	Radiotherapy + chemotherapy (preoperative radiotherapy may be used instead)
Certain sarcomas (Ewing's, osteosarcoma, rhabdomyosarcoma)	Chemotherapy and radiotherapy
Thyroid carcinoma, follicular	^{131}I ablation or hormone suppression

Neoadjuvant (preoperative) therapy may be helpful to reduce tumor bulk and prevent cancer dissemination during surgery. There is no proven benefit for adjuvant therapy after surgical resection of melanoma or prostate cancer.

Improvement in Outcome with Neoadjuvant Therapy

TYPE OF CANCER	NEOADJUVANT THERAPY
Gastric carcinoma	Chemotherapy and radiotherapy
Rectal adenocarcinoma	Radiotherapy
Squamous cell carcinoma of anus	Chemotherapy and radiotherapy

Chemotherapeutic Agents

Cancer chemotherapy is a term that comprises all of the drugs used in the therapy for cancer. It includes both natural and synthetic substances, hormones and hormone analogs, and biologic response modifiers. The oldest chemotherapy agent used in the treatment of cancer is nitrogen mustard (mechlorethamine), which was developed as an offshoot of World War II experimentation with mustard gas. It is still used today in the treatment of some Hodgkin's lymphomas. Methotrexate was next developed and has been used in the treatment of leukemia since 1948.

The many drugs available can be classified according to their dominant mode of action, as shown in the figure.

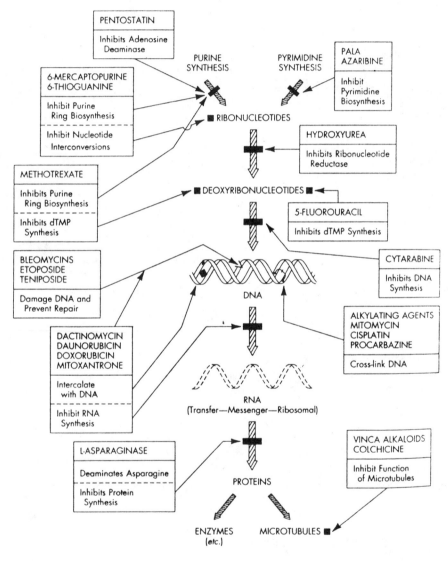

Mechanisms and sites of action of chemotherapeutic agents useful in neoplastic disease. PALA = N-phosphonoacetyl-L-aspartate. (From Calabresi P, et al: Chemotherapy of neoplastic disease. In Goodman-Gilman A, et al: The Pharmacologic Basis of Therapeutics, 8th ed. New York, McGraw-Hill, 1990, p. 1208, with permission.)

The *alkylating agents* interfere with normal mitosis and cell division in rapidly proliferating cells, although they can also damage organs with low mitotic activity. They are not cell cycle specific, but toxicity is usually seen when the cell enters the S phase. The major toxicity of these agents consists of nausea and vomiting, although there are major variations in degree from drug to drug. They also cause leukopenia, and most can cause an occasional maculopapular rash. Thiosulfate is a local antidote for one of these agents- nitrogen mustard. Ifosfamide has severe urinary tract toxicity, which may be decreased with the use of mesna. Melphalan and busulfan are given only orally, unlike most cancer drugs.

The *antimetabolites* act by depleting the tetrahydrofolate cofactors that are required for the synthesis of purines and thymidylate. Depression of blood counts and mucositis are the major clinical toxic effects.

The *pyrimidine analogs* inhibit the biosynthesis of pyrimidine nucleotides or imitate these natural metabolites so that they interfere with essential cellular functions. Toxicities include leukopenia, anorexia, nausea, and sometimes stomatitis and diarrhea.

The *purine analogs* work by converting adenosine or 2'-deoxyribonucleosides of guanine, hypoxanthine, adenine, and their analogs to the matching 5'-monophosphates. The major clinical toxicity is bone marrow depression.

Natural products such as the vinca alkaloids work by blocking mitosis and producing metaphase arrest by binding to tubulin and blocking polymerization into microtubules. The newest vinca is taxol, which also binds to tubules but promotes the assembly of microtubules. Major toxic effects are on nervous tissues, with peripheral neuropathies common. Vinblastine and taxol have myelosuppressive toxicity.

Epipodophyllotoxins block cells at the S-G2 interface of the cell cycle and cause G2 arrest. The major toxicity is myelosuppression.

The *antibiotics* work by binding with double helical DNA. Toxic manifestations are anorexia, nausea, vomiting, and myelosuppression. GI toxicity with proctitis, diarrhea, glossitis, cheilitis, and stomatitis also occur commonly.

Enzymes include L-asparaginase, which catalyzes the hydrolysis of asparaginase to aspartic acid and ammonia and deprives malignant cells of the asparagine needed for protein synthesis. There is minimal toxicity on the bone marrow and GI tract, but pancreatitis and abnormal clotting factors with bleeding can occur.

Miscellaneous agents include platinum compounds, which react with DNA, forming cross-links that interfere with function. Major toxicity includes nephrotoxicity, peripheral neuropathy, and bone marrow suppression. Other agents of unspecified class include hydroxyurea and procarbazine.

Biological response modifiers affect the patient's response to a neoplasm, often by enhancing the immunological response to neoplastic cells. Included in this category are interleukin-2, LAK cells, and interferons. Toxicity includes fever, malaise, myalgias, and cardiovascular collapse.

Hormones used in the treatment of cancer include estrogens, progesterones, testosterone, and their antihormones and analogs.

Mechanism of Action and Toxicities of Chemotherapeutic Agents

DRUG	ACUTE TOXICITY	DELAYED TOXICITY*
Asparaginase Action: Destroys essential amino acid (asparagine)	Nausea/vomiting, fever, chills, headache, hypersensitivity, anaphylaxis, abdominal pain, hyperglycemia	CNS depression or hyperexcitability, hemorrhagic pancreatitis, coagulation defects, thrombosis, renal and hepatic damage

Table continued on next page.

Mechanism of Action and Toxicities of Chemotherapeutic Agents (Cont.)

DRUG	ACUTE TOXICITY	DELAYED TOXICITY*
Bleomycin (Blenoxane) Action: Generates free radicals	Nausea/vomiting, fever, anaphylaxis, other allergic reactions	**Pneumonitis and pulmonary fi- brosis,** rash and hyperpigmenta- tion, stomatitis, alopecia, Raynaud's phenomenon, cavi- tating granulomas
Busulfan (Myleran) Action: Alkylates DNA	Nausea/vomiting, rare diarrhea	**Bone marrow depression, lung infiltrates and fibrosis,** alope- cia, hepatitis, gynecomastia, hy- perpigmentation, cataracts, leuke- mia, seizures and veno-occlusive disease (at high dose)
Carboplatin (Paraplatin) Action: Cross-links DNA	Nausea/vomiting	**Bone marrow depression,** pe- ripheral neuropathy (uncommon), hearing loss, hemolytic anemia, transient cortical blindness
Carmustine (BCNU) Action: Alkylates DNA	Nausea/vomiting, local phlebitis	**Delayed leukopenia, throm- bocytopenia** (may be prolonged), pulmonary fibrosis, renal dam- age, gynecomastia, reversible liver damage, hepatic or pulmo- nary veno-occlusive disease (high dose), leukemia, myocard- ial ischemia
Chlorambucil (Leukeran) Action: Alkylates DNA	Seizures, nausea/vomiting	**Bone marrow depression,** pul- monary infiltrates and fibrosis, leukemia, hepatic toxicity, sterility
Cladribine (2-CdA) Action: Leads to NAD depletion	Fever, nausea/vomiting, rash	**Bone marrow depression**
Cisplatin (Cis-DDP; Plati- nol) Action: Cross-links DNA	Nausea/vomiting, anaphy- lactic reactions	**Renal damage,** ototoxicity, bone marrow depression, hemolysis, ↓Mg++, Ca++, K+, peripheral neu- ropathy, Raynaud's, sterility
Cyclophosphamide (Cy- toxan) Action: Alkylates DNA	Nausea/vomiting, anaphy- laxis, facial burning with IV administration, visual blurring	**Bone marrow depression,** alopecia, hemorrhagic cystitis, sterility (may be temporary), lung infiltrates/fibrosis, ↓Na+, leuke- mia, bladder cancer, SIADH
Cytarabine HCl (Cytosar-U) Action: Inhibits DNA polymerase	Nausea/vomiting, diar- rhea, anaphylaxis	**Bone marrow depression,** oral ulceration, conjunctivitis, hepatic damage, fever, pulmonary edema, neurotoxicity (high dose), rhabdomyolysis, pancreatitis with asparaginase

Table continued on next page.

Mechanism of Action and Toxicities of Chemotherapeutic Agents (Cont.)

DRUG	ACUTE TOXICITY	DELAYED TOXICITY*
Dacarbazine (DTIC-Dome) Action: Alkylates DNA	Nausea/vomiting, diarrhea, anaphylaxis, pain on administration	**Bone marrow depression,** alopecia, flulike syndrome, renal impairment, hepatic necrosis, facial flushing, paresthesias, photosensitivity, urticarial rash
Dactinomycin (Actinomycin D) Action: DNA intercalator	Nausea/vomiting, diarrhea, local reaction and phlebitis, anaphylactoid reaction	**Stomatitis, oral ulceration, bone marrow depression,** alopecia, folliculitis, dermatitis in previously irradiated areas
Daunorubicin HCl (Cerubidine) Action: DNA intercalator	Nausea/vomiting, diarrhea, red urine, severe local tissue damage and necrosis on extravasation, transient ECG changes, anaphylactoid reaction	**Bone marrow depression, cardiotoxicity (may be delayed for years),** alopecia, stomatitis, anorexia, diarrhea, fever and chills, dermatitis in previously irradiated areas, skin and nail pigmentation
Doxorubicin HCl (Adriamycin) Action: DNA intercalator	Nausea/vomiting, red urine, severe local tissue necrosis on extravasation, diarrhea, fever, transient ECG changes, ventricular arrhythmia, anaphylactoid reaction	**Bone marrow depression, cardiotoxicity (may be delayed for years),** alopecia, stomatitis, anorexia, conjunctivitis, acral pigmentation, dermatitis in previously irradiated areas, acral erythrodysesthesia
Estramustine phosphate sodium (Emcyt) Action: Estrogen + DNA alkylator	Nausea/vomiting, diarrhea	Mild gynecomastia, ↑ frequency of CVA, myelosuppression (uncommon), edema, dyspnea, lung infiltrates/fibrosis, leukemia
Etoposide (VP16–213, VePesid) Action: Inhibits Topoisomerase II	Nausea/vomiting, diarrhea, fever, hypotension, allergic reaction	**Bone marrow depression,** alopecia, peripheral neuropathy, mucositis and hepatic damage with high doses, leukemia
Floxuridine (FUDR) Action: Inhibits thymidylate synthetase	Nausea/vomiting, diarrhea	**Oral and GI ulceration, bone marrow depression,** alopecia, dermatitis, hepatic dysfunction with infusion
Fludarabine (Fludara) Action: Inhibits DNA synthesis	Nausea/vomiting	**Bone marrow depression,** CNS effects, visual disturbances, renal damage with high dose, lung infiltrates, immunodeficiency
Fluorouracil (5-FU) Action: Inhibits thymidylate synthetase	Nausea/vomiting, diarrhea, hypersensitivity reactions	**Oral and GI ulcers, bone marrow depression,** diarrhea (esp. with leucovorin), ataxia, arrhythmias, angina, hyperpigmentation, palmar-plantar erythrodysesthesia, conjunctivitis, CHF

Table continued on next page.

Mechanism of Action and Toxicities of Chemotherapeutic Agents (Cont.)

DRUG	ACUTE TOXICITY	DELAYED TOXICITY*
Hydroxyurea (Hydrea) Action: Inhibits ribonucleotide reductase	Nausea/vomiting, allergic reactions to tartrazine dye	**Bone marrow depression,** stomatitis, dysuria, alopecia, rare neurological disturbances
Idarubicin (Idamycin) Action: DNA intercalator	Nausea/vomiting, tissue damage on extravasation	**Bone marrow depression,** alopecia, stomatitis, cardiac toxicity
Ifosfamide (Ifex) Action: Alkylates DNA	Nausea/vomiting, confusion, nephrotoxicity, metabolic acidosis, **cardiac toxicity with high dose**	**Bone marrow depression, hemorrhagic cystitis** (prevented by concurrent mesna), alopecia, SIADH, neurotoxicity (somnolence, hallucinations, blurred vision, coma)
Lomustine (CCNU; CeeNU) Action: Alkylates DNA	Nausea/vomiting	**Delayed (4–6 wks) leukopenia, thrombocytopenia** (may be prolonged), transient ↑ transaminases, neurological reactions, pulmonary fibrosis, renal damage, leukemia
Mechlorethamine HCl (nitrogen mustard, Mustargen) Action: Alkylates DNA	Nausea/vomiting, local reaction and phlebitis	**Bone marrow depression,** alopecia, diarrhea, oral ulcers, leukemia, amenorrhea, sterility
Melphalan (Alkeran) Action: Alkylates DNA	Mild nausea, hypersensitivity reactions	**Bone marrow depression** (esp. platelets), pulmonary infiltrates and fibrosis, amenorrhea, sterility, leukemia
Mercaptopurine (Purinethol) Action: Hypoxanthine analog	Nausea/vomiting, diarrhea	**Bone marrow depression,** cholestasis and rarely hepatic necrosis, oral and intestinal ulcers, pancreatitis; allopurinol + azathioprine increase toxicity
Mesna (Mesnex) Action: Prevents hemorrhagic cystitis	Nausea/vomiting	
Methotrexate (MTX) Action: Inhibits dihydrofolate reductase	Nausea/vomiting, diarrhea, fever, anaphylaxis, hepatic necrosis	**Oral, GI ulceration** ± perforation, **bone marrow depression,** hepatic toxicity, cirrhosis, renal toxicity, **pulmonary infiltrates and fibrosis,** osteoporosis, conjunctivitis, alopecia, depigmentation
Mitomycin (Mutamycin) Action: Crosslinks DNA	Nausea/vomiting, tissue necrosis, fever	**Bone marrow depression** (cumulative), stomatitis, alopecia, pulmonary, hepatic and renal toxicity, pulmonary fibrosis, hemolytic-uremic syndrome, bladder calcification

Table continued on next page.

Mechanisms of Action and Toxicities of Chemotherapeutic Agents (Cont.)

DRUG	ACUTE TOXICITY	DELAYED TOXICITY*
Mitoxantrone HCl (Novantrone) Action: DNA intercalator	Blue-green sclera and pigment in urine, nausea/vomiting, stomatitis	**Bone marrow depression,** cardiotoxicity, alopecia, white hair, skin lesions, hepatic damage, renal failure
Procarbazine HCl Action: Alkylates DNA	Nausea/vomiting, CNS depression, disulfiramlike effect with alcohol	**Bone marrow depression,** stomatitis, peripheral neuropathy, pneumonitis, leukemia
Streptozocin (Zanosar) Action: Alkylates DNA	Nausea/vomiting, local pain, chills and fever	**Renal damage,** hypoglycemia, hyperglycemia, liver damage, diarrhea, fever, eosinophilia, nephrogenic DI
Teniposide (VM-26) Action: Inhibits Topo- isomerase II	Nausea/vomiting, diarrhea, phlebitis, anaphylactoid symptoms	Bone marrow depression, alopecia, peripheral neuropathy, leukemia
Thioguanine Action: Purine analog	Occasional nausea/vomiting	**Bone marrow depression,** hepatic damage, stomatitis
Thiotepa Action: Alkylates DNA	Nausea/vomiting, rare hypersensitivity reaction	**Bone marrow depression,** menstrual dysfunction, leukemia, mucositis with high doses
Vinblastine sulfate (Velban) Action: Inhibits tubulin function	Nausea/vomiting, local reaction and phlebitis with extravasation	**Bone marrow depression,** alopecia, stomatitis, loss of DTRs, jaw pain, muscle pain, paralytic ileus
Vincristine sulfate (Oncovin) Action: Inhibits tubulin function	Local reaction with extravasation	**Peripheral neuropathy,** alopecia, mild bone marrow depression, constipation, paralytic ileus, jaw pain, SIADH

*Dose-limiting effects are in bold type. Cutaneous reactions (sometimes severe), hyperpigmentation, and ocular toxicity have been reported with virtually all of these drugs.

From Drugs of choice for cancer chemotherapy. Med Lett 35:43–50, 1993, with permission.

Familial Cancer

Hereditary cancer accounts for approximately 5–10% of malignancies. Familial cancers involve a specific tissue or group of organs. Inheritance is generally autosomal dominant, with incomplete penetrance. The chance that a gene will result in cancer varies among families; some carriers may never develop a neoplasm.

The natural history of familial cancers is similar to that of sporadic cancers, except that they typically occur at an earlier age than is usual for the particular type of neoplasm. Affected individuals may develop several primary cancers over the course of a lifetime. Tumors tend to arise from multiple foci within an organ and to be bilateral in paired organs. This suggests a diffuse genetic defect throughout the tissue at risk, which has been confirmed by the demonstration of discrete chromosomal defects.

Some Known Familial Cancers with Their Genetic Defect (if identified)

SYNDROME	TUMORS	CHROMOSOMAL ABNORMALITY
Breast cancer, early onset	Breast cancer	17q21
Dysplastic nevus syndrome	Malignant melanoma	1p36
Gardner's syndrome	Colorectal cancer	5q21
Hemochromatosis	Hepatoma	–
Hereditary nonpolyposis colon cancer*	Colorectal carcinoma	5q22†
Li-Fraumeni syndrome‡	Breast cancer, soft tissue sarcomas, leukemia, brain tumors, lung cancer, laryngeal carcinoma, adrenocortical carcinoma	17p13
Lynch family syndrome II	Adenocarcinomas of breast, colon, ovary, endometrium	–
MEN type I (Wermer syndrome)	Parathyroid, pituitary, islet cell tumors	11q13
MEN type II (Sipple syndrome)	Medullary thyroid carcinoma, pheochromocytoma (parathyroid)	10p11
Multiple polyposis	Colorectal cancer	5q22
Neurofibromatosis	Tumors of brain and peripheral nerves	17q11, 22q11
Ovarian carcinoma, familial	Ovarian carcinoma	–
Pancreatitis, hereditary	Pancreatic cancer	–
Tuberous sclerosis	Tumors of brain and peripheral nerves	–
Tylosis (palmar-plantar keratosis)	Esophageal cancer	–
von Hippel–Lindau syndrome	Renal carcinoma, retinal tumor	3p25
Retinoblastoma	Retinoblastoma, pineal tumors, osteogenic sarcoma	13q14

*Lynch syndrome I.
†In some families.
‡Associated with mutation of p53, a tumor suppressor gene.

Another group of inherited diseases cause a predisposition to cancer because of an abnormal immune system or increased instability of the DNA. Inheritance in this group tends to be X-linked or autosomal recessive.

Inherited Diseases That Cause a Predisposition to Cancer

SYNDROME	INHERITANCE	TUMORS	DEFECT
Agammaglobulinemia	X linked or autosomal recessive	Lymphoma, leukemia	Immunodeficiency
Albinism	Autosomal recessive	Skin cancers	↑ UV damage
Ataxia-telangiectasia	Autosomal recessive	Lymphoma, leukemia, adenocarcinoma, esp. breast	DNA repair
Bloom syndrome	Autosomal recessive	Leukemia, lymphoma, squamous cell carcinoma, adenocarcinoma	Chromosome instability

Table continued on next page.

Inherited Diseases That Cause a Predisposition to Cancer (Cont.)

SYNDROME	INHERITANCE	TUMORS	DEFECT
Fanconi's anemia	Autosomal recessive	Leukemia, hepatoma, squamous cell carcinoma	Chromosome instability
Severe combined immunodeficiency	Autosomal recessive	Lymphoma, leukemia	Immunodeficiency
Werner's syndrome	Autosomal recessive	Skin cancers, sarcomas	Premature aging
Wiskott-Aldrich syndrome	X linked	Lymphoma, leukemia	Immunodeficiency
Xeroderma pigmentosum	Autosomal recessive	Epithelial cancers, leukemia, brain tumors	DNA repair
X-linked lymphoproliferative syndrome	X linked	Lymphoma	Immunodeficiency

Persons known to be genetically at risk for cancer should have careful clinical surveillance. Screening of the involved organ, (e.g., colonoscopy in a kindred with colorectal cancer) should start at the age that is at least 5 years before the age cancer occurred in the earliest affected family member. Some familial cancers have a very high penetrance. For example, the lifetime risk of colon cancer for a gene carrier of multiple polyposis approaches 100%. Persons at extremely high risk may, after consulting with a medical geneticist and oncologist, consider prophylactic surgical removal of the tissue at risk. (See also Oncogenes.)

References: Li FP: Familial cancer syndromes and clusters. Curr Probl Cancer 14:73–114, 1990.

Fitzgibbons RJ, et al: Recognition and treatment of patients with hereditary nonpolyposis colon cancer (Lynch syndromes I and II). Ann Surg 206:289–295, 1987.

Risk Factors

One of every 3 persons in the United States will develop cancer at some time during his or her lifetime. Certain factors increase the likelihood of developing cancer, many of which can be modified by the individual.

Risk Factors for Cancer

RISK FACTOR	TYPES OF ASSOCIATED CANCER	COMMENT
Alcohol	Head and neck carcinoma, esophageal carcinoma, breast cancer, hepatoma	Tobacco acts synergistically as cocarcinogen
Estrogen use	Endometrial carcinoma	—
Family history of cancer	Kindred specific	Up to 10,000-fold
Fibrocystic disease with atypia	Breast cancer	—
High-fat diet	Breast and colon cancer	Moderate increase in risk; soft evidence
Immune suppressants (e.g., azathioprine)	Non-Hodgkin's lymphoma, Kaposi's sarcoma, skin cancer	—
Multiple sexual partners	Cervical carcinoma (also HIV and its associated cancers)	Associated with HPV types 16 and 18
Nulliparity	Breast cancer	—

Table continued on next page.

Risk Factors for Cancer (Cont.)

RISK FACTOR	TYPES OF ASSOCIATED CANCER	COMMENT
Occupational exposure		
Aniline dye	Bladder cancer	
Arsenic	Lung, skin, liver angiosarcoma	Lung cancer risk increased 2–9 times
Asbestos	Lung cancer, mesothelioma	Lung cancer risk up to 50-fold in smokers
Benzene	Leukemia	—
Cadmium	Lung cancer	—
Chloromethyl ether	Lung cancer	—
Chromium	Lung cancer	—
Uranium	Lung cancer	Due to radon daughters; smokers at 10x risk
Old age	Most solid tumors, CLL, multiple myeloma	Incidence increases with age
Pesticides	Non-Hodgkin's lymphoma	—
Radiation exposure	Leukemia, breast cancer, thyroid cancer	—
Sun exposure	Skin cancers (squamous and basal cell carcinoma, melanoma)	Risk increased in areas of previous severe sunburn, ↑ in light-skinned persons
Tobacco	Lung cancer, head and neck carcinoma, esophagus, bladder, pancreas, and kidney cancer	Proportionate to pack-years smoked; risk also increased for those who inhale smoke of others (passive smokers); any form of tobacco can cause cancer; alcohol, asbestos, and radon are co-carcinogens with tobacco
Viruses		
EBV	Burkitt's lymphoma, nasopharyngeal carcinoma	—
Hepatitis B	Hepatocellular carcinoma	—
HIV	Lymphoma, Kaposi's sarcoma	Risk ↑ with length of survival after infection
HTLV I	T-cell leukemia/lymphoma	—

Screening Recommendations

In 1993, more than a million people in the United States were diagnosed with cancer, and 520,000 died of malignancy. Screening for the most common cancers could potentially reduce the number of cancer deaths by one-third. In 1987, the National Cancer Institute, in consultation with professional medical organizations and the American Cancer Society (ACS), developed early detection guidelines for cancers of the skin, oral cavity, breast, colon/rectum, cervix, prostate, and testis. The current recommendations are:

Screening for Breast Cancer

- Women are encouraged to do monthly breast self-examination.
- At age 40, begin annual clinical examination with screening mammography at 1- to 2-year intervals through age 49. (The ACS recommends a baseline mammogram between ages 35–39.)

- Beginning at age 50, clinical examination and mammography should be done every year.
- Special surveillance should be given to women with a personal history of breast cancer or history of breast cancer in a mother or sister. (Usually recommended 5 years before the age that cancer occurred in the earliest affected family member.)
- Suspicious palpable lesions should be biopsied even if not seen with mammography.

Cervical Cancer Screening

- Women who are or have been sexually active or who have reached age 18 should have Pap tests for three years in a row after the initiation of screening.
- After three or more consecutive normal annual examinations, the Pap test may be performed every 2–3 years at the discretion of the physician.

Screening for Colorectal Cancer

- A digital rectal examination should be included as a part of the periodic health examination.
- Beginning at age 50, fecal occult blood testing should be performed once a year. Sigmoidoscopy is recommended every 3–5 years.
- Special surveillance should be given to high-risk patients, including those with a strong family history of colon cancer or with a personal history of adenomas, colon cancer, or inflammatory bowel disease. (Usually recommended 5 years before the age that cancer occurred in the earliest affected family member.)

Screening for Oral Cancer

- Starting at age 50, a complete oral examination should be performed as part of the periodic health examination.
- Special attention should be given to individuals at high risk due to tobacco and alcohol use and socioeconomic status.

Screening for Prostate Cancer

- Annual digital rectal examination of the prostate should be done on all men older than 40 years old.
- At present there is insufficient evidence to recommend routine screening with transrectal ultrasound and serum PSA in asymptomatic men. However, this is currently under evaluation.

Screening for Skin Cancer

- The skin should be examined as part of the periodic health examination.
- All individuals should examine their skin thoroughly on a regular basis.
- Special attention should be given to pigmented nevi and to high-risk individuals with a personal or family history of skin cancer, melanoma, or dysplastic nevi.

Screening for Testicular Cancer

- Periodic testicular self-examination is encouraged.
- Routine palpation of the testicles should be done as part of the physical examination.

- Special attention should be paid to high-risk individuals with a history of cryptorchidism, gonadal dysgenesis, and Kleinfelter's syndrome.

Reference: PDQ Prevention and Screening Editorial Board: National Cancer Institute PDQ Data Base Screening and Prevention Guidelines. Bethesda, MD, National Cancer Institute, March 1993.

Tumor Markers

Tumor markers are substances found in serum that are produced by malignant cells or released from tissues disrupted by cancer. Most tumor markers are not specific for cancer, as many of these substances may be elevated in a wide range of benign and malignant conditions. Interpretation of serum tumor marker levels must be done in the context of an individual patient's clinical situation.

Tumor Markers That Are Useful in Clinical Practice

TYPE OF CANCER	TUMOR MARKER
Breast cancer	CA 15–3,[1,2] CEA[2]
Colorectal carcinoma	CEA[1,3]
Germ cell tumors	αFP,[1,2,4] β-HCG[1,2,4]
Hepatoma	αFP[2,4,5]
Lung cancer	CEA[1]
Ovarian carcinoma	CA 125,[1,2,4] CA 15–3[2,4]
Pancreatic cancer	CA 19–9[1,2,4]
Prostate cancer	PSA[1,2,3,4,5]
Follicular thyroid carcinoma	Thyroglobulin[1,2]

[1]Useful to detect relapse after surgery or radiotherapy.
[2]Useful for diagnostic purposes.
[3]High levels at time of diagnosis correlated with poor prognosis.
[4]Useful to monitor therapeutic response.
[5]Useful for screening in selected populations.

Cancers in Which Individual Tumor Markers May Be Elevated

TUMOR MARKER	TYPE OF MALIGNANCY
αFP	Hepatocellular carcinoma,[1] nonseminomatous germ cell tumors, GI tumors
β-HCG	Gestational trophoblastic tumors,[2] germ cell tumors,[2] pancreatic islet cell tumors, lung cancer
CA 19–9	Pancreatic adenocarcinoma, colorectal carcinoma, gastric adenocarcinoma, mucinous ovarian carcinoma
CA-125	Ovarian carcinoma, endometrial carcinoma, hepatocellular carcinoma, lung and pancreatic cancer
CEA	Breast cancer, colorectal carcinoma, gastric adenocarcinoma, lung cancer, medullary thyroid carcinoma, pancreatic adenocarcinoma
PSA	Prostate adenocarcinoma[3]
Thyroglobulin	Papillary/follicular thyroid carcinoma

[1]Very specific for levels >3,000 ng/ml.
[2]Very sensitive and specific.
[3]Very specific for levels >10 ng/ml.

By knowing the half-life of a serum tumor marker, one can both determine the likelihood of a cancer's having been completely resected and follow the disappearance of a tumor after chemotherapy or radiation treatment. (See also Alpha-Fetoprotein; Carcinoembryonic Antigen; Prostatic Cancer: Diagnostic Use of PSA Levels.)

Half-Lives of Some Tumor Markers

αFP	3.5–6 days	CEA	5 days
βHCG	12–20 hours	PSA	2.2–3 days

Reference: Bates SE: Clinical application of serum tumor markers. Ann Intern Med 115:623–638, 1992.

CANDIDIASIS

In Immunosuppressed Patients

The spectrum of disease caused by candidal organisms seems to be relentlessly expanding since the introduction of systemic antibiotics, through the years of increased use of indwelling IV catheters and intensive chemotherapy, and into the era of organ transplantation and AIDS. Candida are normal flora for humans, usually found in the GI tract and the female genital tract. The normal defenses against Candida involve both the neutrophilic and lymphocytic cell lines, helping to explain why these infections are one of the few for which both HIV patients and neutropenic patients are at high risk.

The most common noncutaneous manifestation of candidal infection is **oropharyngeal candidiasis.** Thrush is one form of this and typically presents as white curdlike patches on mucosal surfaces or the tongue. The lesions can be scraped off with a tongue blade and can leave a raw, reddened area, which may bleed. A KOH prep of the lesion will readily show the organisms. Other appearances include a diffuse or patchy erythematous lesion and angular cheilitis. The finding of oral candidiasis in a patient with no known cause for immunosuppression should raise the issue of potential HIV infection. Oral candidiasis is readily treated either with local medication such as nystatin or clotrimazole or with systemic oral antifungals such as ketoconazole or fluconazole.

Esophageal candidiasis is found fairly frequently in advanced HIV infection and is one of the AIDS-defining conditions. It can be debilitating, with progressive dysphagia, odynophagia, and retrosternal pain. Profound weight loss is often seen. An empirical diagnosis can be made with the presence of oral candidiasis and esophageal symptoms with a clinical trial of oral antifungal therapy. Because other infectious causes can be seen in HIV patients, a more definitive diagnosis may be desirable via endoscopy. The most common infections mimicking esophageal candidiasis are herpes simplex virus and CMV.

One of the more difficult clinical diagnoses remains the diagnosis of **disseminated candidiasis.** This condition does not appear to be increased in HIV patients per se but affects those patients with neutropenia, prolonged multiantibiotic regimens, or prolonged IV catheter use, especially with TPN. Other high-risk categories are postoperative patients and burn victims. Blood cultures are frequently negative, and other cultures such as sputum, urine, and feces may demonstrate the organisms but not reflect disseminated disease. Serologic studies for either the antibody or the antigen have been complicated by high false-negative rates. Once disseminated, candidal infection may involve almost any organ system, but the kidney, brain, liver, and spleen are the more likely sites. Treatment is initiated on an emergent basis with amphotericin B.

CARCINOEMBRYONIC ANTIGEN

CEA is a cell-surface glycoprotein that functions as an intercellular adhesion molecule in GI mucosal cells. Although CEA is present in fetal serum, only very low levels of CEA are detectable in the serum of a healthy adult. When there is destruction of colonic mucosal barriers by tumors or inflammatory states, the antigen is released into the bloodstream, resulting in a rise in serum CEA levels.

CEA is not useful for cancer screening because it is too nonspecific. Many types of cancers, as well as several benign conditions, cause elevation of serum CEA levels.

Benign conditions causing elevated CEA levels: Hepatocellular disease, biliary obstruction, pancreatitis, inflammatory bowel disease, gastritis, bronchitis, heavy smoking, and advanced age.

Cancers causing elevated CEA levels: Breast, colorectal, esophageal, gastric, lung, thyroid, pancreatic, and cervical carcinoma.

If the CEA level is elevated preoperatively, it can be used to detect residual disease after definitive surgery for colorectal carcinoma. With a serum half-life of about 5 days, CEA levels should return to normal by 5–6 weeks postoperatively. CEA is also useful for detecting early recurrence of colon cancer. If exploratory laparotomy is performed as soon as the CEA level begins to rise, 15–60% of recurrent tumors may be completely resectable.

The role of CEA in monitoring therapeutic response in other types of cancer is unproven, because CEA levels may not correlate with clinical progress.

Reference: Woolfson K: Tumor markers in cancer of the colon and rectum. Dis Colon Rectum 34:506–511, 1991.

CARCINOID TUMORS

Carcinoid tumors are a heterogeneous group of neoplasms of neuroectodermal origin. Most carcinoid tumors arise from the GI tract, a lesser number from the bronchi, and rarely from ovarian teratomas. The distribution of carcinoid tumors by primary site is approximately:

Foregut	Respiratory tract	10%
	Stomach	2%
	Duodenum	2%
	Jejunum	1%
	Pancreas	1%
	Small bowel nonspecified	5%
Midgut	Ileum	11%
	Appendix	44%
Hindgut	Colon	8%
	Rectum	15%
Ovarian	Ovaries	2%

Carcinoid tumor cells have the capacity for amine precursor uptake and decarboxylation (APUD) cells. The carcinoid cells synthesize and secrete hormonal peptides. The cytoplasmic granules of midgut carcinoid tumors reduce silver salts, giving a positive argentaffin reaction. Foregut carcinoids are often argentaffin negative but exhibit the argyrophilic reaction (i.e., stain with silver after addition of a reducing agent). Neuron-specific enolase is present in APUD cells, including carcinoid cells. Staining for neuron-specific enolase is a semi-specific marker for carcinoid tumors.

Foregut carcinoid tumors commonly produce multiple hormones. Bronchial carcinoid tumors often metastasize early in the course of the illness. Gastric carcinoid tumors are commonly asymptomatic. Foregut carcinoid tumors may be a part of the MEN syndrome in some patients.

Peptides That May Be Produced by Foregut Carcinoids

PEPTIDE	CLINICAL DISORDER
Serotonin	Carcinoid syndrome
5-Hydroxytryptophan	"Atypical" carcinoid syndrome
Gastrin	Zollinger-Ellison syndrome
Glucagon	Dermatitis, diabetes mellitus
VIP	Watery diarrhea
Insulin	Hypoglycemia
ACTH	Cushing's syndrome
Somatostatin	Steatorrhea, diabetes mellitus
MSH	Hyperpigmentation
GHRH	Acromegaly

Carcinoid tumors of the appendix are usually small in size (less than 1 cm) and of little clinical significance. Larger appendiceal carcinoid tumors (greater than 2 cm) and primary carcinoid tumors of the ileum assume significance because of metastases and potential development of "malignant carcinoid syndrome." The likelihood of metastases from ileal carcinoid tumors is correlated with the size of the primary tumor. Mesenteric lymph nodes and the liver are the main sites of spread of malignant midgut carcinoid tumors. Malignant carcinoid syndrome is usually not clinically evident until the hepatic capacity to inactivate vasoactive peptides from the carcinoid is substantially reduced by hepatic metastases. Although carcinoid tumors of the rectum and colon can produce hormones, such tumors usually are clinically asymptomatic.

Symptoms of Malignant Carcinoid Syndrome

SYMPTOM OR LESION	MEDIATOR
Cutaneous flushing	Bradykinin, substance P
Diarrhea	Serotonin, prostaglandins
Wheezing	Histamine, serotonin
Endocardial fibrosis	Serotonin
Retroperitoneal fibrosis	Serotonin
Edema	Serotonin

CARCINOMA OF UNKNOWN PRIMARY SYNDROME

CUP syndrome is defined as a metastatic cancer whose origin cannot be determined after a complete Hx and PE, CXR, and basic laboratory studies, with further tests only as indicated by clues found in the Hx & PE. Except for a few well-defined treatable syndromes to be detailed later, the prognosis for these patients is invariably poor. Median survival is 3–7 months. In a significant number of such patients, the primary site of cancer may never be found, even at autopsy. To avoid the discomfort and expense of unnecessary diagnostic studies, the focus of investigations should be to evaluate for treatable malignancies.

Treatable Cancers That May Present as Carcinoma of Unknown Primary

POTENTIALLY CURABLE	GOOD PALLIATION
Germ cell tumors	Prostate cancer
Lymphoma	Breast cancer
Ovarian adenocarcinoma	Small-cell lung cancer
Breast cancer	
Thyroid cancer	
Head and neck squamous cell carcinoma	

I. The following diagnostic studies are recommended for patients with carcinoma of unknown primary:
   A. CT scans of the chest, abdomen, and pelvis
   B. Careful evaluation of pathology specimens, with additional biopsies if needed. Appropriate studies are determined by the individual clinical situation but include:
      • Light microscopy
      • Chemical and immunohistochemical stains (mucicarmine, S100, cytokeratin, common leukocyte antigen, αFP, β-HCG, estrogen + progesterone receptors, PSA, CEA)
      • Electron microscopy
      • Cytogenetics or flow cytometry
II. Further studies should be directed by tumor histology:
   A. For adenocarcinoma or poorly differentiated carcinoma:
      • Serum tumor markers (αFP, β-HCG, PSA in men; CA-153, CA-125 in women)
      • Mammogram in women
   B. For squamous cell carcinoma above the clavicle:
      • CT or MRI of head and neck
      • Quadruple endoscopy (pharynx, nasopharynx, esophagus, lung)
      • Multiple blind biopsies if no primary seen (base of tongue, piriform sinus, tonsillectomy)
   C. For squamous cell carcinoma below the clavicle:
      • No further studies are indicated
III. After the above evaluation is completed, if the primary cancer is not found, the recommended therapy is based on tumor histology and site.
   A. Adenocarcinoma or poorly differentiated carcinoma
      1. Lymph node, except axillary node in women: surgical resection followed by radiotherapy

2. Axillary node in women: mastectomy plus axillary node dissection (approximately 50% are occult breast carcinoma)
3. Mediastinal or midline involvement among young men with positive αFP or β-HCG: platinum-based chemotherapy (for treatment of potential mediastinal germ cell tumor)
4. Liver or other visceral organ: palliative care only

B. Squamous cell carcinoma
1. High cervical lymph node
   • Radiotherapy for mass <3 cm
   • Surgery plus radiotherapy for larger mass
2. Other node groups: surgical resection followed by radiotherapy
3. Visceral involvement: palliative care only

C. Lymphoma: chemotherapy and/or radiotherapy depending on histology and location

Note that chemotherapy has not been shown to be beneficial for carcinoma of unknown primary, except in the setting of IIIA3 and IIIC above.

References: Bitran JD, et al: Malignancies of undetermined primary origin. Dis Mon 38:213–260, 1992.

Greenberg BR, et al: Metastatic cancer with unknown primary. Med Clin North Am 72:1055–1065, 1988.

CARDIAC CATHETERIZATION

When and Why?

Cardiac catheterization is indicated in the following clinical situations:

1. Chest pain of unclear etiology, with a 50% or greater likelihood (so-called pretest probability) of CAD.
2. Clinical indications for revascularization such as:
   a. Unstable angina with persistent ischemic cardiac pain during hospitalization despite antiplatelet, anticoagulant, and antianginal drug therapy.
   b. Post-MI ischemia—spontaneous or exercise induced.
   c. Exertional angina refractory to a combination of two or more antianginal drugs in at least moderate doses.
   d. Acute MI complicated by moderate or severe LV systolic dysfunction (LVEF ≤40%) or potentially life-threatening ventricular arrhythmias such as V tach.
3. Clinical indications for valve replacement or balloon valvuloplasty such as moderate or severe stenosis or regurgitation of the aortic or mitral valves.
4. CHF of unclear etiology.

Cardiac catheterization is associated with a risk, albeit small, of complications such as arrhythmias, acute MI, death, or stroke. Thus the decision to perform cardiac catheterization should be based on a careful assessment of anticipated risks and expected benefits in each individual patient. That risk-benefit assessment should be considered whenever an invasive diagnostic procedure is entertained. In the assessment, it is particularly important to be well aware of all of the patient's medical problems—cardiac and noncardiac. Regardless of whether or not the patient has one of the aforementioned common indications for cardiac catheterization, it is essential to recognize that, if no surgical or other interventions are to be considered in a particular patient because of the patient's wishes or because of any other reason, cardiac catheterization may not be desirable.

CARDIAC PACEMAKERS

Types

A nomenclature has been developed for cardiac pacemakers to help improve communication between physicians caring for patients with pacemakers. The three-letter pacemaker code was established to describe the three major functions of a cardiac pacemaker:

First position: Refers to the chamber paced.

Second position: Refers to the chamber sensed.

Third position: Refers to the mode of response.

The chamber paced or sensed by a cardiac pacemaker may be the RV (referred to by the letter *V*), the right atrium (referred to by the letter *A*), or both (referred to by the letter *D*).

There are three distinct modes of response for a cardiac pacemaker:

Inhibited (referred to by the letter *I*): Pacemakers with an inhibited mode of response do not depolarize when a spontaneous depolarization (atrial or ventricular) is sensed by the pacemaker.

Triggered (referred to by the letter *T*): Pacemakers with a triggered mode of response pace shortly after a spontaneous depolarization is sensed. However, if no spontaneous depolarization is sensed after a fixed predetermined interval, the pacemaker will pace at its set pacing rate.

Both inhibited and triggered (referred to by the letter *D*): These pacemakers are usually dual-chamber pacemakers with a sensing wire in the right atrium (to which the mode of response is *triggered*) and with a pacing wire in the RV (to which the mode of response is *inhibited*). Thus, the pacemaker will be *triggered* to pace the RV in response to a sensed atrial depolarization and will be *inhibited* from pacing the RV in response to a sensed ventricular depolarization. This pacemaker will thus be named a *VAD*, for it paces the RV, senses the right atrium, and has both inhibited and triggered modes of response.

Pacemakers with a *fixed rate* (i.e., nondemand pacemakers) do not have any specific mode of response and do not have any sensing capabilities. These pacemakers are thus referred to as *AOO* or *VOO*, depending on whether the pacing wire is located in the right atrium or in the RV, respectively.

The most commonly used pacemakers are *VVI* or *DDD* pacemakers.

Indications

The following are general indications for the use of a permanent cardiac pacemaker:

Heart block: Second-degree AV block (Mobitz II) or third-degree AV block, unlike first-degree AV block, generally requires a cardiac pacemaker.

Sinus node dysfunction: Sinus bradycardia with a rate <40 bpm or asystole with sinus pauses of 1.5 sec or greater often indicates a need for permanent cardiac pacemaker insertion.

Generally, documentation of symptoms of hypoperfusion (such as dizziness, lightheadedness, presyncope, or syncope) concomitantly with ECG evidence of a prolonged sinus pause or high-grade heart block on ambulatory ECG monitoring is necessary to recommend a permanent cardiac pacemaker. It is essential both to withhold all cardiac drugs with possible inhibitory effects on the sinus or AV node (such as beta-blockers or calcium antagonists) and to document objective evidence of hypoperfusion and of concomitant sinus or AV nodal disease while the patient is *off any such cardiac inhibitory drugs* before any decision about the need for placement of a cardiac pacemaker can be made.

CARDIAC TAMPONADE

Physical Findings

The classic clinical triad of cardiac tamponade first described by Claude Beck in 1935 consists of:

1. Decline in BP
2. Elevation in systemic venous pressure (SVP)
3. Small quiet heart

In addition to these classic physical findings, cardiac tamponade is characterized by the presence of pulsus paradoxus, which was first described by Kussmaul. Pulsus paradoxus was then described by Kussmaul as the paradoxical finding of absent peripheral pulses despite the presence of a heartbeat during inspiration. Nowadays it is defined as a drop in systolic BP of >10 mmHg during a normal inspiration and is probably one of the most reliable physical findings in patients with cardiac tamponade. In the presence of severe hypotension, pulsus paradoxus may be difficult to appreciate. Expansion of the intravascular blood volume with intravenous fluids may make pulsus paradoxus more easily detectable in these patients.

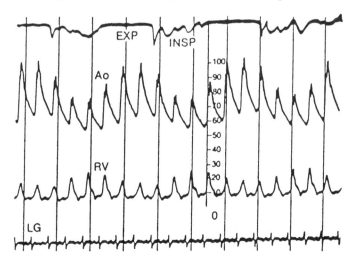

Recording of aortic (Ao) and right ventricular (RV) pressures in a patient with cardiac tamponade complicated by hypovolemia. Pulsus paradoxus is evident as a marked inspiratory decline in aortic systolic and pulse pressures during inspiration (INSP). RV pressure variation is out of phase with aortic pressure. Note that the RV waveform does not show a dip-and-plateau configuration. (From Shabetai R, et al: The hemodynamics of cardiac tamponade and constrictive pericarditis. Am J Cardiol 26:480, 1970, with permission.)

A so-called total paradox refers to the complete disappearance of a palpated peripheral pulse and is indicative of severe cardiac tamponade often with associated hypovolemia.

Differential Diagnosis

Clinical disorders that are characterized by hypotension, pulsus paradoxus, and elevated systemic venous pressure include obstructive pulmonary disease, constrictive pericarditis, restrictive cardiomyopathy, RV infarction, and massive PE. The finding of pulsus paradoxus in the absence of elevated systemic venous pressure is occasionally noted in patients with other causes of shock such as hypovolemia and sepsis.

The presence of other physical, auscultatory, or laboratory findings usually provides important clinical diagnostic clues that help the clinician in making the correct diagnosis. The presence of clinical and ECG evidence of acute inferior wall infarction in a patient presenting with the triad of hypotension (spontaneous or nitroglycerin induced), elevated jugular vein pressure, and clear lungs should raise the possibility of acute RV infarction. A right-sided ECG showing ST segment elevation greater than 1 mm in V3R or V4R and an echocardiogram showing hypokinetic or akinetic RV would make the diagnosis of acute RV infarction very likely.

The clinical diagnosis of massive PE should be entertained in a patient with pulsus paradoxus, hypotension, and elevated jugular venous pressure if arterial hypoxemia, a large alveoloarterial oxygen (A-a O_2) gradient, and/or a wedge-shaped pulmonary infiltrate by chest x-ray are present in a patient known to be at risk for acute PE.

The differentiation of cardiac tamponade from constrictive pericarditis is more difficult. The finding of a Kussmaul sign—the inspiratory increase in systemic venous pressure—generally favors the diagnosis of chronic constrictive pericarditis, whereas pulsus paradoxus is more commonly present in patients with acute cardiac tamponade. However, the distinction between cardiac tamponade and constrictive pericarditis is more difficult in patients with effusive-constrictive pericarditis.

Treatment

The treatment of choice for acute cardiac tamponade is pericardiocentesis. This procedure is performed for two indications: first, to improve cardiac output and second, to establish a definitive diagnosis.

In preparation for pericardiocentesis, patients with acute cardiac tamponade and hypotension should receive IV fluids, blood, plasma, or saline. Intravascular volume expansion is recommended because it has been shown to delay the onset of hemodynamic compromise in these patients.

CARDIOMYOPATHIES

Classification and Pathophysiology

Cardiomyopathies are a unique group of primary myocardial diseases, often of unclear etiology, which are not the result of ischemic, hypertensive, valvular, or pericardial disease. They are characterized by distinctive clinical, pathophysiologic, and hemodynamic features. They can be broadly classified into the three major categories of dilated or congestive, hypertrophic, and restrictive.

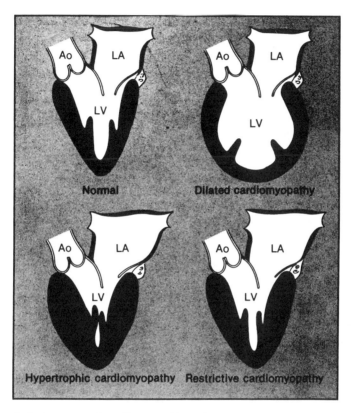

Three morphologic types of cardiomyopathies of unknown cause. (From Waller BF: Pathology of the cardiomyopathies. J Am Soc Echocardiog 1:4, 1988, with permission.)

Dilated cardiomyopathy is characterized by LV dilatation, contractile dysfunction, and CHF. **Hypertrophic cardiomyopathy** is characterized by inappropriate often severe LVH, commonly accompanied by asymmetric septal hypertrophy. LV systolic function is usually normal, but diastolic function (i.e., LV relaxation) is almost always impaired. **Restrictive cardiomyopathy** is most distinctively recognized by normal LV size and systolic function, dilated atria, and impaired diastolic function. Unlike hypertrophic cardiomyopathy, restrictive cardiomyopathy is often caused by an infiltrative process, such as amyloidosis, sarcoidosis, inherited infiltrative disorders (such as Fabry's disease, Gaucher's disease, or hemochromatosis), or endomyocardial disease (such as hypereosinophilic syndrome).

CAROTID ENDARTERECTOMY

Patient Selection

The purpose of carotid endarterectomy is to reduce the risk of stroke in patients with atherosclerotic carotid stenosis. In order to select patients most likely to benefit and least likely to be harmed from this procedure, it is necessary to know the answers to three questions.

1. What is the likelihood of a stroke in a patient with carotid artery disease?

Carotid artery stenosis can be asymptomatic—manifested only by a carotid bruit—or symptomatic—manifested by TIA or stroke. In patients with an asymptomatic carotid bruit, the likelihood of a completed stroke seems to depend on the severity of the carotid stenosis. The incidence of stroke within 1 year is about 5% in patients with severe stenosis (>75%). Some but not all of these strokes will be preceded by a TIA. When persons with severe stenosis have symptomatic carotid disease (i.e., a history of TIA or nondisabling stroke), the risk of stroke within 2 years is 20–28%. When symptomatic carotid artery disease exists but the degree of stenosis is mild (<30%), the risk of stroke within 2 years is only about 5%. Comparable information on patients with symptomatic moderate stenosis (30–70%) is not yet available.

2. What is the morbidity/mortality rate associated with carotid endarterectomy?

Under optimal circumstances (i.e., in randomized, controlled trials), the 30-day postoperative incidence of stroke is 5–8% (however, not all are major), and the 30-day all-cause mortality is 1%. Postoperative stroke and death rates can be expected to be higher under conditions of everyday practice and there is probably significant variation by hospital.

3. What is the magnitude of the reduction of the risk of stroke after carotid endarterectomy?

Two recent trials have demonstrated convincingly that carotid endarterectomy significantly reduces the risk of stroke in patients with severe stenosis who have *symptomatic* (TIA or nondisabling stroke) carotid artery disease. In a 50-center trial in the United States and Canada, at 2 years patients treated surgically had a 3% risk of major or fatal ipsilateral stroke compared to 13% in patients treated medically. In an 80-center European trial, at 3 years surgically treated patients had a 1% incidence of disabling or fatal stroke compared to 8% in medically treated patients. A recent multicenter trial in patients with *asymptomatic* stenosis of >50% showed that surgically treated patients had a 4.7% incidence of fatal and nonfatal ipsilateral stroke at an average of 48 months of follow-up compared to a 9.4% incidence in medically treated patients. There were no significant differences between groups in the combined incidence of stroke and death.

In summary, it seems clear that endarterectomy reduces the risk of major or fatal ipsilateral stroke in patients with high-grade *symptomatic* stenosis who are otherwise fit to undergo surgery. On the other hand, surgery does not appear to be superior to medical therapy in symptomatic patients with mild stenosis, because the risk of stroke is low anyway. In addition, patients with *asymptomatic* carotid bruits do not appear to benefit from endarterectomy, though those with high-grade stenosis need to be monitored regularly for development of symptomatic disease. Answers are not yet in for the large group of patients who are symptomatic but have moderate stenosis.

References: Chambers BR, et al: Outcome in patients with asymptomatic neck bruits. N Engl J Med 315:860–865, 1986.

North American Symptomatic Carotid Endarterectomy Trial Collaborators: Beneficial effect of carotid endarterectomy in symptomatic patients with high-grade carotid stenosis. N Engl J Med 325:445–453, 1991.

European Carotid Surgery Trialists' Collaborative Group: MRC European Carotid Surgery Trial: Interim results for symptomatic patients with severe (70–99%) or with mild (0–29%) carotid stenosis. Lancet 337(8752):1235–1243, 1991.

CARPAL TUNNEL SYNDROME

Carpal tunnel syndrome, also called brachialgia paresthetica nocturna (BPN), the most frequently encountered peripheral nerve lesion in clinical practice, results from entrapment of the median nerve in the carpal tunnel. The carpal tunnel is a fibro-osseous canal at the wrist, which is bounded on the palmar aspect by the flexor retinaculum (transverse carpal ligament), on the dorsal aspect by the carpal bones, and on the canal floor by the ligaments. Through the canal pass the tendons of the deep flexors of the digits—enclosed in a common tendon sheath—and the median nerve. In the hand, the median nerve supplies five muscles (three thenars and two lumbricals) and cutaneous sensation to $3^{1}/_{2}$ digits (thumb, index, middle, and half of the fourth finger).

The history is characteristic. There is the gradual onset of numbness and tingling of the fingers (the little finger is spared), especially at night. These sensations may be accompanied by pain, and symptoms at times extend above the wrist. Weakness may occur. BPN—"waking up at night due to unpleasant sensations in the fingers"—is a common symptom. BPN is also a useful screening device with a high diagnostic value. Patients often say they wring the hand, shake it, or hang it over the side of the bed for relief. Paresthesia may be reproduced by tapping over the nerve (Tinel's sign). There may be sensory deficits over the distribution of the median nerve in the hand and, occasionally, weakness of the thenar muscles. Although the Hx & PE are diagnostic, questionable cases can be resolved by electro-diagnostic tests to determine whether median nerve conduction is slowed at the wrist.

Mild cases can be treated with a wrist splint at night. Severe cases require surgical decompression, which is now commonly done on an outpatient basis. Weakness and wasted thenar muscles may not recover after treatment.

Reference: DeKrom MC, et al: Carpal tunnel syndrome: Prevalence in the general population. J Clin Epidemiol 45:373–376, 1992.

CAVITARY LUNG LESIONS

There are numerous causes of cavitary lesions of the lungs. Most causes are infectious organisms, but cavitary lesions may occur with neoplastic, vascular, or autoimmune disorders.

Causes of Cavitary Lesions of the Lungs

Mycobacterial organisms
  Mycobacterium tuberculosis — Unilateral or bilateral upper lobe cavities
  Mycobacterium kansasii — Cavities indistinguishable from those of *M. tuberculosis*
  Mycobacterium avium-intracellulare — Usually an indolent to slowly progressive pulmonary disease

Fungal organisms
  Histoplasma capsulatum — Cavities are usually unilateral and upper lobe; indicates chronic histoplasmosis
  Blastomyces dermatitidis — Pulmonary disease is generally nodules or infiltrates in lower lobes
  Coccidioides immitis — Thin-walled cavities in the upper lobes are the hallmark
  Sporothrix schenckii — Pulmonary disease is rare; may show thin-walled, upper lobe cavities
  Cryptococcus neoformans — Necrotizing pneumonia with nodular infiltrates, sometimes with cavitation, mainly in immunocompromised hosts

Actinomycetes organisms
  Nocardia asteroides — Usually pneumonic appearance, with late cavitation of lesions
  Actinomyces israelii — Rare cause of pulmonary cavities
Bacterial organisms
  Staphylococcus aureus — Cavitation in necrotizing pneumonia
  Septic pulmonary emboli — *S. aureus* most common organism, multiple bilateral nodular and cavitary lesions, often with air-fluid levels
  Anaerobic organisms — Infection related to aspiration, lower lobe involvement, lung abscesses with cavitary lesions containing air-fluid levels
  Klebsiella pneumoniae — Cavitation in a pneumonic infiltrate
  Pseudomonas aeruginosa — Microcavitation in pneumonic infiltrate
  Pseudomonas pseudomallei — Melioidosis with pneumonia and nodular lesions followed by upper lobe cavitary lesions
  Francisella tularensis — Rarely lung abscess progressive to cavitation
Parasitic organisms
  Entamoeba histolytica — Pulmonary amebiasis with lung abscesses that may cavitate
  Paragonimus westermani — The lung fluke infection, leading to nodular, cystic, and bronchiectatic lesions of the lungs
  Echinococcus granulosus — Cystic lesions of the liver and lungs
Malignancies
  Squamous cell carcinoma — Primary lung tumor may cavitate
  Metastatic tumors — Occasionally cavitate
Autoimmune disorders
  Rheumatoid arthritis — Pulmonary nodules may cavitate
  Wegener's granulomatosis — Cavities within nodules or infiltrates or thin-walled cavities

Vascular disorders
  Pulmonary emboli — Cavitation within pulmonary infarcts
Anatomic abnormalities
  Blebs and bullae — Recognized as cavity when infected
  Bronchiectatic cysts — Appearance as infected cavity
  Bronchogenic cysts — Appearance as infected cavity

CELIAC DISEASE

Synonyms: Adult celiac disease, idiopathic steatorrhea, nontropical sprue, gluten-induced enteropathy

Celiac sprue is defined as a disease in which there is malabsorption of nutrients in an affected portion of the small intestine. The characteristic but nonspecific lesion of the mucosa consists of complete villous flattening and loss of absorptive surface. It appears that interaction between the water-insoluble protein component (gluten) of certain cereal grains and the mucosa of the small intestine is crucial for the development of celiac sprue. There is generally prompt clinical improvement when gluten-containing foods are withdrawn from the diet. The result of gluten exposure in sensitive individuals is loss of the normal small-intestinal villous structure and increase in cellularity of the lamina propria—primarily plasma cells and lymphocytes. Clinically, this results in malabsorption of nutrients, gas, bloating, and diarrhea.

Symptoms of Celiac Disease

MILD DISEASE	SEVERE DISEASE
No symptoms	Panmalabsorption
Iron deficiency anemia	Diarrhea
Folate deficiency	Flatulence
Osteopenic bone disease	Weight loss
	Weakness

Physical findings range from none to pallor due to anemia, emaciation, clubbing, edema, ecchymosis (vitamin K deficiency), hyperkeratosis follicularis (vitamin A deficiency), dermatitis herpetiformis (seen in association with celiac sprue), cheilosis, glossitis, and Chvostek's or Trousseau's sign (with hypocalcemia or hypomagnesemia).

The diagnosis is based on:

1. Evidence of generalized malabsorption: decreased D-xylose absorption, steatorrhea, hypocalcemia, iron deficiency, hypoalbuminemia, hypocholesterolemia, reduced serum carotene, and occasional decreased vitamin B_{12}
2. Abnormal small-bowel biopsy (the most valuable single diagnostic test for the diagnosis)
3. Clinical improvement with gluten-free diet
4. Return of symptoms and small-bowel lesion with gluten challenge

Treatment consists of a gluten-free diet. Removal of gluten from the diet is essential for the successful treatment of patients with celiac sprue. Complete removal of all cereal grains known to contain toxic gluten (wheat, barley, rye, and possibly oats) is important but may in reality be difficult for some patients to achieve.

Failure to respond to a gluten-free diet may indicate:

1. Incomplete removal of gluten from the diet (most common)
2. Incorrect diagnosis
3. Development of intestinal lymphoma as a complication of celiac sprue

CENTRAL NERVOUS SYSTEM INFECTIONS

Spinal Fluid Findings in Central Nervous System Infections

	CELL COUNT (µl)	CSF PRESSURE (mmH$_2$O)	CELL TYPE	GLUCOSE (mg/dl)	PROTEIN (mg/dl)	MICROSCOPIC EXAMINATION	CULTURE
Normal	0–5	50–180	Mononuclear	40–80 or 1/2 serum level	10–45	Negative	Negative
Meningitis Viral	10–2,000	Normal or slight elevation	Early, mostly PMNs; late, mostly mononuclear cells	Normal	Normal to 100	Negative	Sometimes positive
Untreated bacterial	10–100,000	Usually elevated, average = 300	Predominantly PMNs	Low	Normal to 600, usually increased	90% positive	90% positive
Partially treated bacterial	10–10,000	Usually elevated, average = 300	Predominantly PMNs	Low to normal	Usually increased	Positive or negative; bacteria may stain poorly	Frequently negative
Tuberculosis	10–1,000	Usually elevated	30–100% mononuclear	Low, may be normal early	Elevated, 100–500	Rarely positive	Usually positive
Fungal	5–1,000	Usually elevated	Predominantly mononuclear	Low, occas. normal	Normal to 500	India ink positive for *Cryptococci*	Usually positive
Encephalitis	0–2,000	Usually elevated	Early, mostly PMNs; late, mostly mononuclear	Normal	Normal to 120	Negative	Negative
Brain abscess	5–500	Usually elevated	Mixture of PMNs and mononuclear	Normal	Normal to 500	Negative	Negative

Modified from Griffin DE: Infections of central nervous system. In Harvey AM, et al (eds): The Principles and Practice of Medicine, 22nd ed. Norwalk, CT, Appleton & Lange, 1988, p 637.

CELLULITIS

Cellulitis and Skin Infections

Cellulitis is an acute skin infection that spreads into the subcutaneous tissues, usually beginning in a traumatized area or an ulcer or furuncle. Cellulitis also occurs more commonly in areas with damaged lymphatic, venous, or arterial circulation or with foreign bodies. Unlike erysipelas, there is no clearly demarcated border with uninvolved tissues. Classic signs are redness, heat, swelling, and tenderness.

The major causative organisms are group A streptococci and *Staphylococcus aureus.* In immunocompromised patients, consideration must be given to gram-negative bacteria and fungi. *Vibrio* species may cause a severe bullous cellulitis associated with saltwater trauma. Gram stain and culture of a needle aspirate of the advancing border of infection may be very helpful, as may similar studies obtained from a site of origin. Antibiotic therapy is dictated by the identified or suspected causative organism, with penicillin or erythromycin usually the agents of choice (or a penicillinase-resistant penicillin if staphylococcal infection is suspected). IV vancomycin may be used in cases of penicillin allergy. Additional management aims include elevation and appropriate cleansing of the involved area. Incision and drainage, if appropriate, should be delayed until the area has matured. Gangrenous cellulitis may result from infection with anaerobic organisms.

Other significant categories of skin infection are:

1. **Impetigo:** A superficial infection caused by group A hemolytic streptococci and/or *S. aureus.* Erythromycin and cephalexin are the drugs of choice.

2. **Erysipelas:** A well-demarcated and intensely erythematous and raised skin infection, usually on the face (20%) or extremities (70%), acute in onset with systemic toxic symptoms, and usually caused by group A streptococci. Mild cases may be treated with oral penicillin V or erythromycin, but more severe cases require hospitalization for parenteral aqueous penicillin G 600,000–2,000,000 units Q 6 hr.

3. **Chronic cutaneous ulcers:** Associated with impaired circulation, burns, frostbite, decubiti, or neuropathy and usually involving many different organisms.

4. **Folliculitis:** Infection of hair follicles.

5. **Furuncles:** Infection of sebaceous glands, usually on the face, axilla, buttocks, thighs, or labia.

6. **Carbuncle:** Infection of inelastic skin on neck or upper back.

7. **Exfoliative staphylococcal pyoderma**

CHEST PAIN

Patients may describe chest pain as any pain located on the anterior chest between the diaphragm and shoulder, yet attribute the source of pain to the heart. Chest pain has many causes, including pain referred from other body areas. A quick review of chest anatomy will indicate the various sources of chest discomfort.

In evaluation of a patient with chest pain, it is important to search quickly for potentially life-threatening disorders such as dissecting aortic aneurysm, MI, PE, spontaneous pneumothorax, Mallory-Weiss tear, and esophageal rupture. The Hx & PE can quickly begin to differentiate these illnesses, but laboratory tests, including CXR, ECG, hemoglobin, LFT, and lipase, may also be helpful.

Causes of Chest Pain

A. Originating from the chest
  1. Skin
    Herpes zoster (frequently presents with pain *before* any vesicles appear)
  2. Musculoskeletal
    Anterior chest wall muscle sprain
    Tietze's syndrome (inflammation of the costochondral junction)
    Rib fracture
    Metastatic bone disease
    Precordial catch syndrome
  3. Nerve
    Nerve root compression
  4. Vascular
    Dissecting aortic aneurysm
  5. Esophageal
    Gastroesophageal reflux
    Esophageal spasm (frequently relieved by nitroglycerin)
    Esophageal rupture (Boerhaave's syndrome)
    Esophageal tear (Mallory-Weiss tear)
    Other esophageal motility disorders
  6. Pulmonary
    Spontaneous pneumothorax
    Pulmonary embolism
    Pneumonia with pleuritis
  7. Cardiac
    CAD: acute MI, angina
    Valvular: mitral valve prolapse, aortic stenosis
    Pericarditis
B. Originating from adjacent structures
  1. Thoracic and cervical spine
    Metastatic bone disease
    Nerve compression
  2. Gastrointestinal
    Pancreatitis
    Peptic ulcer disease
    Cholecystitis
C. Associated with psychiatric disorders
  1. Depression
  2. Panic attacks
  3. Hypochondriasis
  4. Somatization disorder

CHOLELITHIASIS

Cholelithiasis, or gallstones, affects as many as 20 million people in the United States. Gallstones are frequently composed of cholesterol, but 20% may be pigment gallstones, which contain calcium and are therefore radiopaque. Gallstones are most common in women over the age of 60. Other risk factors for gallstone development include previous childbearing, estrogen therapy, and oral contraceptive use. Gallstone prevalence is particularly high in Scandinavians and Native Americans.

Signs and Symptoms: Most gallstones are asymptomatic and are found incidentally during radiologic procedures done for other reasons. When symptoms develop, patients present with biliary colic resulting from passage of gallstones from the cystic duct. The pain typically begins in the epigastrium and radiates to the right upper quadrant but may also be felt in the back, the right shoulder, or the scapula. The pain is usually aching but also may be sharp and lancinating, lasting for 15–60 minutes. Some patients may have chronic, steady pain lasting several hours. Biliary colic has a diurnal variation, with peak intensity at midnight.

When a gallstone impacts in the cystic duct, cholecystitis occurs and the patient has intense pain, high fever, nausea, and vomiting. The gallbladder is exquisitely tender when palpated, and patients complain of right subcostal pain and tenderness on inspiration (Murphy's sign).

Diagnosis: Gallstones are suspected from the patient's history (see earlier) and can be confirmed through several techniques including plain radiographs, ultrasound, oral cholecystogram, and cholescintigraphy (nuclear scanning). Ultrasound and cholescintigraphy are the most useful (see next topic).

Patients with asymptomatic gallstones frequently have normal laboratory values. During acute cholecystitis, the WBC is markedly elevated above $15,000/mm^3$. Bilirubin and alkaline phosphatase are elevated in one-third of patients, and amylase may also be elevated.

Treatment: Most patients with asymptomatic gallstones do not require any therapy. Prophylactic cholecystectomy may be indicated for asymptomatic patients with sickle-cell disease. Native Americans with gallbladder disease have a high incidence of gallbladder cancer and may require cholecystectomy.

Patients with acute cholecystitis require cholecystectomy, either emergently or shortly after the resolution of symptoms. Patients with recurrent biliary colic also benefit from cholecystectomy. Currently, laparoscopic cholecystectomy is preferred for most patients because of the reduced postoperative morbidity, although the overall operative risks are similar for laparoscopic and open cholecystectomy. The actual operating room time is greater for laparoscopic cholecystectomy, and one always needs to be prepared to convert to an open procedure if complications develop. Open cholecystectomy may be required for patients with unusual anatomy or extensive scarring. Nonsurgical therapies include oral dissolution with bile salts and extracorporeal lithotripsy, but these should be reserved only for patients who are extremely poor risks for surgery.

Reference: Johnston DE, et al: Pathogenesis and treatment of gallstones. N Engl J Med 328:412–421, 1993.

CHOLELITHIASIS AND CHOLECYSTITIS

Diagnosis of Cholelithiasis

1. **Plain film** of the abdomen will visualize stones that contain enough calcium to be seen on x-ray (about 15%).
2. **Ultrasonography** is the preferred test given its lack of radiation exposure and high sensitivity (90–95%).

3. **Oral cholecystogram** (OCG) is an excellent method for the diagnosis of gallstones if the cystic duct is patent. About 40% of gallbladders fail to opacify after the initial dose of contrast and require a double-dose study for visualization.
4. **ERCP** may occasionally be useful to detect stones in patients in whom ultrasound and OCG are negative.

Diagnosis of Cholecystitis

1. **Ultrasonography** is felt to be the most useful test in the diagnosis of acute cholecystitis. The sensitivity for the diagnosis approaches 90%; the specificity is 95%. Ultrasonographic findings include the following:
   a. Presence of stones in the gallbladder.
   b. Tenderness over the gallbladder with palpation using the ultrasound probe.
   c. Thickening of the gallbladder wall >3 mm in diameter.
   d. Gallbladder distention and/or sludge in the gallbladder.
   e. Luminal irregularity or membranes within the gallbladder lumen suggesting the possibility of gangrenous cholecystitis.
   f. Pericholecystic fluid collection.
   (False negatives may occur in the presence of acalculous cholecystitis. False positives may occur when chronic cholecystitis exists.)
2. **Biliary scintigraphy** (HIDA, DiSIDA) with ^{99m}Tc-6-labeled derivatives of iminodiacetic acid. The sensitivity of scintigraphy for the diagnosis of acute cholecystitis approaches 97%; the specificity is approximately 90%. This test primarily allows determination of cystic duct patency. It is positive if there is nonfilling of the gallbladder by 4 hours and negative if filling occurs within 4 hours. False positives can occur in the presence of acute pancreatitis, chronic cholecystitis, alcoholism, and neoplasms of the gallbladder or liver, as well as in patients on long-standing TPN. False negatives occur in the presence of acute acalculous cholecystitis.
3. **MRI and CT scan** are generally not useful unless a pericholecystic abscess is considered.
4. **OCG** is not recommended for evaluation of acute cholecystitis.
5. **Plain films** of the abdomen may reveal gallstones in 15% of patients in whom stones are radiopaque. Plain films tend to be most useful, however, in ruling out other associated disease processes that may result in a similar clinical picture.

CHOLESTEROL

Embolism

The appearance of blue toes, livedo reticularis, or unexplained eosinophilia in a patient with arterial emboli should suggest cholesterol emboli. Atheromatous plaques are rich in crystalline cholesterol, which can be dislodged after manipulation during vascular surgery or angiography and after fibrinolytic therapy for MI.

Chronic anticoagulation with warfarin may also be associated with blue toes and other evidence for cholesterol emboli. In severe atherosclerotic disease of the aorta, cholesterol embolism may occur spontaneously. Such patients typically have elevated blood cholesterol levels and long-standing, significant HTN. Cholesterol emboli may affect the small arteries of organs more important than the toes. Stroke, MI, bowel infarction, pancreatitis, renal failure, and spinal cord infarction have been reported in this syndrome. The cholesterol crystals incite a vasculitis that produces a local inflammatory reaction. Systemic eosinophilia and hypocomplementemia are also observed. Biopsy of involved skin or other tissue shows the presence of cholesterol clefts that remain after the cholesterol has been removed during fixation.

On physical examination, digital ischemia and livedo reticularis are observed, most often with normal peripheral pulses. In some individuals, a palpable abdominal aortic aneurysm is found. Cholesterol embolization should be strongly considered if a Hollenhorst cholesterol plaque is identified in the retina.

Atheromatous renal disease may be more frequent than previously realized and may be diagnosed on renal biopsy. In patients with lower limb microembolism, the removal of a localized source of the emboli is worth considering. The management of more extensive disease is problematic. Medical management with aspirin is successful in some patients, but warfarin is not recommended.

Although cholesterol embolism is an important cause of digital ischemia, other etiologies should be considered. These were recently reviewed by O'Keeffe et al. as follows.

Causes of Blue Toe Syndrome

Atheroembolism	
Fibrinoplatelet aggregates	Warfarin related
Cholesterol crystal embolism	
Cardiac embolism	
Infective endocarditis	Nonbacterial (marantic) endocarditis
Cardiac myxoma	
Hyperviscosity syndromes	
Cryoglobulinemia	Polycythemia rubra vera
Cryofibrinogenemia	Leukemias
Cold agglutinins	Macroglobulinemia
Hypercoagulable states	
Malignancy	Erythromelalgia
Diabetes mellitus	DIC
Antiphospholipid syndrome	DVT
Essential thrombocythemia	Protein C or S deficiency
Vasculitis	
Polyarteritis	SLE
Miscellaneous	
Calciphylaxis	Steroid associated

From O'Keeffe ST, et al: Blue toe syndrome: Causes and management. Arch Intern Med 152:2197–2202, 1992, p 2198, with permission.

Hypercholesterolemia

Elevated levels of LDL cholesterol and low levels of HDL cholesterol are associated with an increased risk of atherosclerotic disease and its associated consequences, including MI, peripheral vascular disease, and cerebrovascular disease. Therapies for these conditions now involve secondary prevention, or disease detection and treatment for elevated cholesterol, before symptoms of atherosclerosis occur. The National Cholesterol Education Program (NCEP) recommends screening for all adults to detect both elevated LDL and low HDL. The available medications for treatment of elevated cholesterol is outlined in the following table.

Cholesterol-lowering Medications

MEDICATION	INDICATIONS	DOSAGE	SIDE EFFECTS
Bile sequestrants	↑ LDL with → TG		Constipation, elevated LFTs, abdominal pain, elevated TG
Cholestyramine		1 scoop BID or TID	
Colestipol		1 scoop BID or TID	
Nicotinic acid (niacin)	↑ LDL or TG or both	Start at 50–100 mg BID or TID and ↑ to 1.5–3.0 gm/d	Flushing, pruritus, abdominal pain, nausea, vomiting, malaise, elevated LFTs
HMG-CoA reductase	↑ LDL		Elevated LFTs, myopathy, elevated CK, rash, headache, insomnia
Lovastatin		20–80 mg/d	
Simvastatin		10–40 mg/d	
Pravastatin		20–40 mg/d	
Fibric acid derivatives Gemfibrozil	↑ TG ± ↑ LDL	600 mg BID	Stomach discomfort, rash, blurred vision, muscle pain, elevated LFTs, increased incidence of gallstones
Clofibrate	Severely ↑ TG		**Use of clofibrate associated with higher mortality**
Other Probucol	↑ LDL	500 mg BID	Diarrhea, stomach discomfort, prolonged QT interval on ECG that may cause arrhythmias

CHRONIC FATIGUE SYNDROME

CFS is a multifaceted, unexplained illness that has become prominent in the 1990s. Although probably present for years and described as neurasthenia or attributed to psychological dysfunction, it is now recognized as a prevalent disease requiring further research. The hallmark of the illness is profound fatigue above and beyond what is usually experienced by most patients as tiredness. Patients with CFS describe overwhelming fatigue occurring even after minimal exertion, which is not relieved by bed rest.

Signs and symptoms: CFS usually begins with a flulike illness with myalgia, low-grade fever, headache, and fatigue. Instead of improving after several weeks, though, the symptoms only worsen. Other accompanying symptoms include sore throat, painful axillary or cervical lymph nodes, muscle weakness, noninflammatory arthralgia, forgetfulness, confusion, irritability, depressed mood, and concentration difficulty. Physical examination usually finds a nonexudative pharyngitis, low-grade fever, and lymphadenopathy (<2 cm) in the anterior or posterior cervical or axillary chains. Patients may have symptoms for years before CFS is diagnosed. Frequently, they have been told the symptoms are "all in your head." These patients are usually frustrated with physicians because of those physicians' inability either to help their symptoms or provide a definitive diagnosis.

Diagnosis: There are no diagnostic tests to confirm CFS. Therefore, the physician must rely on the patient's Hx & PE findings to make the diagnosis. Although a positive titer to Epstein-Barr virus (EBV) is frequently found in patients with CFS, its prevalence is no greater in these patients than in the general population. A positive EBV titer does not confirm the diagnosis, and a negative EBV titer does not refute the diagnosis. Other diagnoses with symptoms similar to CFS include endocrinopathies (hypothyroidism, adrenal insufficiency, DM, Cushing's disease, hyperthyroidism), infections (tuberculosis, influenza, HIV, brucellosis, Lyme disease), hematologic disorders (anemia, lymphoma), occult malignancy, rheumatologic disorders (fibromyalgia, Sjögren's syndrome, polymyalgia rheumatica, polymyositis), and psychiatric disorders (major depression, hypochondriasis, somatization disorder). The diagnosis of CFS involves ruling out these disorders. Case definitions have been developed for CFS for research purposes, but these are not helpful for the practicing clinician.

Treatment: Therapy for CFS is supportive. Patients need counseling about their illness and necessary lifestyle adjustment. Usually, patients with CFS have been hard-working, successful professionals and may find daily rest and limited activity stressful. CFS has been associated with psychiatric disorders, most notably anxiety and depression. Most likely, these symptoms represent secondary adjustments to the illness. Therapy with NSAIDs may be helpful in relieving joint symptoms. Antidepressant therapy, such as doxepin for patients with insomnia and desipramine for patients without sleep disturbance, aid in both mood management and chronic pain management. Antidepressants should be started in low doses (25 mg/day) and increased over several days to full doses of 150 mg/day. Doses of sedating medications are given at bedtime (see table on antidepressant medication in Depression). For severely depressed and anxious patients, psychiatric consultation and therapy may also be helpful.

Reference: Matthews DA, et al: Evaluation and management of patients with chronic fatigue. Am J Med Sci 302:269–277, 1992.

CHURG-STRAUSS VASCULITIS

Churg-Strauss vasculopathy is a distinct subset of clinical vasculitis, associated with intense eosinophilia and allergic phenomena. Clinically, the disease usually begins with an allergy—often intense or intractable allergic rhinitis—followed by asthma. Up to 70% of patients have had some evidence of upper airway allergic disease. Pansinusitis can also be present. The allergic manifestations differ somewhat from more standard atopic disease in that onset is late in life, with no previous or family history. In addition, most patients seem to have progression from rhinitis to asthma, and both phenomena are difficult to control.

Peripheral eosinophilia is a feature of disease, and the level of eosinophilia at least initially is not significantly different from that of patients with purely atopic disease. Ultimately, however, the eosinophilia becomes more marked, and tissue infiltration may develop. Löffler's syndrome describes patients with a peripheral blood eosinophilia associated with asthma and fleeting pulmonary infiltrates. Lung biopsies show tissue infiltration of eosinophils but no vasculopathy. GI involvement in the form of eosinophilic gastroenteritis can occur. Submucosal infiltrates can produce obstructive nodular masses, and mucosal involvement may lead to diarrhea and bleeding.

Ultimately, the vasculitis becomes apparent, and classic Churg-Strauss syndrome can be diagnosed. The asthma may actually improve once the vasculitic component develops. Fever, malaise, weight loss, and leg cramps are common features. Cardiac disease occurs in a majority of patients and is a major cause of death from the condition. Pulmonary disease can occur as pleural effusions, parenchymal pulmonary infiltrates, or nodular densities (which, in contrast to those in patients with Wegener's granulomatosis, rarely cavitate). Nervous system disease occurred in up to 75% of patients in one study, with the most common lesion being mononeuritis multiplex. Rash (usually as urticaria or nodules) is a common feature of the vasculitic phase and occurs in about 70% of patients. Severe renal disease is uncommon.

Glucocorticoids are the cornerstone of treatment. High doses are often required, and only when remission is obtained can taper occur gradually. Major organ involvement or neurologic involvement requires higher doses for longer periods with slower reductions. Occasionally, when disease progresses despite aggressive therapy, immunosuppressives are recommended. Azathioprine, chlorambucil, and cyclophosphamide have been used.

CIGARETTE SMOKING

Sequelae and Risks

More than 2.3 million in the United States have died from lung cancer since the Surgeon General's 1964 report on the hazards of tobacco use. Of all lung cancers, 87% are caused by smoking. Tobacco is responsible for more deaths per year than all of the U.S. military fatalities in World War I, World War II, and Vietnam combined. The following diseases are caused or worsened by tobacco use:

1. Cardiovascular
   - Coronary artery disease
   - Cerebrovascular disease
   - Abdominal aortic aneurysm
   - Peripheral vascular disease
   - Arteriosclerosis obliterans and thromboangiitis obliterans
2. Malignancy
   - Lung cancer
   - Head and neck cancer (oropharynx, larynx)

- Esophageal cancer
- Bladder cancer
- Kidney cancer
- Pancreatic cancer
- Stomach cancer
- Cervical cancer

3. Respiratory disease
   - Chronic bronchitis and emphysema
   - ↑ risk of spontaneous pneumothorax
   - Chronic stomatitis or laryngitis
4. Gastrointestinal disorders
   - Gastric and duodenal ulcers
5. Pregnancy complications
   - Delayed conception
   - Low birth weight
   - ↑ risk of spontaneous abortion
   - ↑ risk of fetal or neonatal death (SIDS)
   - Long-term impairment of infant's physical or intellectual development

All forms of tobacco are harmful, including chewing tobacco, snuff, cigars, and pipe tobacco. About 21% of coronary deaths, 18% of stroke deaths, and 30% of all cancer deaths are attributable to tobacco. It is thought that about a third of lung cancer in nonsmokers is due to inhaling the smoke of others.

The effects of tobacco are dose related, increasing with the number of cigarettes smoked. For men who smoke more than 25 cigarettes a day, the risk of death from lung cancer is 25 times that of a nonsmoker. The risk is even higher in smokers who are exposed to certain cocarcinogens (asbestos, radon daughters).

Improvements in cardiac mortality and pulmonary function can be seen within the first year after quitting smoking. It takes about 10–15 years for the chance of developing lung cancer to revert to baseline levels for light to moderate smokers. The increased risk of cancer never completely reverts to normal in very heavy smokers who quit.

References: Holbrook JH: Tobacco. In Wilson JD, et al (eds): Harrison's Principles of Internal Medicine, 12th ed. New York, McGraw-Hill, 1991.

Novello AC: The slowing of the lung cancer and the need for continued vigilance. CA 3:133–136, 1991.

CIRRHOSIS

Cirrhosis is defined as diffuse fibrosis and nodularity of the liver. The liver's response to injury is strictly limited, and the end stage of any liver disease is cirrhosis. Cirrhosis is a histologic diagnosis that is characterized by the collapse of hepatic lobules, formation of diffuse fibrotic septa, and nodular growth of the cells. Cirrhosis is divided into three types: micronodular, macronodular, and mixed. Micronodular cirrhosis is characterized by thick, regular septa, by regenerating small nodules varying little in size, and by involvement of every lobule. Macronodular cirrhosis is characterized by septa and nodules of variable size, and by normal lobules in the larger nodules.

Etiology, History, and Treatment of Cirrhosis

ETIOLOGY	MORPHOLOGIC PATTERN	TREATMENT
Viral hepatitis (B and C)	Macro or micronodular	Antivirals: interferon
Alcohol	Micro or macronodular	Abstinence
Iron overload	Micronodular	Venous section, deferoxamine
Copper overload (Wilson's disease)	Macronodular	Penicillamine
Alpha-1-antitrypsin deficiency	Micro or macronodular	Transplant or supplement with α-1-antitrypsin
Type IV glycogenosis	Macronodular	Question transplant
Galactosemia	Macronodular	Withdrawal of milk
Tyrosinemia	Macronodular	Withdraw dietary tyrosine, question transplant
Primary biliary cirrhosis	Biliary, macronodular	Ursodeoxycholic acid, methotrexate, transplant
Primary sclerosing cholangitis, morphologic pattern biliary	Micronodular	Balloon dilatation, ursodeoxycholic acid, or transplant
Hepatic venous outflow block (Budd-Chiari syndrome)	Hepatic necrosis	Relieve main vein block or transplant
Heart failure	Hepatic congestion with end-stage cirrhosis	Treat cardiac disease
Autoimmune hepatitis	Micronodular	Steroids
Toxin and drugs	Macro or micronodular	Identify and stop
Cryptogenic cirrhosis	Macro or micronodular	?

Cirrhosis and Liver Disease

Physical Examination Findings

- **Encephalopathy:** fetor hepaticus (sweetish breath), paranoia, stupor, tremor, asterixis
- **Skin:** jaundice, spider nevi above the nipple area, purpura, increased pigmentation, white nails, palmar erythema, gynecomastia, testicular atrophy, decreased body hair, parotid enlargement, Dupuytren's contracture
- **Abdomen:** ascites, distended abdominal wall veins, splenomegaly, large or small liver
- **Extremities:** finger clubbing, white nails, peripheral edema
- **Eye signs:** lid retraction, lid lag, icterus
- **Nutrition:** wasting of muscles

COAGULATION

Hemostasis is a complex system involving interplay between vascular endothelium, circulating proteins, and platelets. Most of the coagulation proteins are produced by the liver and circulate in inactive forms, undergoing activation via either the intrinsic or extrinsic pathways.

The completed enzymatic structure, attached to the surface of platelets activated by exposure to vascular subendothelium, accelerates the conversion of prothrombin to thrombin, which in turn cleaves fibrinogen to allow its polymerization into an insoluble fibrin clot. Thrombin also activates platelets and stimulates release of von Willebrand factor from the vascular endothelium, which stabilizes the platelet plug against the shearing force of flowing blood. On the other hand, thrombin contributes to the activation of protein C (which in turn works with protein S to inactivate factors Va and VIIIa) and stimulates endothelial cell contraction, thus contributing to fibrinolysis, the final component of the coagulation system. Plasmin, a protease generated from plasminogen by the activity of tissue activators, begins to digest the fibrin clot, and plasma protease inhibitors (including alpha-1-antitrypsin) and antithrombin III inactivate and bind procoagulant factors.

The presence of a coagulation disorder should be suspected if review of a patient's past medical history reveals episodes of prior bleeding inappropriate to the degree of trauma or surgery, heavy nosebleeds, easy bruising, or bleeding into a muscle or joint. There are two general types of laboratory tests for measuring coagulation: those that measure the effectiveness of the clotting system (i.e., bleeding time, APTT, PT, and thrombin time) and those that measure the levels of individual clotting factors.

INTRINSIC PATHWAY

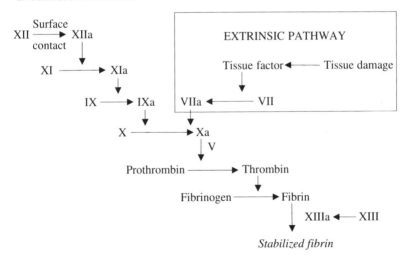

Simplified pathways of blood coagulation. The a denotes the activated form of the circulating inactive zymogen. (From Andreoli TE, et al (eds): Cecil Essentials of Medicine, 2nd ed. Philadelphia, W.B. Saunders, 1990, p 395, with permission.)

Major Inherited Coagulopathies

	HEMOPHILIA A	HEMOPHILIA B	VON WILLEBRAND'S DISEASE
Inheritance	X-linked	X-linked	Autosomal dominant or recessive
Factor deficiency	VIII (coagulant) (= VIII:AHF)	IX	vWF and VIII:AHF
Bleeding sites	Muscle, joints, surgical	Muscle, joints, surgical	Mucous membranes, skin, surgical
Prothrombin time	Normal	Normal	Normal
Partial thromboplastin time	Prolonged	Prolonged	Prolonged or normal
Bleeding time	Normal	Normal	Prolonged
Factor VIII coagulant activity	Low	Normal	Low
Factor VIII antigen (VIII:VWF)	Normal	Normal	Low
Factor IX	Normal	Low	Normal
Platelet aggregation	Normal	Normal	Normal
Ristocetin-induced platelet agglutination	Normal	Normal	Impaired

AHF = antihemophilic factor, vWF = von Willebrand factor. (From Andreoli TE, et al (eds): Cecil Essentials of Medicine, 2nd ed. Philadelphia, W.B. Saunders, 1990, p 397, with permission.)

Replacement therapy is used for management of the hemophilias, as are joint immobilization and ice packs. One unit of factor VIII increases the factor's percent activity by 2% per kg of body weight. The level of replacement depends on the site of bleeding, with 30–60% factor activity required for hemarthroses (excluding 100% for hip), 30–60% for mucous membrane bleeding, and 100% in cases involving head trauma. Treatment should be instituted at the onset of symptoms, as delay may prove less effective and even life threatening. Factor VIII concentrate has a short half-life and must be reinfused every 12 hr until bleeding is stabilized (7–10 days for CNS, nerve entrapment, or airways compression). Factor IX, with its longer half-life, should be infused every 16–24 hr. Epsilon-aminocaproic acid is used to inhibit fibrinolysis and decrease bleeding after dental procedures. Inhibitor antibodies develop in 10–20% of hemophiliacs after repeated infusions and may complicate the computation of correct replacement doses. Bleeding in patients with von Willebrand's disease is managed with normal plasma or cryoprecipitate if severe and with desmopressin if bleeding is mild or for dental prophylaxis. Avoidance of aspirin and NSAIDs should be advised in all cases of inherited coagulation disorders. Other factor deficiencies (V, VII, X, XI, prothrombin) as well as afibrinogenemia and dysfibrinogenemia occur and may be managed, if symptomatic, with fresh-frozen plasma.

There are multiple etiologies of acquired coagulopathies, including the following.

1. **Vitamin K deficiency:** Causes functional abnormalities in prothrombin; Factors VII, IX, and X; and proteins C and S. Occurs secondary to low dietary levels, intestinal malabsorption, or hepatic disease. Manage bleeding with fresh-frozen plasma; monthly injections if necessary.

2. **DIC:** Has multiple causes, including neoplasms, fat embolism, extensive tissue damage (burns, gunshot wounds), infections, liver disease, and various obstetrical syndromes. Laboratory testing reveals low platelet count, schistocytes on peripheral

blood smear, high levels of fibrin degradation products, and prolonged PT, PTT, and thrombin times. Management includes correction of the instigating factors, replacement of clotting factors with fresh-frozen plasma, and platelet transfusions. Heparin anticoagulation is used for thrombotic events such as distal gangrene.

3. **Liver disease:** Is usually related to anatomic abnormalities (varices, associated peptic ulceration) complicated by decreased levels of procoagulant proteins and coagulation inhibitors (secondary to hepatocellular disease and low vitamin K levels) and thrombocytopenia (secondary to hypersplenism). Managed with vitamin K, 10–15 mg IV or SC daily for 3 days (in spite of low response rate), and fresh-frozen plasma (for bleeding).

4. **Vascular purpura (nonthrombocytopenic purpura):** Is a hemostatic defect related to blood vessel dysfunction. Includes Henoch-Schönlein purpura, dysproteinemia related to multiple myeloma or amyloidosis, drug-induced scurvy, and hereditary connective tissue disorders (Ehlers-Danlos, Marfan syndrome), cryoglobulinemia.

5. **Quantitative and qualitative disorders of platelet function:** Are associated with prolonged bleeding time. May be congenital (von Willebrand's disease, inherited platelet defects) or acquired (secondary to medications, leukemia, uremia, paraproteinemia, DIC). Managed by careful surgical hemostatic technique, correction of the underlying cause if possible (hemodialysis, plasmapheresis, discontinuation of responsible drug), and platelet transfusion if necessary.

COCAINE

Cocaine is a naturally occurring alkaloid obtained from the leaves of *Erythroxylon coca,* a plant cultivated in the Andes Mountains. In 1985, it was estimated that 30 million in the United States had used cocaine; 6 million were classified as regular users.

Cocaine may be administered in several forms: Crystallized powder extracted from the plant is used for nasal inhalation or IV administration. Crack cocaine and freebase, made by treatment of cocaine HCl with alkali and solvents, are inhaled while smoking. The intensity and peak of the stimulant effects of cocaine depend on the route of administration.

ROUTE OF ADMINISTRATION	ONSET OF ACTION	PEAK INTENSITY
Chewing coca leaves	5–10 min	45–90 minutes
Intranasal ("snorting")	2–3 min	30–45 minutes
Intravenous	30–45 seconds	10–20 minutes
Intrapulmonary (smoking)	8–10 seconds	5–10 minutes

Adverse Effects

Cocaine has multiple adverse systemic effects, some of which can be lethal. Because it blocks the uptake of several neurotransmitters, many of the side effects of cocaine are due to excess norepinephrine, which results in tachycardia, vasoconstriction, and an acute rise in BP. The following disorders have been associated with cocaine use, with the route of administration in parentheses if the effect is route-specific.

1. Cardiovascular disease
   - Myocardial ischemia and/or infarction
   - Arrhythmias, including sudden death
   - Ruptured aortic aneurysm
   - Infective endocarditis, vascular thrombosis of upper extremity (IV injection)
   - Myocarditis, dilated cardiomyopathy
   - Focal myocardial fibrosis
2. Cerebrovascular disorders
   - Cerebral ischemia or infarction
   - Subarachnoid or intracerebral hemorrhage
   - Rupture of AV malformation or mycotic aneurysm
   - Cerebral atrophy, seizures
3. Pulmonary disease
   - Acute pulmonary edema
   - Hemoptysis (smoking)
   - Pneumomediastinum, pneumothorax, pneumopericardium (inhalation with Valsalva)
   - Septic emboli (IV injection)
   - Asthma or bronchospasm
   - Pulmonary vascular fibrosis and parenchymal granulomas (IV injection)
4. GI disease
   - Ischemic bowel
   - Hepatotoxicity
5. Head and neck complications
   - Atrophy of nasal mucosa/necrosis of turbinates (nasal inhalation)
   - Epistaxis, perforation of nasal septum (nasal inhalation)
   - Chronic sinusitis (nasal inhalation)
6. Autonomic effects
   - Autonomic instability
   - Hyperthermia
7. Acute psychiatric illness
   - Low dose: hyperarousal, elation, euphoria, suspiciousness
   - High dose: anxiety, dysphoria, affect instability, paranoia
   - Toxic dose: catatonic excitement
8. Psychiatric illness in chronic users
   - Paranoid psychosis, hallucinations ("coke bugs")
   - Abnormal involuntary movements, cataleptic-like behavior
   - Depression, social withdrawal
   - Criminal behavior to finance drug habit
9. Other systemic effects
   - Decreased need for sleep, decreased sexuality, poor concentration
   - Susceptibility to infection with HIV and hepatitis viruses
10. Obstetric complications
    - Abruptio placenta
    - Spontaneous abortion, premature labor, fetal death
    - Microcephaly, intrauterine growth retardation
    - Fetal malformations, especially genitourinary system
11. Neonatal complications in infants exposed in utero
    - Intraventricular and intraparenchymal brain hemorrhages
    - Increased irritability, withdrawal syndrome
    - Increased incidence of SIDS (controversial)
    - Developmental delays

Treatment of Drug Abusers

Patients with chest pain, lateralizing CNS findings, hyperthermia, mydriasis, or autonomic instability need immediate, close medical observation. Cardiac arrhythmias and hypertension due to cocaine abuse can be managed with IV beta-blockers. Agitated or anxious patients often respond to IV benzodiazepine. For psychotic symptoms, patients may be treated with low doses of a high-potency neuroleptic, such as 2–10 mg haloperidol. Antipsychotics should be used cautiously in patients with hyperthermia. Hyperthermic patients may be sponged with tepid water or placed under cooling blankets. Psychiatric hospitalization is indicated when a patient remains persistently psychotic, is a significant suicide risk, or needs medical detoxification for other drugs such as opiates or barbiturates. Medications helpful in the chronic treatment of cocaine dependence include amantadine, bromocriptine, desipramine, and flupentixol (the last is not currently available in the United States).

References: Cregler LL: Cocaine: The newest risk factor for cardiovascular disease. Clin Cardiol 14:449–456, 1991.

Mendoza R, et al: Emergency room evaluation of cocaine-associated neuropsychiatric disorders. In Galanter M (ed): Recent Developments in Alcoholism, vol. 10: Alcohol and Cocaine: Similarities and Differences. New York, Plenum Press, 1992, pp 73–87.

COLON CANCER

Colon cancer is a leading cause of cancer deaths in the United States, with approximately 140,000 new cases and 60,000 deaths per year. Risk factors include age, family history, previous adenomatous polyps, history of familial polyposis, and ulcerative colitis. A gene for familial polyposis is located on chromosome 5, and studies suggest that most sporadic adenomatous polyps and perhaps most colorectal cancers may be genetically determined. Screening with yearly fecal occult blood tests and periodic endoscopy after the age of 40 is most appropriate in patients who have two or more first-degree relatives with colorectal cancer. Although adenomatous polyps are considered a risk factor for cancer (up to 95% of colorectal cancers arise from adenomatous polyps), they also increase with age, so that 55% of people over age 80 have at least one polyp. Only 5.5% of this group have a polyp over 1 cm in size. Environment and diet are considered factors in 85–90% of all cases.

Epidemiologic, animal, and biochemical studies suggest that diets high in total calories and fat and low in various dietary fibers (especially insoluble fibers such as wheat bran), vegetables, and micronutrients (such as iodine, iron, vitamins A and D, and calcium) are associated with an increased incidence of colon cancer. A recent study showed the regular use of aspirin to be protective against colon cancer. One study showed that beer drinking in women increased the cancer risk, whereas wine drinking was associated with a decreased cancer risk.

The tumor marker CEA has been used extensively in this disease but has not proved consistently reliable enough to use for screening. Its main roles are as a marker of response to therapy and as an indicator of recurrence.

Once the diagnosis of colon cancer has been made, staging dictates therapy. For early-stage disease, surgery may be curative. About 87% of all cases have primary surgical treatment, which carries a 3% operative mortality. The Dukes system is used for classifying colon cancers.

Dukes System for Staging Colon Cancer

STAGE	DESCRIPTION	% OF CASES	5-YEAR SURVIVAL
A	Infiltration no deeper than submucosa	22	75–90%
B	Infiltration deeper than submucosa, no lymph node involvement	28	40–60%
C	Infiltration deeper than submucosa, with lymph node involvement	34	10–20%
D	Distant metastases	16	<5%

Adjuvant therapy studies in this disease show some benefit when certain subgroups of patients with Dukes C cancer are offered levamisole and 5-fluorouracil, which have been shown by the National Cancer Institute phase III studies to increase survival from 37% to 49%. Systemic therapy of colon cancer for advanced or recurrent disease usually involves systemic chemotherapy including 5-fluorouracil and leucovorin. This results in palliation of symptoms in up to 75% of patients.

COMA

There are only two locations in the brain that can be damaged to cause loss of consciousness: bilateral cerebral hemispheres (both sides must be affected simultaneously) and reticular formation of the brain stem. The task of evaluating a comatose patient is therefore simplified into a determination of whether the patient has bilateral hemisphere disease or brain stem disease.

The commonest causes of coma are not primarily neurologic, but rather reflect loss of brain function due to severe systemic derangements. The most frequent causes of coma, other than the usually obvious situation of head trauma, are:

1. **Drugs:** These can include drug abuse such as with opiates or alcohol, accidental overdose of prescription drugs, and intentional overdose (suicide).

2. **Hypoxia:** This can result from an MI, arrhythmia, pulmonary embolus, COPD, pneumonia, and the like.

3. **Metabolic derangements:** Hypoglycemia is the commonest metabolic cause of coma, but hyperglycemia is also frequent. Sepsis is another common metabolic cause.

Primary neurologic lesions, such as intracerebral hemorrhage, subarachnoid hemorrhage, seizures, and mass lesions, account for only 25–35% of all patients in coma. Most comas are due to medical, not neurologic, problems.

Basic management of the comatose patient includes the following.

1. **ABCs:** Maintain the airway, support breathing, and stabilize the circulation. Vital signs are vital.

2. An **IV line** should be started, with blood drawn and sent for CBC, glucose and electrolytes, ABGs, and a toxicology screen (which may require urine specimens as well).

3. **IV glucose** should be infused. It is impossible to hurt anybody by infusing IV glucose. Many physicians also infuse thiamine, since Werknicke's encephalopathy from thiamine deficiency is a surprisingly frequent cause of coma. Naloxone

(Narcan) is also commonly given because of the importance of opiate drugs as producers of coma.

4. **Rapid Hx & PE:** An adequate history is seldom available. The physical examination should focus on determining whether the process causing the coma is affecting both hemispheres simultaneously, or the brain stem. Most causes of coma, such as drugs, hypoxia, and metabolic derangements, affect both hemispheres simultaneously. A brain stem localization implies a focal neurologic deficit involving the substance of the brain stem itself. If the physical examination can localize the lesion to one area, a structural neurological cause should be suspected. For example, a patient with irregular breathing, pinpoint pupils, abnormal doll's eyes, and decerebrate posturing probably has a brain stem lesion, such as a hemorrhage or infarct. If the examination does not conform to a clear, localizing pattern, then metabolic or systemic causes for coma should be suspected.

5. **Brain imaging:** CT scan or MRI can exclude most structural causes of coma and are especially useful when the physical examination suggests a localized lesion.

Coma is a medical emergency with a grim prognosis. Almost 70% of patients admitted to the hospital in coma die. Brain stem deficits predict an especially grave outcome, and recovery to meaningful function is rare in patients with absent extraocular movements, pupillary responses, or gag reflex.

Reference: Plum F, Posner JB: The Diagnosis of Stupor and Coma, 3rd ed. Philadelphia, F.A. Davis, 1986.

CONGESTIVE HEART FAILURE

CHF is a pathophysiologic state in which an abnormality of cardiac function leads to failure to maintain sufficient cardiac output to meet the demands of metabolizing tissues and/or to do so only in the face of elevated filling pressures. This results in a clinical syndrome characterized by abnormal LV function and neurohumoral regulation, which are accompanied by effort intolerance, fluid retention, and reduced longevity.

Framingham Criteria for Congestive Heart Failure

The diagnosis of CHF requires either one major and one minor or two major criteria.

A. Major criteria
1. Paroxysmal nocturnal dyspnea or orthopnea
2. Neck vein distension
3. Rales
4. Cardiomegaly
5. Acute pulmonary edema
6. S_3 gallop
7. Increased venous pressure >16 cm H_2O
8. Circulation time >25 sec
9. Hepatojugular reflex

B. Minor criteria
1. Ankle edema
2. Night cough
3. Dyspnea on exertion

Table continued on next page.

Framingham Criteria for Congestive Heart Failure (Cont.)

    4. Hepatomegaly
    5. Pleural effusion
    6. Vital capacity decreased 1/3 from maximum
    7. Tachycardia with heart rate >120/bpm
  C. Major or minor criteria
    1. Weight loss >4.5 kg within 5 days in response to treatment

Etiology of Congestive Heart Failure

  A. Diseases of the myocardium
    1. CAD: acute MI, chronic ischemic heart disease, ventricular aneurysm
    2. Hypertensive heart disease
    3. Myocarditis: infectious myocarditis, rheumatic fever, SLE
    4. Congestive cardiomyopathy: idiopathic, alcoholic, sarcoidosis, hemochromatosis, myxedema
    5. Hypertrophic cardiomyopathy: IHSS
    6. Restrictive cardiomyopathy: idiopathic, amyloidosis, endocardial fibroelastosis
  B. Valvular disease
    1. Rheumatic heart disease: mitral stenosis/regurgitation, aortic stenosis/regurgitation
    2. Calcific aortic stenosis
    3. Infectious endocarditis: aortic regurgitation, mitral regurgitation, tricuspid regurgitation
    4. Mitral valve prolapse, which may be complicated by rupture of chordae tendineae
  C. Pericardial diseases
    1. Constrictive pericarditis
    2. Cardiac tamponade
  D. Congenital heart disease: ASD, VSD
  E. Pulmonary disease: cor pulmonale
  F. Arrhythmias
    1. Complete heart block
    2. Tachyarrhythmias: A fib with rapid ventricular response
  G. High-output CHF: thyrotoxicosis, severe anemia, systemic AV fistula, beriberi

Components of CHF Treatment

  1. Treatment of acute episodes versus prevention of further exacerbations.
  2. Treatment must differentiate between *low* LVEF (systolic dysfunction) and normal LVEF (diastolic dysfunction).
  3. Decrease Na^+ intake.
  4. Diuretics: Furosemide (may exacerbate incontinence): First dose should be small. Double dose until response. Give IV doses slowly to avoid ototoxicity; do not dry out patients with diastolic dysfunction, as they need adequate filling pressures to maintain cardiac output.

Table continued on next page.

Components of CHF Treatment (Cont.)

5. ACE inhibitors: Provide afterload reduction, increase CHF survival. Antici-pate first-dose hypotension (hold one dose of diuretic if patient may be intravascularly volume depleted or euvolemic).
6. Digoxin: May be helpful in low LVEF CHF or in A fib. If patient has normal LVEF and A fib, then a calcium channel blocker like verapamil may be a better choice. If the patient is in sinus rhythm and has a normal LVEF, digoxin may be harmful. Maintenance dose may be 0.125 mg/day in older people (maximum ↑ in LVEF seen at digoxin level 0.8 ng/ml).
7. Calcium channel blockers: Patients with normal LVEF may benefit from verapamil or diltiazem.

Reference: Luchi RJ, et al: CHF in the elderly. J Am Geriatr Soc 39:810–825, 1991.

Differentiating Left from Right Ventricular Failure

CHF is a complex clinical syndrome characterized by abnormalities of LV function and neurohormonal regulation, which are accompanied by effort intoler-ance, fluid retention, and reduced longevity.[1] CHF is the single most common cause of hospitalization in the United States. It is thus conceivable that effective diagnosis, early treatment, and prevention will have a drastic, favorable impact on total health care costs.

The signs and symptoms depend to a great extent on which ventricle is primarily involved. Thus, CHF may manifest with signs and symptoms of either LV or RV failure or both. Predominant failure of either ventricle may help the clinician determine the most likely underlying etiology of CHF. For example, ischemic heart disease is most often complicated by LV failure, whereas long-standing severe pulmonary hypertension results in RV failure. However, it is important to recognize the concept of ventricular interdependence. Since all cardiac chambers are enclosed and share space within the pericardial sac, as one ventricle dilates, the other ventricle is compressed and its filling is impaired. Thus, long-standing failure of the LV is often complicated by eventual development of RV failure.

Common Signs and Symptoms of CHF Involving the Left or Right Ventricle

LV FAILURE	RV FAILURE
Pulmonary rales	Jugular venous distention
Third heart sound	Hepatomegaly
Paroxysmal nocturnal dyspnea	Hepatojugular reflux
Orthopnea	Abnormal liver function tests
Exertional dyspnea	Peripheral edema
Fatigue	Ascites
Pleural effusion	Abdominal discomfort
	Anorexia
	Proteinuria

Reference: Packer M: Survival in patients with chronic heart failure and its potential modification by drug therapy. In Cohn JN (ed): Drug Treatment of Heart Failure, 2nd ed. Secaucus, NJ, ATC International, 1988, p 273.

Etiologies of Acute Exacerbations

CHF affects over a million in the United States and is the single most common cause of hospitalization. It is always essential to identify, whenever possible, the underlying precipitating cause for exacerbation of CHF because:

1. Some precipitating factors for acute exacerbations of CHF are life-threatening and potentially fatal if unrecognized and untreated. The best example of a potentially life-threatening precipitating factor is acute PE. Patients with CHF, particularly in advanced stages of the disease, are at greater risk for PE. Moreover, the signs and symptoms of acute PE can be difficult to differentiate from those of CHF.

2. Recognition of the precipitating factor may result in effective prevention of subsequent recurrences of the exacerbations of CHF. Patient education regarding salt intake and compliance with cardiac medications is a simple measure that can, when enforced by the caring physician, substantially reduce the recurrence of an exacerbation of CHF.

3. Treatment aimed at effective treatment of the specific precipitating factor may have long-lasting effects on the patient's general state of health. For example, early diagnosis and specific treatment of hypothyroidism or of hyperthyroidism may have a major impact on the function of many organ systems, such as hematologic, gastrointestinal, endocrine, and cardiovascular.

The most common precipitating factors for exacerbations of CHF are as follows:

1. Increased salt consumption
2. Noncompliance with cardiac medications
3. Pulmonary embolism
4. Infections such as pneumonia or urosepsis
5. Chronic or acute renal failure
6. Paget's disease of bone
7. Anemia
8. Active bleeding
9. Myocardial ischemia or acute myocardial infarction
10. Uncontrolled hypertension
11. High environmental temperatures; physical or emotional stress
12. Thyrotoxicosis
13. Unsuspected pregnancy
14. Cardiac arrhythmias such as A fib or flutter with a fast ventricular response, bradycardia of any cause, or V tach
15. Cardiac depressant or salt-retaining medications (e.g., alcohol, beta-blockers, antiarrhythmic agents, steroids)

CONSTIPATION

Constipation is a very common complaint, especially in the elderly. It is defined as a change in bowel habits from baseline. Most constipated patients have fewer than three bowel movements (BMs) per week. For some patients, one BM per week is baseline, and if there are no complaints of bloating or painful defecation, then this is *not* constipation.

Laxative use is very frequent in the elderly and often leads to dependence on laxatives. Stimulant laxatives destroy the enteric nervous system, setting up a vicious cycle of decreased motility and leading to increased colon diameter, increased constipation, and increased laxative use.

Causes of Constipation

Drugs that cause constipation

Antacids	Antidepressants
Iron	NSAIDs
Psychotropics	Calcium channel blockers
Anticholinergics	Clonidinc
Narcotics	Pseudoephedrine

Diseases associated with constipation

Hypothyroidism	Scleroderma
Stroke	Hyperparathyroidism
Parkinsonism	Diabetic neuropathy
Hyperthyroidism	Volvulus
Tumors	Constricting lesions

The evaluation should start with a rectal exam. If anal tone is decreased, the physician should consider neurologic causes. If the stool is positive for occult blood, further evaluation is needed.

Therapy consists of:

- Hydration (6–8 glasses of liquid per day)
- Bulk agents/lactulose; suppositories and enemas as needed
- Encouragement of physical activity
- Discouragement of frequent use of stimulant laxatives

With aging, the call to defecate may be somewhat decreased, and it is easy to ignore the need. The patient should compensate by setting a regular toilet time in the morning or shortly after meals to take advantage of active peristalsis times.

When the chronically constipated person has sudden abdominal distention and fecal incontinence, fecal impaction and toxic megacolon must be ruled out. Megacolon will have markedly dilated loops of transverse colon on abdominal x-ray.

Types of Laxatives

TYPE	EXAMPLE	MECHANISM	USE	POTENTIAL PROBLEMS
Bulk	Metamucil	↑ stool water	Well tolerated, may be used chronically	Avoid in those with diverticula
Emollient	Colace	↑ water content of stool	Well tolerated, may be used chronically	
Saline	"Magcitrate"	↑ fluid in colon	Not for chronic use	Risk of electrolyte abnormalities
Hyperosmolar	Lactulose	↑ fluid in colon	May use chronically	Bloating
Stimulant	Dulcolax	Direct stimulation of myenteric plexus	Not for chronic use	Dependency

Reference: Castle SC: Constipation in the elderly. Med Clin North Am 73:1497–1509, 1989.

COPD: BRONCHITIS AND EMPHYSEMA

Chronic obstructive pulmonary disease (COPD) is characterized by airflow obstruction and is often classified as being either emphysema or chronic bronchitis. Chronic bronchitis, the "blue bloater," is defined by *symptoms*. Chronic bronchitis is a condition associated with a productive cough on most mornings, for 3 or more consecutive months during 2 or more consecutive years. Unlike bronchitis, emphysema, the "pink puffer," is an *anatomical/structural* term. Emphysema is an abnormal enlargement of air-containing space distal to the terminal bronchioles accompanied by destruction of alveolar tissue. Usually, there is overlap of these two entities, with patients presenting with findings of both processes.

Treatment of COPD

1. **Removal of risk factors:** The most important components are cessation of smoking and removal of any other risk factors (e.g., environmental precipitators, occupational risks).

2. **Bronchodilators:** Although in COPD the airway obstruction is largely fixed, with only a small reversible component, most patients experience a small improvement in their symptoms with the use of bronchodilator therapy. Several classes of bronchodilators are available for the treatment of obstructive airway diseases (both acute and chronic).

a. *Methylxanthines:* These agents, available for oral and parenteral use, include aminophylline, theophylline, and related compounds. It was previously taught that the bronchodilation produced by this class of drugs was due only to their inhibition of phosphodiesterase, an enzyme involved in the conversion of cAMP to noncyclic 5'AMP. That inhibition of the breakdown of cAMP leads to increased levels of cAMP, which in turn leads to bronchial smooth muscle relaxation and bronchodilation. In fact, it has been shown that at pharmacologic doses, less than 10% of phosphodiesterase activity is inhibited. Therefore, other mechanisms are likely responsible for bronchodilation and improvement in symptoms.

Because most patients with COPD have "irreversible" obstruction, the significance of the bronchodilating effect of theophylline has been questioned. However, a variety of beneficial effects other than bronchodilation have been attributed to theophylline and include the following.

- Increased mucociliary clearance
- Increased respiratory drive
- Improved cardiovascular function
- Increased diaphragmatic contractility
- Decreased dyspnea
- Improved exercise capacity

The toxic side effects of theophylline occur with increasing frequency as the serum level exceeds 20 g/ml, although they can be seen even within the therapeutic range of 10–20 g/ml. Serious toxicity (causing seizures and cardiac arrhythmias) is usually not seen until the serum level rises above 30 g/ml; however, it can be seen at lower levels and often is not preceded by less severe signs of toxicity. The common side effects are:

GI: nausea, vomiting, diarrhea, abdominal pain

Cardiac: arrhythmias (sinus tachycardia, multifocal atrial tachycardia, extrasystoles)

Neurologic: headache, nervousness, insomnia, tremor, seizures

Table continued on next page.

Treatment of COPD (Cont.)

Factors affecting theophylline clearance include:
Clearance increased (increased maintenance dose)
- Cigarette and marijuana smoking
- Therapy with phenytoin, phenobarbital, rifampin, carbamazepine
- Ingestion of charcoal-broiled and barbecued meats
- Children (>1 year old)

Clearance decreased (decreased maintenance dose)
- Congestive heart failure
- Hepatic dysfunction
- Elderly patients and infants (<1 year old)
- Viral or bacterial infections with fever
- Therapy with cimetidine, oral contraceptives, erythromycin, ciprofloxacin (and other quinolone antibiotics), allopurinol, propranolol

   b. *Beta-adrenergic agonists:* These agents, available for oral, parenteral, and inhalational use, produce bronchodilation by directly stimulating the β_2-receptors on the bronchial smooth muscle. Epinephrine was the first available agent, but newer agents have been developed that offer increased duration of action and increased β_2 selectivity.

   c. *Anticholinergic agents:* Anticholinergic agents, which can be given via parenteral or inhalational routes, compete with acetylcholine at its receptors. Ipratropium bromide is currently available for inhalational use and causes far fewer systemic side effects than atropine. It also has an extended duration over that of atropine.

   3. **Corticosteroids:** Corticosteroids are available for oral and inhalational use. Patients most likely to respond include those with recurrent attacks of wheezing and a relatively significant response to inhaled bronchodilators (FEV_1 increases >20%). Inhaled steroids have little systemic absorption and therefore fewer systemic side effects. Due to the risk of side effects with use of chronic oral steroids, patient response to their use should be critically evaluated and the lowest possible dose should be used.

   4. **Diuretics:** Indicated for symptomatic relief of symptoms of cor pulmonale.

   5. **Vasodilators:** Studies have shown that long-term vasodilator therapy may decrease pulmonary HTN in some COPD patients, but it is not certain that it improves morbidity or mortality.

   6. **Antibiotics:** Indications for a course of antibiotic therapy for a patient presenting with an acute exacerbation of COPD include increasing dyspnea, increased sputum production, and purulent sputum.

   7. **Continuous oxygen therapy:** In patients for whom it is indicated, long-term O_2 therapy has been shown to decrease the morbidity and mortality of COPD. (See Hypoxemia.)

   8. **Phlebotomy:** In the past, phlebotomy was commonly performed for patients with COPD and secondary erythrocytosis. Today, with the use of O_2 therapy, phlebotomy is rarely indicated.

References: Anthonisen NR, et al: Antibiotic therapy in exacerbations of COPD. Ann Intern Med 106:196–204, 1987.

Goodnight-White S, et al: Pulmonary secrets. In Zollo AJ (ed): Medical Secrets. Philadelphia, Hanley & Belfus, 1991, p 325, with permission.

Meneely GR, et al: Chronic bronchitis, asthma, and pulmonary emphysema: A statement by the committee on diagnostic standards for non-tuberculosis respiratory disease. Am Rev Respir Dis 85:762–768, 1962.

Preoperative Management

The preoperative management of COPD involves a careful Hx & PE to detect a change in pulmonary symptoms. The purpose of the evaluation is to identify factors that are modifiable before surgery. For the pulmonary patient, the main processes to identify are recent infection (including upper respiratory illness) or exacerbation of underlying lung diseases such as bronchitis or asthma.

The history should identify:

1. Current and past tobacco abuse.
2. Level of exercise that can be done without dyspnea.
3. Cough and sputum production.
4. Shortness of breath.
5. Recent hospitalizations for pulmonary disease.
6. Prior general anesthesia.
7. Recent upper respiratory symptoms (fever, nasal congestion, and sore throat).
8. Past and current use of pulmonary medications, including any side effects or adverse reactions.
9. Specific inquiry about corticosteroid use within the past year; any patient who has taken the equivalent of 10 mg of prednisone or more for as long as 2 weeks in the previous year is likely to have adrenocortical suppression and needs stress doses of IV hydrocortisone (100 mg TID) during the perioperative, stressful period.

The physical examination should emphasize:

1. Lungs to detect wheezes and crackles.
2. Extremities to detect nail clubbing, peripheral cyanosis, and peripheral edema.
3. A general inspection to detect a "barrel" chest suggestive of emphysema.
4. Ears, nose, and throat to detect current viral infection.

Some diagnostic tests will be useful such as:

1. CXR
2. PFTs; many patients with severe obstructive disease may have few signs and symptoms, and PFTs are helpful in identifying patients at risk of postoperative complications who may require careful monitoring.
3. Theophylline level for patients receiving that medication.

Patient education before surgery should include:

1. Advice to stop smoking before surgery.
2. Proper technique for handheld inhalers.
3. Incentive spirometry that will be used after surgery to aid in clearing secretions.
4. Deep breathing and coughing.

Patients with signs, symptoms, and PFT results consistent with obstruction who are not receiving inhaled bronchodilators should be started on these before surgery.

Bronchodilator use can be continued throughout the perioperative period via inhalation devices if the patient is unable to use a handheld inhaler.

In general, patients with P_aCO_2 >50 mm Hg and/or an FEV_1 <1.5 L are at highest risk of postoperative pulmonary complications. Patients with an FEV_1 <500 cc and an FVC of <1 L are unlikely to safely tolerate general anesthesia. Other predictors of postoperative pulmonary complications include age older than 70 years, obesity, surgical procedure requiring more than 2 hours of general anesthesia, thoracic or abdominal procedures, and more than one general anesthetic within the preceding year.

Reference: Trautlein JJ: Preoperative pulmonary function. In Kammerer WS, et al (eds): Medical Consultation: The Internist on Surgical, Obstetric, and Psychiatric Services, 2nd ed. Baltimore, Williams & Wilkins, 1990.

CORD COMPRESSION, SPINAL

Epidural spinal cord compression from metastatic cancer is an urgent medical crisis. Spinal cord compression usually causes a triad of signs and symptoms.

1. **Sensory level:** This is often described as a band around the body, usually in the thoracic or abdominal region, below which there is a diminution of sensation.

2. **Weakness:** Usually, cord compression is a symmetric problem, with weakness in both lower extremities approximately equally. The weakness is accompanied by increased reflexes, increased tone, and Babinski signs.

3. **Bowel and bladder difficulties:** Disruption of autonomic fibers in the spinal cord leads to bowel and bladder problems—either incontinence or retention.

Not all patients have all the features of complete cord compression. Generally, the subjective sensory change is the earliest symptom patients report, and a sensory level or band should always be taken very seriously, even when no other accompanying deficits are present. In addition to these signs of spinal cord damage, 80% or more of patients with cord compression from epidural metastases have pain at the site of the lesion. The metastasis generally involves the vertebral body itself and then grows to compress the spinal cord. The commonest locations are cervical, 10%; lumbar, 20%; and thoracic, 70%.

Diagnostically, the most urgent requirement is for imaging of the spine. Plain X-rays are accurate for detecting metastases to the vertebral column that cause epidural cord compression. Cancer patients with back pain should receive X-rays of the painful region. If no lytic lesions or other abnormalities are detected, it is unlikely that the pain is due to metastases, especially if the neurological examination is also normal. Plain X-rays are probably superior to bone scans when screening for cancer.

There is still controversy regarding the optimal imaging procedure for patients with signs of a myelopathy. Traditionally, myelography has been performed, with placement of water-soluble contrast that can be run the entire length of the cord, thus identifying any block that may be present and outlining any small deposits of neoplastic cells. However, this procedure is invasive, uncomfortable, and not without risks, and so it is rapidly being supplanted by MRIs of the spine. MRIs provide excellent visualization but have the disadvantage of requiring more time (thorough screening of the entire spine is much more time-consuming than the rapid assessment that can be made by myelography). In good hands, either technique is quite adequate.

Commonest Tumors Metastasizing to the Spine

1. Breast	4. Renal
2. Lung	5. Lymphoma
3. Prostate	6. Myeloma

Therapeutically, initial treatment begins with 100 mg of dexamethasone as an IV bolus, followed by 4–24 mg QID. Radiation therapy is the preferred method of treatment for most metastases. Surgical decompression, once common, has not been proven superior to radiation therapy alone in several controlled trials, so the role of the neurosurgeon in the management of cord compression has diminished considerably. Currently, the main indication for surgical management of cancerous cord compression is in the patient in whom the primary tumor is unknown. Finding a presumably cancerous lesion in a patient not known to have cancer should initiate a biopsy and decompression.

Reference: Byrne TN: Spinal cord compression from epidural metastases. N Engl J Med 327:614–619, 1992.

CORONARY ARTERY DISEASE

Aspirin in Prevention

It is important to differentiate between primary and secondary prevention of CAD. Primary prevention refers to a strategy aimed at reducing the new development (or incidence) of morbid and fatal clinical manifestations of CAD in subjects initially *free* of CAD. Examples of primary prevention studies are the Coronary Drug Project (CDP), the Physician's Health Study, the Lipid Research Clinics–Coronary Primary Prevention Trial (LRC-CPPT), and the Helsinki Heart Study, to name only a few.

Secondary prevention of CAD refers to a strategy aimed at reducing the clinical manifestations of CAD in patients with *documented CAD*. Examples of secondary prevention studies are the Aspirin in Myocardial Infarction Study (AMIS), the Cardiac Arrhythmia Prevention Study (CAPS), the Cardiac Arrhythmia Suppression Trial (CAST), and the Thrombolysis in Myocardial Infarction trial (TIMI), to name only a few.

It is important to recognize that primary prevention trials are more difficult to perform because of the following factors:

1. Need for longer duration of follow-up
2. More infrequent clinical events (recurrent manifestations of CAD are more common in patients with CAD than in healthy and asymptomatic subjects)
3. Need for larger number of research patients

The role of aspirin in primary prevention of CAD: Several clinical trials have attempted to examine this issue. The Physicians' Health Study[1] is the most recently reported primary prevention trial using aspirin. A total of 22,071 male physicians in the United States were randomized to one of two treatments—aspirin 325 mg every other day or placebo—and were followed for 5 years. In that study, those who received aspirin experienced a statistically significant, 44% reduction in the incidence of a first MI compared to physicians who received placebo.

The role of aspirin in secondary prevention of CAD: Secondary prevention trials have targeted primarily patients with acute MI, unstable angina, or stable exertional angina. In the ISIS-2 trial, a large, randomized clinical trial of patients presenting with a suspected acute MI, aspirin (160 mg/day) reduced 5-week vascular mortality from 11.8% to 9.4% (a 20% decrease), a reduction similar to that achieved with acute administration of IV streptokinase, which resulted in a reduction in 5-week vascular mortality from 12% to 9.2% (a 23% decrease).[2] However, combining both aspirin and IV streptokinase caused a greater reduction in 5-week vascular mortality, from 13.2% to 8% (a 39% decrease), compared to either drug alone.

In patients hospitalized with acute unstable angina, aspirin (325 mg BID) reduced the incidence of fatal and nonfatal MI during hospitalization from 11.9% to 3.3% (a 72% decrease).[3] In a more recent report,[4] aspirin was effective in preventing the reactivation of unstable angina and MI following the abrupt discontinuation of heparin therapy in these patients.

In a subgroup analysis of 333 men with stable angina in the Physicians' Health Study, aspirin reduced the incidence of first MI by 87%, whereas in asymptomatic men, aspirin reduced the occurrence of a first MI by 44%. Based on these results, aspirin is currently recommended in asymptomatic subjects as well as in patients with stable exertional angina.[5]

---

1. Steering Committee of the Physicians' Health Study Research Group: Final report on the aspirin component of the ongoing Physicians' Health Study. N Engl J Med 321:129–135, 1989.

2. The ISIS-2 Collaborative Group: Randomized trial of intravenous streptokinase, oral aspirin, or neither among 17,187 cases of suspected acute myocardial infarction. Lancet 1:349–360, 1988.

3. Theroux PT, et al: Aspirin, heparin, or both to treat acute unstable angina. N Engl J Med 319:1105–1111, 1988.

4. Theroux PT, et al: Reactivation of unstable angina after the discontinuation of heparin. N Engl J Med 327:141–145, 1992.

5. Willard JE, et al: The use of aspirin in ischemic heart disease. N Engl J Med 327: 175–181, 1992.

Percutaneous Transluminal Coronary Angioplasty

Andreas Gruentzig performed the first percutaneous transluminal coronary angioplasty (PTCA) in a human coronary artery in 1974, using a balloon-tipped catheter. Since then, the number of PTCAs performed in the United States has grown to such proportions that it nearly equals the number of CABG procedures.

It is clear that the role of PTCA as a revascularization procedure has grown rapidly. Two major factors contribute to that fast-growing role of PTCA in the United States: First, major technical advances have minimized the risk of complications. Second, the safety of PTCA has clearly stood the test of time.

Indications For and Contraindications To PTCA

Clinical indications for PTCA

Significant stenosis of one or more major epicardial arteries, which subtend at least a moderate-sized area of viable myocardium, in a patient who has:

1. Recurrent ischemic episodes after myocardial infarction or major ventricular arrhythmia,
2. Angina that has not responded adequately to medical therapy.
3. Clear evidence of myocardial ischemia on resting, ambulatory, or exercise electrocardiography, or
4. Objective evidence of myocardial ischemia that increases the overall risk of required noncardiac surgery.

Absolute or relative contraindications to PTCA

High-risk anatomy (including significant left main artery disease) in which vessel closure would likely result in hemodynamic collapse,

Severe, diffuse, and/or extensive CAD better treated surgically,

Target lesion morphology (type C) associated with an anticipated success <60%, unless PTCA is the only reasonable treatment option,

No coronary stenosis >50% diameter reduction,

No objective or compelling clinical evidence of myocardial ischemia, or

Absence of on-site surgical backup, qualified PTCA operators, or adequate radiographic imaging equipment.

From Baim DS: Interventional catheterization techniques: Percutaneous transluminal balloon angioplasty, valvuloplasty and related procedures. In Braunwald E (ed): Heart Disease, 4th ed. Philadelphia, W.B. Saunders, 1992, p 1367, with permission.

Preoperative Management

The assessment of risks from noncardiac surgery in the patient with CAD is challenging to the internist. Although anesthetic agents and techniques have improved dramatically during the recent decades, the risk of intraoperative and perioperative death, MI, and arrhythmia remains in patients with CAD.

The preoperative evaluation must identify and treat any modifiable risk factors. For assessing that risk, Detsky et al. have devised a point system, which includes the complexity and complications of the planned surgical procedure and the patient's current symptoms (see table). As noted in the table, unstable or new symptoms suggest a higher risk of complications than does stable disease. This score is combined with the probability of complications from the surgical procedure itself to determine the overall probability of a complication.

The main tools in a preoperative evaluation are the Hx & PE. The history should inquire specifically about:

1. Symptoms of angina (chest pain on exertion or rest), CHF (shortness of breath, dyspnea on exertion, orthopnea, nocturia, leg swelling), arrhythmias (palpitations), and syncope.

2. Recent hospitalizations for cardiac disease.

3. Past and present use of cardiac medications, including antihypertensives and aspirin, and any side effects or adverse reactions.

The physical examination should be directed toward the cardiovascular and pulmonary systems and include evaluation of:

1. BP measurement in both arms.

2. Carotid upstroke (slow and decreased in aortic stenosis).

3. LV impulse for displacement and hypertrophy.

4. Heart for murmurs of aortic stenosis and S_3.

5. Jugular vein for distension, including detection of hepatojugular reflux.

Modified Multifactorial Index for Prediction of Cardiac Complications in Patients Undergoing Noncardiac Surgery[1]

	POINTS
Coronary artery disease	
MI within 6 months	10
MI more than 6 months	5
Canadian Cardiovascular Society angina	
Class III	10
Class IV	20
Unstable angina within 6 months	10
Alveolar pulmonary edema	
Within 1 week	10
Ever	5
Valvular disease	
Suspected critical aortic stenosis	20
Arrhythmias	
Rhythm other than sinus or sinus rhythm plus APBs[2] on last preoperative ECG	5
More than five PVCs at any time prior to surgery	5
Poor general medical status[3]	5
Age over 70	5
Emergency operation	5

[1] See article for details on application of this model to specific patients.

[2] APB = atrial premature beat

[3] P_aO_2 <60 mm Hg, P_aCO_2 >50 mmHg, K <3.0 mEq/L, HCO_3^- <20 mEq/L, BUN >50 mg/dl, creatinine >3 mg/dl, abnormal SGOT, signs of chronic liver disease, bedridden from noncardiac causes.

From Detsky AS, et al: Predicting cardiac complications in patients undergoing noncardiac surgery. J Gen Intern Med 1986:1:211, p 213, with permission.

6. Lungs for crackles of pulmonary edema and dullness to percussion, suggesting pleural effusion.

7. Liver for enlargement.

8. Lower extremities for edema.

The initial diagnostic tests needed for a preoperative evaluation include:

1. CXR to evaluate cardiac size and pulmonary vasculature.

2. ECG to evaluate for prior MI, ischemia, LVH, conduction disorders, and arrhythmias.

3. Electrolyte measurement, creatinine, glucose, and liver function tests.

Additional testing such as echocardiogram—to detect aortic stenosis or evaluate LV function—and stress testing—to detect ischemia—will be dictated by the Hx & PE and initial laboratory evaluation. (Texts on preoperative evaluation are listed in the references for more detailed discussion of this evaluation.)

References: Detsky AS, et al: Predicting cardiac complications in patients undergoing non-cardiac surgery. J Gen Intern Med 1:211–219, 1986.

Detsky AS, et al: Cardiac assessment for patients undergoing noncardiac surgery: A multifactorial clinical risk index. Arch Intern Med 146:2131–2134, 1986.

Gross RJ, et al: Cardiovascular disease and hypertension. In Kammerer WS, et al (eds): Medical Consultation: The Internist on Surgical, Obstetric, and Psychiatric Services, 2nd ed. Baltimore, Williams & Wilkins, 1990.

Silent Myocardial Ischemia

The term "silent myocardial ischemia" can best be defined as the objective evidence for ischemia in the absence of angina or equivalent symptoms. The potential public health impact of early recognition and effective treatment of silent myocardial ischemia can be best appreciated by examining the estimated prevalence of silent MI. The following table shows the projected prevalence of silent myocardial ischemia in the U.S. population: based on these projections, more than 5 million, or 2% of the population, have silent ischemia, of which 1–2 million are totally asymptomatic.

Estimated Prevalence of Silent Myocardial Ischemia in the
United States by General Type

Totally asymptomatic subjects
- At least 2–4% of asymptomatic middle-aged men (1–2 million men)

Patients with signs and/or symptoms of CAD or coronary spasm
- Old MI, now asymptomatic: 20–30% of asymptomatic, post-MI patients (50,000–100,000 persons per year)
- Angina at other times: 80–90% of patients with angina
- Sudden or near-death episode: unknown prevalence of sudden death victims

Modified from Pepine CJ: Silent myocardial ischemia. Cardiol Clin 4:577–584, 1986.

Insight into the pathophysiology of silent myocardial ischemia can be gained from evaluation of the time sequence of physiologic events in an episode of angina pectoris as illustrated in the following table. According to this scheme, a substantial portion of the ischemic event is silent. In fact, ambulatory ECG monitoring in patients with stable exertional angina pectoris and angiographically documented CAD has clearly shown that three quarters of all ischemic events during daily life are silent. Thus, silent regional ischemia is much more prevalent than symptomatic ischemia.

Sequence of Events in an Episode of Angina Pectoris

1. Decrease in myocardial regional flow/demand ratio
2. Critical decrease in regional PO_2
3. Decrease in regional relaxation and contraction
4. Regional myocardial metabolic changes
5. Electrocardiographic changes
6. Chest discomfort

From Pepine CJ: Silent myocardial ischemia. Cardiol Clin 4:577–584, 1986, with permission.

Silent myocardial ischemia can be documented using one of the following tests.

1. Treadmill exercise test showing transient, exercise-induced horizontal or downsloping ST segment depression of ≥1 mm in the absence of symptoms suggestive of angina pectoris.

2. Transient ST segment depression ≥1 mm during ambulatory ECG monitoring during daily life in the absence of any reported symptoms of angina pectoris.

3. Transient, asymptomatic, exercise-induced episodes of regional wall motion abnormality by echocardiography or radionuclide ventriculography.

4. Transient, asymptomatic episodes of reduced perfusion (called perfusion defect) measured using thallium-201 myocardial scintigraphy during exercise.

The prognostic significance of silent myocardial ischemia has been evaluated in a large number of clinical studies and in different clinical subsets, such as patients recovering from acute MI, stable angina pectoris, and unstable angina. These studies showed that the presence of silent myocardial ischemia, assessed by stress testing or ambulatory ECG monitoring, is highly predictive of future adverse clinical events. However, the impact of therapy with antianginal medications or with revascularization (such as CABG or coronary balloon angioplasty) on the unfavorable clinical outcome of patients with silent myocardial ischemia remains unknown.

Reference: Pepine CJ: Silent myocardial ischemia. Cardiol Clin 4:577–581, 1986.

CORONARY VASOSPASM AND VASOSPASTIC ANGINA

Pathophysiology of coronary vasospasm: The classic clinical manifestations of coronary vasospasm are recurrent episodes of oppressive chest pain at rest associated with ST segment elevation, both of which resolve completely after administration of sublingual nitroglycerin. The first report of a patient with spasm was published by Prinzmetal in 1959, hence the term ''Prinzmetal's angina.'' The concept of coronary vasospasm was a revolutionary concept because it had been widely accepted that angina is consistently associated with either fixed coronary obstruction or other organic disease in which the oxygen demand outstrips the capacity of the coronary vascular bed. Another major breakthrough was the demonstration by Maseri of the temporal sequence between angiographically demonstrable spontaneous spasm and the hemodynamic, ECG, and echocardiographic manifestations of acute myocardial ischemia. An elevation in LVEDP—a sign of acute increase in LV stiffness (or a decrease in compliance)—was clearly shown to precede the appearance of wall motion abnormality by echocardiography. Thus, ischemia causes an impairment of diastolic function before systolic function is affected.

There are four types of coronary vasospasm:

1. Iatrogenically induced vasospasm: spasm induced by catheter manipulation inside a coronary artery, which occurs most commonly during cannulation of the right coronary artery.
2. Spasm due to nitrate withdrawal, as in factory workers.
3. Spontaneous vasospasm in the absence of fixed CAD, which is often called variant angina and which can be induced by the administration of the serotonin inhibitor ergonovine.
4. Vasospasm superimposed on fixed coronary artery obstructive atherosclerotic disease.

It was thought in the early 1980s that coronary vasospasm accounts for a substantial portion of all patients presenting with acute MI, sudden cardiac death, or angina pectoris. Recent acute angiographic and autopsy studies in victims of acute MI or sudden cardiac death indicate that over 95% of these patients have fixed atherosclerotic disease. Moreover, over two-thirds of patients with vasospastic angina have coronary vasospasm superimposed on fixed CAD, and they present with mixed angina, which refers to the presence of both increased demand and decreased supply in patients with angina. These patients classically present with *variable threshold angina,* or *breakthrough angina.* In the morning hours, such patients experience angina at rest or during mild exertion such as shaving or walking a few steps at home upon arising but are able to tolerate walking several miles in the afternoon without any limitation by angina.

Diagnosis and therapy of coronary vasospasm: A rational therapeutic approach in patients with angina pectoris is only possible if the pathophysiologic mechanisms of angina are clearly elucidated. In patients with stable exertional angina with a fixed anginal threshold by clinical history, angina is mediated by an imbalance between oxygen supply and demand due to an increase in demand. The most rational therapeutic regimen in these patients is beta-blocker therapy, particularly in survivors of MI, a subset of patients with CAD who are expected to experience a decrease in cardiovascular mortality of about 20% with beta-blocker therapy. Moreover, beta-blockers are effective in reducing both the number of recurrent episodes of spontaneous exertional angina and the consumption of sublingual nitroglycerin for chest pain while they increase the anginal exercise threshold (that is, the exercise level or duration at which angina first appears). In those patients, the addition of the coronary vasodilator nitroglycerin would also contribute to a reduction in the number of episodes of spontaneous exertional angina and to an increase in the anginal exercise threshold.

The therapeutic approach is different in patients suspected clinically to have vasospastic angina. Vasospastic angina is most effectively controlled with calcium antagonists. The three prototype calcium antagonists are nifedipine, diltiazem, and verapamil. Nitrates are also effective inhibitors of spasm and are effective adjunctive therapeutic drugs in these patients, reducing the number of episodes of exertional as well as rest angina. Beta-blockers have been reported in isolated case reports to exacerbate vasospastic angina and should not be routinely used in patients suspected or proven to have coronary vasospasm.

It is extremely important, in patients suspected to have coronary vasospasm, to document the presence or absence of spasm. Unfortunately, treadmill exercise ECG tests are commonly negative in patients with vasospastic angina and are not helpful to either confirm or exclude spasm. Moreover, coronary angiography may not document vasospasm except in the rare instance in which the patient is experiencing spontaneous vasospastic angina. The serotonin inhibitor ergonovine maleate can provoke vasospasm in patients with vasospastic angina. The induction of *focal coronary artery narrowing* after *low doses* of ergonovine maleate during coronary angiography and its rapid resolution with intracoronary nitroglycerin is the single most reliable diagnostic test for vasospasm. It is important in this setting to realize that normal subjects may develop *diffuse coronary vasospasm* during administration of *high doses* of ergonovine maleate. Unlike focal spasm, the finding of diffuse spasm after large doses of ergonovine maleate is neither specific nor pathognomonic of Prinzmetal's angina, since it may occur in a large number of healthy and asymptomatic subjects.

CORTICOSTEROID THERAPY

Weaning Off Steroids

There are two important considerations when trying to wean a patient off corticosteroids: avoid precipitating adrenal insufficiency, and avoid exacerbating the disease process under treatment. Patients who have been on therapy for less than 3 weeks do not need to be tapered. The course can be ended abruptly without precipitating adrenal insufficiency.

For persons with asthma or COPD, inhaled steroids may be key in decreasing the systemic steroid dose without exacerbations. A gradual taper (over 7 weeks) of oral prednisone did *not* decrease frequency of exacerbations in COPD compared to a quicker, 1-week taper from 60 mg/day (45-, 30-, 25-, 20-, 15-, 10-, and 5-mg daily doses) plus inhaled beclomethasone (two puffs QID) in a 12-week study period. However, if corticosteroids are administered for an exacerbation of asthma in the ED setting, an 8-day prednisone taper (40 mg, decreasing by 5 mg/day until 0 mg) does prevent relapse within the next 3 weeks. Alternate-day prednisone preserves the adrenal response to ACTH in normal situations; however, major stresses such as surgery may require supplemental steroids. Once alternate-day therapy has been instituted, the dose should be decreased slowly (i.e., 5-mg decrease every 2 weeks).

The major complications of long-term steroid therapy include osteoporosis, cushingoid appearance, cataract formation, glucose intolerance, and immunosuppression. Minor complications include easy bruisability, weight gain, edema, and acne.

Reference: Chapman KR, et al: Effect of a short course of prednisone in the prevention of early relapse. N Engl J Med 324:788–794, 1991.

COUGH, CHRONIC

Evaluation of Chronic or Persistent Cough

History
Description of cough
Color and appearance of sputum, if produced
Hoarseness
Occurrence of cough at night or morning
Associated chest pain, dyspnea on exertion, shortness of breath, substernal burning, orthopnea, paroxysmal nocturnal dyspnea
Household pets
Prior history of pulmonary or sinus problems
Recent travel
Exposure to TB
Sore throat
Temporal relation of cough to exercise, work, hobbies
Seasonal occurrence of cough
Cigarette, pipe, cigar, chewing tobacco, or snuff use
Occupation
Irritant exposure
History of allergies
Family history of atopic disease

Physical examination
Vital signs: BP, temperature
Skin: Cyanosis
Pharynx: Postnasal discharge
Nose: Nasal polyps, obstruction, discharge
Ears: Impacted cerumen, inflammation of ear canal, inflamed tympanic membrane
Neck: Thyroid enlargement, nodules, lymphadenopathy (including supraclavicular)
Lungs: Localized and diffuse wheezing, crackles, effusions, signs of consolidation
Heart: Jugular venous distension, displaced point of maximum impulse (PMI), murmurs, gallops (S$_3$)
Extremities: Peripheral edema

Differential Diagnosis of Chronic or Persistent Cough

Environmental irritants
  Cigarette smoking
  Pollutants (sulphur dioxide, nitrous oxide, particulate matter)
  Dusts (all agents capable of producing pneumoconioses)
  Lack of humidity
Lower respiratory tract problems
  Lung cancer
  Asthma and COPD (especially bronchitis)
  Interstitial lung disease
  CHF (chronic interstitial pulmonary edema)
  Pneumonitis
  Bronchiectasis
Upper respiratory tract problems
  Chronic rhinitis, pharyngitis, and sinusitis
  Disease of the external auditory canal (i.e., impacted cerumen)
Extrinsic compressive lesions
  Adenopathy
  Malignancy
  Aortic aneurysm
Gastrointestinal problems
  Reflux esophagitis
Psychogenic factors

From Goroll AH, et al (eds): Primary Care Medicine: Office Evaluation and Management of the Adult Patient, 2nd ed. Philadelphia, J.B. Lippincott, 1987, p 185, with permission.

CROHN'S DISEASE

Crohn's disease is a chronic inflammatory disease of unknown etiology that may involve the entire GI tract, from mouth to anus. It is characterized histologically by inflammation that may extend through the intestinal wall from the mucosa to the serosa and may contain noncaseating granulomas within areas of chronic inflammation. Because of the diversity of anatomic locations in which the disease may occur, the clinical presentation, course, and therapeutic options vary. The three major patterns of disease distribution are ileocecal involvement (40%), disease confined to the small intestine (30%), and disease confined to the colon (25%).

Symptoms of Crohn's Disease

Diarrhea	Abdominal pain
Bleeding	Weight loss
Intestinal obstruction	Perianal disease
Intestinal fistulae	

Complications of Crohn's Disease

1. Abscesses and fistulae
2. Obstruction (small bowel more common than large bowel)
3. Perianal disease
4. Probable increased risk of colon cancer in patients with colitis

Table continued on next page.

Complications of Crohn's Disease (Cont.)

5. Extraintestinal manifestations (arthritis, spondylitis, erythema nodosum, pyoderma gangrenosum, mouth ulcers, iritis, episcleritis)
6. Hepatic complications (fatty liver, pericholangitis, chronic active hepatitis, cirrhosis, sclerosing cholangitis, gallstones)
7. Toxic megacolon (with colitis)

Diagnosis: The two major diagnostic techniques used are colonoscopy and barium studies (small-bowel series or barium enema). Both studies are complementary and the decision as to which is indicated depends on the question being addressed. Radiography is best for identifying small bowel disease, bowel strictures and the presence of fistulae. Endoscopy is best for defining the extent of mucosal disease, for determining the presence of superficial mucosal abnormalities, and for obtaining tissue for histologic examination.

CRYPTOCOCCOSIS AND CRYPTOCOCCAL MENINGITIS

Prior to the HIV epidemic, cryptococcal disease was relatively rare and occurred in immunosuppressed patients, diabetics, and some with no clear predisposition. Patients with HIV infection now represent the vast majority of cases, and HIV-related cryptococcal disease now dominates the literature. A few points need to be kept in mind when one reads the literature and tries to generalize to non-HIV cases. First, cryptococcal disease in the HIV patient is rarely, if ever, curable. Thus many treatment regimens are directed toward control and suppression of the infection and may be inappropriate for those non-HIV patients who may be curable. Second, the manifestations of disease appear different in HIV patients due to the advanced state of immunosuppression. CSF findings are typically abnormal in non-HIV patients, but often totally normal in HIV infection. Also, the presenting symptoms may be more nonspecific, because a severe inflammatory meningitis is often not present.

Until the prevalence of HIV infection increases in areas of the country with a high prevalence of *Histoplasma capsulatum, Cryptococcus neoformans* will remain the most important severe fungal infection in patients with HIV infection. Between 6% and 14% of all AIDS patients develop cryptococcal disease during the course of their HIV infection. Cryptococcal meningitis is the most common manifestation of this infection, occurring in approximately 90% of those infected.

Features of Meningeal Cryptococcosis in 89 Patients

FEATURE	NO.(%)
*Pneumocystis carinii**	12 (13)
Cryptococcosis as initial manifestation of AIDS	40 (45)
Symptoms	
Fever	58 (65)
Malaise	68 (76)
Headaches	65 (73)
Stiff neck	20 (22)
Nausea or vomiting	37 (42)
Photophobia	16 (18)
Altered mentation	25 (28)
Focal deficits	5 (6)

Table continued on next page.

Features of Meningeal Cryptococcosis in 89 Patients (Cont.)

FEATURE	NO.(%)
Seizures	4 (4)
Cough or dyspnea	28 (31)
Diarrhea	19 (21)
Signs	
Temperature >38.4°C	50 (56)
Meningeal signs	24 (27)
Altered mentation	15 (17)
Focal deficits	13 (15)

*Concurrent pneumonia due to *P. carinii.* From Chuck S: Infections with *Cryptococcus neoformans* in AIDS. N Engl J Med 321:795, 1989, with permission.

The diagnosis of cryptococcosis is made by culture of the organism. In AIDS patients, the disease is generally disseminated, and multiple specimens yield the organism. When the diagnosis is considered, CSF, blood, urine, and sputum may be sent for culture. CSF and blood provide the best results. Also important is the identification of cryptococcal polysaccharide capsular antigen in either CSF or blood. Other CSF findings may or may not be helpful in HIV-infected patients. As shown in the following table, CSF findings may be strikingly normal, except for the India ink study and the antigen test.

Laboratory Findings in Patients Presenting with Cryptococcal Meningitis

FINDING	NO. WITH FINDING/NO. TESTED (%)	RANGE
Blood		
WBC <4000/mm^3	44/89 (49)	1300–27,900
Albumin <3.0 g/dl	17/89 (19)	1.8–4.5
Sodium <135 mmol/L	20/89 (22)	
Liver function abnormal	24/89 (27)	
Extrameningeal-source culture positive	54/79 (68)	
Cryptococcal antigen titer		
Negative	1.71 (1)	
≥1:32	62/71 (87)	
≥1:1024	48/71 (68)	
≥1:10,000	15/71 (21)	
Cerebrospinal fluid		
Opening pressure ≥200 mm H$_2$O	33/50 (66)	80–555
Glucose <2.2 mmol/L (40 mg/dl)	21/89 (24)	7–114
Protein >45 mg/dl	49/89 (55)	14–300
White cell count ≥20	19/89 (21)	0–700
PMN count ≥10%	14/89 (16)	
India-ink test positive	64/87 (74)	
Cryptococcal antigen titer		
Negative	8/88 (9)	
≥1:32	63/88 (72)	
≥1:1024	34/88 (39)	
>10,000	5/88 (6)	

From Chuck S: Infections with *Cryptococcus neoformans* in AIDS. N Engl J Med 321:796, 1989, with permission.

Treatment of cryptococcal disease is currently a topic of great discussion, if not debate. Many authorities would prescribe a curative course of amphotericin B in those patients without HIV infection. Again, this reflects the proven efficacy of that regimen and the possibility of cure in such patients. However, in HIV infection, cure is not felt to be possible, so a compromise between efficacy and quality of life is made. Studies of initial therapy with fluconazole alone have raised the issue of early treatment failures. Most authorities now prescribe an initial 2-week course of amphotericin with or without 5-flucytosine followed by lifelong fluconazole therapy at a dose of 200–400 mg per day.

CRYSTALLINE ARTHROPATHY

The syndrome of acute gout was recognized in the 17th century, but it took another 350 years to identify the source and etiology. The presence of monosodium urate crystals in high concentration in the joints and the production of disease by intra-articular urate injection provided the key to understanding. As time progressed, patients with similar syndromes without intra-articular monosodium urate crystals were noted. Eventually, calcium pyrophosphate crystals and basic calcium phosphate (BCP) deposits were detected, in association with painful articular syndromes.

Gout

The presence of uric acid in the body comes primarily from foods containing purines and pyrimidines. Most patients with hyperuricemia have a relative deficit in renal excretion of uric acid, which results in an increase in total body urate. A minority of patients with various genetic deficits or high nucleic acid turnover (patients with myeloproliferative disease and psoriasis) actually overproduce urate and excrete it in increased amounts.

Classic gout is divided into four stages. The first is **asymptomatic hyperuricemia.** All patients who ultimately develop gout have a stage of asymptomatic hyperuricemia, but not all patients with hyperuricemia develop gout. Thus, the diagnosis should await an acute articular disease and demonstration of uric acid crystals in the joint. The second stage, **acute gout,** is the most typically recognizable clinical stage. The metatarsophalangeal (MTP) joint of the great toe is the most commonly affected joint, but ankles, knees, and even the tarsal joints can be affected. Less commonly, the upper limbs are involved. The skin over the involved joint often becomes red and may subsequently peel. Patients may have fever, especially when multiple joints are affected. It is rare that the initial attack of gout will be poly-articular. Little improvement can be made to Sir Thomas Sydenham's description of the disease:

> The victim goes to bed and sleeps in good health. About two o'clock in the morning he is awakened by a severe pain in the great toe; more rarely in the heel, ankle, or instep. The pain is like that of a dislocation and yet the parts feel as if cold water was poured over them. Then follows chills and shivers and a little fever. The pain which was at first moderate, becomes more intense, . . . violent stretching and tearing of the ligaments—now it is a gnawing pain and now a pressure and tightening. So exquisite and lively meanwhile is the feeling of the part affected that it cannot bear the weight of the bed clothes nor the jar of a person walking in the room. The night is passed in torture, sleeplessness . . .

From Major RH: Classic Descriptions of Disease, 3rd ed. Springfield, IL, Charles C Thomas, 1978, pp 288–289, with permission.

Once the attack subsides, the patients enter the period of **intercritical gout**—characterized by elevated serum urate—without articular pain. Ultimately, recurrent acute attacks occur, usually within one year. In one study, only 7% of patients had no recurrence 10 years after their first attack. The frequency, severity, and number of joints involved with each attack increase as time goes by. Finally, usually at least 10 years after the initial attack, the fourth stage, **tophaceous gout,** develops. Urate builds up in the joint and forms deposits of crystalline uric acid (tophi). These are most commonly found in the synovium and olecranon bursa but have been found in the pinnae of the ears, on the walls of blood vessels, and on heart valves.

Serum urate values are occasionally normal at the time of an acute attack of gout and thus do not rule out the diagnosis. Conversely, an elevated serum urate value in the presence of acute arthritis does not establish a diagnosis of gout. Synovial fluid evaluation shows marked elevation of WBCs. Identification of intracellular, needle-shaped, negatively birefringent (yellow parallel to the axis of the red compensator lens when viewed under polarized light) crystals establishes the diagnosis.

The treatment of gout is two pronged: Immediate concern is for quick reduction in inflammation and pain. The long-term goal is a reduction in serum uric acid and thus prevention of further acute attacks. Classically, NSAIDs are effective when given early in the course of acute gout. Traditionally, indomethacin is used, although other NSAIDs have also been shown to have efficacy.

Alternatively, colchicine, a drug known to be effective in acute gout since the late 1800s, can be used. It is given in small doses (0.6 mg) every 2 hours until the patient's attack is relieved or GI side effects develop (most commonly diarrhea). A total of no more than 6–8 mg should be given in 24 hours. Colchicine can also be given IV (in lower doses of 2 mg, with no more than 4 mg/24 hr), with a lower likelihood of GI side effects. Mixing the oral and IV routes increases the risk of toxicity and is contraindicated. Caution must be used in patients who have renal or hepatic dysfunction.

Another treatment option for an acute attack is the use of glucocorticoids. In general, 30 mg of prednisone will suppress an acute attack. Intra-articular steroids can also effectively quiet an attack and provide a particularly useful mode of treatment in patients at risk for toxicity from NSAIDs, colchicine, or systemically administered glucocorticoids.

For prevention of further acute attacks and joint destruction, serum urate must consistently be lowered. Probenecid and sulfinpyrazone effectively increase renal urate excretion. Conversely, allopurinol, a xanthine oxidase inhibitor, allows the excretion of the uric acid precursors xanthine and hypoxanthine. Production of urate is reduced, resulting in a lower serum level. Initiation of these medications proximate to an acute attack may result in a recrudescence or worsening of the attack. Classically, NSAIDs or colchicine over a period of 1–3 months is recommended before initiating the urate-lowering medication.

Calcium Pyrophosphate and Other Crystalline Deposits

As noted, uric acid is not the only crystal capable of inducing arthritis. Calcium pyrophosphate deposition disease (CPDD) is not uncommon (a prevalence of 0.9 per 1,000 population), and the frequency increases with age. CPDD has a hereditary form, which, although transmitted as autosomal dominant with incomplete penetrance, likely represents several different genetic defects. CPDD can be associated with several conditions, including hyperparathyroidism, hemochromatosis, and hypomagnesemia. Finally, cases in which no underlying or hereditary association can be found are termed "idiopathic."

Some Conditions Associated with CPDD

Group A: True association—high probability

Primary hyperparathyroidism	Familial hypocalciuric hypercalcemia
Hemochromatosis	Hemosiderosis
Hypophosphatasia	Hypomagnesemia
Bartter's syndrome	Hypothyroidism
Gout	Neuroarthropathy
Amyloidosis	Localized trauma (surgery for osteochondritis
Corticosteroid therapy (long term)	dissecans, hypermobility syndrome)
Aging	

Group B: True association—modest probability

Hyperthyroidism	Nephrolithiasis
Ochronosis	Diffuse idiopathic skeletal hyperostosis
Wilson's disease	Hemophilia arthritis

Group C: True association unlikely

Diabetes mellitus	Hypertension
Azotemia	Hyperuricemia
Gynecomastia	Inflammatory bowel disease
Rheumatoid arthritis	Paget's disease of bone
Acromegaly	

From McCarty D: The Heberden Oration. Ann Rheum Dis 42:234, 1983, with permission.

Type A: This is the classic presentation of pseudogout. Acute attacks can last from days to weeks, mimicking acute gout. Attacks are more commonly monarticular (most common in the knees), although polyarticular attacks are described. Fever may be present, and postoperative flares are very common.

Type B: This is so-called pseudorheumatoid arthritis, because it mimics RA, causing morning stiffness and synovial swelling. Patients have a history of acute intermittent attacks prior to the onset of chronic disease. Occasionally, RA and CPDD can occur coincidentally. However, as with classic gout, the incidence of this crystalline arthropathy is less in RA than in control populations.

Types C and D: These occur in patients with underlying OA. Low-grade synovitis and pain, out of proportion to the degenerative changes seen on x-rays, should raise a suspicion of crystalline arthropathy (type D). If acute attacks are also seen at intervals (type C), the diagnosis can be a bit easier.

Type E: Lanthanic CPDD is the most common form of the disease, representing chondrocalcinosis.

Type F: This form can mimic neuropathic destruction. It is rare but has been reported to affect the knee more than other joints. There may be no associated neurologic deficit.

Laboratory Findings: Laboratory data in CPDD are generally normal unless there is an underlying metabolic disease present. Thus, abnormalities of calcium, magnesium, glucose, or iron can be suggestive. The diagnosis is based not only on clinical presentation but also on identification of calcium pyrophosphate crystals by examination of synovial fluid under polarized light with first-order rose compensator. Synovial fluid samples should be evaluated promptly because the crystals become less evident over time. The crystals are generally rhomboidal and, in contrast to urate crystals, are only weakly positively birefringent under polarized light (appearing blue when parallel to the axis of the rose compensator). During an acute attack, the synovial fluid has a high WBC count (commonly up to 50,000 cells). Synovial fluid glucose may be low, reflecting the high metabolic activity. Chondrocalcinosis may be demonstrated radiographically. It is most commonly seen in the fibrocartilage of the knee, wrist, and pubic symphysis.

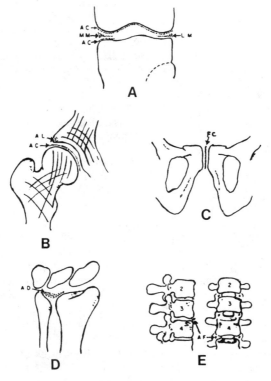

Diagrammatic representation of characteristic sites of CPDD crystal deposition. **A,** A.C. = articular cartilage; L.M. and M.M. = lateral and medial meniscus in knee joint shown in anteroposterior projection. **B,** A.L. = acetabular labrum in anteroposterior projection of hip joint. **C,** F.C. = fibrocartilaginous symphysis pubis in anteroposterior projection of pelvis. **D,** A.D. = articular disc of the wrist in anteroposterior projection. **E,** A.F. = anulus fibrosus of intervertebral discs in anteroposterior and lateral views. (From Schumacher HR (ed): Primer on Rheumatic Disease, 9th ed. Atlanta, Arthritis Foundation, 1988, p 208, with permission.

Hydroxyapatite (also called BCP) deposition is associated with a number of painful articular syndromes. The most common is calcification at tendinous insertions. So-called calcific periarthritis can occur in any age group without sexual predisposition. Onset is abrupt and can sometimes follow trauma. The pain is severe and there is often concomitant limitation of motion and evidence of local inflammation. Calcific deposits may be seen on plain x-rays as fluffy or dense areas. Shoulder disease (more common in elderly women) defines the Milwaukee shoulder syndrome. Rotator cuff arthropathy is associated, and x-rays often show superior migration of the humeral head. Although the shoulder was originally described, other joints can become involved. Intra-articular deposition of hydroxyapatite can lead to acute arthritis as well, which can be progressive and destructive. Finally, BCP deposition has been seen in patients undergoing renal hemodialysis.

Treatment is primarily with NSAIDs for both CPDD and apatite deposition. Colchicine can sometimes be effective in CPDD although rarely as dramatically as when used in acute gout. Intra-articular glucocorticoids are useful, especially in patients in whom NSAIDs are contraindicated. If periarticular deposits are large, surgical removal is occasionally required.

References: Kelly WN, et al: Gout. In Kelly WN, et al (eds): Textbook of Rheumatology, 4th ed. Philadelphia, W.B. Saunders, pp 1291–1336, 1993.

Ryan LM, et al: Calcium pyrophosphate crystal deposition disease; pseudogout; articular chondrocalcinosis. In McCarty DJ (ed): Arthritis and Allied Conditions, 11th ed. Philadelphia, Lea & Febiger, pp 1711–1736, 1989.

CUSHING'S SYNDROME

The most common cause of Cushing's syndrome is iatrogenic due to therapeutic doses of synthetic glucocorticoids.

Causes of Cushing's Syndrome

CAUSES	RELATIVE INCIDENCE
ACTH dependent	75%
Cushing's disease	60%
Ectopic ACTH secretion	15%
Ectopic CRH secretion	Rare
ACTH independent	25%
Adrenal cancer	15%
Adrenal adenoma	10%
Micronodular adrenal disease	Rare
Factitious or iatrogenic	Very common

Cushing's disease (excess ACTH production from a pituitary microadenoma) is four times more common in women than men, and often occurs between the ages of 20 and 40 years. A pituitary tumor is often responsible and is usually very small. However, CT scan or MRI of the pituitary reveals a pituitary adenoma in only 50% of patients.

Adrenal tumors causing Cushing's syndrome may occur at any age, but they predominate in children (particularly carcinoma). Carcinomas are usually aggressive and large, and they may be palpable. In contrast, adenomas are slow growing and usually of moderate size (1.5–6 cm in diameter at presentation). An adrenal adenoma rarely occurs in the context of MEN type I. Micronodular adrenal disease occurs in children and younger adults. The biochemical pathogenesis of the disorder is not clear. It can occur in sporadic or familial forms.

Tumors Associated with the Ectopic ACTH Syndrome

1. Oat cell carcinoma		50%
2. Tumors of foregut origin		35%
Thymic carcinoma	Islet cell tumor	
Medullary carcinoma of the thyroid	Bronchial carcinoid	
3. Pheochromocytoma		5%
4. Other		10%
Gonadal		
Prostate and cervical carcinoma		
Tumors of unknown origin		

Common manifestations of Cushing's syndrome—central obesity, acne, mild hirsutism, HTN, irregular menstruation, and impaired glucose tolerance—are nonspecific (i.e., found in polycystic ovary disease). More characteristic features of Cushing's syndrome are not as common—proximal muscle weakness, large wide stria, thin skin, and fullness of the supraclavicular fossa). Other clinical features are osteoporosis, vertebral collapse, rib fractures, avascular bone necrosis, depression, psychosis, and increased susceptibility to infection. Benign intracranial HTN glaucoma, cataracts, pancreatitis, and avascular necrosis of the head of the femur frequently occur in iatrogenic Cushing's syndrome, but infrequently in endogenous Cushing's syndrome.

Diagnostic Tests

1. **Measurement of 24-hour urine free cortisol excretion:** This is the most useful diagnostic test for Cushing's syndrome. Values in excess of 100 µg/24 hrs are suggestive of Cushing's syndrome. Values in excess of 250 µg/24 hrs are diagnostic of Cushing's syndrome. However, transient elevation of urinary cortisol excretion (100–250 µg/day) is seen in patients with pseudo-Cushing's syndrome due to alcohol, hypoglycemia, depression, and psychological or physical stress.

2. **Loss of normal diurnal variation of cortisol secretion:** In Cushing's syndrome, average morning cortisol and evening cortisol levels are similar. Patients with pseudo-Cushing's maintain a normal diurnal variation.

3. **Overnight 1-mg dexamethasone suppression test:** This is considered a screening test for Cushing's. It is performed on an outpatient basis and requires 8 AM cortisol suppression to <5 µg/dl after PO administration of 1 mg dexamethasone at midnight. Many patients with depression, obesity, alcoholism, and stress have a false-positive test. Therefore, a normal suppression allows the exclusion of Cushing's and an abnormal response does not necessarily imply the presence of Cushing's.

4. **High-dose dexamethasone suppression test:** This test uses a dose of 8 mg of dexamethasone per day. In 80–90% of patients with Cushing's disease, the 24-hour urinary excretion of 17-hydroxy and 17-keto steroids is suppressed by more than 50% of baseline. Lack of suppression leads to the search for an adrenal tumor or an ectopic source of ACTH. If the adrenal CT scan is negative, a CT scan of the chest should be performed to search for a lesion causing ectopic Cushing's.

Diagnostic Difficulties

1. Cushing's disease (suppression may not occur)
2. Bronchial carcinoids suppressed in 40% of cases
3. Periodic hormone production (cyclical or intermittent)

These difficulties can be overcome by the measurement of plasma ACTH, the response of ACTH to corticotropin-releasing factor, and petrosal sinus sampling of ACTH during corticotropin-releasing-factor stimulation test. About 90% of pituitary ACTH-secreting adenomas respond to exogenous administration of corticotropin-releasing factor with an increase in ACTH secretion; Cushing's syndrome due to an ectopic source of ACTH responds less than 10% of the time. Petrosal sinus sampling of plasma ACTH allows confirmation or exclusion of the diagnosis of Cushing's disease and helps identify the site of secretion of ACTH. A right-to-left gradient of >1.5 has been associated with correct localization confirmed surgically in 85% of cases. Primary adrenal disease is suspected in patients with undetectable ACTH and no response to corticotropin-releasing factor.

Treatment

The therapeutic procedure of choice in Cushing's disease has become the transphenoidal removal of a microadenoma (success rate may exceed 90% on the first attempt). If hypercortisolism persists, a second attempt is justifiable (50% success rate). If a pituitary tumor cannot be found, a hemihypophysectomy is often performed. Adverse effects of surgery include CSF leak, sinusitis, and diabetes insipidus.

An alternative to surgery may be a combination of external irradiation (4,500 rads over 6 weeks) and mitotane (Lysodren) (3 gm/day), which results in adequate control of hypercortisolism in 85% of cases.

If the previous two methods have failed, bilateral adrenalectomy should be considered. However, the procedure is associated with a high mortality rate (5%), a lifelong requirement for glucocorticoid and mineralocorticoid replacement, and Nelson's syndrome (5–10% of patients). Nelson's syndrome is characterized by pituitary tumor enlargement and pigmentation. Full recovery from the effects of hypercortisolism may take up to 1 year regardless of the therapy used.

The management of ectopic Cushing's should be addressed to the source of ACTH secretion. If the source cannot be localized or controlled, ketoconazole (400–1,000 mg/day) may be effective in blocking the hypercortisolism. Adverse effects of ketoconazole include hepatocellular damage, which dictates discontinuation of the drug. Metyrapone, aminoglutethemide, and trisolane may be alternative medications when liver damage occurs from ketoconazole.

Surgical removal is the main form of therapy for adrenal adenomas and carcinomas (unilateral flank excision for benign lesions and anterior transabdominal approach for malignant lesions). In malignant adrenal masses, mitotane at high doses is often given after the surgery. Mitotane causes shrinkage of malignant lesions and results in an objective remission in 25% of patients. Continuing removal of malignant adrenal lesions significantly improves survival.

Micronodular adrenal disease is managed with bilateral adrenalectomy.

CYSTIC DISEASES OF THE KIDNEY

Renal cysts are defined as cavities within the kidneys, lined with epithelium and filled with fluid and/or semisolid debris. The cysts may be single or multiple, inherited or acquired, symptomatic or silent, benign or malignant and may present in childhood or older age. The differential characteristics of the major renal cystic disorders are described in the following table.

Characteristics of Renal Cystic Disorders

FEATURE	SIMPLE CYSTS	ADPKD	ARPKD	ACKD	MCD	MSK
Inheritance pattern	None	Autosomal dominant	Autosomal recessive	None	Often present, variable pattern	None
Incidence or prevalence	Common, increasing with age	1/200–1/1000	Rare	40% in dialysis patients	Rare	Common
Age of onset	Adult	Usually adults	Neonates, children	Older adults	Adolescents, young adults	Adults
Presenting symptom	Incidental finding, hematuria	Pain, hematuria, infection, family screening	Abdominal mass, renal failure, FTT	Hematuria	Polyuria, polydipsia, enuresis, renal failure, FTT	Incidental, UTI, hematuria, renal calculi
Hematuria	Occurs	Common	Occurs	Occurs	Rare	Common
Recurrent infections	Rare	Common	Occurs	No	Rare	Common
Renal calculi	No	Common	No	No	No	Common
Hypertension	Rare	Common	Common	Present from underlying disease	Rare	No
Method of diagnosis	Ultrasound	Ultrasound, gene linkage analysis	Ultrasound	CT scan	None reliable	Excretory urogram
Renal size	Normal	Normal to very large	Large initially	Small to normal, occasionally large	Small	Normal

ADPKD = autosomal-dominant polycystic kidney disease; ARPKD = autosomal-recessive polycystic kidney disease; ACKD = acquired cystic kidney disease; MCD = medullary cystic disease; MSK = medullary sponge kidney; FTT = failure to thrive; UTI = urinary tract infection.

From Gabow PA: Cystic disease of the kidney. In Wyngaarden JB, et al (eds): Cecil Textbook of Medicine, 19th ed. Philadelphia, W.B. Saunders, 1992, p 609, with permission.

I. Simple renal cysts: Simple cysts constitute the most common and benign of all the renal cystic disorders. The incidence ranges from 1–5% in children to as high as 50% in people over 50 years of age. Usually, these are benign and incidental findings in radiological studies. When pain or hematuria occurs, a malignant change should be excluded. As opposed to malignant cysts, these are smooth walled and contain no debris inside the cyst. CT scan is sometimes employed to confirm the diagnosis and has, to a great extent, replaced cyst puncture as a diagnostic procedure. Rarely, simple cysts are associated with renin release and HTN, in which cases they should be treated with sclerotherapy using alcohol instillation into the cysts.

II. Polycystic kidney diseases: This occurs in two types: the **infantile**—or autosomal-recessive—and **adult**—or autosomal-dominant varieties. The autosomal-dominant polycystic kidney disease (ADPKD) is seen in 0.1–0.5% of the general population and is the most frequent inherited disorder in the United States. The gene is carried on chromosome 16. This genetic defect causes cysts not only in the kidneys but also in several other organs in the body. Most often the disease is diagnosed during screening of the family members of an affected person. Common clinical symptoms include flank pain and hematuria, either microscopic or gross. An abdominal mass could be a presenting symptom because these kidneys can enlarge to attain the size of a football. Extrarenal manifestations of this disease are given in the following table.

Systemic Features of Adult Polycystic Kidney Disease

1. Genitourinary	3. Cardiovascular
Polycystic kidney	Hypertension
Renal adenoma/hypernephroma	Cardiac valvular abnormalities
Renal calculi	Intracranial aneurysms
Ovarian cysts	
	4. Musculoskeletal
2. Gastrointestinal	Hernia formation
Hepatic cysts	
Pancreatic cysts	
Diverticular disease	

HTN occurs in 60% of these cases and intracranial aneurysms are seen in 10–40%. Renal failure eventually occurs at a variable age, usually after the age of 50. The diagnosis is made from the Hx & PE and confirmed by ultrasound and/or CT scan. Treatment consists essentially of prevention and treatment of complications.

Hematuria is managed with analgesics, bed rest, and hydration. When urinary infections occur, urine and blood cultures should be obtained. The possibility of cyst infection should be kept in mind in an evaluation of the treatment options, especially in resistant cases. Renal function should be evaluated at least annually because ADPKD accounts for 10% of ESRD. Dialysis and renal transplantations are well tolerated by these patients. The differences between simple cysts and ADPKD are summarized in the following table.

Autosomal-recessive polycystic kidney disease (ARPKD) is a rare disorder that represents the infantile or juvenile form of polycystic kidney disease. The kidneys are large at infancy and cause failure to thrive, urinary infections, and eventually ESRD. Hepatic fibrosis and portal HTN contribute significantly to the morbidity of these patients.

Differences Between Simple Cysts and Polycystic Kidney Disease

FEATURE	MULTIPLE SIMPLE CYSTS	PKD
Family history	No	60%
Ultrasonographically demonstrable cysts in other family member(s)	No	90%
Sex distribution	M > F	M = F
Renal size	Normal	Normal to mildly ↑
Kidneys involved	Usually unilateral, may be bilateral	Usually bilateral, may be unilateral early in course
Cyst distribution	Cortical	Cortical and medullary
Cyst size	Usually <2 cm, occasionally larger	<2 cm early
Blood in cysts	Rare	Common
Hepatic cysts	No	40–60%, likelihood increases with age
Intracranial aneurysm	No	10–40%
Mitral valve prolapse	No	26%
Hypertension	Rare	60%
Gene linkage analysis for chromosome 16	No	Likely

Acquired cystic kidney disease (ACKD) denotes the development of cysts in previously noncystic kidneys. Almost all such patients are on chronic dialysis. The incidence of ACKD ranges from 40% to 100% among dialysis patients. The diagnosis is made when pain or hematuria occurs in these patients or incidentally during imaging procedures. When cysts are large, the chance of malignant transformation is high and hence needs to be surgically treated. About 10% of them may produce erythropoietin and cause polycythemia.

Other renal cystic disorders include medullary cystic disease (MCD) and medullary sponge kidney (MSK). MCD is rare and presents in childhood with polyuria, polydipsia, and growth retardation. Retinitis pigmentosa occurs in some cases. The kidneys are small and demonstrate cysts at the corticomedullary junction. Renal failure and renal salt wasting are the other common features. MSK, in contrast, is relatively common and presents with recurrent hematuria, urinary infections, and renal calculi. IVP demonstrates normal-size kidneys with medullary cysts, an appearance often described as ''bouquet of flowers.'' Other manifestations include renal tubular acidosis and secondary hyperparathyroidism. Treatment consists mainly of management of UTIs and stones.

CYTOMEGALOVIRUS

Cytomegalovirus (CMV) is a member of the Herpesviridae family along with herpes simplex types 1 and 2, varicella-zoster virus, and EBV. These viruses are large and enveloped, and they contain DNA. Like others in this family, CMV can remain dormant within humans for extended periods of time and, when reactivated, cause disease years after the primary infection. Thus, CMV-related illnesses can be divided into primary and secondary infections. Secondary infections usually manifest during periods of profound immunosuppression such as after organ or bone marrow transplantation or in advanced HIV infection.

Primary CMV infections occur in previously uninfected individuals and are frequently asymptomatic. Seroprevalence studies in the United States have shown 10–30% of normal children and 40–80% of normal adults have been infected by CMV. Groups identified as having a higher likelihood of prior infection are children in day care settings, sexually promiscuous persons of both sexes (especially homosexual men), and recipients of blood products or tissue transplants. The symptomatic primary infections in immunologically normal individuals are a mononucleosislike syndrome, hepatitis, and, infrequently, pneumonitis and meningoencephalitis. In an immunosuppressed patient, the primary infection may also cause pneumonitis and encephalitis, as well as GI tract disease (especially colitis) and chorioretinitis.

CMV-related mononucleosis is not readily distinguished from that caused by EBV. Fever is the most prominent symptom. Sore throat is rare, and lymphadenopathy occurs but with less frequency than with EBV. Physical findings include the adenopathy and possible splenomegaly. Laboratory studies reveal lymphocytosis with many atypical lymphs. The heterophile-agglutinin test is negative. Acute and convalescent serologies demonstrate a rise in titer. Commonly seen is a chemical hepatitis that is mild and asymptomatic. Recovery is spontaneous and complete.

Clinical manifestations of CMV pneumonitis range from asymptomatic shedding of the virus to rapidly fatal respiratory failure. Fever, nonproductive cough, and dyspnea are the most common complaints. The physical exam is usually unrevealing except for abnormal breath sounds in heavily involved areas of the lung. CXRs show interstitial infiltrates, usually bilateral and diffuse. Progressive hypoxemia and ventilatory support are grave signs. In the AIDS patient, CMV is not infrequently identified in material obtained during evaluation for PCP but does not usually require specific treatment because therapy directed against the pneumocystis results in clinical response.

GI manifestations of CMV infection in the immunosuppressed patient can involve any portion of the GI tract, from the esophagus to the rectum. Most common is an ulcerative lesion in the mucosa and submucosa that can lead to pain, bleeding, or perforation. Patients with advanced HIV disease can develop a profuse watery diarrhea. These lesions are usually readily identified endoscopically, although a biopsy is often needed to demonstrate the presence of CMV.

CMV retinitis is one of the most feared complications of AIDS. It occurs with the most advanced stages of HIV infection, generally when an individual has had a prolonged survival with fewer than 50 CD4+ lymphocytes. Symptoms may be as nonspecific as decreased visual acuity or blurred vision. Patients often mention increasingly frequent floaters. A complaint of a visual-field cut is most significant and warrants immediate full ophthalmologic evaluation. Because of the clustering in these most advanced cases and the irreversible nature of vision loss due to CMV retinitis, routine screening exams should be performed on HIV-infected patients with less than 50–100 CD4+ lymphocytes regardless of symptoms.

Treatment of CMV infection depends on the type of illness and the type of patient. The immunocompetent patient only rarely needs to be considered for therapy and only then in the most severe cases. CMV disease in immunosuppressed patients has shown response to two agents currently available. Both are fairly toxic and require daily IV administration. Ganciclovir was the first agent available and probably remains the drug of choice for non-AIDS patients. Additionally, ganciclovir is indicated for the prevention of CMV disease in transplant recipients. Foscarnet is also available and may be the drug of choice in AIDS patients due to a different side-effect profile and potential anti-HIV activity. Ganciclovir is associated with severe hematologic toxicities, including leukopenia, thrombocytopenia, and anemia. These toxicities often preclude the concomitant use of zidovudine in AIDS. Foscarnet's toxicities are primarily metabolic and renal in nature and include hypocalcemia, hypomagnesemia, hypophosphatemia, and renal insufficiency. Following higher-dose induction therapy, the AIDS patient is usually continued on a lower-dose suppressive or maintenance dose for life. The least frequent dosing that has been well studied thus far is once daily for 5 days per week.

Reference: Studies of Ocular Complications of AIDS Research Group: Mortality in patients with the acquired immunodeficiency syndrome treated with either foscarnet or ganciclovir for cytomegalovirus retinitis. N Engl J Med 326:213–220, 1992.

D

DEEP VENOUS THROMBOSIS

Deep venous thrombosis (DVT) is a major medical problem and occurs in an estimated 500,000 subjects per year. About 10% (50,000) of patients with DVT develop PE and 10% of these patients will die. Symptoms and signs of DVT are often nonspecific, and clinical judgment may be in error up to 50% of the time.

Symptoms and Signs of DVT

1. Local pain
2. Swelling
3. Erythema
4. Tenderness
5. Positive Homan's sign

Diagnosis: Clinical detection of DVT is not reliable and therefore further diagnostic testing is warranted. Options available for the diagnosis of DVT include:

1. **Contrast venography:** This test serves as the gold standard to which all other techniques are compared. It is invasive, requires the use of IV dye to which reactions can occur, may induce minor thrombi, and may cause local pain, and its use for repetitive exams is not feasible.
2. **Impedance plethysmography:** This test detects 95% of all acute thrombi that involve the popliteal vein or above. It is noninvasive and may be used for repetitive exams to evaluate the possible extension of calf vein thrombi. The test will detect only 30% of thrombi confined to the calf.
3. **Radiofibrinogen leg scan:** Detects all fresh thrombi of the lower extremities, including the calf. However, it is not sensitive in the upper thigh or iliac regions.
4. **Other tests** that may prove useful but currently lack sufficient validation or may be quite technician-dependent include radionuclide venography (85% sensitive and specific), Doppler, and ultrasound.

Treatment: Treatment of DVT is aimed primarily at preventing the most serious complication of DVT, namely PE. Therefore, one must understand the natural history of venous thrombosis and the risk for embolism. Thrombi that remain confined to the calf pose little risk for PE; thrombi that extend into the popliteal vein or above pose significant risk. Over 90% of all PEs arise from the lower extremity (above the knee); 5–10% of all PEs arise in the upper extremities or other venous systems (right heart, hepatic, renal, etc.). The risk is increased with right-sided CHF, indwelling catheters, or trauma. The embolic risk is highest in the first 72 hours. About 10–15% of calf vein thrombi may extend, usually within 48 hours. Therefore, close follow-up is mandatory while these patients are followed.

Considerations in the treatment of DVT: Is anticoagulation feasible? Are there any contraindications to anticoagulation? Have you adequately assessed the risk:benefit ratio? If anticoagulation is not feasible, consider the use of vena caval filtration devices. The usual recommendation is to continue therapy for 3 months if there are no persisting risk factors. The duration of therapy is adjusted for the following factors:

1. Persistence of risk factors
2. Presence of residual venous obstruction
3. Risk:benefit ratio

Complications of DVT

1. PE: the most serious and potentially life-threatening complication of DVT
2. Recurrent DVT
3. Postphlebitic syndrome: thrombosis of the vein, especially repeated thromboses, which may lead to valve incompetence and hemorrhage of small veins with resulting chronic edema and discoloration of the extremity, which may lead to stasis ulcers

References: Moser KM, et al: Clinically suspected deep venous thrombosis of the lower extremities. JAMA 237:2195–2199, 1977.

Moser KM, et al: Is embolic risk conditioned by location of deep venous thrombosis? Ann Intern Med 94:439–444, 1981.

Moser KM: Venous thromboembolism. State of the art. Am Rev Respir Dis 141:235–249, 1990.

Risk Factors and Prevention

Virchow described a triad of risk factors for the development of venous thrombosis: venous stasis, intimal injury, and alteration of coagulation. Currently, less than 10–15% of patients have an identifiable "hypercoagulable" condition, and therefore, a clinical condition such as stasis and/or injury is the more likely risk for venous thromboembolism.

Risk Factors for Deep Venous Thrombosis

1. Age older than 70 years
2. Obesity
3. Sedentary, bed rest
4. Trauma
5. Chronic illness
6. Pelvic surgery/trauma
7. Prolonged anesthesia (longer than 1 hour)
8. Surgery of the lower extremities
9. Hip fracture/replacement
10. Right ventricular failure
11. Pregnancy/postpartum
12. Oral contraceptives (5–10 fold increase)
13. Underlying malignancy
14. Inherited/acquired deficiency of naturally occurring anticoagulants: protein C, protein S, antithrombin III, dysfibrinogenemia, antiphospholipid antibody
15. Others: homocystinuria, polycythemia, thrombocytosis

Prevention: Because DVT remains a major medical problem and this problem may lead to PE, prophylactic treatment of patients at risk is warranted. Several prophylactic modalities are available.

1. *Intermittent venous compression pneumatic devices:* These devices repetitively apply pressure to the calf, which enhances venous blood flow. The devices are well tolerated and offer no risk for bleeding. They are best applied prior to surgical procedures and at the onset of immobilization.

2. *Passive compression stockings:* Stockings must be designed to exert graduated compression from the calf upward and must be individually fitted to provide protection. These reasons often limit the feasibility and reliability of their use. The efficacy of such stockings without the described design and fitting has not had any proven value.

3. *Anticoagulation*
   a. Low-dose heparin
      The standard regimen is 5,000 U of heparin SC every 8–12 hours beginning at the time that risk factor is identified and continuing until the patient is ambulatory. This approach has been repeatedly shown to be safe and effective in preventing venous thrombosis. Bleeding risks are minimal, and this regimen is considered safe in most perioperative situations. Exceptions may include pelvic (prostatic) and neurosurgical procedures in which pneumatic devices may be more appropriate.
   b. Adjusted-dose heparin
      In certain clinical conditions, the risk for DVT is quite high (fractured hip, total hip replacement, total knee replacement). Various approaches are used. One is to use SC heparin and adjust the dose to prolong the APTT by 4–5 sec.
   c. Warfarin
      In very high risk patients, warfarin is given on the day of surgery and the dose escalated to achieve therapeutic range after surgery.

Although various "recipes" exist for venous thromboembolism prophylaxis, all studies indicate that prophylaxis is warranted in certain clinical settings. Unfortunately, prophylaxis is still not widely applied in patients at risk.

Reference: Anderson FA Jr, et al: Physician practices in the prevention of venous thromboembolism. Ann Intern Med 115:591–595, 1991.

DELIRIUM

Delirium occurs with increased frequency in older patients, males, and those with preexisting cerebral damage, including preexisting dementia. Its prevalence is very high (14–30%) in elderly patients with significant medical illnesses. It occurs in up to 60% of elderly patients after a major operation, and is associated with significant mortality.

Delirium Defined by DSM-III-R

A. Decreased ability to maintain attention: Patient is unable to count backward.
B. Disorganized thinking: Rambling, cannot follow directions

   C. Must have two of the following six diagnostic points:
     1. Depressed level of consciousness
     2. Perceptual disturbances, hallucinations, or delusions
     3. Altered sleep-wake cycle
     4. ↑ or ↓ psychomotor activity
     5. Disoriented to time, place, or person
     6. Impaired memory; some confabulate
   D. Onset over short period of time, fluctuating in severity, usually worse at night, with lucid periods
   E. Organic factor implicated
   F. Remember: Acuteness parallels reversibility

From American Psychiatric Association: Diagnostic and Statistical Manual of Mental Disorders, 3rd ed., revised. Washington, DC, American Psychiatric Association, 1987, with permission.

Not all delirious patients are yellers; beware of the quiet, agitated patient who is too scared to move. Myoclonus or asterixis is pathognomonic for delirium but is seen infrequently.

Keys to Diagnosis

   1. Get information on nocturnal behavior from nurses or caregivers.
   2. Determine premorbid mental status from family or history.
   3. Use standardized serial mental status exam to follow course.
   4. Keep pictures drawn and sentences written by patient in order to document course and progress.
   5. New-onset urinary incontinence is a frequent sign of delirium.

Potential Causes of Delirium in Hospitalized Patients

Fluid electrolyte imbalances (↑ or ↓ Na^+ or Ca^{++})	Metabolic disturbances (uremia, dehydration, hypoglycemia)
Hypoxia	Drugs with anti-cholinergic activity: antipsychotic, antidepressants, anti-parkinsonism, antiarrhythmics, antihistamines, antispasmodics
Infections (CNS or systemic)	
Hypotension	
Intoxication	
Small cortical strokes	Sedative-hypnotics, narcotics (and withdrawal)
Endocrinopathies	
Subdural hematoma, contusion	Sensory deprivation (sun-downing)
	↓ Cardiac output (including acute MI)
	Thiamine deficiency
	Nonconvulsive status epilepticus and postictal states

Management

   1. Treat underlying conditions.
   2. Review medications and eliminate those that can produce delirium.

3. Correct metabolic and electrolyte abnormalities.
4. Toxin screen sometimes helpful.
5. Short-term control of agitation with haloperidol 0.5 mg IM, repeated as needed. (If possible, wait until cause of delirium is known.)
6. Avoid sedative-hypnotics, neuroleptics, and benzodiazepines; all three groups have lower therapeutic dosage in elderly and further impair mental state of patient.
7. Keep orienting patient. Use sitters whom the patient knows rather than restraints. Use night-light, familiar objects from home.
8. Try not to disturb sleep. Restore day/night cycle, especially in "ICU psychosis."
9. Anticipate and prevent falls and fractures.

Reference: Liston: Delirium in the aged. Psychiatr Clin North Am 5(1):49–66, 1982.

DEMENTIA

Dementia is defined as a progressive, gradual deterioration in cognitive function over a period of at least 6 months. The patient demonstrates prominent impairment in both short- and long-term memory but without any disorder of alertness (in contrast to delerium). In addition, one or more of the following elements are seen:

1. Impaired abstract thinking
2. Impaired judgment
3. Disturbed cortical function: aphasia (impaired language use), apraxia (impaired purposeful movements), agnosia (impaired recognition of familiar objects), construction difficulties
4. Personality change

The Folstein Mini Mental Status Exam can be used not only to screen for dementia but also to follow the course of the illness. (However, use of Folstein serially has not been rigorously validated.)

Etiologies of Dementia

Senile dementia of Alzheimer's type	50–60%
Multi-infarct dementia (MID)	10–20%
Combination Alzheimer's and MID	10–20%
Other disorders	5–10%
Reversible or partially reversible	20–30%

Winograd CH, et al: Physician management of the demented patient. J Am Geriatr Soc 34:295–308, 1986.

Treatable Dementia

Studies of treatable dementias have yielded very disparate statistics, indicating that anywhere between 10% and 80% of demented patients have a treatable cause, with the true figure probably lying closer to 10%. The probability of reversibility decreases with increasing age.

Reversible Causes of Dementia

D	Drugs
E	Emotional disorders (pseudodementia or depression)
M	Metabolic and endocrine disorders (hepatic encephaolpthy, hypothyroidism, chronic renal failure)
E	Eye and Ear dysfunction
N	Nutritional deficiencies, Normal pressure hydrocephalus (NPH)
T	Tumor, Trauma (including chronic subdural hematoma)
I	Infections (neurosyphilis, chronic meningitis)
A	Alcohol, Arteriosclerotic complications

Screening for Reversible Dementias in Addition to Hx & PE

Thyroid function tests	Vitamin B_{12} level
Serum chemistries (including Ca^{++})	Head CT or MRI
Examination of CSF for possible NPH or if RPR positive or if cranial nerve abnormalities are present (consistent with meningitis)	Syphilis serology
	CBC
	Serum folate level

Depression that is masquerading as an organic dementia, or *pseudodementia,* is perhaps the most frequently seen and most readily reversible dementia, even in patients without a prior history of depression. Diagnostic clues include "I don't know" answers and relatively rapid onset. Complaints about memory loss are greater than objective findings, and the functional defect is often worse in the morning, improving throughout the day. Even in patients with underlying Alzheimer or multi-infarct dementia, treatment of coexistent depression may improve the patient's functional status. Aggressive use of antidepressant medications and psychotherapy are indicated. All demented patients should undergo neuropsychiatric testing to rule out pseudodementia.

Normal-pressure hydrocephalus is a treatable, potentially reversible cause of dementia (see Normal Pressure Hydrocephalus). It causes not only dementia but also urinary incontinence and a peculiar, shuffling, magnetic-gait apraxia. Relief of the hydrocephalus by shunting produces only variable results.

Drug use is another common cause of dementia. Alcohol frequently causes a chronic dementia, which is poorly reversible, but some of the accompanying complications of alcoholism, such as Wernicke-Korsakoff syndrome and thiamine deficiency, may be reversible to a certain extent by vitamin replacement. The use of other drugs, especially in elderly patients, can often lead to confusion and cognitive impairment, a situation that can arise even from the most seemingly benign use of over-the-counter medications.

Neurosyphilis has surged in frequency recently, again assuming a major role as a cause of dementia. Other infectious causes are *fungal meningitis* (crypto, histo, etc.) and *TB.*

Metabolic encephalopathies mimicking dementia include decreased function of the thyroid, liver, kidneys, and even lung (chronic hypoxia or CO_2 retention).

The evaluation of any patient presenting with dementia generally focuses on these treatable causes, even though they are uncommon. Demented patients thus undergo MRI, EEG, blood work to exclude metabolic causes, and often lumbar puncture. A toxicology screen and drug history are also appropriate. Then, if no treatable cause is found, a diagnosis of Alzheimer's disease is often assumed.

Reference: Barry PP, et al: The diagnosis of reversible dementia in the elderly. Arch Intern Med 148:1914–1918, 1988.

DEPRESSION

DSM-III-R Criteria for Major Depression

A. At least five of the following symptoms have been present during the same 2-week period nearly every day and represent a change from previous functioning. At least one of the symptoms is either (1) depressed mood or (2) loss of interest in pleasurable activities:
  1. Depressed mood most of the day as indicated either by subjective account or by observations by others
  2. Markedly diminished interest or pleasure in all, or almost all, activities most of the day
  3. Significant weight loss or weight gain when not dieting (e.g., more than 5% of body weight in a month) or decreased or increased appetite
  4. Insomnia or hypersomnia
  5. Psychomotor agitation or retardation
  6. Fatigue or loss of energy
  7. Feelings of worthlessness or excessive or inappropriate guilt
  8. Diminished ability to think or concentrate, or indecisiveness
  9. Recurrent thoughts of death (not just fear of dying), recurrent suicidal ideation without a specific plan, a suicide attempt, or a specific plan for committing suicide
B. 1. It cannot be established that an organic factor initiated and maintained the disturbance.
  2. The disturbance is not a normal reaction to the death of a loved one.

Adapted from American Psychiatric Association: Diagnostic and Statistical Manual of Mental Disorders, 3rd ed., rev. Washington DC, American Psychiatric Association, 1987, pp 128–129.

Organic Causes of Depression

Drugs

ACTH	α-Methyldopa	Barbiturates
Benzodiazepines	β-Blockers	Cholinergic drugs
Corticosteroids	Estrogens	Levodopa
Ranitidine	Cimetidine	Reserpine

Related to drug abuse

Alcohol abuse	Cocaine and other psycho-stimulant withdrawal	Sedative-hypnotic abuse

Endocrine and Metabolism

Hyperthyroidism	Hypothyroidism	Hyperadrenalism
Hypoadrenalism	Hypercalcemia	Hyponatremia
Diabetes mellitus	Lead poisoning	Porphyria

Table continued on next page.

Organic Causes of Depression (Cont.)

Neurologic

Brain tumors	Dementias	Epilepsy, uncontrolled
Huntington's disease	Multiple sclerosis	Parkinson's disease
Stroke	Subdural hematoma	Syphilis
Wilson's disease		

Nutritional

Pellagra   Vitamin B_{12} deficiency

Miscellaneous

Carcinoid syndrome	Pancreatic carcinoma	Polymyalgia rheumatica
Systemic lupus erythematosus	Viral infections (esp. mono-nucleosis and influenza)	

Adapted from Hyman SE, et al: Mood and anxiety disorders. In Rubenstein E, et al (eds): Scientific American Medicine. New York, Scientific American, 1991, 13:II:7.

Selected Characteristics of Antidepressant Drugs

GENERIC NAME	USUAL EFFECTIVE TOTAL DOSE, MG (RANGE)	SIDE EFFECTS		
		Antihistaminic[1]	Antiadrenergic[2]	Anticholinergic[3]
Desipramine	200 (50–300)	+	+ +	+
Nortriptyline	100 (50–150)	+	+	+ +
Amitriptyline	150 (50–300)	+ + +	+ + +	+ + +
Doxepin	150 (50–300)	+ + +	+ + +	+ +
Imipramine	150 (50–300)	+ +	+ + +	+ +

[1]Sedation.
[2]Orthostatic hypotension.
[3]Dry mouth, blurred vision, ↓ intestinal motility, ↓ bladder tone, tachycardia.

Newer Antidepressants

GENERIC NAME	USUAL EFFECTIVE TOTAL DOSE, MG (RANGE)	MAJOR ADVANTAGE	MAJOR DISADVANTAGE
Fluoxetine	20–60	Few anticholinergic effects	Can increase anxiety and insomnia in early treatment
Trazodone	300 (200–600)	Almost no anticholinergic effects	Very sedating; appears to have greater cardiotoxicity; priapism reported
Alprazolam	0.75–4	No anticholinergic effects	Some addictive potential; sedating
Buproprion	300–450	Few anticholinergic effects	May induce seizures; can increase insomnia in early treatment

Adapted from Depaulo JR: Affective disorders. In Barker LR, et al (eds): Principles of Ambulatory Medicine, 3rd ed. Baltimore, Williams & Wilkins, 1991, Table 15.5, p 152.

DERMATITIS, CONTACT

Contact dermatitis can result from skin exposure to any agent that has the potential to cause an allergic or irritant reaction. Irritant contact dermatitis appears as areas of skin necrosis (after strong irritant exposure) or drying or maceration (after weak irritant exposure). Allergic contact dermatitis forms edematous, eczematous lesions with erythematous, scaling papules and plaques. There are usually excoriations from constant scratching. Poison ivy exposure is the only irritant that causes bullae and blister formation.

Diagnosis: Contact dermatitis is diagnosed clinically by the appearance of the lesions in the setting of an appropriate history of irritant exposure. Some exposures may be harder to discover and may be as subtle as nail polish on the fingernails causing a dermatitis around the eyelids when the eye is rubbed. The physician needs to carefully question the patient about possible exposures. The diagnosis is confirmed when removal of the offending agent leads to improvement in the rash.

Treatment: First, the irritant must be identified and future exposure to it by the patient limited. Second, local and systemic symptoms are treated. Irritant dermatitis that causes xerosis (dry skin) can be treated with lubricants and measures to reduce skin drying (see table). Topically applied steroids are useful for allergic dermatitis (see table). Occasionally, steroids are useful for irritant dermatitis. For very severe cases of contact dermatitis, oral steroids in high doses (such as 40–60 mg of prednisone) with rapid taper are sometimes needed. Oral antihistamines may help control itching.

Care of Dry Skin

- Avoid excessive bathing.
- Use tepid, not hot, water for bathing.
- Avoid soap except in axillary or pubic areas. Bath oils can be substituted for soap.
- Pat, rather than rub, skin for drying. Leave a small amount of moisture on skin.
- Apply lubricant such as Eucerin, Keri Lotion, or Lubriderm while skin is still damp. Cream is a better emollient than lotion but is harder to apply.
- Apply lubricant twice a day (more often to hands if frequently exposed to water).

Selected Topical Steroid Preparations[1]

Low potency[2]
0.5–1.0% Hydrocortisone cream (available over the counter)
Mid-potency
0.1% Triamcinolone cream and ointment (Kenalog, Aristocort, generic)
0.1% Betamethasone cream, ointment, and solution (Valisone)
0.25% Desoximetasone cream (Topicort)
High potency
0.05% Fluocinonide cream, ointment, or solution (Lidex)
0.05% Betamethasone ointment (Diprolene)

[1]Steroids can be applied once or twice daily. Lotions are helpful in hairy areas. Ointments can provide extra efficacy. For two weeks of therapy for the feet or hands, 45 grams of steroid are usually adequate. If the whole body requires treatment for two weeks, 120–150 gm should be prescribed.

[2]Only low-potency steroids should be used on the face and intertriginous areas.

Adapted from Lynch PJ: Dermatology for the House Officer, 2nd ed. Baltimore, Williams & Wilkins, 1987, p 25.

DIABETES INSIPIDUS

Diabetes insipidus (DI) is a condition resulting from either low levels of circulating ADH (central DI) or resistance to the action of ADH (nephrogenic DI). Clinically, the condition is characterized by polyuria, hypernatremia, polydipsia, and excretion of very dilute urine.

Causes of Diabetes Insipidus

NEUROGENIC	NEPHROGENIC
Idiopathic (congenital and nonfamilial types)	Chronic renal disease
	Polycystic disease
Infections	Pyelonephritis
Meningitis, encephalitis, Guillain-Barré	Urinary obstruction
	Hypokalemia
Head injury	Hypercalcemia
Posthypophysectomy	Drugs (alcohol, phenytoin, lithium, de-
Suprasellar/intrasellar tumors (cranio-	meclocycline, foscarnet, vinblastine,
pharyngioma, meningioma, glioma,	gentamicin, methicillin, glyburide, to-
metastatic lymphoma, leukemia, or	lazamide, amphotericin, colchicine)
breast cancer)	Miscellaneous
Granulomas	Multiple myeloma, sarcoid, amyloid
Sarcoid, TB, Wegener's, syphilis	
Histiocytosis	
Vascular	
Cerebral aneurysm, thrombosis	
Postpartum necrosis	
Sickle-cell disease	
Autoimmune diseases	

Clinical Features: The polyuria in central DI ranges from 3–15 L/day, and nocturia is often prominent. Polydipsia is a consequence of polyuria and there is a peculiar preference for cold water. But, if the thirst center is also involved, dangerous hypernatremia often develops, especially if the patient has no access to free water. In nephrogenic DI, the polyuria and nocturia are often moderate (<3 L/day). In contrast to central DI, onset is often insidious. Urine is hypotonic in both conditions.

Differential Diagnosis: The most important differential for DI is compulsive water drinking. These conditions can often be differentiated by the fluid deprivation test in which fluids are withheld the night preceding the test to achieve maximal urine osmolality. Serum osmolality should approach 295 mOsm/kg H_2O after fluid deprivation. Urine osmolality is measured at baseline and then hourly until two urine osmolalities vary by <30 mOsm/kg H_2O or 3–5% of body weight is lost. Then 5 units of aqueous ADH are administered subcutaneously and one hour later the final urine osmolality is measured. The differentiation among these conditions can be made from the results as indicated in the following table.

Response to Fluid Deprivation and ADH Administration

CONDITION	UOSM AFTER FLUID DEPRIVATION	UOSM AFTER ADH ADMINISTRATION	% CHANGE
Normal	1,000–1,120	Unchanged	0
Complete CDI	150–180	400–500	>50
Partial CDI	420–480	510–580	>10
Nephrogenic DI	150–200	Unchanged	0
Compulsive water drinking	700–780	700–820	< 5

CDI = central DI, UOSM = urine osmolality.

Therapy: The treatment of central DI is often hormonal replacement. In the acute setting, aqueous vasopressin is preferred; in chronic conditions, Pitressin in oil is preferred. Desmopressin can be given IV, PO, or intranasally. Intranasal desmopressin is the drug of choice for central DI. A number of nonhormonal agents are also useful. Thiazides, by causing chronic Na^+ depletion, achieve a reduction in urine volume. Chlorpropamide and carbamazepine augment the antidiuretic response of ADH, making these agents useful in partial DI. Clofibrate is also useful in the treatment of partial DI. Treatment of nephrogenic DI is primarily that of an underlying disorder. The combination of a low-salt diet and thiazides produces a state of chronic volume depletion, diminishes the GFR, and increases the proximal tubular reabsorption of the filtrate, resulting in decreased urinary volumes. Hypernatremia is often a consequence of diminished thirst sensation in patients with DI. It is frequently corrected by administration of free water (5% dextrose). The exact amount of water deficit can be calculated from the measured serum Na^+ concentration, assuming that total body water is 60% of total body weight. Serum osmolality should decrease by 1–2 mOsm/kg H_2O/hr. Faster rates of correction can result in seizures. If the patient is severely volume depleted, then initial management consists of NS administration.

Treatment of Diabetes Insipidus

DRUGS	USUAL DOSE	DURATION OF ACTION
Hormone replacement		
Aqueous vasopressin	5–10 units SC	3–6 hr
Desmopressin acetate	10–20 μg intranasally	12–24 hr
(dDAVP)	1–2 μg IV	24 hr
	100–400 μg PO	12–24 hr
Lypressin	2–4 units IV	4–6 hr
Vasopressin tannate in oil	5 units IM	24–72 hr
Nonhormonal agents		
Chlorpropamide	200–500 mg daily	–
Clofibrate	500 mg QID	–
Carbamazepine	400–600 mg daily	–

DIABETES MELLITUS

Classification of Types

Classification of Types of Diabetes Mellitus

Type I diabetes
- Minimal endogenous insulin secretion
- Prone to develop ketoacidosis
- Insulin-dependent DM: insulin needed to prevent DKA and needed for survival
- Generally appears in childhood or early adult life
- Genetically linked to the D locus of the histocompatibility antigens on chromosome 6
- Autoimmune destruction of pancreatic islets important in pathogenesis

Type II diabetes
- Patients have considerable capacity for endogenous insulin secretion
- Ketoacidosis is uncommon

Table continued on next page.

Classification of Types of Diabetes Mellitus (Cont.)

- Generally not dependent on insulin for survival (i.e., NIDDM)
- Onset usually in adult life, commonly after the age of 40
- Patients commonly are both insulin deficient and insulin resistant
- A strongly hereditary disease with concordance near 100% for identical twins
- Occurs in two subtypes: obese (70%) and nonobese (30%)

Maturity-onset diabetes of the young
- Clinically similar to type II DM
- However, onset early in life
- Inherited as an autosomal-dominant trait

Pancreatic disease (insulin deficiency)
- Pancreatectomy
- Chronic pancreatitis
- Cystic fibrosis
- Hemochromatosis: Patients also may have cirrhosis, cardiomyopathy, impotence, hyperpigmentation, and arthritis with CPDD

Excess of counterregulatory hormones
- Cushing's syndrome
- Pheochromocytoma
- Corticosteroid therapy
- Acromegaly
- Glucagonoma

Polyglandular autoimmune syndrome type II
- Common manifestations of the syndrome are:
  —Addison's disease
  —Thyroid disease (either hyperthyroidism or hypothyroidism)
  —Type I DM
- Less common manifestations are:
  —Hypogonadism
  —Vitiligo
  —Pernicious anemia

Gestational diabetes
- Glucose intolerance during pregnancy
- Normalization of glucose tolerance after delivery

Drugs that exacerbate DM
- Thiazides
- Adrenergic agents
- Phenytoin
- Corticosteroid hormones

Associations of DM with other disorders
- Acanthosis nigricans: insulin resistance
- Congenital lipodystrophy: insulin resistance
- Ataxia telangiectasia: insulin resistance
- Myotonic dystrophy: insulin resistance
- Muscular dystrophy
- Friedreich's ataxia
- Prader-Willi syndrome
- Turner's syndrome
- Klinefelter's syndrome

Insulin-Dependent Diabetes Mellitus (IDDM)

Characteristic Features of IDDM (Type I)

Ketosis prone
Insulin treatment mandatory
Usually nonobese
Acute onset
Onset younger than 40 years of age in 75% of cases
Onset delayed in patients with polyglandular failure syndrome, type II
HLA associations: HLA DR3 and DR4 common
Frequent presence of islet-cell antibodies
Family history of diabetes present in 10%
50% concordance rate in identical twins
Severe symptoms, especially nocturia, marked weight loss, heavy glycosuria, ketonuria common
Destruction of islet B cells may result from organ-specific autoimmunity or a mixture of
    autoimmune and environmental factors that are mostly viral infections

---

Management of IDDM: Since the issue as to whether strict eumetabolic control of diabetes prevents and/or minimizes the occurrence and acceleration of chronic complications of DM seems to have been definitely settled, one should attempt to achieve and maintain normal or near-normal metabolic control. Insulin therapy is the main component of IDDM management: (1) conventional insulin therapy (a mixture of NPH or Lente insulin with regular insulin given once or twice daily); or (2) intensive insulin therapy (pumps or multiple daily injections); multidose therapy is safer and at least as effective as the pump, and it allows eumetabolic control of IDDM (one or two daily injections of Ultralente, Lente, or NPH and premeal injection of regular insulin).

Guidelines in the Management of IDDM
---

1. Use of human insulin preferred (less lipodystrophy, fewer local and systemic reactions)
2. Diet (exchange techniques: calories adjusted to physical activity; regular, well-balanced meals)
3. Physical fitness and exercise (regular daily exercise)
4. Emotional support (to minimize or prevent serious psychopathology)
5. Use of self-monitoring blood glucose device:
   Goal values for blood sugar:
      80–120 mg/dl preprandial; 180 mg/dl postprandial
6. Use of glycosylated hemoglobin every 3–4 months
7. Urine testing should be abandoned because of the poor correlation between urine sugar and blood levels.
8. Measurement of fasting blood lipid levels at least once a year, including total, LDL, and HDL cholesterol, and TGs. If lipid abnormalities are not fully corrected with glycemic control, then aggressive management of dyslipidemia with a pharmacological agent should be initiated.
9. Therapy should avoid hypoglycemia.
10. Early detection of autoimmune diseases that may be associated with IDDM such as Hashimoto's thyroiditis and Addison's disease, which may alter insulin requirements and may predispose to hypoglycemia.
11. Intensive therapy is associated with some disadvantages, particularly the expense, more frequent hypoglycemia, weight gain, and accelerated microvascular complications. The use of devices has been associated with increased frequency of DKA, infection, unexplained death, suicide, and hyperinsulinemia.

Non–Insulin-Dependent Diabetes Mellitus (NIDDM)

NIDDM is the most frequent form of DM (prevalence 3–4%) and accounts for at least 85% of all patients with DM. The prevalence of NIDDM varies both among different ethnic groups living in the same environment and among people from the same ethnic group living in different environments and is the end result of both genetic and environmental interactions. Obesity is present in 80% of patients with NIDDM. It is among the ten most common causes of mortality in most countries.

The development of NIDDM follows four stages: genetic susceptibility, insulin resistance, impaired glucose tolerance, and, finally, diabetes. Initially, insulin and C-peptide levels are elevated because the main mechanism of glucose intolerance is peripheral insulin resistance; gradually, with worsening hyperglycemia, there is a significant decrease in insulin levels.

Management

1. Diet: Obese patients need a hypocaloric diet. Ideal body weight may be obtained from standard tables. All patients should be maintained on a low-saturated-fat diet (less than 10%), which helps in maintaining low lipid levels. A high-fiber diet may also lower lipid levels.
2. Exercise: Certainly has psychological benefits, and the hypoglycemic effect is related mostly to increased absorption of injected insulin. Intensive exercise increases insulin sensitivity.
3. Oral hypoglycemic agents

Characteristics of Oral Hypoglycemic Agents

GENERIC NAME	BRAND NAME	STRENGTH (MG)	ONSET (HR)	DURATION (HR)	DOSAGE RANGE	MAJOR TOXICITY	EXCRETION/ METABOLISM
Tolbutamide	Orinase	500	0.5	6–12	500–3,000	Photosensitivity	Hepatic
Chlorprop-amide	Diabinese	100, 250	1	60–90	100–500	Hypersensitivity, jaundice, rash, pancytopenia, hyponatremia	Renal
Acetohex-amide	Dymelor	250, 500	0.5	12–24	250–1,500	GI disturbance, headache, rash	Hepatic
Tolazamide	Tolinase	100, 250, 500	4–6	10–18	100–1,000	GI disturbance	Hepatic
Glyburide	Micronase	1.25, 2.5, 5	1	18–24	2.5–20	Hypoglycemia	Hepatic and renal
Glipizide	Glucotrol	5, 10	0.5	12–24	5–40	Hypoglycemia	Hepatic

From Garber AJ: Diabetes Mellitus. In Stein J H (ed): Internal Medicine, 3rd ed. Boston, Little, Brown, 1990, p 2249, with permission.

Drug Interaction with Sulfonylureas

- Potentiating effect (NSAIDs, warfarin, clofibrate, salicylates)
- Antagonizing effect (thiazide diuretics, glucocorticoids, oral contraceptives)

Side Effects of Oral Agents

- Alcohol flush
- Nausea
- Exfoliative dermatitis (rare)
- Skin rash
- Hepatitis

An oral agent should not be used if the fasting plasma glucose level is higher than 180 mg/dl, despite maximal doses of the drug. Insulin should be used when maximal doses of one of the sulfonylurea agents do not achieve control of diabetes (primary or secondary features). Both methods of insulin therapy (i.e., conventional and intensive) may be used in NIDDM as in IDDM, except for insulin pump devices.

Treatment of Diabetes Mellitus

General and Preventive Care

Routine Office Evaluation of the Patient with Diabetes Mellitus

Physical Examination

Vital signs:	Blood pressure
Feet:	Calluses, ulcers, nonhealing lesions, improperly trimmed nails
Optic fundus:	Neovascularization, hemorrhages, cataracts[1]
Heart:	Gallops
Lungs:	Crackles, dullness to percussion (if pleural effusion present)
Extremities:	Edema

Diagnostic tests

Urine for protein and pyuria
Hemoglobin A1C to determine long-term control
Baseline electrocardiogram
Creatinine

Immunizations

Annual influenza vaccination
Tetanus-diphtheria toxoid every 10 years
Pneumococcal pneumonia vaccine once

Patient education

Home glucose monitoring record
Diet and compliance
Symptoms of hypoglycemia and hyperglycemia
Understanding of medications and compliance
Proper foot care (see table on p. 186)

[1] Annual examination by ophthalmologist is also needed to detect retinal changes at earliest stages.

Perioperative Management of Oral Hypoglycemics and Insulin

Decisions about how to manage the diabetic patient undergoing surgery are based on answers to four questions: (1) Is the surgery major or minor? (2) How long will it take for the patient to resume a normal diet postoperatively? (3) How tightly is the blood sugar controlled under usual circumstances? (4) Is the patient a type I or a type II diabetic? No one regimen for perioperative management of a diabetic patient has been shown to be superior to another. Therefore, management is based on the answers to these four questions, experience, and common sense.

Major surgery, performed under general anesthesia, precipitates the stress response by means of an outpouring of catecholamines and cortisol. In addition to their hemodynamic effects, the catecholamines epinephrine and norepinephrine stimulate the pituitary to secrete ACTH. ACTH in turn stimulates the adrenal glands to secrete glucocorticoids, which promote gluconeogenesis, mostly through catabolic mechanisms. Postoperative hyperglycemia is the result and can be observed even in nondiabetics. There is some evidence that the stress response is muted in patients undergoing surgery under spinal anesthesia. Major surgery can be expected to lead to more marked changes in glucose homeostasis than can minor procedures.

Clinical experience suggests that patients who can quickly resume their normal oral intake postoperatively have fewer problems in glycemic control. For example, if scheduled for the early morning, diabetics can eat at least some type of midday meal after almost any joint procedure and any of several urologic procedures. This also means their usual antidiabetic regimen can be restarted promptly.

To some extent, the patient's usual glycemic control dictates the intensity of perioperative insulin or antidiabetic regimens. Because there is more danger from hypoglycemia than hyperglycemia, it is better to use only one-third to one-half the usual subcutaneous intermediate or long-acting insulin dose on the day of surgery in the patient who is ordinarily tightly controlled. On the other hand, two-thirds or even more of the usual insulin dose can be given subcutaneously on the morning of surgery to the patient whose blood sugar is typically higher than 250 mg/dl. The amount of insulin administered the morning of surgery can be based on that morning's blood or capillary glucose level. Some of the oral hypoglycemics have a long half-life, and tightly controlled diabetics using such drugs may need to discontinue them for several doses preoperatively (not just on the morning of surgery).

With regard to the type of DM, type II diabetics secrete sufficient endogenous insulin to prevent the development of postoperative DKA: insulin suppresses some of the catabolic processes in the stress response. Therefore, type II diabetics are prone to develop the hyperglycemic hyperosmolar nonketotic state postoperatively, even after relatively minor operations. On the other hand, type I diabetics can develop full-blown DKA postoperatively if they are not treated with sufficient insulin.

Many clinicians prefer to administer a continuous low-dose infusion of IV insulin intraoperatively and in the immediate postoperative period, especially when the surgery is major and the patient will be unable to resume oral intake promptly. This approach seems especially warranted in the diabetic undergoing emergent or urgent procedures who must undergo operation before the blood sugar, acid-base, and electrolyte status can be optimized. Capillary glucose levels should be measured every 1–2 hours intraoperatively and in the recovery room. An alternative approach to continuous insulin infusion is to give intermittent boluses of insulin based on the capillary glucose level.

A blood sugar below 280 simplifies postoperative fluid and electrolyte management, because osmotic diuresis would not be expected below that level. Good glycemic control postoperatively is believed to aid in wound healing and prevention of infection.

References: Gavin LA: Perioperative management of the diabetic patient. Endocrinol Metab Clin North Am 21:457–475, 1992.

Hirsch IB, et al: Perioperative management of surgical patients with diabetes mellitus. Anesthesiology 74:346–359, 1991.

DIABETIC FOOT ULCERS

Diabetic foot ulcer is the most common abnormality leading to amputation. However, many foot ulcers and their sequelae are preventable. The National Diabetes Advisory Board estimates that over half of the 50,000 lower extremity amputations performed each year in diabetics could have been avoided with appropriate comprehensive care.

Four factors cause or at least contribute to the development of foot ulcers in diabetics: neuropathy, ischemia due to vascular disease, abnormal biomechanics with or without structural changes in the foot, and infection. Neuropathic ulcers can be distinguished from those primarily due to ischemia by their location. Neuropathic ulcers occur at sites of excessive pressure. Ischemic ulcers usually begin as black, dry gangrene of most distal parts of the toes. Approximately 60–70% of diabetic foot ulcers are neuropathic, 15–20% are ischemic, and 15–20% have both neuropathic and ischemic components.

The neuropathic ulcer results from pressure necrosis. Neuropathy leads to a diminution of pain sensation when pressure is increased, and eventually pressure necrosis ensues. Because of the pressure of walking, pressure necrosis usually occurs on the plantar surface, but ill-fitting shoes can cause pressure necrosis of the sides or even the dorsum of the foot. Diabetics have abnormal foot biomechanics, and during walking their plantar surfaces may have 100 times the pressures observed in normals. Increased transmission of pressures occurs because of the reduced cushioning caused by thinned muscle and thinned foot pads. Bony abnormalities such as bunions, hammertoe, and claw foot also contribute to increased pressure transmission.

Ischemic ulcers are the direct result of inadequate blood flow. Macrovascular disease is commonly found at the metatarsal arch and in the digital vessels. Diabetics with ischemic ulcers often have coexisting cardiac dysfunction. This and the pedal edema further decrease tissue perfusion.

Infection can complicate neuropathic as well as ischemic ulcers. Determining causative organisms can be difficult. Organisms obtained by swab or needle aspiration are usually not the same ones found in the deeper tissues at the time of amputation. Culture of tissue obtained by curettage seems much more accurate, and many now suggest that curettage be performed on all ulcers to identify the offending organisms. Appropriate antibiotics are the mainstay of treatment of diabetic foot ulcers, but local care is also important, especially removal of nonviable tissue.

The diagnosis of osteomyelitis under an ulcer can be very difficult. A foot ulcer overlying bone can cause periosteal bone resorption even without extension of infection into the bone. Some have found that this radiographic sign is a false positive in as many as 40% of diabetic foot ulcers. Bone biopsy is the most reliable way to diagnose osteomyelitis, and patients should not be subjected to long-term antibiotic therapy without a confirmed diagnosis.

Prevention of foot ulcers should be the paramount goal. The American Diabetes Association's instructions for patients are summarized in the accompanying table:

Instructions for Patients Who Are Insensate and at Risk for Diabetic Foot Ulcers

Foot care
- Inspect the inside of shoes for foreign objects before putting on the shoes.
- Inspect feet daily for blisters, cuts, scratches, redness, dryness, hot spots, or infection.
- Wash feet daily and dry carefully, especially between the toes.
- Avoid hot temperatures; test water with elbow before bathing.
- If your feet are cold, wear socks; do not use hot water bottles or heating pads.
- Do not cut corns or calluses or use chemical removal agents.
- Do not use adhesive tape on your feet.
- Cut nails in contour with the toes; do not cut deep down the sides or corners.
- Consult your physician before soaking feet or using lubricating creams or oils.
- If your vision is impaired, a family member or friend should be trained in these care items.

Footwear
- Shoes should be measured properly at the time of purchase; do not depend on them to stretch out.
- Break shoes in slowly, wearing them no more than a few hours at a time in the beginning.
- Do not wear the same pair of shoes every day; try to change shoes within the same day.
- Wear shoes of material that breathes.
- Avoid pointed toes and high heels.
- Do not walk barefoot; particularly avoid hot surfaces in the sun, on beaches, and around swimming pools; at night, turn on the lights and do not walk barefoot to the bathroom.
- Wear shoes appropriate to the weather: avoid wearing wet shoes; use thick socks or lined boots in the winter.
- Avoid sandals and thongs.
- Avoid garters, tight elastic bands on socks, and rolled hose; always wear socks or stockings with shoes, but avoid thick seams and mended areas.

Professional care
- See your physician regularly and be sure that your feet are examined at each visit.
- Notify your physician at once if you develop a blister, sore, or crack in the skin of your feet.

Adapted from Committee on Standards of Care, Council on Foot Care, American Diabetes Association: Diabetic Foot Care. Alexandria, Virginia, American Diabetes Association, 1990, pp 1–12.

Grunfeld C: Diabetic foot ulcers: Etiology, treatment and prevention. In Stollerman GH, et al (eds): Advances in Internal Medicine. St. Louis, Mosby–Year Book, 1992, 37:103–132.

DIABETIC KETOACIDOSIS

DKA is defined as severe, uncontrolled DM with elevation of plasma ketones (>2 mmol/L), and metabolic acidosis (pH <7.2) requiring intensive and urgent therapy with insulin and IV fluids. With aggressive therapy, survival has markedly improved. The overall mortality rate ranges between 0 and 20% and depends on quality of patient care and socioeconomic status. It is also higher among older people, possibly due to associated illnesses.

DKA occurs in both IDDM and NIDDM. In NIDDM, a precipitating factor (intercurrent illness) is often present. The pathogenic factors of DKA are insulin deficiency, excess of counterregulatory hormones (i.e., glucagon, cortisol, catecholamines, and GH), and dehydration (due to fever, vomiting, diarrhea, hyperventilation, and osmotic diuresis). Increased lipolysis, glycogenolysis, gluconeogenesis, and ketone body production lead to metabolic acidosis. The end result is the occurrence of hypovolemia, volume contraction, dehydration, hyperglycemia, metabolic acidosis, and electrolyte abnormalities. The three ketone bodies present in the serum of patients with DKA are acetoacetate, acetone, and betahydroxybutyrate.

Predisposing Factors in DKA

1. Insulin-dependent diabetes mellitus
2. Withholding insulin on sick days (for both type I and type II DM)
3. Use of an insulin pump
4. Infections (for both type I and type II DM)
5. Surgery
6. Pancreatitis
7. Any severe intercurrent illness such as MI or stroke

Clinical Presentations of DKA

Vomiting (70%)
Polyuria (40%)
Abdominal pain (15%) (in patients younger than 40 years, or if HCO_3^- <10 mEq)
Dehydration
Warm dry skin
Hypothermia (occasional)
Gastric stasis (often due to depletion of potassium and magnesium and autonomic dysfunction)

Thirst (55%)
Weight loss (20%)
Weakness (20%)
Tachycardia
Hypotension
Prerenal azotemia
Hyperventilation
Impaired consciousness (poor prognosis)

Laboratory Evaluation in DKA

1. Hyperglycemia
2. Blood urea elevated, consistent with prerenal azotemia
3. Electrolytes (potassium may be normal, low, or elevated)
4. WBC elevated (leukocytosis)
5. ABGs consistent with metabolic acidosis
6. Blood ketone bodies: betahydroxybutyric acid to acetoacetic acid ratio normally 3:1 (increases with more severe acidosis); betahydroxybutyric acid is not measured by qualitative methods for ketones.
7. Tests for identification of precipitating factors (CXR, ECG, blood and urine cultures, and a throat swab)

Differential Diagnosis of DKA

1. Lactic acidosis (due to circulatory collapse, alcohol, hepatic and renal disease)
2. Phenformin or salicylate abuse
3. Formaldehyde intoxication
4. Methanol
5. Pancreatitis
6. GI bleeding
7. Ethylene glycol (antifreeze) intoxication

Management

1. *IV fluids:* Infuse 1 L NS (15 ml/kg the first hour). Repeat the same amount in the second hour and then 500 ml/hr. Adjust infusion rate subsequently according to clinical and biochemical parameters. Switch to ½ NS once hypovolemia has been corrected. CVP should be monitored in the elderly. IV fluids should be switched to

D5W when glucose level reaches 300 mg/dl—in order to maintain a blood sugar higher than 250 mg/dl during the first 24 hours (while ketosis is being reversed with appropriate insulin therapy). Rapid drop in osmolality should be avoided.

2. *Insulin therapy:* Initial IV bolus of 0.15 unit/kg followed by continuous IV infusion of 0.1 unit/kg/hour. Insulin infusion rate should be adjusted according to response of acidosis rather than to blood sugar changes.

3. *Bicarbonate therapy:* Should be given only if pH is <7.1. Infuse 1–2 mEq/kg over 2 hours, not to exceed 3 mEq/kg the first 12 hours.

4. *Phosphate therapy:* Beneficial only if severe hypophosphatemia is present.

5. *NG tube:* Indicated only in selected patients (e.g., gastric stasis and severe vomiting).

Complications of DKA

Persistent acidosis	Anuria
Hypokalemia	Hypoxemia
Cerebral edema	Severe acidosis
Gastric dilatation	Severe hypotension
(with or without ileus)	DIC

DIABETIC NEPHROPATHY

Diabetic nephropathy is the leading cause of end-stage renal disease (ESRD). Its incidence is 27% in IDDM and 25% in NIDDM. The diagnosis is based on the presence of persistent proteinuria higher than 0.5 gm/day or albuminuria higher than or equal to 0.3 gm/day in at least three consecutive 24-hour urine collections. Persistent proteinuria in both IDDM and NIDDM predicts the development of clinically significant renal impairment. The risk factors are (1) IDDM, (2) male sex, (3) long duration of DM (10–15 yr), (4) hypertension, (5) urinary infections, and (6) obstruction.

Natural History of Nephropathy Due to IDDM

Stage I: Initial renal hypertrophy and high GFR. Albumin excretion in this stage is variable. Insulin therapy may improve the GFR, but the renal enlargement persists.

Stage II (silent phase): May persist for 2–15 years after the diagnosis of DM. The patient is normotensive. The albumin excretion is normal or increased during stress or poor metabolic control. The GFR is normal or slightly increased. The expansion of mesangium reduces the filtration surface. There is also thickening of the glomerular basement membrane.

Stage III (incipient diabetic nephropathy or microalbuminuria): Approximately 30–40% of IDDM enters this phase after 10–20 years. The microalbuminuria is in the range of 20–200 µg/min (normal is <10 µg/min). Microalbumin is measured by radioimmunoassay or ELISA. It should be confirmed by three urine samples over a period of 6 months, for transient microalbuminuria may occur as a result of poor control, physical exercise, or UTI. In this stage there is an increasing severity in the structural changes in the glomeruli with more mesangial expansion. The GFR is still elevated and the total albumin excretion is in the range of 25–250 mg/24 hr. Patients with microalbuminuria are more likely to have retinal changes due to diabetes, and BP is higher.

Stage IV (overt diabetic nephropathy): The proteinuria is detectable by the dipstick, and total albumin excretion is higher than 250 mg/24 hr. This stage of gross proteinuria is characterized by glomerular closure and a gradual decline in the GFR. Late in the course, the GFR becomes <30 ml/min. There are both a concomitant rising systemic arterial BP and significant retinopathy.

Stage V (uremia): Glomerular closure, decrease in albumin excretion, and a GFR ranging between 0 and 10 ml/min are characteristic.

In NIDDM, ESRD may be present within 5 years of diagnosis, and persistent proteinuria has been observed in 8% and microalbuminuria in 20–40% of patients at the time of diagnosis. In IDDM, the onset of proteinuria predicts clinically significant renal disease. In NIDDM, in contrast to IDDM, an increased urinary albumin excretion rate does not predict retinopathy.

Mechanism of Nephropathy

Several metabolic and hormonal abnormalities have been proposed to induce the glomerular hyperfiltration. They include hyperglycemia, insulinopenia, increased extracellular volume, increased production of vasodilatory prostaglandins, high dietary protein intake, abnormalities of polyol pathway, hereditary susceptibility, diet, coagulation, and platelet factors.

Management of Diabetic Nephropathy

1. Good metabolic control may have a beneficial effect in patients with minimal nephropathy.
2. Dietary protein restriction (0.6 gm/kg/day)
3. Control of systemic HTN
4. ACE inhibitors even in normotensive patients may reduce albuminuria and slow the progression of diabetic nephropathy.
5. IVPs and other radiographic dyes should be avoided, particularly if heavy proteinuria is present.

Therapeutic Options for Uremia

1. *Renal transplantation:* Recommended mostly in uremic children and young adults; patients can survive a decade or longer.
2. *Continuous ambulatory peritoneal dialysis:* Associated with a high dropout rate, a high mortality rate, and progression of retinopathy.
3. *Maintenance home hemodialysis:* IDDM patients usually fail after about 3 years; more effective in NIDDM.

DIABETIC NEUROPATHY

Diabetic neuropathy is the most common peripheral nerve disorder in the Western Hemisphere. It affects nearly half the patients with DM within 25–30 years of the diagnosis. Symptoms of diabetic neuropathy often occur several years after the onset of IDDM; in NIDDM they may coincide with the diagnosis or even precede the onset of diabetes. Slowing of nerve conduction velocity (NCV) usually precedes the signs and symptoms of peripheral neuropathy. Signs of diabetic neuropathy also usually precede the symptoms. Glycemic control correlates very well with the presence or absence of diabetic neuropathy. Three types of peripheral diabetic nephropathies have been defined:

1. *Symmetrical syndrome (polyneuropathy):* Sensory or mixed motor neuropathy (acute or subacute), autonomic neuropathy involving cardiovascular, GI tract

2. *Asymmetrical syndromes:* Limb mononeuropathy and radiculopathy, lumbosacral plexopathy, thoracoabdominal radiculopathy, cranial mononeuropathy, mononeuropathy multiplex

3. *Unique syndromes:* Diabetic pseudotabes, lumbosacral polyradiculopathy, diabetic amyotrophy, neuropathic cachexia

Clinical Presentations

1. *Sensory polyneuropathy* is the most common presentation. It has an insidious onset. Its manifestations are reduced touch and vibratory senses, absent distal reflexes and sensory ataxia, deep burning pain associated with cutaneous hyperesthesia, acral pain, temperature insensitivity, hair loss, discolored shiny skin, brittle nails, and demineralization of bone.

2. *Acute motor neuropathy* (mimics Guillain-Barré syndrome) has a satisfactory outcome.

3. *Diabetic dysautonomic neuropathy* often includes cardiovascular manifestations such as postural hypotension, syncope, and heart rate abnormalities; GI manifestations such as dysphagia, gastric atony and reflux, diabetic diarrhea; urogenital dysfunction (including bladder atony and incontinence and impotence in men); pseudomotor dysfunction such as anhydrosis, heat intolerance, and gustatory hyperhidrosis; and pupillary, lacrimal, and respiratory disorders. Autonomic testing is simple and includes the orthostatic response of BP and heart rate response to valsalva, deep breathing, and hand clenching. These responses are blunted in diabetic dysautonomic neuropathy. The presence of autonomic dysfunction often predicts poor outcome.

4. *Asymmetrical syndromes* (mononeuropathies) may lead to carpal tunnel syndrome and other entrapment syndromes, foot drop, meralgia paresthetica, and cervical and lumbosacral radiculopathies. Diabetic radiculopathy is characterized by an acute or subacute onset of weakness of the hip and thigh muscles, as well as thigh pain followed by weight loss and depression. Unilateral truncal pain may reflect thoracoabdominal radiculopathy. Cranial nerve neuropathies III, IV, VI, and VII are the most frequent.

5. *Mononeuropathy multiplex* implies focal lesions of nerve(s) due to advanced diabetes.

6. *Rare neuropathic conditions* in diabetics: pseudotabes, diabetic neuropathic cachexia (anorexia, profound weight loss, and severe distal neuropathic pain) in older men. The search for malignancy and the treatment of depression are important.

Evaluation

1. Electromyography (EMG) and nerve conduction velocity (NCV)
2. Tests for dysautonomic neuropathy
3. Peripheral nerve biopsy (should not be systematic); may be useful in the differential diagnosis of mononeuropathy multiplex.

The pathophysiology is most likely related to metabolic abnormalities, including increased nerve glucose, fructose, sorbitol, and reduced myoinositol.

Therapy

1. Glycemic control seems to be of benefit and should be stressed in the prevention and management of diabetic neuropathies.
2. Aldose reductase inhibitors reduce sorbitol levels, correct myoinositol levels, and improve neurophysiologic functions.
3. Feeding of myoinositol, gangliosides, and B vitamins is without definite effectiveness.
4. Pain therapies include NSAIDs, tricyclic antidepressants (phenothiazines), carbamazepine, phenytoin, and lidocaine infusion.
5. Capsaicin cream presumably acts as a substance P depleter.

DIARRHEA

ACUTE

Approach and Differential Diagnosis

Acute diarrhea is defined as being less than 2–3 weeks in duration. Acute diarrheas are most commonly a result of infection. However, other environmental factors such as ingested drugs or toxins may also be implicated. The most common mode of transmission for infectious acute diarrheas is the fecal-oral route via contaminated food or water. Person-to-person transmission may also occur as is the case with rotavirus and *Clostridium difficile* infection. High-risk groups for infectious diarrhea include travelers to developing nations, homosexuals and HIV-infected patients (gay bowel syndrome), residents of institutions or nursing homes, children and workers in day care centers and their families, and those ingesting foods likely to be contaminated, including seafood and shellfish, food from restaurants and fast-food chains, and food from banquets and picnics. The approach to the patient with acute diarrhea should include a careful Hx & PE in order to categorize patients falling into one of the aforementioned high-risk groups.

Most patients with infectious diarrhea have nausea, vomiting, and abdominal pain and either watery, malabsorptive, or bloody diarrhea with fever. The nature of the symptoms helps to establish a differential diagnosis as to suspected location of infection and type of organism. Small-intestinal infection tends to lead to a watery secretory diarrhea or malabsorptive-type diarrhea; colonic infections tend to result in bloody diarrhea with abdominal pain. Laboratory diagnosis of acute diarrheal illness may not be necessary in patients in whom there is nonbloody diarrhea without evidence of systemic toxicity. Frequently, the illness runs its course and the high cost of evaluation by means of stool culture, proctoscopy, and antibiotic therapy does not warrant evaluation given the self-limited nature of most illnesses. On the other hand, if the patient appears systemically toxic or has bloody diarrhea, then evaluation may be necessary and hospitalization possible. Fecal leukocyte smear and examination of the rectal mucosa with proctoscopy (stool culture) give the highest yield for establishing a cause.

The differential diagnosis of acute diarrhea includes all of the infectious causes (table follows), food allergies, drug toxicity, medication ingestion, and environmental or food toxins. For acute bloody diarrhea, the differential should also include ischemic colitis, inflammatory bowel disease, and drug-induced colitis.

Correlations Between Pathophysiology and Symptoms of Infectious Diarrhea

PATHOPHYSIOLOGY	MICROORGANISMS	SYMPTOMS
Preformed toxins (food poisonings)	*B. cereus, S. aureus, C. perfringens, C. botulinum*	Nausea, vomiting, watery diarrhea, low-grade fever, mild–moderate pain
Enterotoxin production Adherent organisms:	*V. cholerae,* enterotoxigenic *E. coli, K. pneumoniae*	Watery diarrhea; may contain mucus (i.e., "rice water" stool), low-grade fever, mild–moderate pain
Invading organisms:	*Campylobacter, Aeromonas, Shigella,* noncholera *Vibrio*	Initially watery diarrhea, then bloody; high fever, severe pain
Invasive organisms Enterocyte invasion and destruction Minimal inflammation:	Rotavirus, Norwalk agent	Watery diarrhea and malabsorption, high fever, moderate pain
Severe inflammation:	*Shigella,* enteroinvasive *E. coli, E. histolytica*	Bloody diarrhea, high fever, severe pain
Mucosal penetration with multiplication in lamina propria and inflammation:	*Campylobacter, Salmonella, Aeromonas, ?Plesiomonas, Yersinia, V. parahemolyticus, V. fulnificus, M. avium-intracellulare, M. tuberculosis, Histoplasma*	Either watery or bloody diarrhea depending on degree of mucosal destruction, high fever, severe pain
Attachment or colonization Local cytotoxin and inflammation: Adherent:	Enteropathogenic (enteroadherent) *E. coli, Giardia,* cryptosporidia, helminths	Watery diarrhea, low–moderate fever, moderate–severe pain
Cytotoxic:	*C. difficile*	Usually watery diarrhea, occasionally bloody diarrhea, low–moderate fever, severe pain
	Enterohemorrhagic *E. coli*	Watery diarrhea for short time, then bloody diarrhea; low–moderate fever, severe pain
Systemic infection	Hepatitis, listeriosis, legionelosis, Rocky Mountain spotted fever, psittacosis, otitis media in infants, toxic shock syndrome (*S. aureus*), measles	Watery diarrhea may be initially a part of disease or it may accompany disease; clinical manifestations are overwhelmingly those of the organs and tissues primarily involved by the organisms

From Powell DW: Approach to the patient with diarrhea. In Yamada T, et al (eds): Textbook of Gastroenterology. Philadelphia, J.B. Lippincott, 1991, p 745, with permission.

Treatment of acute diarrhea should be symptomatic (fluids and antidiarrheal agents) for the mild nontoxic cases. Specific antimicrobial therapy may be indicated in some instances, particularly when evidence of toxicity is present. Because of the possibility of worsening the colonization or invasion of organisms when intestinal motility is slowed by anticholinergics, anticholinergics are generally not recommended for severe cases of infectious diarrhea.

CHRONIC DIARRHEA

Classification, Diagnosis, and Management of Chronic Diarrheal Disorders

CAUSE	EXAMPLES	KEY ELEMENTS IN DIAGNOSIS	TREATMENT
Iatrogenic dietary factors	Excess tea, coffee, cola, beverages, simple sugars	Careful history taking	Appropriate dietary modifications
Infectious enteritis	Amebiasis	Demonstrate leukocytes in stool	Metronidazole, diodoquinol antibiotics
	Giardiasis	Identify trophozoites or cysts in stool and duodenal aspirate	Metronidazole
Inflammatory bowel disease	Ulcerative colitis	History: diarrhea, abdominal pain, rectal bleeding	Sulfadiazine Cortiocosteroids
	Regional enteritis	Sigmoidoscopy, barium enema, upper GI and small bowel series	
Irritable bowel syndrome	—	Careful history taking	Dietary modifications Antispasmodics
Lactose intolerance	Milk intolerance	Milk → abdominal pain, diarrhea, gas, bloating. Cessation of milk drinking → amelioration of symptoms Lactose load (1 gm/kg) → exacerbation of symptoms and blood glucose fails to rise > 20 mg/ 100 ml.	Discontinue milk
Laxative abuse	—	Add few drops of NaOH to stool. Because most laxatives contain phenolphthalein, the stool will turn red.	Discontinue laxatives
Drug induced	Antacids, antibiotics (clindamycin, lincomycin, ampicillin, penicillin), colchicine, PAS, lactulose, sorbitol	Careful history taking and review of medication	Discontinue offending drug
Diverticular and prediverticular disease	—	History: intermittent symptoms Physical exam: palpable left colon Barium enema: diverticulosis and/or muscle hypertrophy	High-fiber diet; avoid corn, nuts, peanuts, kernel-containing foods
Malabsorptive disease	Sprue Pancreatic insufficiency	Upper GI plus small bowel x-rays; tests of intestinal absorptive function (D-xylose, stool fat, Schilling test, serum carotenes, calcium, albumin, cholesterol, iron, PT)	Appropriate for the underlying disorder

Table continued on next page.

Classification, Diagnosis, and Management of Chronic Diarrheal Disorders (Cont.)

CAUSE	EXAMPLES	KEY ELEMENTS IN DIAGNOSIS	TREATMENT
Metabolic	Diabetes mellitus	Abnormal blood glucose levels	Appropriate to the underlying disorder
	Hyperthyroidism	↑ T4, ↑ radioiodine uptake	
	Adrenal insufficiency	↓plasma cortisol, ↓ response to synthetic ACTH	
Mechanical	Fecal impaction	Rectal exam	Remove impaction
Neoplastic	Pancreatic carcinoma	Suspect the diagnosis	Surgical
	Carcinoid syndrome		
	Villous adenoma		
	Medullary carcinoma of the thyroid		
	Tumors producing vasoactive intestinal peptide		
	Gastrinoma		

Mnemonic to remember the classification: I, I, I, I, L, L, D, D, M, M, M, N.

From Greenberger NJ: A diagnostic approach to the patient with a chronic diarrheal disorder. J Kansas Med Soc (Jun): 257–263, 1978, with permission.

Infectious Diarrhea

Differential Diagnosis of Infectious Diarrhea

AGENT	EPIDEMIOLOGIC CHARACTERISTICS	CLINICAL CHARACTERISTICS
Viral		
• Rotavirus	Major cause of endemic severe diarrhea in infants and young children worldwide; occurs in winter in temperate zones	24–36 hr incubation; dehydrating diarrhea, vomiting, and fever; lasts 4–6 days
• Enteric adenovirus	Endemic diarrhea of infants and young children	24–36 hr incubation; prolonged diarrhea with vomiting and fever; lasts 4–6 days
• Norwalk virus	Winter epidemics of vomiting and diarrhea in older children and adults; occurs in families, communities, and nursing homes; often associated with shellfish, other food, or water	24–48 hr incubation; acute vomiting, diarrhea, fever, myalgia, and headache; lasts 1–2 days
• Calicivirus	Usually pediatric diarrhea; associated with shellfish and other foods in adults	24–36 hr incubation; rotavirus-like illness in children and Norwalk-like in adults; lasts 4–6 days
• Astrovirus	Pediatric diarrhea; also reported in nursing homes	24–36 hr incubation; watery diarrhea, similar to rotavirus; lasts 2–3 days

Table continued on next page.

Differential Diagnosis of Infectious Diarrhea (Cont.)

AGENT	EPIDEMIOLOGIC CHARACTERISTICS	CLINICAL CHARACTERISTICS
Bacterial		
• Enteropathogenic *E. coli* (EPEC)	Outbreaks of diarrhea in infants <6 mos old; frequently involves hospital nurseries	12–38 hr incubation; profuse, foul-smelling, watery diarrhea without blood or mucus; lasts 1–3 days
• Enteroinvasive *E. coli* (EIEC)	Uncommon cause of foodborne outbreaks	12–72 hr incubation; scant stools containing blood and mucus; fever; lasts 4–10 days
• Enterotoxigenic *E. coli* (ETEC)	Major cause of traveler's diarrhea	24–38 hr incubation; abdominal cramping, profuse watery diarrhea without blood or mucus; nausea and vomiting common; no fever; lasts 1–3 days
• Enterohemorrhagic *E. coli* (EHEC)	Food-borne outbreaks, especially associated with undercooked meat	24–96 hr incubation; cramping, abdominal pain with bloody diarrhea and no fever; lasts 2–9 days
• *Vibrio cholerae*	Outbreaks (epidemics) associated with poor sanitary conditions and ingestion of food or water contaminated with fecal matter	24–72 hr incubation; profuse, "rice-water" diarrhea that results in life-threatening diarrhea without cramping or fever; lasts 1–2 wks
• *Shigella* sp.	Outbreaks occur under poor sanitary conditions resulting in fecal contamination of food; involves primarily children <10 years old and homosexual men; very low inoculum required to cause disease	24–72 hr incubation; early in illness, small bowel is involved resulting in watery diarrhea and high fever; later, colitis develops manifested by urgency, tenesmus, and frequent low-volume stools with blood and mucus; low-grade fever; lasts 2–20 days
• *Salmonella* sp.	Food-borne illness associated with poor sanitary practices, especially associated with dairy products, eggs, poultry, meats, fruits, and vegetables	8–48 hr incubation; cramping, abdominal pain, vomiting, and fever; stools are loose and foul smelling with moderate WBC and rarely bloody; lasts 1–4 days
• *Vibrio parahaemolyticus*	Occurs in outbreaks, frequently in summer months; associated with improperly cooked or stored seafoods	8–24 hr incubation; abdominal cramping, headache, low-grade fevers associated with explosive noninflammatory, watery diarrhea without blood; lasts 1–4 days
• *Campylobacter jejuni*	Food-borne illness associated with raw milk, poultry, and beef	12–24 hr incubation; abdominal pain, nausea, vomiting, and watery diarrhea that sometimes contains blood and pus; lasts 1–4 days.

Table continued on next page.

Differential Diagnosis of Infectious Diarrhea (Cont.)

AGENT	EPIDEMIOLOGIC CHARACTERISTICS	CLINICAL CHARACTERISTICS
• *Clostridium difficile*	Occurs in persons exposed to antimicrobial agents and occasional nosocomial outbreaks	Colitis with fever, abdominal cramping, tenesmus, and diarrhea that may contain blood
• *Staphylococcus aureus*	Very common form of food poisoning due to toxin caused by bacterial growth in improperly prepared or stored foods	1–4 hr incubation; vomiting and noninflammatory diarrhea; lasts <24 hr
• *Bacillus cereus*	Frequent cause of food poisoning, especially associated with refried rice and vegetables; results from ingestion of preformed toxin in improperly prepared or stored foods	8–16 hr incubation; abdominal pain, profuse watery diarrhea without blood or mucus; no fever; lasts <24 hr
• *Clostridium perfringens*	Food-borne outbreaks, which may involve large numbers of persons; follows ingestion of preformed toxin in contaminated foods, especially meats	7–15 hr incubation; cramping, abdominal pain with watery diarrhea that contains no blood or mucus; no fever; lasts <24 hr
Protozoa		
• *Giardia lamblia*	Water- and food-borne illness in travelers (Rocky Mountains, Russia, underdeveloped countries) and those in day care centers	1–4 wk incubation; chronic small bowel symptoms with bloating, flatulence, nausea, anorexia, watery noninflammatory diarrhea, and malabsorption; lasts 1–6 wk
• *Entamoeba histolytica*	Endemic in most parts of the world, most commonly occurring in areas of poor sanitation; institutionalized persons and homosexuals especially at risk	Abdominal pain, cramping, nausea, chills, fever, tenesmus, and liquid stools that may contain mucus or blood; lasts weeks to months
• *Cryptosporidium*	Illness seen in outbreaks associated with consumption of water contaminated with waste from livestock; also seen in day care settings and patients with AIDS	1–3 wk incubation; profuse, noninflammatory diarrhea that is usually self-limited (1–2 wk) except in immunocompromised patients, in whom it can produce chronic wasting

References: Blacklow NR, et al: Viral gastroenteritis. N Engl J Med 325:252–264, 1991. Guerrant RL, et al: Bacterial and protozoal gastroenteritis. N Engl J Med 325:327–340, 1991. Quadri SMH: Infectious diarrhea. Postgrad Med 88(5):169–184, 1990.

DIGITALIS TOXICITY

Digoxin toxicity is a significant problem for the elderly primarily because of the high frequency of digoxin use in older people, added to age- and disease-related changes. Clearly the best way to avoid digoxin toxicity is to avoid digoxin altogether. Only those with a clear indication should be on digoxin. In one study, 80% of nursing home patients on digoxin had no indication for the drug. In all of them, digoxin was discontinued without incident. However, *patients with A fib and prior history of rapid ventricular response should be kept on digoxin.*

Reasons That the Elderly Are Likely to Develop Digoxin Toxicity

- Decrease in lean body weight with age causes decrease in digoxin's volume of distribution.
- Decrease in creatinine clearance with age (normal aging results in a 40% decrease) that is not reflected by an increase in serum creatinine because of a concomitant fall in muscle mass.
- Digoxin excretion is mostly renal, so half-life is prolonged and clearance is reduced.
- Higher likelihood of developing dehydration due to effects of age and diuretics.
- Higher frequency of nephrotoxic drug use (especially NSAIDs).
- Higher frequency of other drug use that interacts with digoxin (hold digoxin dose and check level when instituting these drugs; plan on decreasing maintenance dose).
  —Quinidine doubles digoxin levels.
  —Verapamil increases digoxin levels.
- Higher frequency of cardiac amyloid, which may increase digoxin toxicity.

Digoxin toxicity should not occur, because serum digoxin level measurement is routinely available. The target level in patients with CHF with low LVEF and sinus rhythm is 0.9 ng/ml (this is lower than in younger patients).

Symptoms of Digoxin Toxicity

- Anorexia, nausea, vomiting, diarrhea
- Apathy, depression
- Fatigue, weakness
- Confusion, delirium, nightmares
- Dizziness
- Almost any arrhythmia
  —Increased automaticity: A fib or flutter, bigeminy or trigeminy, multifocal PVCs and V tach (may presage V fib)
  —↓ AV conduction: first-, second- or third-degree AV block
  —Combination of two effects:
  1. If baseline is A fib, you may see regularization of the patient's rhythm.
  2. Paroxysmal atrial tachycardia with block

Treatment of Digoxin Toxicity

- Fab antibodies are very effective in serious toxicities.
- Normalize potassium and magnesium, if low.
- Monitor patient.
- Maintain euvolemia.
- If possible, discontinue other medications that may interact with digoxin.

Reference: Kelly RA, et al: Recognition and management if digitalis toxicity. Am J Cardiol 69:108G-119G, 1992.

DIPLOPIA

Double vision almost always arises from weakness of cranial nerves III (oculo-motor), IV (trochlear), or VI (abducens), which are directly responsible for eye movements. Whenever the two eyes fall out of alignment, double vision results.

Six Syndromes of the VIth Nerve

1. Brain stem
   a. Infarction
   b. Multiple sclerosis
   c. Tumor
2. Subarachnoid space (exiting brain stem)
   a. Carcinomatous meningitis
   b. Basilar meningitis, such as TB
3. Crossing the petrous bone
   a. Osteomyelitis or inflammation
   b. Tumor, especially from increased ICP
4. Cavernous sinus
   a. Thrombosis
   b. Tumor
5. Orbit
   a. Granulomatous inflammation
   b. Tumor
6. Isolated VIth nerve palsy
   a. DM
   b. Postviral syndrome

Six Syndromes of the IIIrd Nerve

1. Brainstem nucleus
   a. Infarction
   b. Multiple sclerosis
   c. Tumor
2. Uncal herniation
3. Posterior communicating artery aneurysm
4. Cavernous sinus
   a. Thrombosis
   b. Tumor
5. Orbit
   a. Granulomatous inflammation
   b. Tumor
6. Pupillary-sparing isolated IIIrd nerve palsy (especially common in diabetes)

Six Syndromes of the IVth Nerve

1. Brain stem
   a. Infarction
   b. Multiple sclerosis
   c. Tumor
2. Subarachnoid space
   a. Carcinomatous meningitis
   b. Basilar meningitis
3. Intracranial (especially ↑ pressure)
4. Cavernous sinus
   a. Thrombosis
   b. Tumor
5. Orbit
   a. Granulomatous inflammation
   b. Tumor
6. Isolated IVth nerve palsy
   a. Congenital = very common
   b. Acquired = especially diabetes

Diseases Causing Diplopia That Mimic Cranial Nerve Palsies

1. Myasthenia gravis
2. Thyroid eye disease
3. Congenital strabismus
4. Ocular trauma

References: Leigh RJ, et al: The Neurology of Eye Movements. Philadelphia, F.A. Davis, 1991.

Rush JA, et al: Paralysis of cranial nerves III, IV and VI. Course and prognosis in 1,000 cases. Arch Ophthalmol 99:66–69, 1981.

DISSEMINATED INTRAVASCULAR COAGULATION

DIC is a pathologic process wherein platelet-fibrin thrombi form widely in the microcirculation, resulting in impaired perfusion and function of various organs and consumption of hemostatic factors. Renal failure, hepatic failure, altered cerebral function, acute adrenal insufficiency, ARDS, GI ulceration, and skin necrosis may occur in acute DIC, related principally to microvascular thrombosis. Prolongation of the PT and PTT, as well as thrombocytopenia results from consumption of platelets and coagulation factors (such as I, II, V, and VIII) in the microthrombi. Compensatory fibrinolysis leads to circulating fibrin degradation products, which exert anticoagulant effects by inhibiting the fibrinogen-to-fibrin reaction and impairing platelet function. Erythrocytic fragmentation is frequently observed in the peripheral blood of patients with DIC. In evaluating patients for DIC, the physician diagnoses based on the appropriate clinical situation coupled with thrombocytopenia, diminished plasma fibrinogen level, prolonged PT and PTT, and elevated fibrin degradation products, or, more specifically, D-dimer. DIC may occur as an acute or as a chronic disorder. In addition, intravascular coagulation may be localized to a particular vascular site and lead to consumptive coagulopathy.

Causes of Intravascular Coagulation

1. Acute DIC	
Infections	Brain trauma
Obstetrical disorders	Hyperthermia
Hemolytic transfusion reaction	Snake venom
Shock	Purpura fulminans
2. Chronic DIC	
Adenocarcinoma	Promyelocytic leukemia
Retained dead fetus	
3. Localized intravascular coagulation	
Aortic aneurysm	Hemangioma

Sepsis with shock due to endotoxin-producing gram-negative bacterial rods is the most common cause of severe acute DIC. In DIC due to meningococcal sepsis, adrenal hemorrhage (Waterhouse-Friderichsen syndrome) is a serious complication. Functional or anatomic asplenia predisposes to DIC in patients with pneumococcal sepsis. Clostridial organisms are important in DIC related to septic abortion. *Mycobacterium tuberculosis* is an infrequent bacterial cause of DIC. Among nonbacterial infections, prominent examples with DIC are Rocky Mountain spotted fever, dengue, falciparum malaria, and the viral exanthems of childhood.

Purpura fulminans is a postinfectious disorder with extensive hemorrhagic necrosis of skin, occurring particularly in children after streptococcal infections. Deficiency of protein C predisposes to purpura fulminans.

Obstetrical disorders resulting in acute DIC are septic abortion, uterine rupture, abruptio placentae, and amniotic fluid emboli. Release into the circulation of thromboplastic material from the amniotic fluid or placenta provokes intravascular coagulation.

In hemolytic transfusion reactions, the lysed stroma of erythrocytes may exert a procoagulant effect. Tissue factor released from brain tissue, infarcted or destroyed by trauma, promotes DIC. Some snake venoms act directly on the coagulation system to promote fibrin formation. Shock that is related to massive trauma or following surgical procedures can cause DIC independent of other etiologies.

Patients with mucin-producing adenocarcinomas are prone to experience chronic DIC. In addition to DIC, such persons may have recurrent migratory venous thromboses (Trousseau's syndrome) and marantic endocarditis. The primary sites of adenocarcinomas most often associated with DIC are pancreas, lung, and prostate. Acute leukemia, particularly promyelocytic leukemia (PML), is associated with DIC. In fact, most patients with PML have clinically important DIC that requires treatment.

A dead fetus retained in the uterus may provoke a slowly developing DIC that resolves with removal of the fetus. Occasionally there is sufficient production of clot within aneurysms and large hemangiomas to consume coagulation factors and platelets.

DIVERTICULITIS

Diverticulitis occurs in 10–25% of patients with diverticulosis and pathologically begins as a microperforation of a diverticulum with a surrounding peridiverticulitis. Symptoms and signs of diverticulitis include local abdominal pain over the area of inflammation (with or without focal peritoneal signs), a palpable mass, fever, nausea, vomiting, and ileus. As the inflammation progresses, abscess formation, free perforation, fistulization, or obstruction may occur. Frank bleeding is rarely associated with acute diverticulitis. The differential diagnosis should include any other cause of peritoneal inflammation such as appendicitis, cholecystitis, inflammatory bowel disease, other colitides, and gynecologic inflammatory or neoplastic processes.

The diagnosis is often made on clinical grounds, and treatment is often initiated before the diagnosis is confirmed. Frequently, diagnostic tests may be postponed if there is a rapid clinical response to allow a "cooling-off period."

In the acute setting, CT scan of the abdomen is often highly useful and may reveal thickening of the colonic wall, pericolic inflammation, fistula, sinus or abscess formation, and evidence of obstruction. Contrast barium enema is more reliable than colonoscopy in documenting diverticulosis and diverticulitis. In the case of diverticulitis, findings include displacement or narrowing of the bowel wall with an altered mucosal pattern or evidence of a soft tissue mass. These findings are indicative of a pericolic inflammatory mass but are not pathognomonic of diverticulitis. It is generally believed that instillation of contrast and air into the colon during acute diverticulitis is contraindicated given the risk of exacerbating an acute attack or leading to barium peritonitis. For this reason, barium enema is usually postponed until there has been clinical improvement. However, should a contrast study be necessary, water-soluble contrast agents may be used safely and with a relatively high degree of accuracy.

Therapy of diverticulitis consists of antibiotics aimed at coverage for the major colonic pathogens including anaerobes, gram-negative bacilli, and gram-positive coliforms. Ampicillin, gentamicin, and metronidazole are a commonly used regimen; however, third-generation cephalosporins and other broad-spectrum antibiotics may be used with success.

Surgical management is necessary in only 15–30% of patients with diverticulitis and generally is indicated in cases of free perforation, suppurative peritonitis secondary to ruptured abscess, fistula formation, obstruction, and recurrent diverticulitis. Recurrent diverticulitis occurs in 30% of patients after successful medical management.

DIVERTICULOSIS

Diverticulosis is an acquired condition caused by herniation of the bowel mucosa through the muscular layer of the colon. It is a common condition in highly industrialized countries and infrequent in economically underdeveloped nations. This may be a reflection of the relatively low dietary fiber intake in industrialized nations. It appears to be dependent upon age as well as possible gut motility disorders and lack of dietary fiber.

Diverticula tend to be distributed unequally throughout the colon, with the sigmoid colon most commonly involved. About 65% of patients have diverticulosis limited to the sigmoid colon, and 24% to the sigmoid and other segments of the colon; 7% have diverticula scattered over the entire length of the colon; only 4% have diverticula limited to a segment of the colon proximal to the sigmoid. In general, right-sided diverticula tend to occur earlier in life than left-sided diverticula for reasons that are unclear.

Approximatley 70% of patients with diverticulosis have uncomplicated disease and no symptoms; 10–25% develop diverticulitis and 5% diverticular hemorrhage, both of which are the two most common complications of diverticular disease.

Diverticulosis per se requires no specific therapy unless complications develop. There is some support for the treatment of uncomplicated but symptomatic (irritable-bowel-type) diverticular disease by use of dietary fiber or fiber supplementation. Additional fiber may result in a reduction of abdominal symptoms and may prevent the development of further diverticula.

DIZZINESS

Dizziness or vertigo is a sudden feeling of rotation or displacement of the environment or of patients themselves. Symptoms can be vague and should not be confused with faintness, which may have a cardiac cause. Pallor suggests impaired blood supply and should lead to investigation of cardiac rather than labyrinthine causes.

The first several days of a labyrinthine disorder may be accompanied by nausea and loss of balance, requiring physical support for balance. It may take up to 6 weeks for enough compensation to occur that the patient does not experience vertigo when quickly changing position of the head or body. Dizzy spells may reoccur for up to 3 years after these attacks.

Trauma, infection, or vascular lesions are the causes of acute unilateral labyrinthine syndrome. Vascular causes tend to be seen in elderly patients with other vascular lesions and are due to compromise in the vertebral basilar system. Occasionally, an infarct in the posterior-inferior cerebellar artery distribution is the etiology. Brain stem function is likely to be compromised, so other symptoms such as dysarthria and unilateral or bilateral sensory symptoms may be found. There is usually neither difficulty swallowing nor weakness in extremities.

Sinus infection near the inner ear is associated, in 25% of cases, with labyrinthine dysfunction. Either x-rays of the sphenoid or maxillary sinuses or a history of postnasal drip may help in the diagnosis. Trauma as an etiology should be elicited in the history.

Examination of a patient with dizziness may be quite normal, unless an attack is occurring at the time. Nystagmus may be gross or fine or elicited by the Barany maneuver, which involves seating the patient on a table, then quickly lowering the patient backwards so that the head is over the edge of the table 30 degrees below the horizontal, with the head turned 45 degrees to one side. This is repeated with the head 45 degrees to the other side and then straight forward. Reproduction of the patient's symptoms or of rotary nystagmus indicates true vertigo.

Many medications can cause dizziness, such as antianxiety agents, sleeping medications, and antihypertensives. If the etiology of the problem is peripheral, tinnitus may be associated, and a perforated tympanic membrane or fluid behind the eardrum may be seen. The seventh and fifth nerves should be carefully tested, and tests for hearing loss should be performed. Although an acoustic neuroma can produce vertigo, it is usually large and has already caused severe deafness, nystagmus, and fifth-cranial-nerve sensory loss prior to vertigo's appearing. Viral infections causing vestibular neuronitis usually spare hearing, affecting the vestibular function bilaterally. Electronystagmograms (ENGs) are positive for bilateral vestibular impairment. MS may present with vestibular dysfunction as the first symptom, but other signs and symptoms of the disease that reflect brain stem dysfunction, as well as a previous history of neurologic problems, are present. Vertigo without other neurologic findings does not support the diagnosis of a brain tumor.

Recurrent attacks occur in some patients. The differential diagnosis includes Meniere's disease, benign recurrent vertigo, or panic disorder. In Meniere's disease, patients have recurrent attacks of hearing loss, tinnitus, and fullness in one ear. Attacks last up to several hours and ENGs are usually abnormal. There may be a positive family history.

In most patients, dizziness is an isolated, nonspecific, and self-limited symptom. Improvement usually occurs within 6 weeks, and reassuring the patient is of primary concern. Antivertigo drugs such as meclizine HCl, dimenhydrinate, diphenidol, diazepam, and transdermal scopolamine are sometimes helpful. (See also Vertigo.)

DRUGS AFFECTING TASTE AND SMELL

Metronidazole, ampicillin, griseofulvin, sulfasalazine, tetracycline, ethambutol, theophylline, codeine and morphine, lithium, trifluoperazine, phenytoin, baclofen, chlormezanone, levodopa, allopurinol, colchicine, phenylbutazone, captopril, ethacrynic acid, and glipizide.

DRUGS AND THE ELDERLY

People older than 65 constitute 10% of the population but spend 35–45% of all the money expended on drugs (almost 40% of this on over-the-counter drugs). Only

10% take no drugs regularly, with an average of 13 prescriptions filled/year for each person over 65. Adverse drug reactions occur in 10% of patients aged 20–30 but in 40% of patients aged 65 and older. They lead to 3–10% of hospital admissions.

Compliance with medications has been estimated to be only 50%. Compliance can be improved by avoiding childproof containers (which are often elder proof as well) and using either charts with the patient's pills attached or divided pillboxes.

Patient instructions are important. They should include a family member if possible and utilize simple schedules. Large labels and ensuring that the patient's color vision is intact (yellow and white pills may look the same) are helpful. Old medications should be destroyed.

Who Is Most Likely to Have an Adverse Drug Reaction?

- Probability increases with the number of drugs a patient is taking.
- Neuroleptics are more frequently used in elderly and lead to drug-induced parkinsonism, orthostatic hypotension, and tardive dyskinesia.
- Antidepressants, antiparkinson agents, and other drugs with anticholinergic activity lead to urinary retention, confusion, and constipation.
- Diuretics lead to dehydration, which is worsened by decreased thirst drive in the elderly.
- Errors in taking drugs are more likely in patients who are older than age 75, taking multiple medications, living alone, having difficulty coping with environs, and having multiple diagnoses.

Factors to Consider in the Use of Drugs in the Elderly

Absorption
A. Age-related changes (generally *not* significant)
  - ↓ stomach acid, absorptive surface, intestinal blood flow and intestinal motility.
B. Drug effect
  - Motility agents may cause rapid delivery and ↓ absorption.
  - Antacids block absorption of many drugs.

Distribution
A. Age-related changes
  - ↓ body water, muscle, serum albumin, and glycoprotein.
  - ↑ body fat.
  - Very lipophilic drugs have prolonged half-life. (Half-life of diazepam increases from 20 hours at age 20 to 90 hours at age 90.)

Metabolism
A. Age-related changes
  - ↓ liver mass, hepatic blood flow, enzyme activity, and inducibility.
B. Drug effect
  - Multiple drugs compete for same enzyme.
  - Loss of protective effect of enzyme induction.

Excretion (most important)
A. Age-related changes
  - ↓ renal blood flow, filtration, and tubular secretion.
  - Creatinine clearance $= \dfrac{(140 - \text{age}) \times (\text{wt in kg})}{72 \times (\text{serum creatinine})}$

    (Multiply by 0.85 for women.)
B. Drug effect
  - Competition for excretion sites.

DYSPHAGIA AND ODYNOPHAGIA

General Causes and Evaluation

The term "dysphagia" refers to the sensation of difficulty in passing food from the mouth into the stomach. Dysphagia can be classified into two distinct types:

1. *Oropharyngeal dysphagia,* in which there is difficulty initiating the act of swallowing and which is typically the result of a transfer problem or impaired ability to transfer food from the mouth into the upper esophagus.

2. *Esophageal dysphagia,* a result of any disorder affecting the smooth muscle of the esophagus that may be motility related or due to a true mechanical obstruction.

Careful history taking often facilitates categorization of the patient into one of these two main groups.

Causes of Oropharyngeal Dysphagia

NEUROMUSCULAR DISEASES	LOCAL STRUCTURAL LESIONS
Stroke	Inflammatory (pharyngitis, abscess)
Parkinson's disease	Neoplastic
Multiple sclerosis	Congenital webs
ALS	Plummer-Vinson syndrome
Brain stem tumors	Extrinsic compression (thyroid, cervical spine,
Syphilis	lymph nodes)
Peripheral neuropathy	Surgical resection of the oropharynx
Myasthenia gravis	Motility disorders of the upper esophageal
Muscular dystrophies	sphincter
Primary myositis	
Amyloidosis	
SLE	

Causes of Esophageal Dysphagia

Motility disorders

Common causes
  Achalasia
  Scleroderma
  Diffuse esophageal spasm

Uncommon causes
  Nutcracker esophagus
  Hypertensive LES
  Other collagen disorders
  Chagas disease

Mechanical obstruction—intrinsic

Common causes
  Peptic stricture
  Lower esophageal ring (B-ring or
    Schatzki's ring)
  Cancer

Uncommon causes
  Webs
  Benign tumors
  Foreign bodies
  Esophageal diverticula

Mechanical lesions—extrinsic

Vascular compression
Mediastinal abnormalities
Cervical osteoarthritis

Odynophagia is defined as pain on swallowing and should not be confused with dysphagia. Odynophagia generally implies that an inflammatory process is involving the esophageal mucosa.

Causes of Odynophagia

1. Infectious esophagitis: *Candida* sp, herpes simplex virus, CMV, varicella-zoster virus, *Aspergillus*
2. Caustic ingestion (lye)
3. Pill esophagitis (antibiotics, potassium chloride, iron preparations, quinidine, NSAIDs)
4. Peptic esophagitis (rarely)

Evaluation of the patient with dysphagia should begin with a careful Hx & PE. Patients with dysphagia to both solids and liquids at the outset are most likely to have a motility disorder, whereas patients with solid food dysphagia progressing to include liquids are more likely to have a mechanical obstructing lesion that has been slowly progressive. On the other hand, patients with oropharyngeal dysphagia typically describe difficulty initiating the swallow; they sometimes have nasal regurgitation, coughing during swallowing and aspiration, and nasal speech due to palatal weakness.

The available diagnostic modalities for evaluation of dysphagia include barium swallow, upper endoscopy with visualization of the mucosa, and esophageal manometry. If a motility disorder is suspected, then manometry is likely to be diagnostic; however, upper endoscopy or barium swallow is often necessary to rule out a true mechanical lesion. Patients with suspected esophageal dysphagia due to a mechanical disorder should undergo upper endoscopy for definition of the lesion and endoscopic dilatation, if possible, to relieve obstruction. Patients with oropharyngeal dysphagia often require a modified barium swallow to fluoroscopically evaluate the swallowing process and determine the exact nature of the lesion. Therapy may then be aimed at the primary cause, or swallowing retraining may be undertaken. In cases of odynophagia, although barium swallow may suggest esophageal ulceration or infectious esophagitis, generally endoscopy is necessary in order to obtain histologic specimens that determine a specific infection source prior to institution of appropriate therapy. In the case of pill-induced esophagitis, generally discontinuation of the offending agent results in rapid improvement; however, endoscopy or barium swallow may be necessary to rule out additional causes.

Reference: Richter JE, et al: A new, common sense approach to dysphagia. Patient Care (Sep 30):87–108, 1992.

DYSPNEA

Dyspnea is a very complex and highly variable symptom. It is a sensation and not a physical finding. The diagnosis may be evident from the Hx & PE in combination with the database including laboratory screening, CXR, ECG, and spirogram. If those tests are nondiagnostic, more elaborate testing may be needed. A step-by-step approach yields a diagnosis in almost all patients. (See also Shortness of Breath.)

Causes of Acute Dyspnea

Anxiety/hyperventilation
Asthma
Chest trauma (pneumothorax, fractured ribs, pulmonary contusion)
Pulmonary edema
Pulmonary embolism
Spontaneous pneumothorax

From Mahler DA: Dyspnea: Diagnosis and management. Clin Chest Med 8:216, 1987, with permission.

Causes of Chronic Dyspnea

Respiratory
  Airway disease
    Upper airway obstruction
    Asthma
    Chronic bronchitis
    Emphysema
    Cystic fibrosis
  Parenchymal lung disease
    Interstitial lung disease
    Malignancy—primary or metastatic
    Pneumonia
  Pulmonary vascular disease
    Arteriovenous malformations
    Intravascular obstruction
    Vasculitis
    Veno-occlusive disease
  Pleural disease
    Effusion
    Fibrosis
    Malignancy
  Chest wall disease
    Deformities (e.g., kyphoscoliosis)
    Abdominal "loading" (e.g., ascites, pregnancy, obesity)
  Respiratory muscle disease
    Neuromuscular disorders (e.g., myasthenia gravis, polio)
    Phrenic nerve dysfunction
    Weakness
Cardiovascular
  Decreased cardiac output
  Elevated pulmonary venous pressure
  Right-to-left shunt
Anemia
Anxiety/psychological
Deconditioning

From Mahler DA: Dyspnea: Diagnosis and management. Clin Chest Med 8:218, 1987, with permission.

Evaluation of Dyspnea

Acute Dyspnea
1. Comprehensive Hx & PE
2. CXR
   Based on the above, further testing may include:
3. Lab screening
   ABGs (evaluate A–a gradient, acidosis)
   CBC (anemia, polycythemia—chronic hypoxemia)
   Electrolytes (metabolic acidosis)
4. ECG
5. Spirogram

Chronic Dyspnea
In addition to the above, a variety of tests may be needed to diagnose and/or confirm the cause of chronic dyspnea. That testing should guided by Hx & PE and performed in a stepwise fashion. Other tests that may be beneficial in evaluating chronic dyspnea include:
1. Complete PFTs
2. Cardiopulmonary exercise testing
3. V/Q scan
4. Specialized PFTs:
   Bronchial inhalation challenge
   Tests of respiratory muscle strength
5. Cardiac testing
6. Other:
   Esophageal evaluation (reflux, aspiration)
   Evaluation of nose and sinuses
   Psychiatric evaluation

References: Pratter MR, et al: Cause and evaluation of chronic dyspnea in a pulmonary disease clinic. Arch Intern Med 149:2277–2282, 1989.
Burki NK: Dyspnea. Lung 165:269–277, 1987.

E

EDEMA

Edema is excess fluid that may be either localized to an extremity or anatomic region, such as the pleural or peritoneal cavity, or generalized over the entire body. Generalized edema typically first manifests in the most dependent area. Thus, pedal edema develops in the ambulatory patient, and presacral edema in the bedridden patient. Many conditions are capable of causing excess fluid accumulation.

Causes of Edema

Localized edema
1. Venous insufficiency
   - Varicose veins
2. Venous obstruction
   - Thrombophlebitis
   - Obstruction of IVC, SVC, or hepatic vein by clot or compression
3. Lymphatic obstruction
   - Filariasis
   - Tumor
   - Fibrosis secondary to radiotherapy
   - Status post lymph node dissection
4. Both venous and lymphatic blockage
   - Obstruction by mass lesion
5. Inflammatory
   - Response to injury or infection

Generalized edema
1. Volume overload
   - Congestive heart failure
   - Renal insufficiency
   - Cirrhosis of the liver
   - Drug induced (estrogens, minoxidil, nifedipine)
   - Hypothyroidism
   - Mineralocorticoid excess
   - Normal pregnancy
   - Toxemia of pregnancy
   - Iatrogenic (IV fluids)
2. Decreased plasma oncotic pressure
   - Hypoalbuminemia (<2.5 gm/dl)
a. Malnutrition
b. Protein loss (nephrotic syndrome, GI tract)
c. Decreased albumin synthesis (hepatic failure, cancer)
3. Increased capillary permeability
   - Sepsis, ARDS
   - Hypersensitivity reactions
   - Drugs (interleukin 2)
4. Idiopathic
   - Cyclic edema of women
   - Obesity

The therapy for edema must be directed at the underlying cause. The use of diuretics is helpful in many conditions, except if the serum albumin is less than 2.5 gm/dl. Diuretics must be used with caution if there is evidence of intravascular volume depletion, such as occurs in cirrhosis of the liver. Edema of the extremities can be treated with compression stockings if the resultant fluid shift to the central compartment will not be a danger to the patient.

ELECTROLYTE CONTENT OF BODY FLUIDS

There are basically two body fluid compartments: the intracellular fluid (ICF) and the extracellular fluid (ECF) compartments. The electrolyte content of ICF varies somewhat according to the organ from which the cells come. For example, thyroid cells have a concentration of inorganic iodide that is 30 times that in plasma. The ECF compartment can be further divided into the interstitial compartment (fluid in spaces between cells), the plasma compartment (the noncellular portion of the blood), and the transcellular compartment, which consists of secretions from epithelial cells. Ionic composition varies depending on the epithelial cell of origin. The GI tract is the great producer of transcellular fluids, secreting 5–8 liters per day. However, most of what is secreted is reabsorbed, helping to keep the body's ionic composition balanced. When there is vomiting, diarrhea, prolonged drainage of the biliary tree, small bowel or pancreatic fistulae, or loss of ileal fluids through an ileostomy, fluid and electrolyte derangements can occur. It is important to know the electrolyte composition of the various transcellular fluids so that the net effect of their losses can be projected and the appropriate replacements given.

Electrolyte Content of Transcellular Fluids

FLUID	Na^+ mEq/L	K^+ mEq/L	Cl^- mEq/L	HCO_3^- mEq/L
Saliva	20–80	10–20	20–40	20–60
Gastric juice	20–100	5–10	120–160	0
Bile	150	5–10	40–80	20–40
Pancreatic juice	120	5–10	10–60	80–120
Ileal fluid	140	5	105	40
Colonic fluid	140	5	85	60
Sweat	65	8	39	16

From Rose BD: Clinical Physiology of Acid-Base and Electrolyte Disorders, 3rd ed. New York, McGraw-Hill, 1989, p 23, with permission.

ENCEPHALITIS

Encephalitis is most commonly viral in origin and presents as a subacute picture of diffuse headache, fever, and altered mental status, sometimes progressing to focal neurologic findings and coma. Lumbar puncture is usually diagnostic, showing a mononuclear pleocytosis with normal glucose, protein, and Gram stain.

The commonest sporadic, isolated cause of encephalitis is herpes simplex virus. This is best recognized by its predilection for the temporal lobe, thereby leading to focal findings such as aphasia or hemiparesis superimposed upon the headache and fever. Imaging of the brain, such as with MRI or CT scan, often shows the temporal lobe destruction. Similarly, an EEG often shows focal temporal slowing, sometimes accompanied by evidence of brain irritation, such as spikes or epileptiform discharges. The CSF may provide additional confirmation, for, unlike most viral infections, it often shows a high percentage of PMNs and often has many RBCs from the focal temporal lobe destruction. A definitive diagnosis depends on brain biopsy, which is actually a rather straightforward procedure with little morbidity. However, at some institutions, cases of presumed herpes simplex encephalitis are treated empirically, without a definitive biopsy.

Therapy for herpes simplex is IV acyclovir 30 mg/kg/day for 14 days. The outcome depends heavily on the patient's mental status at the time treatment is initiated, because mild cases recover well but those with impaired mental status do poorly; there is therefore some urgency to initiate treatment as soon as possible.

Most other common viral encephalitides occur in outbreaks or epidemics, generally spread by vectors such as mosquitoes and generally attributable to arthropod-borne viruses. The commonest arboviral encephalitides in the United States are:

1. California (La Crosse) encephalitis
2. St. Louis encephalitis
3. Venezuelan encephalitis
4. Western equine encephalitis
5. Eastern equine encephalitis

Treatment for these encephalitides is largely supportive, without specific antiviral therapy.

Reference: Whitley RJ: Viral encephalitis. N Engl J Med 323:242–250, 1990.

ENDOCARDITIS, INFECTIVE

In the preantibiotic era, infective endocarditis was a uniformly fatal disease. However, mortality rates are still surprisingly high, and they persist at about 20%. Infective endocarditis is usually divided into native valve endocarditis (NVE) and prosthetic valve endocarditis (PVE). NVE is further categorized as acute (abrupt onset, prediagnosis course of only a few days) and subacute (insidious onset, prediagnosis course of up to 6 weeks). PVE is categorized as early (occurring within 60 days of valve replacement) and late (after 60 days).

Acute NVE can be caused by any microorganism, but the most common causative organism is *Staphylococcus aureus*. Bacteria causing acute NVE tend to be more invasive and can invade normal valves and endocardium. Often the patient gives a history of recent infection (e.g., furunculosis), and even more often nowadays is a history of recent instrumentation (e.g., central or peripheral IV lines) or IV drug abuse. Acute bacterial NVE is rapidly progressive and can be present even without a heart murmur. A new murmur, especially one of valvular insufficiency, which develops within a few days of the onset of a febrile illness is strongly suggestive of the diagnosis. When *S. aureus* is the causative organism, cutaneous manifestations are common and include pustular petechia and purulent purpura. Gram stain of material from these lesions often shows *S. aureus* and can be a help in diagnosis. Embolic events are common. Valvular insufficiency and heart failure often require valve replacement.

Subacute bacterial endocarditis (SBE) is most often caused by streptococcal species (including enterococci). Some sort of preexisting cardiac disease (it need not be a rheumatic valve) is found in about half of the patients. Recent studies suggest that an obvious portal of entry such as dental work is discovered in only a minority of patients, which may reflect the increasing attention to preprocedure antibiotic prophylaxis. The course is indolent. Fever is present in about three-fourths of patients. Anorexia is almost universal, and weight loss is common. Myalgias and arthralgias occur in about half the patients. Petechiae are common (Osler's nodes are not), and splenomegaly is present in about a third of patients. Anemia is common, but the median WBC count is only about 10,000 mm^3. Microscopic hematuria can be seen.

Coagulase-negative staphylococci are the most common causative organisms in early PVE. They are still common in late PVE, though *S. aureus* assumes the dominant role in late PVE.

Establishing a **definite** diagnosis of endocarditis requires histologic confirmation using material obtained at surgery or necropsy. **Probable** endocarditis requires at least two positive blood cultures and three of the following clinical findings: fever, a regurgitant murmur, splenomegaly, embolic lesions, and echocardiographically documented vegetations. It has been shown repeatedly that two-dimensional echocardiography is not a sensitive diagnostic test for endocarditis (one of our cardiologist friends says you can enhance sensitivity by sending the echo tape for culture!). Transesophageal echocardiography is better at showing vegetations.

References: Keys T: Diagnosis and management of infective endocarditis. Cleve Clin J Med 57:558–562, 1990.

Gentry LO, et al: New approaches to the diagnosis and treatment of infective endocarditis. Tex Heart Inst J 16:250–257, 1989.

Subacute Bacterial Endocarditis

SBE is an infection of the endocardium, usually occurring on previously abnormal heart valves. In contrast to acute endocarditis, the infecting organisms in SBE are of low virulence. The infection may go on for weeks or months before it is clinically recognized. The signs and symptoms are nonspecific and may include some or all of the following:

Signs and Symptoms of SBE

Anemia	Malaise	Proteinuria
Embolic episodes	Microscopic hematuria	Roth spots (rare)
Heart failure	Mycotic aneurysms	Splenomegaly
Heart murmurs	Petechiae	Splinter hemorrhages
Low-grade fever	(+) Rheumatoid factor	Weight loss

SBE develops during periods of transient bacteremia, when organisms infect sterile platelet and fibrin thrombi that have formed on valvular lesions.

Conditions Predisposing to SBE

Aortic sclerosis	Patent ductus arteriosus
Rheumatic fever	Mitral valve prolapse
Interventricular septal defects	Prosthetic heart valve
IV drug abuse	Previous history of endocarditis
Severe pulmonary HTN	Other congenital heart disease
Syphilitic aortitis	IHSS

Most Frequent Causes of SBE

ORGANISM	COMMENT
1. *Streptococcus viridans: S. sanguis, S. mutans, S. salivarius*	Normal dental flora
2. *S. bovis*	From GI tract: $^{1}/_{3}$ of patients have colon cancer or polyp
3. Enterococci[1]	From GU or GI tract
4. *Staphylococcus epidermidis*	Normal skin flora

[1]Often associated with acute endocarditis.

However, almost any species of bacteria can cause SBE, including:

Streptococcus pneumoniae	*Serratia marcescens*
Neisseria gonorrhoeae	*Bacteroides*
Enteric gram-negative bacteria	*Hemophilus*
Pseudomonas	*Brucella*
Salmonella	*Mycobacterium*
Streptobacillus	*Listeria*
N. meningiditis	Diphtheroids
Legionella	*Coxiella burnetii*
Spirillum minor	

Nonbacterial organisms may also cause subacute endocarditis, including chlamydiae (*Chlamydia psittaci, C. trachomatis*) and fungi. *Candida* and *Aspergillus* endocarditis occur in patients on long-term broad-spectrum antibiotics, chronic steroids, or cytotoxic chemotherapy.

The diagnosis of SBE is made with blood cultures and echocardiography. Treatment involves antibiotic administration, usually over a period of 4–6 weeks. Surgery is required in cases of fungal endocarditis, resistant organisms, CHF, recurrent septic emboli, or infection of a prosthetic valve. Patients with known valvular heart disease or prior history of endocarditis should receive antibiotic prophylaxis before undergoing procedures that might expose them to bacteremia. This includes dental manipulation and surgery of the respiratory, GI, and GU tracts.

References: Keys TF: Diagnosis and management of infective endocarditis. Cleve Clin J Med 57:558–562, 1990.

Birrer RB, et al: Infective endocarditis. J Fam Pract 24:289–295, 1987.

Prophylaxis in Patients with Valvular Heart Disease

Contaminated surgical procedures, dental procedures, and instrumentations of mucosal surfaces are often associated with transient bacteremia. During such episodes, bacteria may lodge on abnormal heart valves or endocardial surfaces and cause bacterial endocarditis. Preventing such occurrences is based on a strategy of (1) knowing which cardiac abnormalities place patients at risk for endocarditis, (2) knowing which procedures are likely to be associated with transient bacteremia, (3) knowing the bacteria most often implicated in endocarditis acquired in this setting, and (4) providing appropriate antibiotic coverage during the time bacteremia is most likely to occur.

Not all cardiac abnormalities place patients at risk for endocarditis (see following table). Those that do place them at risk include prosthetic heart valves (mechanical and tissue), previous endocarditis, most congenital cardiac malformations, rheumatic and other acquired valvular dysfunction, hypertrophic cardiomyopathy, and MVP with valvular regurgitation. Prophylaxis is not recommended for patients with previous CABG, a pacemaker, MVP when regurgitation or leaflet thickening is absent, or innocent heart murmurs.

The procedures for which persons at risk should receive antibiotic prophylaxis include dental procedures likely to cause bleeding (including cleaning), operations or procedures involving respiratory mucosa, GI mucosa (including sclerotherapy for varices, esophageal dilatation, cholecystectomy, and bile duct procedures), and GU mucosa (including urethral dilatation, urethral catheterization if infection is present, prostatic surgery, vaginal hysterectomy, and vaginal delivery if infection is present). Prophylaxis is not required for cardiac catheterization and is also not currently recommended for fiberoptic bronchoscopy or upper or lower GI endoscopy, with or without biopsy (see following table).

Viridans streptococci are the most common cause of SBE acquired after dental procedures or invasive procedures involving the respiratory mucosa; enterococci are most commonly observed after GI or GU procedures. Amoxicillin (3.0 g orally 1 hr before the procedure, then 1.5 g 6 hr after the initial dose) is the standard prophylactic regimen for dental, oral, and upper respiratory tract procedures. The standard regimen for GU and GI procedures is IV or IM ampicillin 2 g plus gentamicin 1.5 mg/kg (up to 80 mg) 30 minutes before the procedure, followed by amoxicillin 1.5 g 6 hours after the initial antibiotics. Alternatively, the parenteral regimen can be repeated 8 hours after the initial dose.

Recommendations for Endocarditis Prophylaxis
for Cardiac Conditions and Procedures

I. Cardiac Conditions
Endocarditis prophylaxis recommended
- Prosthetic cardiac valves, including bioprosthetic and homograph valves
- Previous infective endocarditis, even in the absence of heart disease
- Surgically constructed systemic-pulmonary shunts or conduits
- Most congenital cardiac malformations
- Rheumatic and other acquired valvular dysfunction, even after valvular surgery
- Hypertrophic cardiomyopathy
- Mitral valve prolapse with valvular regurgitation

Table continued on next page.

*Recommendations for Endocarditis Prophylaxis
for Cardiac Conditions and Procedures (Cont.)*

Endocarditis prophylaxis not recommended
- Isolated secundum atrial septal defect
- Surgical repair without residua beyond 6 months of secundum atrial septal defect, ventricular septal defect, or patent ductus arteriosus
- Previous coronary artery bypass graft surgery
- Mitral valve prolapse without valvular regurgitation
- Physiologic, functional, or innocent heart murmurs
- Previous Kawasaki disease without valvular dysfunction
- Cardiac pacemakers and implanted defibrillators

II. Dental or Surgical Procedures

Endocarditis prophylaxis recommended
- Dental procedures known to induce gingival or mucosal bleeding, including professional cleaning
- Tonsillectomy and/or adenoidectomy
- Surgical operations that involve GI or respiratory mucosa
- Bronchoscopy with a rigid bronchoscope
- Sclerotherapy for esophageal varices
- Esophageal dilatation
- Gallbladder surgery
- Cystoscopy
- Urethral dilatation
- Urethral catheterization or urinary tract surgery if UTI is present
- Prostatic surgery
- Incision and drainage of infected tissue
- Vaginal hysterectomy
- Vaginal delivery in the presence of infection

Endocarditis prophylaxis not recommended
- Dental procedures not likely to induce gingival bleeding, such as simple adjustment of orthodontic appliances or fillings above the gum line
- Injections of local intraoral anesthetic (except intraligamentary injections)
- Shedding of primary teeth
- Tympanostomy tube insertion
- Endotracheal intubation
- Bronchoscopy with a flexible bronchoscope, with or without biopsy
- Cardiac catheterization
- GI endoscopy with or without biopsy
- Caesarean section
- In the absence of infection for urethral catheterization, dilatation and curettage, uncomplicated vaginal delivery, therapeutic abortion, sterilization procedures, or insertion or removal of intrauterine devices

Recommended Standard Prophylactic Regimen for Dental, Oral, or Upper Respiratory Tract Procedures in Patients Who Are at Risk for Infective Endocarditis

Standard regimen

Amoxicillin	3.0 g orally 1 hr before procedure; then 1.5 g 6 hr after initial dose

Amoxicillin/penicillin-allergic patients

Erythromycin	Erythromycin ethylsuccinate 800 mg or erythromycin stearate 1.0 g orally 2 hr before procedure; then half the dose 6 hr after initial dose
or	
Clindamycin	300 mg orally 1 hr before procedure and 150 mg 6 hr after initial dose

Table continued on next page.

*Recommended Standard Prophylactic Regimen for Dental, Oral,
or Upper Respiratory Tract Procedures in Patients Who Are at Risk
for Infective Endocarditis (Cont.)*

Patients unable to take oral medications

Ampicillin IV or IM ampicillin, 2.0 g 30 min before procedure; then 1.0 g IV or IM *or* 1.5 g PO, 6 hr after initial dose

Ampicillin/amoxicillin/penicillin-allergic patients unable to take oral medications

Clindamycin IV clindamycin, 300 mg 30 min before procedure and IV or PO clindamycin 150 mg 6 hr after initial dose

Patients considered high risk and not candidates for standard regimen

Ampicillin, IV or IM administration of ampicillin, 2.0 g plus gentamicin 1.5 mg/kg gentamicin, and (not to exceed 80 mg) 30 min before procedure, followed by and amox- amoxicillin 1.5 g orally 6 hr after initial dose; alternatively, the parenteral icillin regimen may be repeated 8 hr after initial dose

Ampicillin/amoxicillin/penicillin-allergic patients considered high risk

Vancomycin IV vancomycin, 1.0 g over 1 hr, starting 1 hr before procedure; no repeat dose necessary

---

*Regimens for Genitourinary/Gastrointestinal Procedures
for Endocarditis Prophylaxis*

Standard regimen

Ampicillin, IV or IM ampicillin 2.0 g plus gentamicin 1.5 mg/kg (not to exceed 80 gentamcin, mg) 30 min before procedure, followed by amoxicillin, 1.5 g PO 6 hr and amox- after initial dose; alternatively, the parenteral regimen may be repeated icillin once 8 hr after initial dose

Ampicillin/amoxicillin/penicillin-allergic patient regimen

Vancomycin IV vancomycin, 1.0 g over 1 hr plus IV or IM gentamicin 1.5 mg/kg (not andgentami- to exceed 80 mg), 1 hr before procedure; may be repeated once 8 hr after cin initial dose

Alternative low-risk patient regimen

Amoxicillin 3.0 g PO 1 hour before procedure; then 1.5 g 6 hr after initial dose

---

Preceding three tables from Dajani AS, et al: Prevention of bacterial endocarditis. JAMA 264:2919–2922, 1990, with permission.

Kaye D, et al: Prevention of bacterial endocarditis. Ann Intern Med 114:803–804, 1991.

EOSINOPHILIA

Causes

Eosinophilia exists when the absolute number of eosinophils is 500/mm^3 of blood or greater. The principal functions of eosinophils are (1) destruction of the larvae of helminths and (2) modification of hypersensitivity reactions.

Important Causes of Eosinophilia

Parasitic infections
1. Metazoan
   a. Nematodes: strongyloidiasis, visceral larva migrans (toxocariasis), ascariasis, hookworm disease, trichinosis
   b. Cestodes: cysticercosis, echinococcosis, taeniasis
2. Protozoan: pneumocystis, amebiasis, toxoplasmosis

Allergic disorders
1. Asthma
2. Allergic rhinitis
3. Urticaria
4. Eczema

Connective tissue disorders
1. Allergic granulomatosis (Churg-Strauss syndrome)
2. Polyarteritis nodosa
3. Allergic vasculitis
4. Eosinophilic fasciitis
5. Eosinophilic connective tissue disease

Malignancies
1. Eosinophilic leukemia
2. Hodgkin's disease
3. Lymphoid malignancies
4. Carcinomas

Familial

Other
1. Löffler's syndrome
2. Pulmonary infiltrates with eosinophilia
3. Löffler's endocarditis
4. Eosinophilic gastroenteritis
5. Dermatitis herpetiformis
6. Hypereosinophilic syndrome

EPISTAXIS

Epistaxis is a frequent clinical problem; the nasal cavity is often a site of spontaneous hemorrhage, second only to the uterine cervix. The arteries that supply the nasal cavity are the terminal branches of the external and internal carotid systems. The vessels of the nasal cavity have very little surface protection. Directly beneath the mucosa of the nasal cavity is the thin fibrous layer that contains the vascular supply to the septum. These vessels also lack the supporting connective tissue common in other parts of the body, prohibiting the contractile response characteristically seen in traumatized vessels.

Epistaxis may be due to either local or systemic etiologies. Most bleeding results from mechanical factors, such as drying of the nasal mucosa by overheated air or digital trauma. In these instances, bleeding starts from a mucosal vessel in the anterior aspect of the nasal septum (Kiesselbach's plexus). Following trauma, epistaxis may indicate either damage to the orbit or maxillary sinus with bleeding through the sinus ostia or fracture of the temporal bone with blood draining from the middle ear into the nose via the eustachian tube. Children and mentally impaired patients should always be examined for foreign bodies. Spontaneous bleeding from deep in the nasal cavity is most frequent in the elderly population and is usually profuse. The most common associated cause is HTN.

In managing such patients, the practitioner should determine whether the bleeding is anterior or posterior and whether or not the bleeding is life threatening. Anterior bleeding usually ceases spontaneously or with direct pressure. Compressing the nose or applying cotton gauze soaked with epinephrine is usually effective. A clearly defined bleeding point can be cauterized by silver nitrate or electric cautery—after topical nasal anesthesia. If bleeding is vigorous, packing can be used, in either the anterior or posterior position. It is to be noted that posterior bleeding and subsequent packing can be associated with morbidity and mortality due to the significant effect posterior packs have on pulmonary physiology. Most cases have uncomplicated causes, occur in readily accessible sites in the nose, and are easily stopped.

Differential Diagnosis of Epistaxis

LOCAL	SYSTEMIC
Mechanical factors	Inflammatory states
Drying	Acute and chronic rhinitis
Digital trauma	Common cold
Barometric changes	Influenza
Foreign bodies	Mononucleosis
Drug-induced septal perforation	Vascular
Caustic chemical erosion	HTN/atherosclerosis
Trauma	Hereditary telangiectasia
Facial fractures	Menstruation
Iatrogenic causes	Coagulation dysfunction
Septal deformity	Hemophilia
Tumors	Hepatic disease
Benign nasal polyps	Uremia
Malignant neoplasms	Leukemia
Juvenile nasopharyngeal angiofibromas	Drug induced
	Heparin/warfarin
	Aspirin
	Penicillin and analogs

EPSTEIN-BARR VIRUS INFECTION

Serologic Diagnosis

The diagnosis of infection due to EBV depends on clinical presentation of fever, sore throat, lymphadenopathy, and malaise in association with laboratory findings of atypical lymphocytosis. About 90% of patients will have heterophile antibodies present at some point in the illness. Commercially available spot tests are available that are sensitive and specific. In heterophile-negative patients, it may be necessary to evaluate for EBV antibodies in order to establish a diagnosis.

Interpretation of Epstein-Barr Virus Serology

ANTIBODY SPECIFICITY	TIME OF APPEARANCE	% POS. HETEROPHILE SEROLOGY*	LENGTH OF PERSISTENCE	COMMENTS
Viral capsid antigen (VCA)				
IgM	Clinical presentation	100	4–8 wk	Sensitive and specific
IgG	Clinical presentation	100	Lifelong	Most useful as epidemiologic tool but not for diagnosis
Early antigen (EA)				
Anti-D	Peaks 3–4 wk after onset	70	3–6 mo	Correlates with severe disease and nasopharyngeal carcinoma

Table continued on next page.

Interpretation of Epstein-Barr Virus Serology (Cont.)

ANTIBODY SPECIFICITY	TIME OF APPEARANCE	% POS. HETEROPHILE SEROLOGY*	LENGTH OF PERSISTENCE	COMMENTS
Anti-R	Peaks 2 wk to several mo after onset	Low	2 mo to >3 yr	Correlates with African Burkitt's lymphoma
Epstein-Barr nuclear Ag (EBNA)	3–4 wk after onset	100	Lifelong	Late appearance helpful in diagnosis of heterophile-negative cases
Heterophile antibodies	Peak at 2–3 wk	> 90	Gradually disappear over 24 mo.	Most convenient and cost-effective test for acute diagnosis

*Percentage of patients with EBV-associated mononucleosis who have a positive heterophile serology.

Modified from Schooley RT, et al: Epstein-Barr virus (infectious mononucleosis). In Mandell GH, et al (eds): Principles and Practice of Infectious Diseases, 3rd ed. New York, Churchill Livingstone, 1990, p 1179.

ERYTHROCYTOSIS

Causes of Erythrocytosis

I. Primary
  A. Polycythemia vera
  B. Familial polycythemia with normal hemoglobin function
II. Secondary
  A. Physiologic
      1. Altitude (hypobaric)
      2. Sleep apnea
      3. Chronic pulmonary disease with hypoxemia
      4. Right to left shunts
          a. Congenital heart defects
          b. AV malformations
      5. Carboxy hemoglobin
      6. High-affinity hemoglobin
  B. Inappropriate elaboration of erythropoietin
      1. Hepatoma
      2. Renal carcinoma
      3. Cerebellar hemangioma
      4. Leiomyoma of the uterus
      5. Renal cysts
      6. Polycystic kidney disease
      7. Renal allograft rejection
  C. Other
      1. Bartter's syndrome
      2. Cobalt
      3. Anabolic steroids
      4. Danazol
      5. Erythropoietin administration

The approach to the patient with an elevated Hct is a challenge to the internist and often a challenge to the patient, who has difficulty comprehending the problem of "too much blood." The algorithm on p. 220 outlines the approach to such patients.

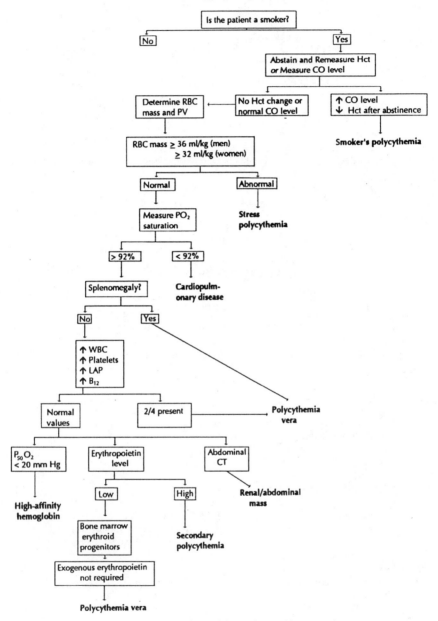

Approach to the patient with an elevated hematocrit.

Two pitfalls must be avoided: First, internists are accustomed to caring for sick patients who are often mildly anemic, so there is sometimes a tendency to overreact to hematocrits in the upper normal range. When the hematocrit is >60% in a man and >55% in a woman, an investigation will be rewarding. Men with hematocrit of 53–60% and women with slightly lower hematocrit should undergo measurement of the RBC mass by a ^{51}Cr-labeled RBC method and plasma volume (PV) determination by dilution of ^{131}I-labeled albumin. An increased RBC mass should be pursued. An RBC mass at the upper limits of normal with a reduced PV is typical of stress polycythemia (Gaisböck's polycythemia). Although patients with stress polycythemia do not require further investigation of their erythrocytosis, their condition should not be dismissed. Such patients may be at high risk for cardiovascular events. The role of phlebotomy has not been clarified in such patients.

The second pitfall concerns the smoking patient. Carbon monoxide generated by cigarette or cigar smoke produces erythrocytosis and may be a significant factor in patients who seem to have stress erythrocytosis. The amount of carbon monoxide correlates with the number of cigarettes consumed. The typical patient with smoker's polycythemia smokes one pack per day or greater. The hematocrit can be repeated a month or so after smoking cessation. If this is not possible, measurement of the carboxy hemoglobin level should be undertaken. In a patient with erythrocytosis with an elevated RBC mass, the workup depends on clues from the patient's Hx & PE and CBC.

Important findings from the history: A family history of polycythemia suggests the presence of a high-affinity hemoglobin. High-affinity hemoglobins show a left-shifted relationship between oxygenation and hemoglobin saturation, which can be ascertained by determining the $P_{50}O_2$. It is important to know that these hemoglobins are often the result of an amino acid substitution that does not alter electrophoretic mobility. Thus, a routine hemoglobin electrophoresis is not as helpful as a determination of the $P_{50}O_2$. Familial erythrocytosis with normal hemoglobin function also occurs. These patients may have erythroid cells that have erythropoietin receptors with increased sensitivity.

Some obvious reasons for a high hematocrit established from a patient's history include residence at high altitude, history of significant pulmonary disease (including sleep apnea), and congenital heart disease. Athletes and body builders should be questioned carefully about use of anabolic steroids or even surreptitious use of recombinant erythropoietin to enhance performance. Occasional patients receiving the attenuated androgen danazol for immune thrombocytopenia have developed erythrocytosis. Rare individuals who are infected with HIV have been reported with erythrocytosis, which, instead of the usual anemia, also occurs while taking AZT.

Important physical findings: During the physical exam, careful attention must be paid to the spleen. If splenomegaly is present, then polycythemia vera is the most important diagnosis to consider. It would be unfortunate to miss enlarged polycystic kidneys, the hepatic bruit of a hepatoma, or the presence of a uterine leiomyoma. Another important indication of myeloproliferative disease is the presence of erythromelalgia, a distinctive syndrome of pain, warmth, redness, or burning of the extremities. These symptoms respond dramatically to tiny doses of aspirin. The presence of gout and hyperuricemia in the patient with erythrocytosis also suggests myeloproliferative disease.

Importance of the laboratory evaluation: The platelet count or WBC count, if elevated, suggests a myeloproliferative disorder. The presence of eosinophilia, basophilia, or atypical platelet morphology may also indicate polycythemia vera. Some patients who have polycythemia vera have a tendency to bleed and may be iron deficient. These patients present with thrombocytosis (often "platelet million-aires") and are labeled as having essential thrombocythemia until iron replacement results in polycythemia. In patients with cardiopulmonary disease, oxygen saturation is a useful determination. If it is <92%, secondary polycythemia is likely.

Recently, erythropoietin radioimmunoassay has been touted as a means to differentiate primary from secondary polycythemic disorders. Unfortunately, there is overlap between the low levels seen in polycythemia vera and the normal range, although a very high erythropoietin level makes the diagnosis of polycythemia vera unlikely. Patients with pulmonary disease and chronic hypoxemia frequently have normal erythropoietin levels. Patients with congenital heart disease and right to left shunts do have elevated levels, but the diagnosis of secondary polycythemia seldom requires the erythropoietin level to be drawn.

Polycythemia Vera

This is a clonal disorder marked by expansion of erythropoiesis and often by leukocytosis and thrombocytosis. The criteria espoused by the Polycythemia Vera Study Group are displayed in the table that follows. These criteria are stringent and intended for use in selecting patients for the study of treatment or natural history. Some patients will not fulfill these requirements but nevertheless have polycythemia vera and are likely to benefit from phlebotomy. Occasionally, CML is associated with erythrocytosis in addition to leukocytosis. Such patients demonstrate the Philadelphia chromosome on cytogenetic analysis of bone marrow or peripheral blood cells.

Polycythemia Study Group Criteria

Polycythemia vera is diagnosed if all three category A criteria or if criteria A1 + A2 and two category B criteria are present.

Category A
1. Increased RBC mass (≥36 ml/kg in men, ≥32 ml/kg in women)
2. Normal oxygen saturation (≥92%)
3. Splenomegaly

Category B
1. Increased platelet count (>400,000/μl)
2. Increased WBC count (>12,000/μl)
3. Elevated leukocyte alkaline phosphatase score (>100)
4. Increased vitamin B_{12}:
   B_{12} >900 pg/ml
   B_{12} binding capacity >2,200 pg/ml

Reference: Berk PD, et al: Therapeutic recommendations in polycythemia vera based on Polycythemia Vera Study Group protocols. Semin Hematol 23:132–143, 1986.

Polycythemia vera sometimes evolves into acute leukemia, usually myelogenous. This tendency is influenced by the treatment of the erythrocytosis. If ^{32}P or alkylating agents are used, then there is a higher transformation rate to leukemia. Most hematologists employ hydroxyurea in the management of patients who require chemotherapy. This form of treatment may have fewer leukemogenic effects than treatment with busulphan. Other patients evolve into a picture resembling myelofibrosis. These patients with "spent polycythemia" may develop anemia, myeloid metaplasia, and troublesome splenomegaly.

Stroke and other thrombotic events are also frequent in polycythemia vera, particularly in patients whose erythrocytosis is poorly controlled. Phlebotomy with a goal of reducing the hematocrit to 45% reduces the risk of thrombosis. When phlebotomy is used as treatment, excessive thrombocytosis may occur. In circumstances when the risk of stroke is high (those who have a history of TIAs or previous strokes or have other risk factors such as HTN), the treatment of polycythemia consists of judicious phlebotomy followed by administration of hydroxyurea.

Like other myeloproliferative disorders, the tendency to thrombosis has an imperfect relationship to the platelet count or to known aspects of platelet function. An early trial of aspirin in asymptomatic patients with polycythemia vera met with failure because bleeding complications far outweighed the benefit of antiplatelet therapy. Patients who show evidence of thrombosis may benefit from antiplatelet drug therapy. Hemorrhage is also a complication of untreated, poorly controlled polycythemia vera. Elective surgery should be deferred in such patients until the blood volume has been adequately controlled.

Renal Causes of Erythrocytosis

Physicians, knowing that the kidney is the major source of erythropoietin, expect to find anemia associated with renal dysfunction. In some renal disorders, erythrocytosis occurs. These include cysts and polycystic disease of the kidney, renal artery stenosis, and renal carcinoma. During allograft rejection, erythropoietin levels may increase dramatically and cause significant erythrocytosis. In the approach to the patient who has erythrocytosis but in whom the diagnosis of polycythemia vera is unlikely, a CT or ultrasound to look at the abdomen can be helpful.

Reference: Cotes PM, et al: Determination of serum immunoreactive erythropoietin in the investigation of erythrocytosis. N Engl J Med 315: 283–287, 1986.

ERYTHROPOIETIN

Indications for Use

The purification of erythropoietin, the localization of its gene, and the clonal expression of this gene to produce a recombinant erythropoietin for clinical use represent one of the triumphs of modern molecular biology and medicine. Initial clinical use was in the treatment of the anemia of chronic renal failure. Other uses of erythropoietin are summarized as follows:

Clinical Applications of Erythropoietin

Treatment of anemia associated with:	.
Chronic renal failure	Chronic disease (RA)
AIDS-related anemia	Malignancy
Prematurity	
Other	
Presurgical patients	Autologous blood donors
Sickle-cell anemia	Myelodysplastic syndromes

Chronic renal failure: The kidneys are the major source of erythropoietin, although extrarenal sources such as the liver may account for 10% of the circulating erythropoietin level. In most ESRD patients, anemia is present and the erythropoietin level is low. In polycystic kidney disease, the degree of anemia may not be as severe as in other forms of renal failure due to the increased production of erythropoietin associated with the renal cysts. Nevertheless, patients on or before dialysis who have significant anemia will respond to IV or SC erythropoietin. Although expensive, the treatment of the anemia has definite advantages. Improvements in exercise tolerance, sense of well-being, and, in some individuals, sexual function have been observed. Chronic renal failure and dialysis patients who had transfusion requirements before treatment no longer required such support while on erythropoietin. The bleeding diathesis of uremia is also improved by an increase in hematocrit during treatment. Response to erythropoietin may be blunted by concomitant iron deficiency, hyperparathyroidism, infection, inflammation, folate deficiency, or aluminum toxicity.

Anemia of chronic disease: The availability of recombinant erythropoietin has also facilitated a generation of better immuno-diagnostic tests for serum erythropoietin levels. As a result, it was noticed that in some circumstances, the erythropoietin level did not seem to be appropriately elevated for the degree of anemia. The anemia of chronic disease associated with RA is just such a disorder, and several reports demonstrate the efficacy of erythropoietin in that condition.

Anemia of AIDS: Anemia is a feature of AIDS. Patients who are receiving zidovudine may require blood transfusions for the associated anemia. Studies of AIDS patients suggest that their erythropoietin level is inappropriately low and that those patients with levels below 500 mU/ml benefit from treatment.

Anemia of malignancy: Surveys of patients with solid tumors, with multiple myeloma, or receiving cisplatinum chemotherapy demonstrated a lower than expected erythropoietin level. Treatment of such patients appears both to reduce the transfusion requirements created by chemotherapy and to improve well-being. It has also been used after bone marrow transplant to hasten the recovery of erythropoiesis by the donor marrow and to reduce the requirement for transfusions.

Anemia of prematurity: The premature infant also has a low level, due presumably to immature kidneys and failure to produce erythropoietin. The anemia of prematurity also responds to erythropoietin treatment.

Other applications: Patients who are about to undergo elective surgery often opt to participate in an autologous blood donation program. The ability to obtain several units of blood before surgery and to undergo surgery with a favorable hematocrit level may be enhanced by use of recombinant erythropoietin. Studies are under way to determine whether some anemic individuals who cannot donate blood preoperatively will be helped by presurgical erythropoietin treatment. An important misuse of erythropoietin that needs to be discouraged by physicians is the self-administration undertaken by endurance athletes—the pharmacological equivalent of "blood doping."

Erythropoietin has received attention from physicians who are interested in the treatment of sickle-cell disease. Alone in high doses or in lower doses in conjunction with hydroxyurea therapy, it appears to increase the hemoglobin F level in such patients. If sufficiently increased, these higher levels of hemoglobin F may ameliorate the sickling of hemoglobin S. Modest success has been achieved by the use of erythropoietin to improve erythropoiesis in myelodysplastic syndromes.

Complications: Initiation of erythropoietin therapy may be associated with a flulike syndrome and mild bone pain. High-dose therapy and rapid increase in the hematocrit in renal failure patients may be accompanied by exacerbation of HTN and seizures. Generally speaking, however, erythropoietin is a safe and well-tolerated therapeutic agent.

Reference: Erslev AJ: Erythropoietin. N Engl J Med 324:1939–1944, 1991.

ESOPHAGEAL CANCER

Risk Factors for Esophageal Squamous Cell Carcinoma

Male sex
Blacks > whites
High-risk geographic location: Iran,
   Northern China, former Soviet Union, South Africa
Low socioeconomic class
Tobacco (smoking and chewing)
Alcoholism
Betel nut chewing
Tylosis
Achalasia
Lye strictures
Squamous cell carcinoma of the head and neck
Plummer-Vinson syndrome

Risk Factors for Adenocarcinoma of the Esophagus

Barrett's esophagus	Male sex
White > black	? Smoking

ESOPHAGEAL VARICES

Treatment and Diagnostic Steps

Portal HTN—the increase in pressure in the portal system—manifests itself clinically by the development of portal-systemic collaterals. One of these collaterals is esophageal varices, which occur in 40% of cirrhotics. About 35% of cirrhotic patients with varices will have bleeding varices over a 2-year period. The chance of a first variceal bleeding can be decreased by propranolol or nadolol in a dose that decreases the resting pulse by 25%.

In the patient with liver disease presenting with an upper GI bleed, endoscopy is needed to confirm the diagnosis, because only 50% will be bleeding from varices. At endoscopy, treatment should be initiated with either sclerotherapy or band ligation of the varices. If this does not control bleeding or is not available, IV vasopressin at 0.4 IU/min with IV nitroglycerin at 40 mg/min or, alternatively, somatostatin at 200 mg/hr can be used. If these steps fail to control bleeding, a Sengstaken-Blakemore tube can be inserted and the patient prepared for a radiologically placed transjugular intrahepatic portosystemic stent (TIPS), repeat efforts at sclerotherapy, or band ligation. If these modalities are unavailable, thought should be given to esophageal transection or surgical portocaval shunting. After the initial bleeding has been controlled, varices should be eradicated by biweekly banding or sclerotherapy. If the patient develops bleeding gastric varices or bleeding portal gastropathy, TIPS or surgical shunting becomes necessary.

ETHANOL ABUSE

Alcohol abuse is a serious medical and psychological problem that most practicing physicians will encounter frequently. It may go unrecognized for long periods of time, with hints to its presence manifesting as employment instability due to absenteeism, recurrent injuries, marital distress, or driver's license suspension. In the United States, nearly 5% of the population abuse this drug, with an associated death rate exceeded only by those of vascular disease and cancer.

Medical Complications of Ethanol Abuse

Heart
   Cardiomyopathy
   Arrhythmia ("holiday heart")
   Hyperlipidemia
   Hypertension

Gastrointestinal
   Gastritis/peptic ulcer disease
   Hepatitis/cirrhosis/fatty liver
   Pancreatitis
   Head/neck/esophageal/liver cancer
   Malabsorption/chronic diarrhea

Blood
   Iron or folate deficiency
   Hypersplenism
   Bone marrow depression and cytopenias
   Prothrombin deficiency

Endocrine
   Male sexual impairment
   Increased fetal risk

Immune system
   Increased susceptibility to infection
   Impaired healing

Electrolyte disturbances
   Hypocalcemia
   Hypomagnesemia
   Hypophosphatemia
   Hypoglycemia
   Acute water intoxication
   Alcoholic hyperosmolality
   Alcoholic ketoacidosis

Neurologic
   Amblyopia and optic atrophy
   Progressive cerebral degeneration
   Peripheral neuropathy/myopathy
   Withdrawal seizures
   Dementia/hallucinosis: Wernicke-Korsakoff disease (confusion, external ophthalmoplegia, and nystagmus)
   Parenchymatous cerebellar degeneration
   Cerebral leukodystrophy

Modified from Andreoli TE, et al (eds): Cecil Essentials of Medicine, 2nd ed. Philadelphia, W. B. Saunders, 1990, pp 701–702.

Alcohol exerts its destructive effects on the body primarily by nutritional deprivation, although direct toxicity may also play a role. It interferes with proper food, vitamin, and trace mineral intake, and it decreases absorption of ingested glucose, amino acids, calcium, folate, and vitamin B_{12} from the gut. Acute severe intoxication (blood alcohol levels greater than 300–500 mg/dl) may result in death from central respiratory depression.

Additional complications of alcohol are related to various withdrawal syndromes, which may make an unexpected appearance during hospitalization for a possibly unrelated cause. Those syndromes may be classified as follows:

1. **Minor withdrawal:** Associated with tremulousness, insomnia, and irritability usually resolving within 48 hours of last ingestion of alcohol but may last for up to 14 days. Managed with reassurance and benzodiazepines—either chlordiazepoxide 25–100 mg PO Q 6–8 hr or diazepam 5–20 mg PO Q 6–8 hr—with the dosage titrated to avoid excessive sedation. Thiamine 100 mg IM or PO plus multivitamins with folic acid must also be administered.

2. **Rum fits:** Withdrawal seizures usually occurring 12–24 hours after the last drink; commonly of the grand mal type. Managed with standard doses of diazepam—with the addition of alternative anticonvulsants (e.g., phenytoin) only if seizures are prolonged or frequent. Consideration should be given to brain CT

scanning and CSF evaluation, especially if there is associated fever, suspected head trauma, or focal seizures.

3. **Delirium tremens:** Associated with marked tremulousness, confusion, fever, tachycardia, and visual hallucinations, usually occurring 3–5 days after the last ingestion of alcohol. Sedation with necessary doses of diazepam, sometimes as much as 1,200 mg during the first 2–3 days (5–10 mg IV initially, followed by 5 mg IV Q 5–10 min to control symptoms, then 5–10 mg IV Q 1–4 hr to maintain sedation, and changing to 5–10 mg PO Q 6–8 hr when appropriate). Close attention must be paid to associated medical conditions (e.g., trauma, infection) by means of proper evaluation, fluid management, and vitamin supplementation with thiamine 100 mg IM or PO daily, multivitamin supplements, and folic acid.

4. **Acute alcoholic hallucinosis:** Usually auditory but may be visual, tactile, or olfactory, occurring 3–5 days after the last ingestion of alcohol. Associated with less autonomic hyperactivity and mental agitation than are DTs.

Outpatient treatment of alcoholism is difficult and may require joint employer/ family confrontation of the alcoholic. Referral to experienced therapists is frequently necessary. Participation in support and reinforcement groups such as AA (Alcoholics Anonymous) can be effective in preventing relapse. The use of disulfiram (Antabuse) may be appropriate in severe, refractory cases.

F

FALLS

One-third of the community-dwelling elderly older than age 75 falls each year, with half of those suffering multiple falls. However, only 5% of falls result in fractures. Wrist fractures are common in patients aged 65–75, whereas hip fractures are most common in those over age 75.

Factors Potentially Contributing to Falls

- Age changes: ↑ sway, ↑ response time to postural challenges, gait alterations
- Neurologic lesions: strokes, CVA, parkinsonism, cerebellar disease, NPH, lumbar stenosis, vitamin B_{12} deficiency
- Premonitory fall: marks presence of otherwise asymptomatic systemic illness such as pneumonia, UTI, MI
- Osteoarthritis of hip/knees/muscular weakness
- Sensory changes: ↓ visual, ↓ proprioception, ↓ vestibular function
- Postural hypotension
- Dementia
- Drugs: antipsychotics, diuretics, anti-HTNs, tricyclic antidepressants, sedatives, oral hypoglycemics, ethanol
- Environment: home visit needed for evaluation

Assessment of the elderly patient who has fallen includes:

- Current medical problems and medications
- Description of prior falls (if applicable)
- Description and circumstances of current fall: time of day, location, specific activity (toileting, stairs, exercise), witnesses, environmental hazards, and associated symptoms
- Did the patient know he or she was going to fall?
- After fall: Inquire whether the patient knew what happened, was able to get up right away, or had any pain or injury.
- If loss of consciousness occurs: Think syncope.
- If loss of bladder or bowel control occurs: Think seizures.
- Complete physical exam (including neurological and mental status)

Causes or Types of Falls

Accident or environment related	36.9%
Weakness, balance/gait	12.3%
Drop attack	11.4%
Dizziness/vertigo	7.7%
Postural change/orthostatic hypotension	5.1%
CNS lesion	1.2%

Table continued on next page.

Causes or Types of Falls (Cont.)

Syncope	1.0%
Unknown	8.0%
Miscellaneous (acute illness, confusion, poor vision, drugs)	18.0%

Percentages total over 100% because some falls were classified as having more than one cause.
Reference: Rubenstein LZ, et al: Falls and instability in the elderly. J Am Geriatr Soc 36:266–278, 1988.

FECAL INCONTINENCE

Fecal incontinence is defined as involuntary leakage of stool. It is very common in demented patients and its most common cause is *fecal impaction,* in which liquid stool leaks around an impacted mass. Neuronal causes may be due to local damage (the effect of a long history of stimulant laxative abuse) or to loss of central inhibition (damage to spinal cord, as in metastases to the spinal cord, or cerebral cortex, as in severe dementia). *Diarrhea* may overwhelm a patient's continence mechanisms. Severely *depressed* persons may not care where they move their bowels.

Evaluation: The history should explore the patient's pattern of incontinence. Frequent or continuous leakage of small amounts of stool is seen in fecal impaction. Less frequent passage of formed stool is characteristic of uninhibited colonic activity or the inability to get to the toilet (functional incontinence). Pain upon defecation points to local processes. Bleeding (either gross blood or positive fecal occult blood test) requires endoscopic evaluation for cancer or angiodysplasia. On examination, there is no correlation between anal tone and the cause of incontinence. The "anal wink" can evaluate sacral reflexes. If stool is not found on digital exam, an abdominal x-ray should be done to evaluate for a higher impaction.

Treatment: The patient should be instructed to avoid both constipating and diarrhea-inducing medications. If there is no mechanical obstruction, then the patient's diet should include fruit, fiber, increased water intake, and lactulose to produce soft, formed, bulky stool. Patients with uninhibited movements may often be very predictable and manageable with a toileting program using suppositories to induce peristalsis, then sitting on the commode approximately 15 minutes later.

Reference: Madoff RD, et al: Fecal incontinence. N Engl J Med 326:1002–1007, 1992.

FEVER OF UNDETERMINED ORIGIN

Diagnostic Criteria

1. Illness of more than 3 weeks' duration
2. Documented fever higher than 101°F (38.3°C) on several occasions
3. Uncertain diagnosis after 1 week of study in the hospital, allowing for the completion and interpretation of routine laboratory studies

Principles for Evaluating FUO

Assemble all available information about the case
- Complete Hx & PE (medical, social, occupational, travel, etc.)
- Routine laboratory studies and initial cultures
- Cross-reference causes of FUO (review of symptoms, disease classification, published lists of FUO causes [see table])

Diagnostic Categories of FUO

CATEGORY	NUMBER OF CASES	
	Second Series[1]	First Series[2]
Infections		
Abdominal abscesses (including liver and biliary tract)	11	11
Subphrenic	3	2
Splenic	2	0
Diverticular	2	0
Liver and biliary tract	3	7
Pelvic	1	2
Mycobacterial	5	11
Cytomegalovirus	4	0
Infection of the urinary tract	3	3
Sinusitis	2	0
Osteomyelitis	2	0
Catheter infections	2	0
Candidiasis	1	0
Amebic hepatitis	1	0
Wound infection	1	0
Endocarditis	0	5
Psittacosis	0	2
Brucellosis	0	1
Cirrhosis with *E. coli* bacteremia	0	1
Gonococcal arthritis	0	1
Malaria	0	1
Total	32	36
Neoplastic diseases		
Lymphoma, leukemia and related malignancies	22	8
Non-Hodgkin's lymphoma	7	4
Leukemia	5	2
Hodgkin's disease	4	2
Other reticuloendothelial malignancies	4	0
Other lymphocytic malignancy	2	0
Solid tumors	11	9
Nonhistologic diagnosis	0	2
Total	33	19
Collagen diseases		
Still's disease	4	2
Polyarteritis nodosa	2	0
Giant-cell arteritis	1	2
Panaortitis and arteritis	1	0
Rheumatic fever	1	6
Systemic lupus erythematosus	0	5
Total	9	15
Granulomatous diseases		
Granulomatous hepatitis	4	2
Crohn's disease	2	0
Sarcoidosis, erythema nodosum	2	2
Total	8	4

Table continued on next page.

Diagnostic Categories of FUO (Cont.)

	NUMBER OF CASES	
CATEGORY	Second Series[1]	First Series[2]
Miscellaneous		
Hematomas	3	0
Pulmonary embolus	1	3
Familial Mediterranean fever	1	0
Myxoma	1	0
Nonspecific pericarditis	1	2
Other	0	6
Total	7	11
Periodic fever	0	5
Factitious fever	3	3
Undiagnosed	13	7
Grand Total	105	100

Modified from [1]Larson EB, et al: Fever of undetermined origin: Diagnosis and follow-up of 105 cases, 1970–1980. Medicine 61:269–292, 1982.
[2]Petersdorf RG, et al: Fever of unexplained origin: Report of 100 cases. Medicine 40:1–30, 1961.

FIBROMYALGIA

Fibromyalgia (FM) is a musculoskeletal pain syndrome associated with a predictable distribution of localized tender points. First described in 1904, it was called fibrositis to describe the putative inflammation of musculature. Although subsequent studies have failed to document any inflammatory changes, the associated pain and areas of localized tenderness remain characteristic. With the development of American College of Rheumatology criteria, FM is increasingly being recognized as a significant cause of pain. The widespread nature of the pain and the characteristic and requisite number of tender points are useful in differentiating FM from other causes of pain.

FM is seen in approximately 2.6% of patients in a family practice setting and 15% of patients in a rheumatology practice setting. Nearly 90% of patients are women with onset in middle age. One-third of patients report onset after a viral illness and another third report trauma as an inciting factor.

Patients commonly present with gradual onset of generalized and chronic muscular achiness. They report morning stiffness with intensification of pain, and they may manifest neuropathic symptoms, irritable bowel syndrome, tension headaches, and bladder irritability. Taken collectively, this has been referred to as "irritable everything syndrome."

Nonrestorative sleep is characteristic. Patients often remark that they are more fatigued and achy on awakening than on retiring. Sleep laboratory studies have shown poor stage IV (nonREM) sleep. Nocturnal myoclonus is another commonly experienced sleep abnormality.

Physical examination shows normal articular function without swelling or range-of-motion limitation. Predictable areas of tenderness with normal control points are present. The evaluation of tender points is usually subjective (palpation with the pulp of the thumb or the first two fingers). Objective data show that tissue tenderness with a pressure of less than 4 kg is abnormal.

American College of Rheumatology 1990 Criteria for the Classification of Fibromyalgia*

1. **History of widespread pain**

   Definition: Pain is considered widespread when all of the following are present: pain in the left side of the body, pain in the right side of the body, pain above the waist, and pain below the waist. In addition, axial skeletal pain (cervical spine or anterior chest or thoracic spine or low back) must be present. In this definition, shoulder and buttock pain in considered as pain for each involved side. "Low back" pain is considered lower segment pain.

2. **Pain in 11 of 18 tender point sites on digital palpation**

   Definition: Pain, on digital palpation, must be present in at least 11 of the following 18 tender point sites:

   Occiput: bilateral, at the suboccipital muscle insertions

   Low cervical: bilateral, at the anterior aspects of the intertransverse spaces at C5–C7

   Trapezius: bilateral, at the midpoint of the upper border

   Supraspinatus: bilateral, at origins, above the scapula spine near the medial border

   Second rib: bilateral, at the second costochondral junctions, just lateral to the junctions on upper surfaces

   Lateral epicondyle: bilateral, 2 cm distal to the epicondyles

   Gluteal: bilateral, in upper outer quadrants of buttocks in anterior fold of muscle

   Greater trochanter: bilateral, posterior to the trochanteric prominence

   Knee: bilateral, at the medial fat pad proximal to the joint line

   Digital palpations should be performed with an approximate force of 4 kg.

   For a tender point to be considered "positive," the subject must state that the palpation was painful. "Tender" is not to be considered "painful."

*For classification purposes, patients will be said to have fibromyalgia if both criteria 1 and 2 are satisfied. Widespread pain must have been present for at least 3 months. The presence of a second clinical disorder does not exclude the diagnosis of fibromyalgia.

From Wolfe F, et al: The American College of Rheumatology 1990 criteria for the classification of fibromyalgia. Arthritis Rheum 33:160–172, 1990, with permission.

There is no clear understanding of the etiology or the pathophysiology of fibromyalgia. Changes have been documented in the muscles of patients with FM, yet it remains possible that such changes are a result of deconditioning. Muscle fiber injury as a cause for tender points is supported by Danneskold-Samsoe et al., who measured an increase in plasma myoglobin after massage of control and tender points. Bennett postulates that repetitive microtrauma of daily living may play a significant role in FM. Fatigue and physical inactivity may lead to unfit muscles, which are susceptible to microtrauma.

Abnormal pain processing has been hypothesized as a problem in FM. Studies have shown elevated levels of substance P and lower levels of 5 hydroxy-indoleacetic acid in CSF. Psychologic dysfunction has also been documented in FM patients, but the extent of dysfunction does not appear to vary from the general population.

Treatment should be directed toward improving sleep and controlling discomfort. Although not dramatically effective, NSAIDs remain important. Tricyclic antidepressants are frequently used because they increase stage IV sleep. Injection of tender points with a mixture of local anesthetic and glucocorticoids has had some success controlling local pain. Focus has also shifted to nonpharmacologic treatment such as fitness training, cognitive behavior training, patient education (avoiding the aggravating and encouraging the beneficial factors), and psychological support.

Finally, a word about the distinction between FM and chronic fatigue syndrome (CFS). There are some striking demographic similarities between FM and CFS. In addition to demographic similarities, patients with CFS have muscle pain and achiness. Those patients with CFS and joint symptoms usually met criteria for FM. Sleep studies have documented similar changes in alpha and delta sleep patterns. Thus the exact relationship between the two entities remains intriguing but unclear.

Reference: Danneskold-Samsoe B, et al: Myofacial pain and the role of myoglobin. Scand J Rheum 15:174–178, 1986.

FUNCTIONAL ASSESSMENT

A systematic assessment of function allows the physician to evaluate the severity of an illness and to measure the impact of illness on a patient's independence and quality of life. Functional assessments are developed independent of underlying diagnoses. They can also be used to evaluate utility of treatment and to follow the response to treatment. Functional assessment can be used to judge the significance of physical findings or lab abnormalities. Individual decisions about the level of care and monitoring required, readiness for discharge, or need for institutionalization can be made using those data.

Components of Functional Assessment

1. Activities of daily living (ADL): Three levels: independent, needs help, can't do. Includes feeding, bathing, dressing, toileting, transferring, and continence. (*Note:* It is usually adequate to ask patients if they can feed themselves, etc.)
2. Independent activities of daily living (IADL): Includes using telephone, preparing meals, housekeeping, taking medicines, managing money, shopping, and transportation. (*Note:* It may be necessary to ask patients to explain how they would "prepare an omelette," "call for a TV repairman," etc.)
3. Cognitive: Mental Status Exam (Folstein)
4. Geriatric Depression Scale

Geriatric Depression Scale

Choose the best answer for how you felt over the past week.

1. Are you basically satisfied with your life?	yes/no
2. Have you dropped many of your activities and interests?	yes/no
3. Do you feel that your life is empty?	yes/no
4. Do you often get bored?	yes/no
5. Are you hopeful about the future?	yes/no
6. Are you bothered by thoughts you can't get out of your head?	yes/no
7. Are you in good spirits most of the time?	yes/no
8. Are you afraid that something bad is going to happen to you?	yes/no
9. Do you feel happy most of the time?	yes/no
10. Do you often feel helpless?	yes/no
11. Do you often get restless and fidgety?	yes/no
12. Do you prefer to stay at home, rather than going out and doing new things?	yes/no
13. Do you frequently worry about the future?	yes/no
14. Do you feel you have more problems with memory than most?	yes/no

Table continued on next page.

Geriatric Depression Scale (Cont.)

15. Do you think it is wonderful to be alive now?	yes/no
16. Do you often feel downhearted and blue?	yes/no
17. Do you feel pretty worthless the way you are now?	yes/no
18. Do you worry a lot about the past?	yes/no
19. Do you find life very exciting?	yes/no
20. Is it hard for you to get started on new projects?	yes/no
21. Do you feel full of energy?	yes/no
22. Do you feel that your situation is hopeless?	yes/no
23. Do you think that most people are better off than you are?	yes/no
24. Do you frequently get upset over little things?	yes/no
25. Do you frequently feel like crying?	yes/no
26. Do you have trouble concentrating?	yes/no
27. Do you enjoy getting up in the morning?	yes/no
28. Do you prefer to avoid social gatherings?	yes/no
29. Is it easy for you to make decisions?	yes/no
30. Is your mind as clear as it used to be?	yes/no

Scoring Details: Score 1 point for "No" answer to Questions 1, 5, 7, 9, 15, 19, 21, 27, 29, 30. Score 1 point for a "Yes" answer to all other questions.

A total score of ≥ 14 indicates definite depression.

A total score of ≤ 6 indicates that depression is very unlikely.

A total score of 7–13 indicates the need for further investigation.

(Note: some investigators use 0–10 as normal and > 10 as depressed. Recently, the scale has been shown to be equally valid in mildly to moderately demented persons as it is in nondemented persons.)

From Yesavage JA, et al: Development and validation of a geriatric depression screening scale. J Psychiatr Res 17:41, 1983, with permission.

GAIT EVALUATION

About 15–20% of the elderly have a very slow or abnormal gait. With age, normal gait changes. Due to muscle weakness, the elderly do not pick up their feet as high as the young. Men develop a wide-based, short-stepped gait; women develop a narrow-based, waddling gait.

Gait assessment should include performance-based gait testing (i.e., have patient get up from chair, walk down hall, turn around, come back, and sit down again), as well as the following.

Parameters in Gait Evaluation

PARAMETERS	ABNORMAL FINDINGS
Step length	At least the foot length
Step symmetry	—
Continuity	—
Path deviation	Deviation to sides
Turning	Struggles, stops, then turns
Get up from chair	Needs arms
Immediate balance	Unsteady, staggering
Standing	Must keep feet apart
Nudge sternum	Needs help, starts to fall
Stand on one leg	Unable to balance
Turn head	Unsteady
Reach up	Unable or unsteady
Bend down	Unable to get up
Sit down	Falls into chair, lands off center

Clues to the Etiology of Gait Disturbances

OBSERVATION	SUGGESTED CONDITIONS
Difficulty getting up and down	Myopathy, arthropathy, parkinsonsim, orthostatic hypotension, deconditioning
Difficulty with neck turn and reach	Cervical spine disease, vertebrobasilar insufficiency
Unsteady gait after sternal nudge	Parkinson's disease, NPH, CNS/back problems
Decreased step height	CNS disease, sensory deficits, fear
Unsteady turning	Parkinson's disease, cerebellar, hemiparesis, visual field deficits
Path deviation	Cerebellar, sensory deficits, sensory or motor ataxia

GAMMOPATHY, MONOCLONAL

The wide availability and routine use of automated batteries of blood chemistry tests has resulted in the frequent identification of increased serum gamma globulins. When submitted for serum electrophoresis, a monoclonal protein (M-spike, M-protein) or monoclonal gammopathy may be discovered. The significance of the monoclonal protein ranges from a benign phenomenon that needs only to be observed, to the malignant disorder multiple myeloma. As people age, the frequency of monoclonal gammopathy increases. Blacks appear to have a higher incidence of such proteins and of multiple myeloma than whites. A working list of entities associated with monoclonal gammopathy is shown in the following table.

Conditions Associated with Monoclonal Gammopathy

Benign monoclonal gammopathy of uncertain significance (MGUS)
Chronic inflammation: osteomyelitis, TB
Collagen vascular disease: SLE, Sjögren's
Cryoglobulinemia
Skin disease (pyoderma gangrenosum, psoriasis, scleromyxedema, urticaria)
Recovery from bone marrow transplantation
Peripheral neuropathy
Angioimmunoblastic lymphadenopathy with dysproteinemia
Amyloidosis
Non-Hodgkin's lymphoma
CLL
Indolent myeloma
Solitary plasmacytoma
Multiple myeloma
Plasma-cell leukemia
Light chain disease
Heavy chain disease
Polyendocrinopathy with myelosclerosis
Waldenström's macroglobulinemia

Differentiation of Multiple Myeloma (MM) from Monoclonal Gammopathy

	MM	MGUS
M-protein	>3.5 g/dl	<3.5 g/dl
Anemia or other cytopenia	Usually present	Usually absent
Urine monoclonal protein	>500 mg/24 h	<500 mg/24 h
Bones	Lytic lesions	Normal
Marrow plasma cells	>10%	<10%
Serum B_2 microglobulin	>3.0	<3.0 mg/L
Calcium	± elevated	Normal
Creatinine	± elevated	Normal
Change in monoclonal protein with time	Increases	No change

Benign monoclonal gammopathy has been studied and reviewed extensively by Kyle. When a large group of MGUS patients is followed for a long period, most have a stable course, whereas about 10% develop multiple myeloma—hence the recommendation for periodic examination of the serum protein electrophoresis.

Reference: Kyle RA: Monoclonal gammopathy of undetermined significance: Natural history in 241 cases. Am J Med 64:814, 1978.

GAS

"Gas" as a complaint by a patient often gives physicians a cause to have the same. It is a mysterious, nebulous symptom, almost always vague, and complicated by subjective feelings and interpretations. Little information can be found in the medical literature, and much of that is conjecture. Nevertheless, some information on the subject may give the physician an element of credibility, because most causes of "gas" are benign and require only reassurance as a treatment.

Ninety-nine percent of intestinal gases are composed of five elements: nitrogen, oxygen, hydrogen, methane, and carbon dioxide. Sources of this gas are swallowing of air, intraluminal production of gas, and diffusion of gases from blood into the intestinal lumen. The usual gas content of the intestinal tract is about 200 ml. Air swallowing probably does not contribute a great deal to intestinal gas, for even if we swallowed as little as 2–3 ml of air with each swallow, we would accumulate many liters of nitrogen in a 24-hour period. On the average, about 400 ml of nitrogen is passed per rectum per day, and there is basically no net absorption of nitrogen in the small bowel. Inspired air is about 80% nitrogen, whereas intestinal gas may range from 10% to 90% nitrogen, suggesting that other contributing factors are more important.

Sources of carbon dioxide in the gut include production of carbon dioxide after meals from the reaction of hydrogen and bicarbonate. About 22 ml of carbon dioxide is produced per 1 mEq of bicarbonate. Hydrogen production after meals may be up to 30 mEq/hr, and TG digestion yields about 100 meq of bicarbonate per 30 g of fat; thus several liters of carbon dioxide may be produced. Fortunately, carbon dioxide is easily absorbed from the intestine. The carbon dioxide in flatus is derived mainly from bacterial fermentation.

Hydrogen production in the colon is due to incomplete absorption of carbohydrate and protein, which then provide substrates for bacteria in the colon. The main source of hydrogen in flatus is bacterial metabolism. Some bacteria consume as well as produce hydrogen, which is why antibiotics may upset that balance. Oligosaccharides and polysaccharides are not digested by small-bowel enzymes but are used by intestinal bacteria for the production of hydrogen. The two oligosaccharides raffinose and stachyose are found in beans, causing the flatus associated with ingestion. The bean that causes the most flatus has been found to be soybeans. Other poorly digested polysaccharides include sorbitol, found both as a sweetener in many sugar-free products and naturally in some fruits.

There is a relatively complicated relationship between the production of gases in the bowel, the absorption of gases from the bowel, and the diffusion of gases back into the bowel. It is thus very difficult to determine which of these factors may be more important in the production of increased gas in any one individual.

The majority of these gases are odorless and colorless. Gases including ammonia, hydrogen sulfide, and short-chain fatty acids, constituting less than 1% of bowel gas production, usually cause the social problems. Both dietary intake and makeup of the bacteria of the colon contribute to the composition of these gases.

Studies on the production of gas in patients with complaints of increased gas do not elucidate the subject, because there is no difference in amount of gas in those with and those without symptoms. It has been suggested that a motility disorder might interfere with passage of the gas. However, anticholinergics have not been useful in most patients. Metoclopramide has had some success.

It has been determined that the number of times that a normal person passes flatus per day is 13.6 ± 5.6 times. Elimination diets are often helpful in determining the foods that are contributing to symptoms in some patients. Lactose intolerance and lactase deficiency, however, are probably the most important causes of functional GI complaints. Legumes, wheat flour, and oat flour are frequent offenders.

It has also been shown that methane production in the gut is a familial trait. Methane can be found in the fasting state and may be the result of catabolism of endogenous glycoproteins.

The differential diagnosis of gas includes:

1. Increased air swallowing due to nervous habit, poor dentition, rapid eating, or chronic postnasal discharge.
2. Diet including milk products used by those with lactase deficiency; sorbitol-containing foods—either fruits or additives; legumes; wheat or oat flour; beer and other carbonated beverages; nuts; onions; and leafy green vegetables.
3. Malabsorption.
4. Gastric outlet obstruction.
5. Familial tendency.
6. Iatrogenic changes in colonic bacteria due to antibiotics.

GASTRIC CANCER

The incidence of gastric cancer has been decreasing in the United States since 1930, when it was the most frequent cause of cancer death. However, it is still a frequent killer in other areas of the world, such as Japan, Chile, and Iceland. Nevertheless, no etiologic factors have been clearly defined. It appears to occur more often in lower socioeconomic classes, but no specific occupational or rural versus urban differences have been discovered. Familial gastric cancer has been found, and there is an increase in incidence among close relatives of patients with gastric cancer. Type A blood has been implicated in some studies as a risk factor, although this may be a confounding factor. Diet or environmental exposures early in life have been supported by other epidemiologic studies. Pernicious anemia, hypochlorhydria, and achlorhydria have also been implicated. Atrophic gastritis and intestinal metaplasia are felt to be precursor lesions. Diets in areas of high prevalence have been examined; salted meats, corn, talc-dusted rice, smoked meats, and nitrates have been suspected. The protective effects of lettuce and vitamin C have also been suggested by these dietary studies. Lab studies show that nitrosamines can produce gastric cancer in experimental animals. Recent studies have shown a significant correlation with infection with *Helicobacter pylori* at a young age.

Gastric cancer is difficult to diagnose at an early stage because most early signs are nonspecific. About 10% of patients present with anemia, weakness, and weight loss. Occasionally, patients present with acute abdominal emergencies such as GI bleeding, acute obstruction of the lower esophagus or pylorus, or gastric perforation. Early physical findings are lacking, with the exception of positive stool guaiac. All other findings indicate late disease, such as palpable supraclavicular lymph nodes, rectal shclf, ovarian mass, hepatomegaly, abdominal mass, ascites, jaundice, and cachexia.

The widespread availability of upper GI endoscopy has contributed greatly to the ease of diagnosis, and much discussion has been devoted to the use of that tool for screening. However, due to the low incidence, extensive screening is not cost-effective.

A five-level American Joint Committee (AJC) staging system is used. The stages vary from stage 0, which is limited to mucosa, to stage IV, which includes distant metastasis. The majority of gastric cancers are adenocarcinomas.

Surgical resection, first performed by Billroth in 1881, is still the only useful method of treatment for this disease. Long-term (5-year) survival rates for successful complete resection are approximately 25% for distal lesions and less than 10% for proximal lesions. Chemotherapy for advanced disease has been tried with only minimal impact. Complete response is unlikely, and less than 50% of patients have subjective or objective partial responses.

GASTROESOPHAGEAL REFLUX DISEASE

Treatment Methods

Phase I: Lifestyle Modifications to Reduce Reflux

1. Elevate head of bed 6 inches (reverse Trendelenburg)
2. Quit smoking
3. Reduce alcohol intake
4. Reduce dietary fat intake
5. Remain upright for 2 hours after eating or drinking
6. Lose weight if obese
7. Avoid chocolate, spearmint, peppermint, coffee, tea, cola
8. Discontinue anticholinergics, theophylline, diazepam, narcotics, calcium channel blockers, beta-adrenergic drugs, progesterone, alpha-adrenergic blockers

Phase II: Drug Therapy for GERD

1. Antacids
2. H_2 receptor antagonist
3. Bethanechol
4. Cisapride or metoclopramide
5. Sucralfate
6. Omeprazole (if above fail)

GIANT-CELL TUMOR OF THE TENDON SHEATH

Benign giant-cell tumors of the tendon sheath occur on the index and middle fingers of adults aged 40–60 years. They are usually painless, but impingement on local joints may create discomfort with movement. The patient usually complains of a swelling in the involved area. On physical exam, the nodules are firm, nontender, and nonmobile. There are no characteristic x-ray findings.

The only therapy for these tumors is resection, and they may recur after surgery. Xanthofibromas, xanthomas, and benign fibrous histiocytomas are the types of giant-cell tumors frequently found.

Reference: Dick HM: Tumors of the hand and wrist. In Dee R, et al (eds): Principles of Orthopedic Practice. New York, McGraw-Hill, 1988.

GI BLEEDING, LOWER

Common Causes

1. Diverticulosis
2. Angiodysplasia
3. Neoplasms—benign or malignant
4. Perianal disease (hemorrhoids, fissures)
5. Meckel's diverticulum
6. Inflammatory bowel disease
7. Ischemic, infectious, or radiation colitis
8. Intussusception

Rare Causes

1. Ileal or colonic varices
2. Solitary rectal or cecal ulcer
3. Aortoenteric fistula

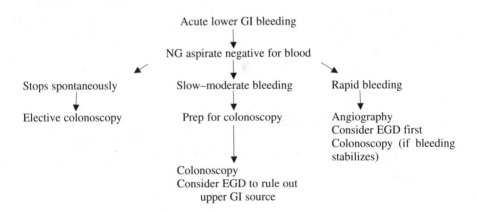

Diagnostic algorithm for lower GI bleeding. There is no present role for barium studies, and the value of radionuclide scans is currently questionable. (EGD = esophagogastroduodenoscopy.)

GI BLEEDING, UPPER

Causes of Acute Upper GI Bleeding

Duodenal ulcer	Gastric ulcer
Gastric erosion	Esophageal/gastric varices
Mallory-Weiss tear	Esophagitis
Neoplasm	Anastomotic ulcer
Esophageal ulcer	Angiodysplasia
Aortoenteric fistula	Hematobilia
Dieulafoy's lesion (gastric)	

Diagnostic Steps

Patients with self-limited minor bleeding and serious medical problems may not require endoscopy, for endoscopy has not been shown to alter prognosis. However, in the majority of patients, accurate diagnosis leads to appropriate clinical management and allows endoscopic therapy if needed.

Aggressive initial resuscitation should be undertaken to stabilize the patient prior to instituting specific diagnostic steps. Most patients with significant upper GI bleeding should be placed in an ICU setting for hemodynamic monitoring and transfusion if needed. NG lavage may help to access ongoing blood loss as well as cleanse the stomach of blood and debris in preparation for upper endoscopy. Gastric lavage can be undertaken using a large-bore NG tube flushed with tap water or saline. Iced-water lavage has not been shown to be any more useful than lavage with room temperature solutions.

Once the patient has been resuscitated, the diagnostic procedure of choice for localization of upper GI bleeding is endoscopy. There is virtually no role for barium studies in the evaluation of acute upper GI hemorrhage. Endoscopy allows not only accurate diagnosis but the additional benefit of directed endoscopic therapy should a lesion be identified.

Radionuclide scanning is of questionable value in precisely locating bleeding sites and is unable to provide an exact diagnosis. Angiography of the superior mesenteric artery may be useful when endoscopy has failed to localize a bleeding site. Bleeding should be arterial and active at a rate of 0.5–0.6 ml per min. Angiography also provides a therapeutic alternative and can deliver intra-arterial vasopressin or allow embolization of bleeding vessels.

GLOMERULONEPHRITIS, ACUTE

Acute GN, often referred to as acute nephritic syndrome, refers to the abrupt onset of hematuria and proteinuria along with variable impairment of renal function. It is often associated with salt and water retention resulting in HTN and edema. The proteinuria rarely exceeds 3 g in 24 hrs. The HTN is volume dependent and can often be controlled by salt restriction alone.

Etiology: Although poststreptococcal GN is the prototype of acute GN, there are several primary and secondary glomerular diseases that present as acute GN. They include:

- Poststreptococcal GN
- Other postinfectious (e.g., infective endocarditis, infected ventriculoatrial shunt)
- SLE
- Membranoproliferative GN (type I and type II)
- Idiopathic crescentic nephritis
- IgA nephropathy
- Essential mixed cryoglobulinemia
- Anti-glomerular basement membrane disease (Goodpasture's syndrome)
- Wegener's granulomatosis
- Microscopic polyarteritis

Clinical features: Acute poststreptococcal GN results following a pharyngeal infection with a nephritogenic (type 12) strain of group A beta-hemolytic streptococci. There is usually a latent period of 6–20 days before nephritis is seen. Granular immune complex deposits in the glomeruli are characteristic, histologically diffuse, glomerular hypercellularity along with proliferation of epithelial cells and subepithelial electron-dense nodules under the electron microscopy. The disease is common in children and rare over the age of 50. Abrupt onset of hematuria, malaise, nausea, edema, HTN, and renal failure are components of the syndrome. Complement levels are decreased in the acute phase and return to normal within 8 weeks. The pattern of complement activation involves the alternate pathway. Increases in antistreptolysin O (ASO) titer and other antistreptococcal antibodies are diagnostic. UA reveals hematuria, proteinuria, and RBC casts.

The treatment is often symptomatic. Salt restriction is usually sufficient to control HTN and edema. However, diuretics and antihypertensives may be needed if CHF and/or resistant HTN are present. Temporary dialysis may be needed under some circumstances. In more than 90% of cases, complete recovery occurs, although abnormal urinary sediment may persist for as long as 2 years. In less than 5% of cases, patients have prolonged oliguria, and recovery is prolonged and partial. In a very small group of patients, the disease progresses relentlessly (as in crescentic nephritis), necessitating permanent dialytic support. Patients with oliguria for more than a week should undergo a renal biopsy, and if extensive crescents are present, they should be treated as having rapidly progressive GN, with steroids and/or immunosuppressive agents.

Other disorders: There are several other diseases, both primary and secondary glomerulopathies, that present as acute GN. Some of these disorders are listed in the previous table. IgA nephropathy (Berger's disease) is regarded as a monosymptomatic form of Henoch-Schönlein purpura, which is the most common cause of primary glomerular disease in the world. Histologically, it is characterized by the presence of mesangial deposits of IgA and C3. Clinically, the disease is characterized by recurrent episodes of gross hematuria occurring in young males, coincident with a URI in 50–75% of cases. The disease is therefore referred to as synpharyngitic nephritis. Complement levels are normal. Proteinuria rarely exceeds 1 g/day. Only 25% of patients have renal failure. There is no specific therapy, and progression to renal failure is seen in 25% of cases.

The clinical and laboratory features of some of the other conditions resulting in acute GN syndrome are discussed in the accompanying table. Rapidly progressive GN is characterized by formation of epithelial crescents in the biopsy and rapid deterioration of renal function clinically. This disease is often due to Goodpasture's syndrome, which is characterized by the presence of anti-glomerular basement membrane antibody, which cross-reacts with alveolar basement membrane and

Summary of Primary Renal Diseases that Present as Acute Glomerulonephritis

	POSTSTREPTOCOCCAL GN	IgA NEPHROPATHY	GOODPASTURE'S SYNDROME	IDIOPATHIC RAPIDLY PROGRESSIVE GN (RPGN)
Clinical manifestations				
Age and sex	All ages, mean 7 yrs; 2:1 male	15–35 yrs, 2:1 male	15–30 yrs, 6:1 male	Mean 58 yrs, 2:1 male
Acute nephritic syndrome	90%	50%	90%	90%
Asymptomatic hematuria	Occasionally	50%	Rare	Rare
Nephrotic syndrome	10–20%	Rare	Rare	10–20%
HTN	70%	30–50%	Rare	25%
ARF	50% (transient)	Very rare	50%	60%
Other	Latent period of 1–3 wks	Follows viral syndromes	Pulmonary hemorrhage; iron deficiency anemia	None
Laboratory findings	↑ ASO titers (70%) Positive streptozyme (95%) ↓ C3–C9; normal CI, C4	↑ Serum IgA (50%) IgA in dermal capillaries	Positive anti-GBM antibody	Positive ANCA
Immunogenetics	IILA-B12, D "EN" (9)*	HLA-Bw 35, DR4 (4)*	HLA-DR2 (16)*	None established
Renal pathology				
Light microscopy	Diffuse proliferation	Focal proliferation	Focal→diffuse proliferation with crescents	Crescentic GN
Immunofluorescence	Granular IgG, C3	Diffuse mesangial IgA	Linear IgG, C3	No immune deposits
Electron microscopy	Subepithelial humps	Mesangial deposits	No deposits	No deposits
Prognosis	95% resolve spontaneously 5% RPGN or slowly progressive	Slow progression in 25–50%	75% stabilize or improve if treated early	75% stabilize or improve treated early
Treatment	Supportive	None established	Plasma exchange, steroids, cyclophosphamide	Steroid pulse therapy

*Relative risk.

From Couser WG: Glomerular disorders. In Wyngaarden JB, et al (eds): Cecil Textbook of Medicine, 19th ed. Philadelphia, W. B. Saunders, 1992, p 553, with permission.

causes pulmonary hemorrhage. Treatment with pulsed methylprednisone and cytotoxic agents, along with plasma exchange therapy, improves the prognosis, especially in those with milder forms of renal failure.

Reference: Glassock RJ: Clinical aspects of glomerular disease. Am J Kidney Dis 10:157, 1987.

GLOSSODYNIA

Glossodynia is also known as burning mouth or burning tongue syndrome. Patients complain of *severe* burning pain of the tongue and oral mucosa. On exam, the mouth and tongue frequently appear normal. This is a frustrating illness for both patient and physician; frequently, the physician is unable to detect an etiology of the symptom, and therapy is sometimes ineffective.

The disorder occurs most frequently in postmenopausal women. In addition to burning sensations, patients frequently describe altered taste sensations and mouth dryness. Hot and spicy foods and chewing may exacerbate the symptoms.

Physicians should look carefully for other etiologies such as oral candidiasis, poorly fitting dentures, dry mouth (xerostomia), nutritional deficiencies (niacin and folic acid), DM, and aphthous stomatitis. If found, the underlying disorder should be treated.

Therapies should attempt to relieve the painful symptoms. If dry mouth is present, artificial lubricants may be helpful. Patients should also use "sensitive" toothpastes and pay strict attention to good oral hygiene. The pain may respond to medications that work for neuralgia, such as antidepressants (amitriptyline) or carbamazepine.

GONORRHEA

Gonorrhea is a bacterial illness causing a purulent exudate involving the lower GU tract, rectum, oropharynx, or conjunctivae. The causative organism, *Neisseria gonorrhoeae,* is a nonmotile gram-negative coccus that is spread sexually or perinatally. The incubation period ranges from 1 to 10 days. Genital infection in men usually presents with dysuria and a grossly purulent urethral discharge that, when tested by Gram staining, reveals the typical gram-negative diplococci in association with neutrophils. Uncomplicated genital infection in women presents as cervicitis and/or urethritis with symptoms of prominent vaginal discharge, dysuria, irregular menstrual bleeding, and pelvic pain. Rectal infection, which is often associated with genital disease, is usually asymptomatic but may present with pruritus, discharge, local pain, or bleeding. Oropharyngeal infection is also usually asymptomatic but may present with pharyngitis and associated lymphadenitis. Progression to PID (endometritis, salpingitis, pelvic peritonitis) occurs in 10–20% of cases and is usually associated with progressive lower abdominal pain, fever, and systemic toxicity. Following a single episode of PID, 15–20% of women develop fallopian tube obstruction and secondary infertility; the percentage rises to 50–80% following three or more episodes. Fitz-Hugh and Curtis syndrome, or acute perihepatitis, may be the cause of RUQ pain and guarding in association with acute genital infection.

Multiple complications of the primary gonococcal infection may occur. Acute conjunctivitis usually results from autoinoculation from a genital source. Dissemination via gonococcal bacteremia occurs in up to 3% of patients and presents as an arthritis-dermatitis syndrome, which may progress to septic arthritis. During the arthritis-dermatitis phase, blood or synovial fluid cultures are positive in only 50% of cases. Alternatively, in the septic joint phase, synovial fluid cultures are usually positive while most blood cultures are negative. Infrequent consequences of bacterial dissemination may include endocarditis, meningitis, osteomyelitis, and overwhelming sepsis or pneumonia.

Definitive diagnosis rests on culture, the choice of culture sites depending on the clinical situation. In women, endocervical and rectal cultures should be taken, as most rectal infections in this group probably result from spontaneous peritoneal contamination and not from anal intercourse. In heterosexual men, urethral cultures are usually adequate. In homosexual males, all symptomatic areas as well as rectal and pharyngeal cultures should be taken. After 4–7 days following completion of treatment, all previously infected sites should be recultured. Preferably, cultures should be inoculated onto selective growth medium immediately after collection, but nonnutrient transport media may be used if the specimen remains at room temperature and is inoculated onto growth medium within 6 hours. Serologic tests remain under investigation. Attention should also be paid to the risk of coexistent chlamydial infection (15–25% in heterosexual males, 35–50% females), syphilis, and possible HIV infection.

Treatment: Treatment schedules have been outlined as follows. Ceftriaxone is the agent of choice for all anatomic sites. It has no known teratogenic properties and is believed to cure incubating syphilis (unlike spectinomycin, following which serologic tests for syphilis should be repeated at 6 and 12 wk). The routine use of aqueous procaine penicillin G is no longer encouraged due to the high incidence of penicillin resistance in many strains. Oral therapy with amoxicillin 3.0 g plus probenecid 1.0 g may be effective in areas where penicillin resistance is not a common problem, but it is often ineffective for eradication of pharyngeal and rectal

---

Recommended Treatment of Uncomplicated Gonorrhea

Initial treatment
  Ceftriaxone 250 mg IM[a]
    or
  Spectinomycin 2.0 g IM[b]
Plus continuing treatment[c] with
  Doxycycline 100 mg PO BID for 7 days
    or
  Tetracycline HCl 500 mg PO QID for 7 days
    or
  Erythromycin 2.0 g PO per day in divided doses for 7–10 days[d]

---

[a]Single doses of 125 mg have proved effective and are used in some clinics, but 250 mg is the smallest commercially available unit dose. Ceftriaxone should be dissolved in 1% lidocaine.

[b]Should be restricted to patients who cannot tolerate ceftriaxone and to those with persistent infection after treatment with ceftriaxone. Not effective for pharyngeal infection.

[c]Optional for homosexually active men with gonorrhea.

[d]Should be used only for patients who cannot take doxycycline or tetracycline HCl.

Recommended Treatments for Acute Pelvic Inflammatory Disease

Hospitalized patients

Regimen A   Doxycycline 100 mg IV Q 12 hr   *plus*
                Cefoxitin 2.0 g IV Q 6 hr.
                (Continue both drugs for >4 days and >48 hr after patient improves; then continue doxycycline 100 mg PO BID to complete 10–14 days' total therapy.)
                                        OR

Regimen B   Clindamycin 900 mg IV Q 8 hr   *plus*
                Gentamicin 2.0 mg/kg IV once, followed by 1.5 mg/kg Q 8 hr[a]
                (Continue both drugs for >4 days and >48 hr after patient improves; then continue clindamycin 450 mg PO QID to complete 10–14 days' total therapy.)

Outpatients   Ceftriaxone 250 mg IM[b]   *plus*
                Doxycycline 100 mg PO BID for 10–14 days

---

[a]Adjust dose if renal function is abnormal or if indicated by serum gentamicin levels.

[b]Cefoxitin 2.0 g IM may be substituted for ceftriaxone in locales where antibiotic-resistant strains of *N. gonorrhoeae* are known to be uncommon.

From Handsfield HH: *Neisseria gonorrhoeae.* In Mandell G, et al (eds): Principles and Practice of Infectious Disease, 3rd ed. New York, Churchill Livingstone, 1990, pp 1627–1628, with permission.

reservoirs. Investigations are ongoing into the use of single-dose quinolones, but these cannot be given either to patients younger than age 18 or to pregnant patients. Spectinomycin is probably safe for use during pregnancy but will not eradicate pharyngeal disease.

Patients with PID should be hospitalized if markedly toxic; if concerns about possible pelvic abscess, ectopic pregnancy, or appendicitis exist; or if the patient is pregnant or prepubertal. Any IUD should be promptly removed. Failure to respond to therapy within 3 days may be an indication for laparoscopy.

Disseminated infection is best treated with a 7 to 10 day course of ceftriaxone, 1.0 g once daily IM or IV. If clinical response occurs within 3 days and the organism is shown by culture and sensitivity to be sensitive to penicillin or tetracycline, some patients may be changed to oral therapy with amoxicillin, doxycycline, or tetracycline for a 7 to 10 day course.

Completion of therapy requires notification, examination, and treatment of all sexual partners. Counseling in safe sex practices, including the use of condoms and the avoidance of symptomatic partners, is critically important.

GRANULOMATOUS LIVER DISEASE

Often, when liver biopsy is taken for abnormal liver function tests or fever, the report says that the patient's liver contains granulomas. Usually, granulomas do not cause marked liver disease, but they point to another underlying disorder which must be diagnosed. Hepatic granulomas are found in 4–10% of needle liver biopsies. They are reticuloendothelial reactions to a multitude of diseases. Sarcoidosis and TB account for 50–65% of hepatic granulomas.

Causes of Granulomatous Liver Disease

DISEASE	CLINICAL ACCOMPANIMENT	DIAGNOSTIC AIDS
Sarcoidosis	Lung changes, uveitis, lymph-adenopathy	CXR, ACE level, Kveim test
TB	Pulmonary disease	CXR, PPD, liver biopsy
Brucellosis	Fever	Complement fixation test, blood cultures
Berylliosis	Industrial exposure	CXR
Syphilis	Skin lesions	VDRL
Leprosy	Skin, nerve lesions	Lepro skin test
Histoplasmosis	Fever	CXR, histoplasmosis skin test, complement fixation
Ascariasis	GI and pulmonary symptoms	Eosinophilia, fecal examination
Tularemia	Septicemia	Complement fixation test
Lymphoma	Lymphadenopathy, splenomegaly	Lymph node biopsy
Primary biliary cirrhosis	Jaundice	Antimitochondrial antibody, liver biopsy
Hypogammaglobulinemia	Recurrent bacterial infections	Serum Ig
Drug reactions	Allopurinol, sulfonamides, hydralazine, procainamide	—
M. avium-intracellulare	Fever	Biopsy, HIV test

Others include schistosomiasis, SLE, psittacosis, coccidiomycosis, listeriosis, CMV.

GYNECOMASTIA

Gynecomastia is defined as enlargement of the male breast. It results from either excessive estrogens or deficient androgens. Evaluation of patients with gynecomastia should include:

1. A thorough drug history to exclude causative drugs.
2. A testicular examination to look for atrophy or masses.
3. An evaluation of the adequacy of liver function.
4. An endocrine evaluation consisting of:
    a. Androstenedione or 24-hr urinary 17-ketosteroids
    b. Estradiol
    c. β-HCG
    d. Luteinizing hormone
    e. Testosterone

Classification of the Causes of Gynecomastia

Physiologic: newborn, puberty, senescence
Pathologic
   A. Increased estrogen secretion
      1. Hermaphroditism
      2. Klinefelter's syndrome

Table continued on next page.

Classification of the Causes of Gynecomastia (Cont.)

3. Congenital adrenal hyperplasia
4. Neoplastic
   a. Adrenal adenoma or carcinoma
   b. Testicular tumor (Sertoli cell, Leydig cell, or germ cell)
   c. Neoplasms secreting HCG (lung, liver, kidney, stomach, lymphopoietic system)
B. Increased conversion of androgens to estrogens
   1. Adrenal carcinoma
   2. Liver disorders (failure secondary to infectious or nutritional causes, carcinoma)
   3. Nutritional (refeeding after starvation)
   4. Hyperthyroidism
C. Decreased androgen secretion
   1. Primary testicular failure: anorchia, Klinefelter's syndrome, enzymatic defects in testosterone synthesis
   2. Secondary testicular failure: castration, infectious orchitis (mumps and other viruses, leproma, TB), neurologic disorders (paraplegia, muscular dystrophy), renal failure, panhypopituitarism, prolactin-secreting tumors
D. Decreased androgen activity due to abnormal receptor protein
   1. Complete testicular feminization
   2. Incomplete testicular feminization
   3. Reifenstein's syndrome

Drug related
A. Hormones: androgens and anabolic steroids, HCG, estrogens, and estrogen agonists
B. Antiandrogens or inhibitors of androgen synthesis: cyproterone, flutamide
C. Antibiotics: isoniazid, ketoconazole, itraconazole, metronidazole
D. Antiulcer medications: cimetidine, omeprazole, ranitidine
E. Cancer chemotherapeutic agents (especially alkylating agents): cyclophosphamide, mechlorethamine, vincristine, mitotane, busulfan
F. Cardiovascular drugs: amiodarone, captopril, digitoxin, enalapril, methyldopa, nifedipine, reserpine, verapamil
G. Psychoactive agents: diazepam, haloperidol, phenothiazines, tricyclic antidepressants
H. Drugs of abuse: alcohol, amphetamines, heroin, marijuana
I. Others: phenytoin, penicillamine, spironolactone

Idiopathic

Reference: Braunstein GD: Gynecomastia. N Engl J Med 328:490–495, 1993.

H

HEADACHE

Because the brain itself is anesthetic, head pain arises from other cranial structures, especially from the blood vessels and from the musculoskeletal system of the head and neck. Some important clinical points about headache are the following.

1. The more severe the headache, the more benign the disease. The one exception to this rule occurs with intracranial hemorrhages, since bleeding inside the skull can cause "the worst headache of my life."

2. Eye problems and sinus problems seldom cause headaches. Most laypersons attribute their headaches to eye strain or sinusitis, but this is a setting in which the physician should ignore Osler's advice and *not* listen to the patient.

Serious causes of headaches include the following.

1. **Brain tumor, abscess,** or other intracranial mass that causes headache is generally diffuse and of moderate intensity. The best clue to the presence of a mass lesion is an abnormal neurologic examination. Any mass large enough to cause pain will also cause other disturbances of the nervous system.

2. **Temporal arteritis** is a granulomatous giant-cell arteritis involving systemic vessels and often accompanied by fevers, malaise, polymyalgia rheumatica, and elevated LFTs. It is not, as the name might suggest, an inflammation of only the temporal arteries. The headache may not even be temporal or primarily frontal but is usually diffuse. The vasculitis may choke off blood vessels—especially the ophthalmic arteries—causing permanent blindness. Elderly patients with a headache should always have a measurement of their ESR, which is almost invariably elevated with temporal arteritis. A definitive diagnosis may require biopsy of a substantial length of the temporal artery. Treatment should be with high-dose oral steroids for 1–2 years to prevent the visual complications.

3. **Intracranial hemorrhage** causes an abrupt, excruciating headache. If the hemorrhage is within the substance of the brain itself, there are almost always focal neurological signs. If the hemorrhage is around the brain—a subarachnoid hemorrhage—there may be little focality, although mental status is usually diminished. Intracranial hemorrhages are neurologic catastrophes that require expert neurologic and neurosurgical management to deal with the many nuances of care that arise.

4. **Infections** such as meningitis and encephalitis can present with headache, but patients are usually febrile, appear acutely ill, and often have altered mental status and a stiff neck. Definitive diagnosis usually requires CSF examination.

The most common causes of headache are:

- Migraine (see Migraine)
- Tension headache
- Cluster headache.

Tension headaches produce a generalized pain, are often described as a band encircling the head, and usually cause the greatest pain posteriorly. Although seldom severe, the pain can be agonizing. Tension headaches generally occur daily or almost daily, persisting throughout most of the day, with few other accompanying signs or symptoms. They appear early in life and women are affected more than men. The cause of tension headaches is unclear. Although frequently ascribed to psychological stress, no definitive data support such an association. Similarly, the pain has been ascribed to chronic tension in the cervical and cephalic muscles, but again, that theory, although still viable, has been difficult to substantiate.

Treatment of tension headache is controversial, but amitriptyline is probably the most useful therapy, in doses of 50–200 mg daily. NSAIDs, muscle relaxants, and physical therapy (including biofeedback) are often also employed, but with surprisingly little scientific data about their effectiveness.

Cluster headaches occur almost exclusively in 20- to 40-year-old men. They begin with little warning and build rapidly to a severe pain localized behind the eye or in the temporal region, sometimes with an accompanying Horner's syndrome (ptosis and miosis). The pain lasts 20–45 minutes and then resolves quickly. "Cluster" refers to the pattern of headaches that occur once or twice daily for several weeks. Such headaches then cease, only to appear again many months or years later. Thus, the pain occurs in clusters through the years.

Therapy for cluster headaches requires "breaking the cluster," which can usually be accomplished by oral steroids, such as 60 mg of prednisone daily for several days. Should steroids fail, lithium is an excellent therapy, usually in doses of 300 mg BID, although blood levels must be followed closely.

Reference: Saper JR, et al: Handbook of Headache Management: A Practical Guide to Diagnosis and Treatment of Head, Neck and Facial Pain. Baltimore, Williams & Wilkins, 1993.

HEARING LOSS, AGE-RELATED

Presbycusis is the age-related, gradual, progressive, and bilateral hearing loss involving predominantly the higher frequencies (where consonant sounds are found). It is due to atrophy of the organ of Corti, with a decreased number of sensory cells. This is superimposed on the damage due to a lifetime of excess noise. It is more severe in men than women. About 30% of patients over age 65 have decreased hearing; this increases to 50% in those over age 85.

Two components are identified: (1) peripheral, which results in decreased pure tone discrimination; and (2) central, which results in impaired speech understanding even when correcting for peripheral loss.

Treatable causes of hearing loss need to be ruled out, including drug effects, Paget's disease, cholesteatoma, otosclerosis, and cerumen impaction. Audiograms measure the patient's pure tone thresholds, but the ability to hear a whisper is still the best functional (and clinically relevant) test for hearing loss. The physician should stand to the patient's side so the patient cannot lip-read. ("I can't hear without my glasses" is a common complaint of lip-readers).

Treatment involves hearing aids. These may be refused for many reasons including the expense, dexterity requirements, amplification of background noise, and association with "feeling old."

Audiogram Thresholds for Pure Tone

<25 dB	Normal
26–40 dB	Difficulty with first sounds
41–60 dB	Difficulty with normal speech
61–80 dB	Difficulty with loud speech
>81 dB	Difficulty with amplification

HEART BLOCK

Classification and Etiologies

AV block is classified—according to its severity—into three general categories:
1. **First-degree AV block** is characterized by a fixed prolongation of the P-R interval in excess of 200 msec (or 0.2 sec). First-degree AV block is almost always due to a delayed conduction in the atrioventricular node, rather than in His bundle.
2. **Second-degree AV block** is characterized by dropped or nonconducted P waves, that is, P waves not followed by a QRS complex. It is important to differentiate between the following two types of second-degree AV block:
   a. **Mobitz I (type 1 second-degree AV block)** is also referred to as the Wenckebach phenomenon and is characterized by a gradual lengthening of the P-R interval followed by a nonconducted P wave. The P-R interval after a nonconducted P wave is typically shorter than the P-R interval of the last conducted P wave. Wenckebach phenomenon is often suspected by the finding of group beating, i.e., the finding of a fixed number of ventricular complexes separated by a pause. Like first-degree AV block, Mobitz I is commonly due to delayed conduction in the AV node rather than in His bundle and can be induced by drugs such as digoxin, beta-blockers, or nondihydropyridine calcium channel blockers.
   b. **Mobitz II (type 2 second-degree AV block)** is characterized by the sudden appearance of a nonconducted P wave not preceded by any prolongation of the P-R interval. Unlike first-degree or type 1 second-degree AV block, Mobitz II is most commonly due to structural or organic disease of the cardiac conduction system, such as coronary artery disease, degeneration, or calcification, as occurs in elderly subjects.
3. **Third-degree AV block** is characterized by the absence of any conduction from the atrium to the ventricle. It is also referred to as **complete heart block** and is commonly manifested by atrioventricular dissociation—the absence of any relationship between atrial and ventricular depolarizations. Third-degree AV block may, rarely, be due to drugs that slow AV conduction, but it is more commonly due to severe underlying organic or structural heart disease.

HEART SOUNDS

Pathophysiology and Significance of S_3 and S_4

Third and fourth heart sounds (S_3 and S_4, respectively), also referred to as ventricular and atrial gallops, are low-frequency heart sounds that may be normally

HEART SOUNDS AND HEART MURMURS

Response of Heart Sounds and Murmurs to Physiologic and Pharmacologic Interventions

CLINICAL CONDITION	AMYL NITRITE	VALSALVA STRAIN	ISOMETRIC HANDGRIP	STANDING	SQUATTING	INSPIRATION	PAUSE AFTER PREMATURE BEAT
Aortic stenosis	←	←	→	←	←	—	
Obstructive cardiomyopathy	←	←	→	←	→	—	↑
Mitral valve prolapse	Click moves toward S_1; murmur starts earlier	Click moves toward S_1; murmur starts earlier		Click moves toward S_1; murmur starts earlier	Click moves toward S_2; murmur starts later	Click occurs earlier	Click moves toward S_2; murmur starts later
Mitral stenosis	←		←				
Tricuspid insufficiency	←	—				←	
Aortic insufficiency	→		←		←		
Mitral insufficiency	→	→	←		←		
Tetralogy of Fallot						—	
Ventricular septal defect with pulmonary hypertension							
Small defect	→		←				
Large defect	←		→				
Pulmonic stenosis	←	↑ after release					

Reference: Criscitiello MG: Physiologic and pharmacologic aids in cardiac auscultation. In Fowler NO (ed): Cardiac Ddiagnosis and Treatment. Hagerstown, MD, Harper and Row, 1980.

present in infants and children; they are called physiologic S_3 and S_4 in the pediatric age group. However, the finding of an S_3 or S_4 in an adult usually suggests the presence of organic heart disease.

An S_3 results from an increase in the velocity of blood entering the LV during the early rapid filling phase of ventricular diastole, whereas an S_4 results from decreased compliance of the LV, resulting in an increased resistance to filling of the LV during the late active atrial contraction phase of ventricular diastole.

Conditions Associated with the Finding of S_3

1. Congestive heart failure	5. Aortic regurgitation
2. Coronary artery disease	6. Mitral valve prolapse
3. Cardiomyopathies	7. Constrictive pericarditis
4. Mitral regurgitation	8. Thyrotoxicosis

Conditions Associated with the Finding of S_4

1. Hypertension	4. Aortic valve stenosis
2. Coronary artery disease	5. Pulmonary valve stenosis
3. LV or RV hypertrophy regardless of etiology	

HEAT ILLNESS

Heat illness results from disordered thermoregulation secondary to exposure to high environmental temperatures. Heat gain results from a combination of basal metabolism, physical work, catecholamine effects, certain drugs, hormones (thyroid and others), and irradiation from the sun. Heat loss in humans is regulated primarily by sweating, with lesser benefits from redistribution of circulation to the skin and cardiac output. A disturbance in the ratio of heat-gained-to-lost by the body may result in one of the following syndromes:

1. **Heat edema:** Swelling in the distal extremities during the first few days of heat exposure and acclimatization; resolves spontaneously.

2. **Heat cramps:** Painful muscle cramps usually of the extremities and secondary to inadequate sodium replacement in acclimatized individuals.

3. **Heat syncope:** Orthostatic symptoms following exposure to high heat and humidity; usually associated with inadequate acclimatization.

4. **Heat tetany:** Hyperventilation secondary to exposure to environmental heat.

5. **Heat exhaustion:** Associated with headache, weakness, nausea, and vomiting; differs from heat stroke in that there is no serious impairment of mental function, and core temperature is usually less than 39°C (102°F). There are two forms, which frequently overlap:

    a. *Water depletion:* Seen in infants and impaired adults or laborers in hot climates, secondary to salt ingestion without adequate water.

    b. *Salt depletion:* Seen in individuals who consume water without adequate sodium chloride to replace large volumes of fluid lost in heavy sweating.

6. **Heat stroke:** Results from impaired sweating associated with exposure to high temperatures (>90°F) for several days combined with high humidity (60–75%). Usually seen in elderly patients, often in conjunction with CHF, DM, or alcoholism. There are few warning symptoms, and either loss of consciousness or seizures may occur first. Multiple-organ-system failure may occur with rhabdomyolysis and DIC. Classic findings include a rectal temperature >105°F (40.6°C), hot and dry skin with absent sweating, tachycardia, tachypnea, and hypotension. Differential diagnosis includes:

- Hyperthermia secondary to delirium tremens.
- Hypothalamic hyperthermia secondary to damage or mass.
- Neuroleptic malignant syndrome (seen with haloperidol, phenothiazines, and thioxanthenes).
- Malignant hyperthermia secondary to anesthesia.
- Hyperthermia with sepsis.
- Endocrine disorders (hyperthyroidism, adrenocortical insufficiency, pheochromocytoma, and diabetic ketoacidosis, following insulinoma resection).

Management: Whereas milder forms of heat illness may be managed conservatively by relocation to a cool area and oral rehydration with appropriate salt and water replacement, heat stroke must be managed aggressively to reduce the 70% mortality rate associated with delay of treatment beyond 1–2 hours. Immediate cooling must be accomplished, whatever the cause of hyperthermia. The most effective means of dissipating heat in the emergency setting is by evaporation utilizing a lukewarm water spray and fans that blow air at room temperature over the patient. Many emergency centers rely on an ice-water bath for cooling. However, that method makes it difficult to handle and monitor the patient during the process, in addition to which studies have demonstrated that heat is consumed only 14% as efficiently with this technique as with the water spray method. Iced peritoneal lavage and cardiopulmonary bypass have proven effective as well. Antipyretics are of no use, as they require intact hypothalamic function to be effective. During the cooling process, a rectal thermistor probe inserted to a depth of 20 cm should be used to measure core temperature. Cooling should continue at a rate greater than 0.1–0.2°C per minute until rectal temperature drops to less than 102°F (39°C).

Baseline laboratory studies should include:

- CBC and coagulation studies
- Urinalysis
- CPK level
- CXR
- Electrolytes, BUN, and creatinine
- Liver enzymes
- Arterial blood gases
- ECG
- CSF analysis and brain CT scan (if intracranial bleed or meningitis is suspected)

Because most patients are relatively normovolemic, hypotension should be managed with gentle replacement of IV fluids (usually D5 1/2 NS) under central venous monitoring, using dopamine as needed. Seizures may be managed with IV diazepam. Traditional management of rhabdomyolysis and DIC should be employed. Hypocalcemia should be managed conservatively, because calcium that has been deposited in injured muscle will be released 2–3 days following successful therapy, resulting in rebound hypercalcemia. Shivering during cooling (which limits the effectiveness of the cooling technique employed) may be managed with 25–50 mg IV chlorpromazine. Patients should be monitored for recurrent hyperthermia 3–4 hours later. (See also Heat Stroke.)

References: Tek D, et al: Heat illness. Emerg Med Clin North Am 10:299–310, 1992. Knochel JP: Heat stroke and related heat stress disorders. DM 35(5):301 377, 1989.

HEAT STROKE

Heat stroke is the most serious of the three major heat-related disorders. The other two are heat cramps and heat exhaustion, and in contrast to heat stroke, in those two conditions the body's thermoregulatory ability is preserved. Heat cramps are muscle cramps, usually of the calves, in people who have exercised vigorously. Heat exhaustion is a syndrome resulting from excessive loss of body water and electrolytes. Victims may have headache, lightheadedness, malaise, nausea, vomiting, and muscle pain. Mental status is normal, however, and body temperature is less than 39°C. These last two features help to distinguish heat exhaustion from heat stroke.

Heat stroke is a true medical emergency. **Exertional heat stroke** can occur in healthy persons who exercise vigorously under conditions of extreme heat and humidity. **Classic heat stroke** occurs in patients who have been exposed to high ambient temperatures for at least 2 days and who have disordered homeostatic mechanisms, because of either age, medications (e.g., anticholinergics, phenothiazines), or chronic illness (e.g., cardiovascular disease, autonomic neuropathy, psychosis). Urban-dwelling, poor, elderly persons who live in poorly ventilated dwellings without air-conditioning during hot, humid summers are the most common victims of classic heat stroke. Once body temperature exceeds 42°C, enzyme systems and oxidative phosphorylation begin to fail, membrane permeability increases, ionic composition of the intracellular milieu becomes deranged, proteins denature, and cellular dysfunction leads to multiple-organ-system failure.

Neurologic dysfunction is the hallmark of heat stroke. Such dysfunction can range from mental status changes (obtundation, delirium) to seizures, to focal or lateral deficits, or to posturing. Tachycardia is present, and tachypnea may be extreme. Hypotension may exist or there may be normotension with a wide pulse pressure. In about half the cases, the skin is warm and dry; in the other half, cool and clammy. Pulmonary edema may be present. Mortality increases exponentially with delays in diagnosis and cooling, and therefore when a diagnosis of heat stroke is entertained, cooling procedures should begin immediately while both the laboratory tests are pending and the differential diagnosis is explored. There is less harm in cooling a patient who turns out not to have heat stroke than in delaying the start of cooling in a patient who does have heat stroke.

Many methods of cooling have been tried. Immersion in an ice bath or cold-water bath is effective but makes it difficult to perform the other diagnostic, therapeutic, or resuscitative procedures the patient needs. Packing the patient in slush or ice on a stretcher is easier; ice bags laid across the neck, axilla, and groins are also somewhat effective. The currently preferred method is to place the patient nude on a stretcher, spray the patient with tepid water, and blow air at room temperature over the patient by means of powerful fans. Ice-water lavage is minimally effective, and ice-water enemas may cause further electrolyte derangement. Iced peritoneal lavage seems to be effective and may be used in refractory cases. The target temperature is 39°C; once it has been reached, cooling procedures should stop so that overshoot does not occur, causing its own set of problems.

Neurologic abnormalities often, but not always, clear once the body is cooled. Cardiac dysfunction, cardiogenic or noncardiogenic pulmonary edema, acute renal failure, rhabdomyolysis, and DIC often complicate heat stroke.

Reference: Tek D, et al: Heat illness. Emerg Med Clin North Am 10:299–310, 1992.

HEMATEMESIS

Hematemesis is one of the most disconcerting symptoms for both patient and physician alike. The differential diagnosis includes an acutely bleeding ulcer or cancer, Mallory-Weiss tear, bleeding esophageal varices, and acute gastritis. A careful history often discloses symptoms differentiating these diagnoses. Patients with ulcers have a history of epigastric pain with melena. Patients with cancer may have associated weight loss, pain, and/or early satiety. A history of severe retching prior to hematemesis is elicited in most patients with Mallory-Weiss tears. A history of heavy ethanol intake or regular use of aspirin or NSAIDs is obtained from patients with the diagnosis of acute hemorrhagic gastritis. A long history of heavy ethanol use or chronic liver disease is obtained from patients with bleeding esophageal varices. About 25% of patients are diagnosed with duodenal ulcers, 25% with gastritis, and approximately 15% with varices, depending on the patient population.

It is important to quickly assess and stabilize a patient with hematemesis. In the presence of hypotension, most patients have a hematocrit of less than 30%. Very early in the course, the hematocrit may be close to normal before the vascular compartments compensate. In brisk and significant bleeding, the BUN usually rises to greater than 40 mg/dL because of the absorption of nitrogen from the small bowel. Shock, secondary to bleeding, can cause damage to the liver, with SGPT and SGOT rising to ten times their normal values. Renal failure from shock can also occur, so it is important to replace vascular volume as quickly as possible.

Surgical intervention may be needed to control bleeding. Although most cases are self-limited, diagnostic studies to determine the source should be done as soon as the patient is stabilized. Upper endoscopy gives the most information, and its only limitation is in the patient whose bleeding is so profuse as to preclude visualization. Endoscopy may also be therapeutic, as epinephrine or sclerotherapy with ethanol or other agents can be administered in patients with bleeding ulcers or esophageal varices; it has a reported success rate of up to 90%.

Nd-YAG surgical laser treatment and multipolar and heater probes have also been used and are quite effective in controlling bleeding in more than 80% of patients. Nevertheless, perforations are possible and occur in about 3% of these patients. Mesenteric angiography is also a useful diagnostic tool in massive upper GI bleeding, successful only when bleeding occurs at rate of at least 2 ml/min or more. Embolization of feeding arteries can be accomplished with particulate agents, or intra-arterial vasopressin may be used.

Unfortunately, rebleeding occurs in 5–30% of patients even after surgery. For this reason, surgery is not the treatment of first choice and should be used only in those patients who lose more than 6 units of blood in the first 24 hours and who fail endoscopic therapy.

HEMATOPOIETIC SYSTEM

A multipotential hematopoietic stem cell is the progenitor of two cell lines—the myeloid line and the lymphoid line—as shown in the accompanying figure. The pluripotent myeloid stem cell possesses extensive capabilities to give rise to new hematopoietic stem cells (self-renewal) and to generate primitive specific progenitors that differentiate.

The existence of the pluripotent myeloid stem cell (CFU-S) was first demonstrated in experiments in which bone marrow cells from mice were injected intravenously into other, heavily irradiated, syngeneic mice. Discrete nodules (colonies) of hematopoietic cells appeared in the spleens of the recipient mice 8–10 days after injection. These nodules showed microscopically erythroid, granulocytic, and megakaryocytic cells. Each colony was the product of proliferation and maturation of a single stem cell, termed a spleen colony-forming unit (CFU-S).

The pluripotent stem cell (CFU-S) is capable of differentiation into unipotent stem cells of a specific lineage (erythroid, granulocytic, megakaryocytic). Knowledge about the characteristics of committed (unipotent) hematopoietic stem cells has been derived principally by observations of the growth of specific colonies (erythroid, neutrophilic-macrophage, megakaryocytic, eosinophilic, and basophilic) when stem cells are cultured in semisolid media in vitro. The specific terms for unipotent stem cells responsible for the colonies are:

CFU-NM	Neutrophil-macrophage colony-forming unit
CFU-G	Granulocyte colony-forming unit
CFU-M	Macrophage colony-forming unit
CFU-EOS	Eosinophil colony-forming unit
CFU-BAS	Basophil colony-forming unit
CFU-MEG	Megakaryocytic colony-forming unit
CFU-E	Erythroid colony-forming unit
BFU-E	Erythroid burst-forming unit—a primitive erythroid progenitor and the precursor of CFU-E

The earliest cells recognizable morphologically in the development of blood cells are the pronormoblast, myeloblast, monoblast, eosinophilic promyelocyte, basophilic myelocyte, and megakaryoblast. Stem cells cannot be specifically identified morphologically.

In each specific lineage (erythroid, neutrophilic, monocytic, eosinophilic, basophilic and megakaryocytic) there is progressive maturation of cells in the marrow from the unipotent stem cells leading to the mature functional cells, which are then released from the marrow into the circulation. This maturation is under the control of hematopoietic growth factors.

Hierarchy of the Hematopoietic Stem Cell and Progenitor System

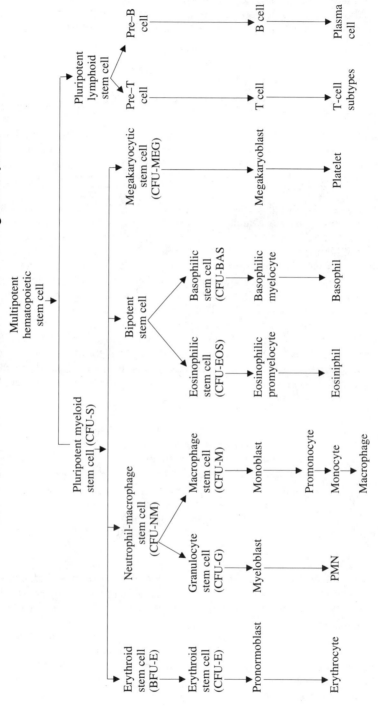

HEMATURIA

Hematuria is defined as the presence of abnormal quantities of RBCs in the urinary sediment. Normally, urine shows 2 or 3 RBCs per high-power field (HPF) in freshly voided urine. Persistent or recurrent presence of >3 RBC/HPF warrants further evaluation.

Gross hematuria is obvious on visual examination of freshly voided urine. Microscopic hematuria is detected by examination of urinary sediment under the microscope or by using orthotoluidine-impregnated paper strips (dipsticks) in the urine. Calcium oxalate crystals and air bubbles are often mistaken as RBCs under the microscope. A urine dipstick is positive with as little as 3–5 RBC/HPF, although hemoglobin and myoglobin also give positive reactions.

Approach to patients with hematuria: The following table gives a correlation between the clinical features and localization of the site of bleeding. In all patients, the initial laboratory studies should include coagulation tests, UA, and cultures. Sterile pyuria with hematuria is seen with renal TB and analgesic use. Plain abdominal films should be taken to rule out renal and pelvic calcifications and masses. In younger patients, the evaluation of hematuria includes renal ultrasound or IVP to rule out polycystic or medullary sponge kidney and urolithiasis. Hypercalciuria is present in 35% of children with isolated hematuria in the absence of visible stones. In older patients (>40 yr), evaluation includes renal imaging studies and cystoscopy with biopsy of all suspected masses. If cystoscopy is negative, further imaging studies such as retrograde or antegrade pyelography, CT scan, and angiography should be considered (depending on the clinical profile of the patient). Even after all studies, however, the cause remains unknown in about 10% of cases.

Clinicoanatomic Correlation of Hematuria

	RENAL PARENCHYMA	URINARY TRACT
Pain	Usually dull flank pain	Commonly either suprapubic pain with dysuria or colicky flank pain
Blood clots	Absent in glomerular diseases; may occur with trauma, tumors, and vascular anomalies	Commonly present
Cellular casts	Commonly present in glomerular diseases	Absent
Proteinuria >150 mg/dl	Commonly present	Absent
RBC shape	Usually distorted	Normal

Glomerular bleeding accounts for 35% of cases of isolated hematuria. Presence of RBC casts and dysmorphic RBCs indicates glomerular origin of blood. A variety of glomerulonephritides present as isolated hematuria and later develop into the full-blown clinical picture. Persistent and recurrent isolated hematuria is characteristic of IgA nephropathy and thin basement membrane disease. When urological and radiological evaluation fails to reveal a definite source of hematuria, renal biopsy should be considered, especially if other features of glomerular disease are also present.

Common Causes of Hematuria

I. **Renal parenchyma**
  A. Glomerular diseases
    • Primary glomerulonephritis
    • Glomerulopathies associated with systemic diseases: SLE, vasculitis, Wegener's granulomatosis, Goodpasture's syndrome, Henoch-Schönlein purpura, diabetic nephropathy, thrombotic microangiopathies
    • Infectious: postinfectious glomerulonephritis, infective endocarditis, shunt nephritis
    • Hereditary: Alport's syndrome
  B. Vascular
    • Malignant hypertension
    • Renal thromboembolism
    • Loin-pain hematuria syndrome
    • Vascular anomalies
  C. Tubulointerstitial
    • Hereditary: polycystic and medullary cystic diseases
    • Allergic interstitial nephritis
    • Renal papillary necrosis
    • Acute bacterial pyelonephritis
  D. Renal tumors
    • Renal cell carcinoma
    • Wilms's tumor
II. **Urinary tract disorders**
    • Renal pelvis: calculi, trauma, transitional cell carcinoma
    • Ureter: calculi, tumors, retroperitoneal fibrosis
    • Bladder: cystitis, tumors, trauma, vascular, schistosomiasis
    • Prostate: benign hypertrophy, carcinoma, prostatitis
    • Urethra: trauma, polyps, urethritis, tumors, foreign bodies
III. **Systemic coagulopathies**
IV. **Renal trauma**

Treatment: The treatment in most cases of hematuria is that of the underlying disorder. The blood loss from hematuria is often not major enough to require blood transfusions. Occasionally, the passing of a blood clot may produce severe pain and urinary obstruction (''clot colic''), which may require urethral catheterization and saline irrigation. In patients with hypercalciuria, a therapeutic trial with thiazide diuretics resolves the hematuria in 60% of cases and is useful as a ''therapeutic test.''

HEMOCHROMATOSIS

Hemochromatosis is a disorder associated with increased iron absorption and/or storage resulting in:

• Skin pigmentation
• Liver dysfunction/cirrhosis/hepatocellular carcinoma
• Arthritis
• Gonadal failure and loss of libido
• Diabetes mellitus
• Congestive heart failure
• Cardiac arrhythmias

Classification of Iron Overload

Genetic
  Frequency of 2:1,000 of the white population
  Male:female ratio of 5:1
  Recessive transmission
  Heterozygotes may develop manifestations of the disease when exposed to alcohol or
    increased oral iron intake.
Secondary
  Refractory anemias, including thalassemia and sideroblastic
  Chronic liver disease
  Prolonged dietary overload
  Inherited disorders, including porphyria cutanea tarda, atransferrinemia, and neonatal iron
    overload
Parenteral iron overload
  Multiple blood transfusions
  Excessive parenteral iron
  Hemodialysis

Adapted from Hauser SC, et al: Spotlight on hemochromatosis and its treatment. Contemp Intern Med (Nov/Dec):71, 1992.

The diagnosis is based on suspicious clinical findings and abnormal serum iron studies (see table following). A liver biopsy is necessary for definitive diagnosis.

Representative Iron Values in Normal Subjects, Hemochromatosis,
and Alcoholic Liver Disease

	NORMAL	SYMPTOMATIC HEMOCHROMA-TOSIS	EARLY ASYMPTOMATIC HEMOCHROMA-TOSIS	ALCOHOLIC LIVER DISEASE
Plasma iron, µmol/L (µg/dl)	9–27 (50–150)	32–54 (180–300)	Usually elevated	Often elevated
TIBC, µmol/L (µg/dl)	45–66 (250–370)	36–54 (200–300)	36–54 (200–300)	45–66 (250–370)
Transferrin saturation, %	22–46	50–100	50–100	27–60
Serum ferritin, µg/L	10–200	900–6000	200–500	10–500
Urinary iron,* mg/24 h	0–2	9–23	2.5	Usually <5
Liver iron, µg/100 ng dry wt	30–140	600–1800	200–400	30–200

*After IM administration of 0.5 g deferoxamine.

From Powell LW, et al: Hemochromatosis. In Wilson JD, et al (eds): Harrison's Principles of Internal Medicine, 12th ed. New York, McGraw-Hill, 1991, p 1827, with permission.

Primary hemochromatosis is treated with lifelong repeated phlebotomy, beginning with 1 unit/wk and continuing until Hct falls to 36% or 38% and a repeat liver biopsy demonstrates depleted hepatic iron stores. Then maintenance phlebotomy at approximately 3-month intervals is continued indefinitely. Chelation therapy with deferoxamine can reduce iron loads in cases of secondary hemochromatosis related to chronic anemia.

HEMODYNAMIC MONITORING

Pulmonary Artery Catheters

The clinical use of the pulmonary artery catheter was first introduced by Swan and Ganz in 1970. Since that time its use has become common to help diagnose, treat, and manage patients in the ICU setting. Information obtained, including cardiac output, filling pressures, and systemic and pulmonary resistance, can help guide the use of IV fluids, inotropic agents, and afterload-reducing drugs.

Indications for Use of Pulmonary Artery Catheterization

Severe myocardial dysfunction
    Cardiogenic shock/pump failure
    Refractory CHF
    MI with CHF, VSD, mitral regurgitation
    Management of afterload reduction
    Pericardial tamponade
    Acute mitral regurgitation
    Constrictive pericarditis
Hypovolemic shock not responsive to volume resuscitation
Hypotension
Sepsis with hypotension and/or poor urine output
Pulmonary edema (cardiac versus noncardiac)
Unexplained oliguria
Management of ARDS
Suspected pulmonary hypertension
Prior to procedures requiring large-volume administration, fluid shifts (aortic surgery, cardiac surgery, etc.)

Complications Associated with Pulmonary Artery Catheters

Complications associated with central venous puncture
    Catheter-related infection
    Pneumothorax
    Puncture of the subclavian vein
    Intrapleural infusion of fluids
    Injury to the brachial plexus
    Subcutaneous emphysema
    Damage to the thoracic duct (leading to chylothorax, with left internal jugular approach)
    Accidental shearing of the catheter/catheter emboli
    Arterial puncture
Complications unique to the pulmonary artery catheter
    Ventricular arrhythmias
    Premature ventricular contractions
    Atrial fibrillation, flutter
    Ventricular tachycardia, fibrillation
    Right bundle branch block
    Balloon rupture

Table continued on next page.

Complications Associated with Pulmonary Artery Catheters (Cont.)

Ventricular rupture
Endocardial damage
Valvular damage
Chordae tendineae and/or papillary muscle damage
Intracardiac knotting of the catheter
Pulmonary infarction
Pulmonary artery rupture
Predisposition to right-sided endocarditis

RIGHT HEART PRESSURES

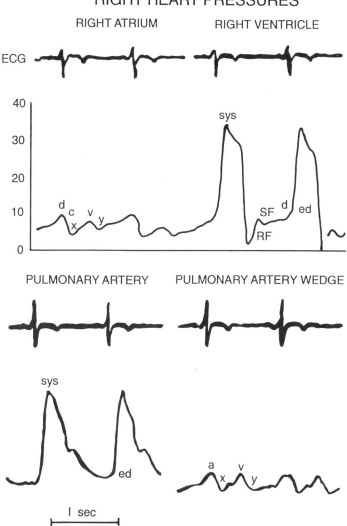

Above, Normal pressure waveforms measured through a PA catheter. *Below,* PA systolic, diastolic, and wedge (PAO) pressures. (From Braunwald E (ed): Heart Disease: A Textbook of Cardiovascular Medicine. Philadelphia, WB Saunders, 1980, with permission.)

Range of Normal Resting Hemodynamic Values (mm Hg)

PRESSURES	a WAVE	v WAVE	MEAN	SYSTOLIC	END-DIASTOLIC	MEAN
Right atrium	2–10	2–10	0–8			
Right ventricle				1–30	0–8	
Pulmonary artery				5–30	3–12	9–16
Pulmonary artery wedge and left atrium		3–15	3–12	1–10		
Left ventricle				100–140	3–12	
Systemic arteries				100–140	60–90	70–105

Equations Useful in Hemodynamic Monitoring

Mean Arterial Pressure

MAP = (systolic BP – diastolic BP) 1/3 + diastolic BP
(Normal = 85–95 mm Hg)

Systemic Vascular Resistance

$$SVR = \frac{MAP \ (mm \ Hg) - CVP \ (mm \ Hg)}{Cardiac \ output \ (L/min)} \times 79.9$$

(Normal = 770 – 1500 dynes·sec·cm^{-5})

Pulmonary Vascular Resistance

$$PVR = \frac{MPAP \ (mm \ Hg) - PAOP \ (mm \ Hg)}{Cardiac \ output \ (L/min)} \times 79.9$$

(MPAP = mean pulmonary artery pressure; PAOP = pulmonary artery output pressure)
(Normal = 20–120 dynes·sec·cm^{-5})

Arterial O_2 Content

$C_aO_2 = (Hb \times 1.34) \ S_aO_2 + (P_aO_2 \times 0.0031)$
(S_aO_2 = percent saturation of arterial blood)

Mixed Venous O_2 Content

$C\bar{v}O_2 = (Hb) \ (1.34) \ S\bar{v}O_2 + (P\bar{v}O_2 \times 0.0031)$
($S\bar{v}O_2$ = percent saturation of mixed venous blood)

Shunt Fraction

$$\frac{\dot{Q}s = Cc'O_2 - CaO_2}{\dot{Q}t = Cc'O_2 - C\bar{v}O_2}$$

$Cc'O_2 = (1.34) \ (Hb) \ 100\% \ saturation + 0.0031 \ P_aO_2$

$$P_AO_2 = (P_B - P_{H_2O}) \ F_IO_2 - \frac{PCO_2}{0.8}$$

(P_B = barometric pressure; P_{H_2O} = water vapor pressure)
(Normal shunt ≤ 0.05 [5%])

Reference: Swan HJC, Ganz W, Forrester J, et al: Catheterization of the heart in man with use of a flow-directed balloon-tipped catheter. N Engl J Med 283:447, 1970.

HEMOLYSIS

Hemolysis is defined as destruction of RBCs before their normal 120-day life span. Hemolytic anemia occurs when the body's ability to produce RBCs cannot keep up with the rate at which they are being destroyed. The diagnosis of hemolytic anemia is made by the peripheral blood smear and reticulocyte count. The latter is elevated in hemolytic anemias, unless there is also impaired RBC production.

Causes of Hemolysis

A. Congenital hemolytic anemias
  1. Defects in hemoglobin structure or synthesis
     - Sickle-cell anemia, hemoglobin C disease
     - Thalassemia
     - Unstable hemoglobins (Heinz body anemia)
  2. Defects in red cell membrane
     - Hereditary spherocytosis, hereditary elliptocytosis
  3. Defects in RBC metabolic pathways
     - Hexokinase, phosphofructokinase, pyruvate kinase deficiency
     - G6PD deficiency
     - Deficiency in glutathione synthesis

B. Acquired hemolytic anemias
  1. Autoimmune
     a. Warm reactive antibodies
        - Idiopathic
        - Secondary
          — Lymphoproliferative diseases (CLL, lymphoma)
          — Connective tissue diseases
          — Drugs (hapten type, immune complex type, autoantibody type)
     b. Cold reactive antibodies (cold agglutinin disease)
        - Idiopathic
        - Secondary
          — Lymphoproliferative diseases
          — Infections
            Mycoplasma pneumoniae,
            infectious mononucleosis
     c. Paroxysmal cold hemoglobinuria
        - Associated with tertiary syphilis
        - Postviral infection (self-limited)
  2. Other immune hemolysis
     - Incompatible blood transfusion
     - Hemolytic disease of the newborn
  3. Mechanical hemolysis
     - Prosthetic heart valves
     - Microangiopathic hemolytic anemia, DIC
     - Hemolytic-uremic syndrome, TTP
     - Cardiopulmonary bypass

Table continued on next page.

Causes of Hemolysis (Cont.)

---

4. Acquired membrane defects
   - Paroxysmal nocturnal hemoglobinuria
   - Spur cell anemia (cirrhosis)
5. Direct destruction by infectious agent or septic state
   - Malaria, babesiosis, bartonellosis
   - *Clostridium*
6. Metabolic depletion
   - Prolonged storage of RBCs

Adapted from Greenberger NJ, et al: Differential diagnosis of hemolytic anemias. In The Medical Book of Lists, 3rd ed. Chicago, Year Book Medical Publishers, 1990, pp 131–132, with permission.

Schwartz RS, et al: The autoimmune hemolytic anemias. In Hoffman R, et al (eds): Hematology: Basic Principles and Practice. New York, Churchill Livingstone, 1991, pp 422–441.

HEMOPTYSIS

Hemoptysis refers to blood in the sputum and includes the full range of bloody sputum from minimal blood streaking to frank blood. Massive hemoptysis implies copious bleeding and has been defined as the expectoration of greater than 600 cc of blood in a 24-hour period. This potentially lethal and alarming clinical situation requires expeditious evaluation, close observation, and possible surgical intervention.

In addition to Hx & PE, all patients should have a CXR. Further diagnostic procedures should be guided by these findings. Patients with hemoptysis may present with a normal CXR (up to 50%). In several large series, hemoptysis with a normal CXR was the indication for outpatient bronchoscopy in 20% of cases.

Causes of Hemoptysis with Normal CXR

---

1. Nonpulmonary source
   Nosebleed
   Hematemesis
2. Systemic coagulation disorder
3. Pulmonary vascular disease
   Occult pulmonary emboli
   Mitral stenosis
4. Benign endobronchial lesions
   Chronic bronchitis   Bronchiectasis
   Bronchial adenoma   Foreign bodies
   Inflammatory polyps   Endobronchial TB
   Hereditary pulmonary hemosiderosis
5. Bronchogenic carcinoma
6. Miscellaneous
   Congestive heart failure
   Idiopathic pulmonary hemosiderosis
   Fractured bronchus

Adapted from Chang S-W, et al.: Hemoptysis with a normal chest roentgenogram. In Schwarz MI (ed): Pulmonary Grand Rounds. Toronto, BC Decker, 1990, p 123.

Causes of Hemoptysis with Abnormal CXR

Airway diseases
Acute or chronic bronchitis
Bronchieclasis, including cystic fibrosis
Bronchogenic carcinoma
Bronchial adenoma or hamartoma
Endobronchial tuberculosis
Broncholithiasis
Foreign body aspiration
Bronchial endometriosis

Parenchymal diseases
Tuberculosis
Pneumonia
Lung abscess
Aspergilloma
Alveolar hemorrhage syndromes
Wegener's granulomatosis
Paragonomiasis

Vascular diseases
Pulmonary embolism
Elevated pulmonary wedge pressure
Mitral stenosis
Left ventricular failure
Pulmonary hypertension
Pulmonary arteriovenous malformations

Other causes
Anticoagulant therapy
Bleeding diathesis
Iatrogenic
Bronchoscopy
Swan-Ganz catheterization
Idiopathic

From McDonnell TJ: Hemoptysis with localized pulmonary infiltrates. In Schwarz MI (ed.): Pulmonary Grand Rounds. Toronto, BC Decker, 1990, p 131, with permission.

Comparison of Causes of "Ordinary" and "Massive" Hemoptysis

DIAGNOSIS	ORDINARY*	MASSIVE†
Active pulmonary tuberculosis	4	47
Bronchiectasis	52	37
Chronic necrotizing pneumonia	4	11
Lung abscess	—	6
Cancer of the lung	31	6
Bronchovascular fistula	—	5
Fungal infections	—	4
Bleeding diathesis	4	3
Congestive heart failure	5	—
Pulmonary infarction	2	—
Miscellaneous	13	4
No diagnosis	14	—
Total	129	123

*Gong H Jr, Salvatierra C: Clinical efficacy of early and delayed fiberoptic bronchoscopy in patients with hemoptysis. Am Rev Respir Dis 124:221–225, 1981.

†Conlan AA, Hurwitz SS, Kriege L, et al: Massive hemoptysis. Review of 123 cases. J Thorac Cardiovasc Surg 85:120–124, 1983.

From Murray JF: Diagnostic evaluation: History and physical exam. In Murray JF, Nadel JA: Textbook of Respiratory Medicine. Philadelphia, W.B. Saunders, 1988, p 435, with permission.

Reference: Adelman M, et al: Cryptogenic hemoptysis. Ann Intern Med 102:829–834, 1985.

HEMORRHOIDS

The anal canal is approximately 4 cm long and has an important mucocutaneous landmark, the dentate line, located about midway. Proximal to the dentate line, the canal is lined with a mixture of columnar and squamous epithelium and has longitudinal ridges, which terminate at the line in the crescent-shaped anal valves. The anal canal, distal to the dentate line, is lined by stratified squamous epithelium. The dentate line marks the boundary between two venous plexuses and therefore between internal and external hemorrhoids. Above the dentate line the superior hemorrhoidal veins (which drain the mucosa of the rectum) carry blood predominantly into the portal system. Below the line the inferior hemorrhoidal plexus drains eventually into the caval circulation. The pressure is therefore higher in the superior hemorrhoidal plexus than in the lower. Also, internal hemorrhoids are covered with mucous membrane, and external hemorrhoids are covered with skin.

Internal hemorrhoids have four grades:

Grade 1: Hemorrhoids bulge excessively but remain proximal to the dentate line.
Grade 2: Hemorrhoids prolapse below the dentate line with defecation but reduce spontaneously.
Grade 3: Hemorrhoids require manual reduction.
Grade 4: Hemorrhoids cannot be manually reduced.

Bleeding from internal hemorrhoids is usually mild, and anemia from bleeding hemorrhoids is uncommon enough to be a diagnosis of exclusion. However, because of their connection to the portal system, bleeding from internal hemorrhoids in a patient with portal hypertension can be dramatic. Internal hemorrhoids are only mildly painful, unless they thrombose, an uncommon but extremely painful situation. This pain lasts for as long as a week.

In contrast to the anal mucosa above the dentate line, which is innervated by the autonomic nervous system, the mucosa distal to the line is innervated by somatic nerves. As a consequence, external hemorrhoids, while smaller, tend to be much more painful than internal hemorrhoids. They also are more likely to thrombose than internal hemorrhoids, but pain from acute thrombosis disappears in two or three days.

Patients with hemorrhoids are generally counseled to avoid having to strain at stool. This is most successfully accomplished by increasing the bulk of stool by increasing fiber in the diet or by use of a hydrophilic laxative. In those patients thought to need definitive correction, many techniques are now available, including infrared coagulation, elastic band ligation, and cryotherapy. Hemorrhoidectomy, often performed in the outpatient setting, is required by only 5 to 10% of patients.

Reference: Smith LE: Hemorrhoidectomy with lasers and other contemporary modalities. Surg Clin North Am 72:665–79, 1992.

HEPATIC DISEASE

Child-Turcotte-Pugh Classification

The Child-Turcotte-Pugh classification was created to assess a cirrhotic patient's surgical risk. However, it is now used as a general measure of severity of liver disease.

Child-Turcotte-Pugh Classification of Liver Disease

ABNORMALITY	POINT SCORE ACCORDING TO ABNORMALITY		
	1	2	3
Ascites	Absent	Slight	Moderate
Encephalopathy grade	None	1–2	3–4
Bilirubin	<3.4	3.4–5.1	>5.1
Albumin	>3.5	2.8–3.5	<2.8
Prothrombin time (sec prolonged)	1–4	4–6	>6

(Grade A = 5–6; Grade B = 7–9; Grade C = 10–15)

LFT Patterns

Elevated liver tests are often the first detected abnormality that points to liver disease. Liver tests usually include albumin, PT, SGOT (AST), SGPT (ALT), alkaline phosphatase, GGT, and bilirubin.

Liver Disease	LFT Patterns
Alcohol related	AST <400 and two times ALT
Cholestatic	Elevated bilirubin and alkaline phosphatase; minor elevations of ALT and AST
Infiltrating tumor	Elevated alkaline phosphatase and GGT with minor elevation of other tests
Acute hepatitis	Elevation of ALT and AST ≥1,000
End-stage disease	Increased PT not corrected with vitamin K and low albumin
Drug reaction	Any pattern

HEPATIC ENCEPHALOPATHY

Hepatic encephalopathy is a reversible state of impaired cognitive function and altered consciousness that occurs in subjects with liver disease or portal systemic shunts. Encephalopathy is probably due entirely to shunting of blood away from the liver into the systemic circulation. Such blood has not been detoxified and contains ammonia, bacterial particles, and other substances that impair the nervous system. Most cases of hepatic encephalopathy occur in patients with cirrhosis; only 5% occur in patients with noncirrhotic portal hypertension. In patients with hepatic encephalopathy, the most important precipitating factors are renal impairment, overdiureses, protein consumption, infection, GI bleed, benzodiazepine use, or other analgesic/sedative use. In the patient who presents with hepatic encephalopathy, precipitating causes should be looked for.

Clinical Features of Hepatic Encephalopathy

Monotonous speech flat affect	Metabolic tremor
Muscular inclination	Impaired handwriting
Asterixis	Fetor hepaticus
Coma	Upgoing plantar responses
Hypoactive or hyperactive reflexes	Decerebrate posture
Paranoia	Sleeplessness
Hyperventilation	Respiratory depression
Seizures	

Stages of Hepatic Encephalopathy

Stage 1:	Subtle alterations in personality, sleep disturbance, lethargy	Stage 3:	Stupor
Stage 2:	Somnolence	Stage 4:	Coma

Treatment of hepatic encephalopathy: Treatment of hepatic encephalopathy remains empirical and relies largely on establishing the correct diagnosis, identifying and treating precipitating factors, emptying the bowels of blood, protein and stool, and attending to electrolyte and acid-base disturbances and the use of benzodiazepine antagonists in patients who have taken benzodiazepines in the preceding weeks. Nonabsorbable disaccharides such as lactulose remain the mainstay of therapy. The postulated mechanism of action of these agents includes acidification of colonic contents with reduced absorption of ammonia and change in the colonic bacterial flora in favor of forms that utilize ammonia. Lactulose more than doubles fecal bacterial output, causing a marked reduction in colonic absorption of soluble nitrogen. The dose is usually titrated to give two or three loose stools per day. Therapy is usually started at 30 cc QID. If this is not possible, enemas may be used with 500 cc of lactulose with 500 ml of water TID.

If lactulose is not helpful alone, neomycin may be used (1 gm QID). This drug appears to kill the colonic bacteria that secretes the toxic products that cause encephalopathy. Alternatively, metronidazole (250 mg QID) may be used. Other therapies include decreasing the amount of protein intake or the form of protein intake. Branch chain amino acids or vegetable protein, as opposed to meat protein, appears to cause less confusion. Strict protein restriction is often helpful for the encephalopathy but harmful to the patient. One should always strive to give patients as much protein as possible without compromising their mental status.

HEPATITIS

Chronic

Evaluation: Patients often present with asymptomatic elevated liver enzymes, fatigue, hepatomegaly, or signs of chronic liver disease. These patients usually have one of the following disorders: alcohol-induced liver disease, chronic viral hepatitis, autoimmune hepatitis, hepatic steatosis, Wilson's disease, hemochromatosis, α-1-antitrypsin deficiency, drug-induced liver disease, primary biliary cirrhosis (PBC), primary sclerosing cholangitis (PSC), granulomatous liver disease, or idiopathic etiology.

The first step consists of a detailed Hx & PE with specific reference to viral exposure risk factors and alcohol and drug use. If the enzymes are more than twice normal, tests should be done to exclude autoimmune or chronic hepatitis. These tests include anti-HCV, HBsAg, anti-HBcAg, antimitochondrial antibody (AMA), and ESR. If the patient is over 40 years of age, elevated iron saturation and ferritin are suggestive of hemochromatosis. If under 40, a low serum ceruloplasmin and an elevated 24-hour urinary excretion of copper are suggestive of Wilson's disease. If the cause of the disease is still unclear, an ultrasound can suggest hepatic steatosis (usually a benign condition) or hepatic tumors. If the picture is mainly cholestatic (elevated alkaline phosphatase and bilirubin), then an AMA will usually diagnose PBC and an ERCP will diagnose PSC. If the patient has liver enzyme elevations greater than three times normal for longer than four months, a liver biopsy should be done to help establish the diagnosis and stage the disease. The table outlines treatment of the disorders mentioned.

Treatment of Chronic Liver Diseases

DISORDER	TREATMENT
Chronic hepatitis C	α-Interferon
Chronic hepatitis B (HBeAg +)	α-Interferon
PSC + PBC	Ursodeoxycholic acid
Wilson's disease	Penicillamine
Hemochromatosis	Phlebotomy
Autoimmune hepatitis	Steroids
All diseases (end stage)	Transplantation

Drug-induced and Toxic

Patients with toxic or drug-induced liver disease can present with cirrhosis, acute or chronic hepatitis, hepatomegaly, or elevated liver enzymes. Over 600 drugs have been shown to induce liver injury. The swift recognition of a drug-induced liver disease is of paramount importance, because in many cases, continued administration can be fatal and specific antidotes are sometimes required. Drug-induced injury may occur either as an unexpected idiosyncratic reaction to a therapeutic dose of a drug or as an expected consequence of an intrinsically hepatotoxic drug taken in a sufficiently large dose.

When faced with a patient with evidence of acute or chronic liver injury, the clinician must always ask if a drug or toxin could be involved. The patient should stop all suspected drugs and be given any specific antidote, and a complete workup for other causes should be done. Toxic screen of blood and urine can be helpful. If the patient has allergic phenomena, such as fever, rash, or eosinophilia, this is supportive of a drug reaction, but most drugs do not cause these phenomena. If the etiology remains unclear, a liver biopsy might be helpful. The table lists some of the most frequent drugs and toxins encountered.

Drug-induced Liver Disease

CATEGORY	EXAMPLE	TREATMENT
Histologic zonal necrosis	Acetaminophen Carbon tetrachloride	N-acetylcysteine
Viral-like	Amanita mushrooms	Silymarin (not available in U.S.)
Cholestasis	Halothane, isoniazid, phenytoin	Steroids
	Estrogens, NSAIDs, chlorpromazine, erythromycin	

Table continued on next page.

Drug-induced Liver Disease (Cont.)

Fatty Liver	
Large droplet	Ethanol, amiodarone
Small droplet	Tetracycline, valproic acid
Granulomas	Allopurinol, phenylbutazone
Fibrosis	Vitamin A, methotrexate
Tumors	Estrogens
Vascular lesions	Anabolic steroids

Viral

Acute

Acute hepatitis presents with change in sleep patterns, fatigue, jaundice, anorexia, and hepatomegaly. Laboratory tests reveal elevation of the SGPT and SGOT into the thousands, with variable elevations of bilirubin and modest elevations of the alkaline phosphatase (<400). Any patient presenting with these symptoms should have the following laboratory tests: IgM anti-HAV, HBsAg, IgG anti-HBcAg, and anti-HCV. If the IgG anti-HBcAg is positive and HBsAg is negative, then an IgM anti-HBcAg should be obtained. The most common causes of viral hepatitis are A, B, C, E, CMV, and EBV.

Clinical Features of Viral Hepatitis

	TYPE OF VIRAL HEPATITIS				
FEATURES	A	B	C	D	E
General					
Age at onset	Childhood	All	All	All	Adulthood
Mean incubation (days)	30	50	50	?	40
Clinical					
Rash	–	+	–	–	+
Arthralgia	–	+	–	–	+
Nausea	+	+	+	+	+
Vomiting	+	+	+	+	+
Jaundice	–	+/–	–	+	+
Virologic					
Type of virus	RNA	DNA	RNA	RNA	?RNA
Viremia	Transient	Prolonged	Prolonged	Prolonged	?Transient
Fecal excretion of virus	+	–	–	–	+
Severity of disease	Mild	Moderate	Mild	Moderate	Moderate
Mortality	Low	Low	Low	High	Moderate (↑ in pregnant women)
Chronic carrier state	–	+	+	+	–
Chronic disease	–	+	+	+	–

Table continued on next page.

Clinical Features of Viral Hepatitis (Cont.)

	TYPE OF VIRAL HEPATITIS				
FEATURES	A	B	C	D	E
Transmission routes					
Oral	+	?	?	?	+ (contaminated water)
Percutaneous	Rare	+	+	+	–
Sexual	+	+	–	+	?
Perinatal	–	+	?	–	?
Hepatocellular carcinoma	–	+	+	–	–
Other					
Special features	Disease more virulent in older individuals	—	—	Infects only hepatitis B carriers	Rare in U.S.
Diagnosis	IgM anti-HAV	IgM, anti-HCV, HBsAg	Anti-HCV, HCV RNA	HBsAg, IgM anti-HDV	Anti-HEV
Prognosis	99% recovery	95% recovery 1% death 4% chronic	50% recovery 50% chronic 25% cirrhosis	Over 25% chronic	95% recovery
Vaccine	Yes	Yes	No	No	No
Indication of immunity	IgG anti-HAV	Anti-HBs IgG anti-HBC (with negative HBsAg)	Unknown	IgG anti-HDV	Unknown

Modified from Ergun GA, et al: Viral hepatitis. Postgrad Med 88(Oct):70, 1990.

Serologies for hepatitis C usually become positive three months after initial infection. Therefore, it may be difficult to diagnosis acute hepatitis C if HCV-RNA tests are not available. If hepatitis A, B, C, D, and E have been excluded, one must consider autoimmune hepatitis, Wilson's disease, drug reaction, or viral hepatitis secondary to CMV or EBV. One can obtain IgM and IgG tests for these viruses. A positive IgM indicates acute infection, as does a fourfold rise in IgG antibodies over 4 weeks.

Hepatitis B

Hepatitis B Serologic Markers in Different Stages of Infection and Convalescence

			ANTI-HBc			
STAGE OF INFECTION	HBsAg	ANTI-HBs	IgG	IgM	HBeAg	ANTI-HBe
Late incubation period of hepatitis B	+	–	–	–	+ or –	–
Acute hepatitis B	+	–	+	+	+	–
HBsAg-negative acute hepatitis B	–	–	+	+	–	–

Table continued on next page.

Hepatitis B Serologic Markets in Different Stages of Infection and Convalescence (Cont.)

STAGE OF INFECTION	HBsAg	ANTI-HBs	ANTI-HBc IgG	ANTI-HBc IgM	HBeAg	ANTI-HBe
Healthy HBsAg carrier	+	−	+++	+ or −	−	+
Chronic hepatitis B	+	−	+++	+ or −	+	−
HBV infection in recent past	−	++	++	+ or −	−	+
HBV infection in distant past	−	+ or −	+ or −	−	−	−
Present HBV vaccination	−	++	−	−	−	−

Modified from Robinson WS: Hepatitis B virus and hepatitis delta virus. In Mandell GL, et al (eds): Principles and Practice of Infectious Diseases. New York, Churchill Livingstone, 1990, p 1219, with permission.

Hepatitis C

Hepatitis C is an RNA virus that is responsible for most of the cases of community-acquired hepatitis that were previously classified as non-A, non-B hepatitis. Viral transmission occurs through blood or blood product transfusion, needle sharing among IV drug abusers, hemodialysis, or sexual contact. Many patients with hepatitis C infection have no identifiable risk factors for transmission. Hepatitis C can also be transmitted from mother to fetus. Patients infected with hepatitis C may develop chronic hepatitis and hepatocellular carcinoma, although fulminant hepatitis during the acute infection is rare. The prevalence of hepatitis C infection in the United States is approximately 1%.

Signs and symptoms: The clinical presentation of hepatitis C infection is similar to that of other hepatitides: jaundice, nausea, right upper quadrant pain, and elevated liver enzyme tests. The infection may be asymptomatic.

Diagnosis: Hepatitis C infection can be detected through the use of an assay for antibody to hepatitis C. Second-generation forms of this test are more specific and sensitive than earlier preparations. There may be a serologic window of up to a year between acute infection and antibody detection, so the tests are not as useful for the detection of acute illness.

Therapy: There is no specific therapy for acute hepatitis C other than avoidance of hepatotoxic agents and careful LFT monitoring. Infected patients should be counseled about sexual contacts and sharing of any utensils potentially contaminated with blood (such as razors). Chronic hepatitis C may be treated with recombinant α-interferon for 6 weeks. About 50% of treated patients show improvement in their symptoms and LFTs. Approximately 50% of those who do respond are able to sustain the remission. Studies are still ongoing to determine which patients with HCV infection are most likely to respond to treatment.

HEPATOMEGALY AND HEPATIC MASSES

When hepatomegaly or a liver mass is discovered on physical examination or on a scan performed for another reason, an etiology must be found. If the patient has elevated liver enzymes, positive anti-HCV, positive HBsAg, or elevated αFP, a CT-guided, fine-needle biopsy or a liver biopsy is needed. If none of these tests is positive, an ultrasound can be done and the following chart used to decide on therapy.

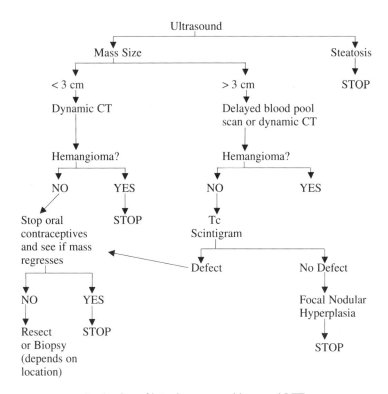

Evaluation of hepatic masses with normal LFTs.

HEPATORENAL SYNDROME

ARF occurs with increased frequency in patients with liver disease and is usually secondary to acute tubular necrosis (ATN) or hepatorenal syndrome. Because hepatorenal syndrome is usually fatal without a transplant, it is important to distinguish it from other causes of renal impairment. Hepatorenal syndrome is defined as unexplained renal failure in patients with liver disease in the absence of another cause of renal failure. Drugs, sepsis, dehydration, infection, circulatory failure, and other causes should be excluded. Laboratory tests can suggest the diagnosis of hepatorenal syndrome.

Urinalysis in Renal Failure Accompanying Liver Disease

LAB TEST	PRERENAL AZOTEMIA	HEPATORENAL	ATN
Urine Na$^+$, mEq/L	<10	<10	>30
Urine sediment	Normal	Nonspecific	Casts
Urine Osm, mOsm/L	>100	>100	Equal to plasma
Urine to plasma urea nitrogen	>8	>8	<3
Renal failure index	<1	<1	>1

Renal failure index = urine Na$^+$/urine creatinine/plasma creatinine.

HERPES SIMPLEX

The herpes simplex virus (HSV) is a member of the group of viruses sharing a core of double-stranded DNA, including varicella-zoster, EBV, and CMV. By newer technological developments, HSV types 1 and 2 can be differentiated serologically and biochemically. However, the classic means of differentiating the two types lies in attention to epidemiologic and clinical presentations. These viruses are characterized by latency and frequent recurrences.

Differences Between HSV-1 and HSV-2*

CHARACTERISTICS	HSV-1	HSV-2
Urogenital infections	– (10–30%)	+ (70–90%)
Nongenital infections		
Labialis	+ (80–90%)	– (10–20%)
Keratitis	+	–
Whitlow (hand)	+	+
Encephalitis (adult)	+	–
Neonatal infection	– (≈30%)	+ (≈70%)
Transmission (primary route)	Nongenital	Genital
Mice-genital or intramuscular	Less neurotropic	More neurotropic
Pock size on chorioallantoic membranes	Small	Large
Plaques in chick embryo monolayers	–	+
Temperature sensitivity (40°C)	–	+
Heparin sensitivity	+	–
Syncytium formation in human embryonic kidney cells	–	+

*Antigenic differences between HSV-1 and HSV-2 can be detected by a variety of serologic techniques, including immunofluorescence, immunoperoxidation, microneutralization and enzyme-linked immunoadsorption.

From Hirsch MS: Herpes simplex virus. In Mandell GL, et al (eds): Principles and Practice of Infectious Diseases, 3rd ed. New York, Churchill Livingstone, 1990, p 1145, with permission.

Life-threatening HSV infections include encephalitis, neonatal infections, and infections in immunocompromised hosts. Encephalitis is most commonly associated with HSV-1, but only a third of patients have concurrent fever blisters. The diagnosis rests on brain biopsy after localization by EEG or MRI scanning. The CSF is usually normal. Mortality may be as high as 60 to 80% in untreated cases. Most neonatal infections are caused by HSV-2 via retrograde spread of maternal genital infection or exposure during vaginal delivery. Such infections may be either localized or systemic, with the mortality rate in the latter approaching 85%.

The diagnosis is most rapidly made by staining scrapings from skin or mucous membrane lesions with Giemsa or Wright stain and searching for multinucleated giant cells. Serologic studies are rarely helpful. Treatment involves the use of nucleoside derivatives that interrupt DNA synthesis. Topical preparations of idoxuridine and vidarabine are used for herpes keratitis. IV vidarabine or acyclovir is used in the treatment of herpes encephalitis and neonatal infections, with the latter having a far lower incidence of side effects. Acyclovir has also demonstrated efficacy in the management of genital herpes and oral-labial infections. Its use in recurrent disease in the immunocompetent host is discouraged due to the appearance in recent years of resistant viral strains. However, in the immunocompromised host, acyclovir is used successfully for both treatment and suppression of herpetic recurrences.

HISTOPLASMOSIS

Infection by *Histoplasma capsulatum* is the most common systemic fungal infection in the United States, with an estimated 500,000 new cases each year. Most cases occur in areas known to be endemic for the organism, primarily the large river valleys of the Mississippi and Ohio rivers, but also extending into eastern Kansas, Oklahoma, and Texas (see map that follows). Other cases can arise in persons who previously lived in an endemic area but now develop illness associated with decreasing cellular immunity while living in nonendemic areas. A typical example would be an HIV-infected Indianapolis native now living in New York City.

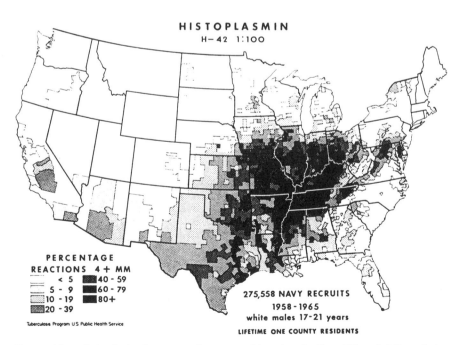

Geographic variation in the frequency of reactors to histoplasmin. From Edwards LB, et al: An atlas of sensitivity to tuberculin, PPD-D and histoplasmin in the United States. Am Rev Respir Dis 99(Suppl):1–132, 1969, with permission.

Whereas the majority of infections are asymptomatic, the likelihood of developing symptoms following infection is dependent upon the inoculum size. Persons exposed to a small inoculum have only a 1% chance of developing symptomatic disease. In contrast, 50–100% of persons experience symptoms after a heavy exposure. In some instances, a thorough history will elicit a potential exposure because the organism inhabits areas with humid, organic material often frequented by birds or bats. Examples include cave exploration, working with rotten wood, cleaning chimneys or eaves soiled with bird droppings, and digging in areas near bird roosts.

Of those individuals developing symptoms, the vast majority present with an acute self-limited illness characterized by fever, chills, headache, myalgias, and cough with or without pleuritic or retrosternal chest pain. Physical exam is usually unrevealing but may reveal rales on lung exam and cervical or supraclavicular adenopathy. Hepatosplenomegaly is found infrequently. Symptomatic patients may also have pulmonary infiltrates on CXR with hilar and/or mediastinal adenopathy. One out of 10 patients may develop an inflammatory pericarditis. This is not an extension of histoplasma infection, but an inflammatory reaction to the infected mediastinal nodes. Pericardial tamponade can occur.

Disseminated histoplasmosis was a rare clinical entity prior to the HIV era. It was estimated to occur in 1 of 2,000 to 5,000 acute infections. As HIV became more prevalent in areas endemic for histoplasmosis, however, it became clear that HIV was a strong promoter for dissemination as a result of individuals' impaired cellular immunity. Three patterns of disseminated disease have been described: acute, subacute, and chronic. Patients with AIDS or other causes of immunosuppression typically follow the acute course and are characterized by fever, weight loss, hepatosplenomegaly, and bone marrow suppression with pancytopenia. This development of new or newly severe pancytopenia can be an important diagnostic clue in the evaluation of an AIDS patient, and histoplasmosis should be strongly considered in all such patients. Both the subacute and chronic forms are characterized by an increased incidence of focal organ involvement with such complications as adrenalitis, endocarditis, or meningitis.

Diagnosis of histoplasmosis is usually by culture. However, in acute pulmonary disease following initial exposure, cultures will most likely be negative and the diagnosis made clinically. In chronic pulmonary disease, the sputum cultures will be positive in over half the cases. Disseminated disease is readily documented if it is included in the differential diagnosis and pursued. Both bone marrow and blood cultures will be positive in upwards of 75% of cases. Urine and sputum cultures have yields of over 50% in disseminated disease and should be submitted. If neurologic involvement is suspected, CSF should also be cultured and will be positive in 50% of those with meningitis.

A radioimmunoassay has been developed for identification of histoplasma antigen, but this test is not generally available. Tests for antibody are more readily available and are useful with the following caveats: False negatives are often seen in early disease and in the immunosuppressed patient. False positives are possible in patients with other fungal infections. Antibody clearance is relatively slow and a positive test may result from a prior exposure and not represent the etiology of the patient's current condition. Skin testing is of no use in the diagnosis of histoplasmosis and is used only as an epidemiologic tool.

Treatment of acute histoplasmosis is not indicated unless it is an unusually severe case. These cases are usually self-limited and resolve spontaneously. Chronic pulmonary disease and all disseminated disease should receive antifungal therapy.

Traditionally, treatment has meant amphotericin B. However, development of the oral azole antifungals has brought some flexibility into treatment decision making. In the instance of chronic pulmonary disease, these agents may be the drugs of choice. In disseminated disease it may still be most prudent to initiate therapy with amphotericin B and then complete the course with oral azoles. In disseminated histoplasmosis in HIV infection, itraconazole has been clearly shown to be effective therapy for the prevention of relapse, and trials under way are evaluating its place as initial therapy.

References: Wheat LJ: Histoplasmosis. Infect Dis Clin North Am 2:841–859, 1988.

Wheat LJ, et al: Disseminated histoplasmosis in the acquired immune deficiency syndrome: Clinical findings, diagnosis and treatment, and review of the literature. Medicine 69:361–374, 1990.

HIV INFECTION AND AIDS

Acute HIV Infection Syndrome

HIV infection is recognized to have three distinct phases: (1) primary HIV infection—an acute illness occurring with initial infection; (2) asymptomatic phase or clinical latency; and (3) immune deficiency accompanied by clinically apparent disease.

Primary HIV infection was initially recognized retrospectively as a mononucleosis or flulike viral syndrome. Now the manifestations have been more fully characterized and should not be misdiagnosed as influenza or mononucleosis. Thus, it is likely that the syndrome can be recognized in 50–90% of persons infected with HIV.

The onset of symptoms occurs 1–3 weeks after initial infection and lasts 1 to 2 weeks. Fever, a nonexudative pharyngitis, headache, and a diffuse, erythematous maculopapular rash are characteristic findings. Lymphadenopathy is also frequent and may abate after the initial infection or persist into the asymptomatic phase of the illness. Splenomegaly may also occur. In some patients, the headache is severe and accompanied by retro-orbital pain, photophobia, and a meningoencephalitis. Mouth ulcers and *Candida* esophagitis have also been described.

The illness is marked by a transient, but sometimes profound, lymphopenia with inversion of the CD4/CD8 ratio. During this period, there are anergy and poor response to mitogens. Recently, episodes of PCP have been recognized during this initial profound lymphopenia. A mild thrombocytopenia may also occur. Lymphopenia is succeeded by a lymphocytosis of CD8 cells. On the peripheral blood film, atypical lymphocytes are recognized. A mild increase in the alkaline phosphatase may also be seen.

IgM antibodies may be detected by immunofluorescent assay or ELISA tests during the first 2 weeks and peak by the end of 5 weeks. IgG antibodies are subsequently detected. Early in the course of infection, even before antibodies are detected, the p24 antigen can be seen. The virus can also be isolated early from blood or CSF.

The differential diagnosis of the acute febrile illness of primary HIV infection is summarized below. The distinguishing features of acute HIV infection are the rash, the nonexudative pharyngitis, and the presence of mucocutaneous ulcers. Unfortunately, acute HIV infection is often overlooked.

Differential Diagnosis of Primary HIV Infection

Primary HIV	EBV
CMV	Toxoplasmosis
Rubella	Viral hepatitis
Secondary syphilis	Disseminated gonococcal infection
Drug reaction	Primary herpes simplex virus

From Tindall B, et al: Primary HIV infection. In Sande MA, et al (eds): The Medical Management of AIDS, 3rd ed. Philadelphia, W.B. Saunders, 1992, with permission.

Once the primary HIV infection has been recognized, management is largely supportive. To date, the role of zidovudine (AZT) therapy has not been clarified for the treatment of a person who has had intense viremia for 1 to 3 weeks before presentation. In some case reports, zidovudine was unable to abort HIV infection in the setting of the acute retroviral syndrome. It is essential to counsel patients to avoid further spread of the disease and to initiate a program of careful follow-up and monitoring of symptoms and immunological status. Some investigators believe that progression to AIDS is likely to occur earlier in those individuals who have had a severe, prolonged (>2 weeks) episode of primary HIV infection.

Reference: Gaines H, et al: Clinical picture of primary HIV infection presenting as a glandular-fever-like illness. BMJ 297:1363–1368, 1988.

Antiretroviral Therapy

Therapy directed against HIV dates only to late 1986, when zidovudine first became available to patients not enrolled in research protocols. FDA approval of this drug in March, 1987 set the stage for more rapid approval of other drugs in following years. At that time, zidovudine had been evaluated in only one, single, phase II/III trial with 282 enrolled participants, 145 of whom received active drug. When the study was terminated early for reason of the clear superiority of zidovudine, only 27 participants had completed 24 weeks of the study. Although there was little question that zidovudine was beneficial in that trial, to this day our knowledge of the use of zidovudine and other antiretroviral agents is hampered by the use of small, nonrandomized trials, premature termination of larger trials, or approval of drugs based on scant clinical information or trial endpoints. As a result, therapy recommendations are relatively soft and undergo continual reevaluation.

Currently Available Antiretroviral Agents (1994)

Zidovudine (ZDV, AZT, Retrovir)
- For initial monotherapy against all stages of HIV with CD4+ lymphocytes <500/mm^3
- Best dose interval unknown
- Plasma half-life 1 hour, intracellular half-life 3 hours
- Commonly prescribed doses: 100 mg every 4 hours while awake (500 mg/day), 200 mg every 8 hours (600 mg/day)
- Toxicities: anemia, leukopenia, myopathy
- Decreasing viral susceptibility seen within weeks to months

Didanosine (ddI, Videx)
- For therapy in those intolerant of or failing on zidovudine, and also for those with "prolonged" prior zidovudine use

Table continued on next page.

Currently Available Antiretroviral Agents (1994) (Cont.)

- Administered avoiding food twice per day: buffered tablets to neutralize gastric acid, plasma half-life 0.5 hours, intracellular half-life 12 hours
- Prescribed based on body weight: 300 mg BID if >75 kg, 200 mg BID if 50–75 kg, 125 mg BID if <50 kg
- Toxicities: peripheral neuropathy, pancreatitis, diarrhea
- Decreasing viral susceptibility also described

Zalcitabine (ddC, HIVID)
- For therapy in those with <300 CD4+ lymphocytes/mm^3 who have clinical or immunologic progression
- Administered every 8 hours with zidovudine every 8 hours
- Plasma half-life 0.3 hours, intracellular half-life 2.5 hours
- Dosed at 0.75 mg every 8 hours
- Toxicities: peripheral neuropathy, stomatitis, pancreatitis
- Cross-resistance seen with didanosine-resistant strains of HIV

Stavudine (d4T)
- Indications as for ddC

Reference: Hirsch MS, et al: Therapy for human immunodeficiency virus infection. N Engl J Med 328:1686–1695, 1993.

Complications

The primary medical complications of HIV infection result from the progressive decline in immunologic status. As such, these complications are primarily infectious in nature. Organisms that are pathogenic to non-HIV-infected individuals (*Mycobacterium tuberculosis, Histoplasma capsulatum*) retain their pathogenicity, may have their clinical presentations altered by the lack of a normal immune response, and tend to present earlier in the course of HIV infection. Other organisms, which may be nonpathogenic in non-HIV-infected individuals, present as causes of illness in HIV patients at various levels of immunosuppression. A broad list of the most frequent infectious complications in HIV infection follows.

Infectious Complications of AIDS

INFECTING ORGANISM		TYPE OF INFECTION
Viruses	Cytomegalovirus	Pneumonia, disseminated infection, retinitis, encephalitis, gastrointestinal ulcerations
	Epstein-Barr virus	Important pathogenic factor in B-cell lymphoproliferative disorders and Burkitt's lymphoma, oral hairy leukoplakia
	Herpes simplex virus	Recurrent severe localized infection
	Papovavirus	Progressive multifocal leukoencephalopathy
	Varicella-zoster virus	Localized or disseminated infection
Fungi	*Aspergillus*	Invasive pulmonary infection with potential for dissemination
	Candida albicans	Mucocutaneous infection, esophagitis, disseminated infection
	Coccidioides immitis	Disseminated infection

Table continued on next page.

Infectious Complications of AIDS (Cont.)

INFECTING ORGANISM	TYPE OF INFECTION
Cryptococcus neoformans	Meningitis, disseminated infection
Histoplasma capsulatum	Disseminated infection
Petriellidium boydii	Pneumonia
Protozoa *Pneumocystis carinii*	Pneumonia, retinal infection
Cryptosporidium	Enteritis
Isospora belli	Enteritis
Toxoplasma gondii	Encephalitis
Myco- *M. avium-intracellulare*	Pulmonary, extrapulmonary, or disseminated infection
bacteria *M. tuberculosis*	Pulmonary, extrapulmonary, or disseminated infection
Atypical mycobacteria (e.g., *M. kansasii, M. haemophilum*)	Pulmonary, extrapulmonary, or disseminated infection
Bacteria *Haemophilus influenzae* type b	Pneumonia, disseminated infection
Legionella	Pneumonia
Listeria monocytogenes	Bacteremia, meningitis, meningo-encephalitis
Nocardia	Pneumonia, disseminated infection
Pseudomonas aeruginosa	Bacteremia, pneumonia
Salmonella	Gastroenteritis, disseminated infection
Streptococcus pneumoniae	Pneumonia, disseminated infection

From Rubin RH: Acquired immunodeficiency syndrome. In Rubenstein E, et al (eds): Scientific American Medicine. New York, Scientific American, 1993, with permission.

The relative likelihood of these infective agents causing disease as related to CD4+ lymphocyte count is presented in the following graph.

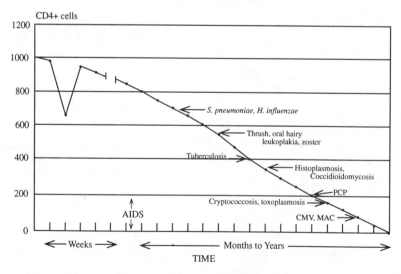

The natural history of HIV infection.

An important complication of HIV infection that may lead to an earlier diagnosis of HIV is the frequent presentation of dermatologic manifestations. Although conditions such as herpes zoster, psoriasis, and dermatitis are relatively common in the general public, their frequency, severity, and recurrence rate are greater in individuals with HIV infection. Patients with the following conditions should be assessed for HIV infection in the case of unusual courses.

Skin Conditions Commonly Seen with HIV Infection

CONDITION	MORPHOLOGY	LOCATION
Staphylococcal folliculitis	Erythematous follicular pustules or papules; may be pruritus	Face, trunk, groin
Bacillary angiomatosis	Friable, vascular papules, cellulitic plaques, subcutaneous nodules	Skin, bone, liver, spleen, lymph node
Herpes zoster (shingles)	Grouped vesicles on erythematous bases	Dermatomal distribution, may spill onto adjacent dermatomes
Herpes simplex	Grouped vesicles on erythematous bases, rapidly evolving into superficial mucocutaneous ulcerations or fissures; necrotizing ulcers may be seen when chronic	Face, hand, anogenital area
Molluscum contagiosum	2–5-mm, pearly, flesh-colored papules often with central umbilication	Face, anogenital area
Insect bite reactions	Erythematous, urticarial papules	Scabies: axillae, groin, finger webs. Fleas: lower legs. Mosquitoes: upper and lower extremities
Photosensitivity	Eczematous eruption	Face (tip of the nose), extensor forearms, neck
Eosinophilic folliculitis	Urticarial follicular papules	Trunk, face
Seborrheic dermatitis	Fine, white scaling without erythema (dandruff) to patches and plaques of erythema with indistinct margins and yellowish, greasy scale	Scalp, central face, eyebrows, nasolabial and retroauricular folds, chest, upper back, axillae, groin
Psoriasis	Sharply marginated plaques with a silvery scale	Elbows, knees, lumbosacral area
Kaposi's sarcoma	Palpable, firm, cutaneous nodules 0.5–2.0 cm, violaceous to dark brown	Head and neck, oral cavity, soles of feet

Adapted from Berger TG: Dermatologic care in the AIDS patient. In Sande MA, et al (eds): The Medical Management of AIDS, 3rd ed. Philadelphia, W.B. Saunders, 1992, with permission.

Neurologic complications are also frequent in HIV infection. Many of them are infections (cryptococcal meningitis, herpes zoster), but many are poorly understood. Neurologic manifestations include meningitis, encephalopathy, myelopathy, peripheral neuropathy, and myopathy.

Definition and Diagnositic Criteria

The syndrome designated as AIDS has had several definitions since the first cases were described in 1981. The definition was established by the CDC to facilitate reporting of cases to public health authorities. As such, it is not, and never was, intended to assess disability or eligibility for social benefits. The definition has been changed to reflect increased understanding of the spectrum of disease caused by the HIV. The most recent revision of the AIDS case definition became effective January 1, 1993, replacing the 1987 version. The major differences between the two definitions is the new use of a T-laboratory test, the CD4+ lymphocyte count, to establish a diagnosis of AIDS and the addition of three clinical manifestations of the disease to the list of AIDS-indicator illnesses. The three conditions added are pulmonary TB (extrapulmonary TB was already on the list), recurrent pneumonia within a one-year period, and invasive cervical cancer.

The following table below gives the relationship between the clinical categories and the CD4+ categories. The second table lists the conditions that are included under clinical Category C—AIDS-indicator conditions. Under the 1993 classification system, HIV-positive persons (over age 13 yrs) with any one of the Category C conditions, or with a CD4+ count <200/μL, are considered to have AIDS. Infants and children, because of their variable CD4+ counts, are classified under a separate system.

1993 Revised Classification System for HIV Infection and Expanded AIDS Surveillance Case Definition for Adolescents and Adults*

| | CLINICAL CATEGORIES | | |
CD4 + T-CELL CATEGORIES	(A) Asymptomatic, Acute (Primary) HIV or PGL†	(B) Symptomatic, not (A) or (C) Conditions	(C) AIDS-Indicator Conditions
(1) ≥500/μl	A1	B1	**C1**
(2) 200–499/μl	A2	B2	**C2**
(3) <200/μl AIDS-indicator T-cell count	**A3**	**B3**	**C3**

*Categories A3, B3, C1, C2, C3 (boldface) illustrate the expanded AIDS surveillance case definition. Persons with AIDS-indicator conditions (Category C) as well as those with CD4+ T-lymphocyte counts <200/μl (Categories A3 or B3) are reportable as AIDS cases in the United States and Territories.

†PGL = persistent generalized lymphadenopathy. Clinical Category A includes acute (primary) HIV infection.

AIDS-Indicator Conditions in the 1993 AIDS Surveillance Case Definition

- Candidiasis of bronchi, trachea, or lungs
- Candidiasis, esophageal
- Cervical cancer, invasive*
- Coccidioidomycosis, disseminated or extrapulmonary
- Cryptococcosis, extrapulmonary
- Cryptosporidiosis, chronic intestinal (>1 month's duration)
- Cytomegalovirus disease (other than liver, spleen, or nodes)
- Cytomegalovirus retinitis (with loss of vision)
- Encephalopathy, HIV-related
- Herpes simplex: chronic ulcer(s) (>1 month's duration); or bronchitis, pneumonitis, or esophagitis
- Histoplasmosis, disseminated or extrapulmonary
- Isosporiasis, chronic intestinal (>1 month's duration)

Table continued on next page.

*AIDS-Indicator Conditions in the 1993 AIDS Surveillance
Case Definition (Cont.)*

- Kaposi's sarcoma
- Lymphoma, Burkitt's (or equivalent term)
- Lymphoma, immunoblastic (or equivalent term)
- Lymphoma, primary, of brain
- *M. avium* complex or *M. kansasii,* disseminated or extrapulmonary
- *M. tuberculosis,* any site (pulmonary* or extrapulmonary)
- *Mycobacterium,* other species or unidentified species, disseminated or extrapulmonary
- *Pneumocystis carinii* pneumonia
- Pneumonia, recurrent*
- Progressive multifocal leukoencephalopathy
- *Salmonella* septicemia, recurrent
- Toxoplasmosis of brain
- Wasting syndrome due to HIV

*Newly added in the 1993 expansion of the AIDS surveillance case definition.

Reference: CDC: 1993 revised classification system for HIV infection and expanded surveillance case definition for AIDS among adolescents and adults. MMWR 41(RR-17):1–19, 1992.

Diagnostic Testing

The diagnosis of infection by HIV has been dependent upon tests demonstrating the presence of specific antibodies to HIV as a sign of prior infection. Because infection is believed to be lifelong, all those found to have anti-HIV antibody also harbor virus and remain infected and infectious. The most common screening test for anti-HIV antibodies is the enzyme-linked immunosorbent assay (ELISA). The test is performed with microtiter plates having wells coated with HIV antigen harvested from cell cultures. Antibodies in serum samples placed in the wells then react with the coated antigens and result in a positive ELISA test when a detecting system of an enzyme-labeled anti-human globulin is added and attaches to the antibody-antigen complex. This test is extremely sensitive, with a large standardized national program showing 99.7%. Specificity in this same national program was 98.5%. However, despite these high figures, in a population with a low prevalence of HIV infection, most of the positive results will be false positives. Therefore, a positive ELISA is repeated, and if positive again, a confirmatory test, usually the Western blot, is performed.

Western blot testing is performed by obtaining HIV viral proteins and glycoproteins from cell culture and separating them by molecular weight electrophoretically onto a detection system, usually filter paper. This detection system is then exposed to serum for testing, and specific antibodies, if present, react with specific HIV antigens, causing a characteristic band pattern on the detection system when exposed to anti–human antibodies. A standardized combination and number of bands must be present for HIV infection to be diagnosed. Unfortunately, a large number of persons will have some nonspecific pattern of bands on Western blot testing and will be labeled "indeterminate." In this instance, testing needs to be repeated periodically.

Tests for HIV viral antigen are now more readily available, as is the capability for direct viral culture from clinical specimens and the demonstration of viral genetic material via polymerase chain reaction (PCR). The sensitivity of antigen testing has been variable, making interpretation of results difficult. What is desired is a way to assay potential viral burden to help make prognostic projections, to assist in the evaluation of antiviral therapy, and to diagnose neonatal infection. Recently described is a procedure for causing dissociation of HIV antigen-antibody complexes. Following the dissociation, a separate assay for antigen can be performed.

How this procedure may assist in the clinical management of HIV-infected individuals is unclear at this time. It does, however, hold great promise in the early detection of HIV infection in newborns, for the passively transferred maternal antibodies can be dissociated and antigen circulating in the newborn identified.

Diarrhea in Infected Patients

The evaluation of diarrhea in patients with HIV infection should take a stepwise course. The patient should be evaluated for the continued severity of symptoms prior to advancing to the next step. There remains much diagnostic and therapeutic uncertainty because organisms previously believed to be nonpathogenic and known pathogens for which there is no effective therapy may be involved.

Causes of Diarrhea in HIV-infected Patients

Proctitis
- *Neisseria gonorrhoeae*
- *Chlamydia trachomatis*
- Cytomegalovirus
- Herpes simplex virus
- *Treponema pallidum*

Enterocolitis
- *Giardia lamblia*
- *Cryptosporidium*
- *Campylobacter jejuni*
- *Clostridium difficile*
- Cytomegalovirus
- Microsporidia
- Non-Hodgkin's lymphoma
- *Entamoeba histolytica*
- *Shigella flexneri*
- *Salmonella* species
- *Mycobacterium avium* complex
- *Isospora belli*
- *Strongyloides stercoralis*

Approach to the HIV-infected Patient with Diarrhea

Initial evaluation and therapy
- Dietary history for intolerance
- Stool cultures for bacterial enteric pathogens
- Stool exam for ova and parasites
- Stool for *Clostridium difficile* toxin
- Stool cultures for acid-fast bacilli smear
- Nonspecific antidiarrheal medication
- Specific therapy as indicated by above tests

Nonresponse to initial steps
- Upper and lower endoscopy for visual examination, small and large bowel biopsies
- Culture of biopsy material for acid-fast bacilli and viral enteric pathogens
- Duodenal aspirate for parasites

Continued symptoms with no etiologic agent identified
- Electron microscopy of biopsy specimens (microsporidia, adenovirus)

Reference: Rabeneck L: Diagnostic workup strategies for patients with HIV-related chronic diarrhea. What is the end result? J Clin Gastroenterol 16:245–250, 1993.

Epidemiology and Prevention

Epidemiology: The epidemiology of HIV infection has shown dramatic evolution during the past 5 years. Initially, two patterns of HIV infection in various populations were described. They resulted from differing types of sexual activity and times of entry of HIV into the populations.

Pattern I infection is the one initially common in the United States and Canada, Western Europe, and Australia/New Zealand. Its pattern is characterized by transmission through sexual contact of homosexual and bisexual men. The male-to-female ratio is disproportionately male due to the much smaller contribution by bisexual men and IV drug use. As a result, children are relatively infrequently affected.

Pattern II HIV infection is the one found in the Caribbean islands and sub-Saharan Africa. Transmission is primarily through heterosexual contact, and men and women are equally affected. Due to the large number of infected women of childbearing age, children are frequently infected.

Although these two patterns continue to exist, some areas are evolving from one to another. In Latin America, the initial spread of HIV was typical of pattern I. Due to the relatively larger involvement of bisexual men and IV drug abusers, the characteristics of pattern II are becoming more prominent. Additionally, there has been a dramatic entry of HIV into populations previously only minimally affected, particularly in Asia and India; it appears the HIV epidemic is poised to explode in those areas of the world. Estimates of worldwide HIV infection by 1995 range from 15 to 20 million infected persons and from 30 to 110 million by the year 2000.

Another evolution of the epidemic is that occurring in the United States. Initially a disease of relatively affluent white homosexuals, HIV has increasingly become a disease of inner-city minorities. African-Americans and Hispanics are more heavily represented in currently reported cases than their proportion in the general population would suggest. This is the result of heterosexual contact with infected IV drug users. Within these groups in the United States, a pattern II transmission is becoming predominant. This will have a significant impact upon the ways HIV care is provided and funded, for most of these individuals are medically indigent.

Transmission: As opposed to the epidemiology of HIV infection, the routes of transmission remain unchanged since first hypothesized in the early to mid 1980s.

Homosexual contact remains a more efficient transmitter of infection than heterosexual contact. Male-to-female heterosexual contact is more efficient than

Known Routes of HIV Transmission

1. Sexual exposure
   - Male homosexual
   - Heterosexual
2. Blood exposure
   - Contaminated needles in IV drug use
   - Blood or blood product transfusion
   - Infected organ transplantation
   - Occupational exposure
     —Needle stick
     —Mucous membrane exposure
     —Open wound/sore exposure
3. Perinatal exposure
   - Intrauterine/peripartum
   - Breast-feeding

female-to-male. IV drug use and associated HIV infection remains a major mode of transmission and is the bridge into the heterosexual population in pattern I countries.

Infection through transfusion or transplantation has been greatly reduced by routine testing of products for HIV infection. Rarely, infection is transmitted due to lack of anti-HIV antibodies in donors with early infection or those donating organs following major trauma and with resuscitation attempts including large-volume transfusions. Occupational exposure represents a small but real risk and depends on the severity of the exposure, with higher risk associated with larger inoculations, hollow-bore needles, and patient sources with viremia or advanced disease. Only one health care worker, a dentist, has been identified with transmission of infection to patients.

Perinatal infection remains problematic. The timing of infection is not clear, but both early and late infection have been documented. Differing prevalences of infection have now been described in infants delivered by C-section versus those delivered vaginally, with C-section babies having a lower rate in some studies.

Prevention: Prevention of HIV infection revolves around knowledge of the routes of transmission. Sexual abstinence or a mutually monogamous sexual relationship between uninfected partners will reduce to zero the risk of infection by this route. Absent these interventions, the routine and correct use of condoms will help decrease the rate of transmission but will not eliminate it. Alteration of sexual practices to minimize genital and oral exposure to blood, semen, and cervical and vaginal secretions will also help minimize exposure.

In the developed world, blood products are no longer a primary source of HIV infection due to both routine testing for HIV and voluntary deferral of donation by those at highest risk of prior infection. IV drug use as a means of transmission can be potentially minimized through the cleansing of needles with bleach, the use of new needles, or exclusive use by a single user; however this group of high-risk individuals is difficult to reach with educational efforts. Optimally, opportunities for drug rehabilitation would address the size of this high-risk population, and the social circumstances contributing to continuing drug use could be interrupted.

Transmission in the health care setting will remain a distinct possibility but already is a minuscule portion of the HIV epidemic and is adequately addressed through universal precautions and continuing efforts to adapt instruments for safer use. Perinatal transmission could be eliminated through a combination of full birth control or abstinence. In HIV-positive pregnant women, zidovudine has been found to be effective in decreasing the rate of perinatal transmission. This implies a strong effort at continuous counseling for women at risk throughout their childbearing years. Educational efforts must be directed toward both (1) increasing people's awareness of those behaviors in their own lives that have placed them at higher risk for infection and (2) the encouragement of HIV testing.

General Care Guidelines

General care of the HIV-infected patient must begin with counseling and education. Specific attention must be paid to the patient's anxiety upon initial diagnosis and continuing exacerbations of anxiety during the course of illness. Also of utmost importance is education on the need to inform those potentially exposed and on the methods to prevent further exposures in the future.

Medical care begins with a thorough Hx & PE. Included in the history should be all known or potential exposures in an attempt to date the time of infection. Use of licit and illicit drugs will have great bearing on potential compliance. A history of all STDs and their treatment, as well as any history of PPD testing, TB exposure, or clinical TB is very important due to the consideration of both the need for further therapy and future reactivation and complications. A vaccination history should be obtained. Finally, a travel and residence history should be obtained to anticipate possible infectious complications that have a geographical component (coccidioidomycosis, histoplasmosis).

Baseline Laboratory Evaluation in HIV Infection

CBC with differential	Platelet count
Complete chemistry panel	RPR
Hepatitis B serology	Toxoplasma IgG titer
T-lymphocyte subsets	PPD and control reactions
CXR	

Immunization of HIV-infected adults has been recommended by the CDC. The following vaccines should be administered.

VACCINE	FREQUENCY	COMMENTS
Diphtheria/tetanus	Every 10 years	
Polio	Once	Only inactivated
MMR	Once	If born after 1956
Pneumococcal	Once	
Influenza	Annually	
Hepatitis B	One complete series	If serology negative
Haemophilus influenzae type B	Once	No formal CDC recommendation

The frequency of clinic visits and laboratory monitoring should be individualized, but based upon expected rates of progression and current recommendations for medical intervention, the following suggestions can be made.

CD4+ COUNT	VISIT/TEST	COMMENTS
>600	every 6–12 mos	No therapy; health maintenance exams
500–600	every 3 mos	Anti-HIV therapy may soon be utilized
300–500	every 6 mos	Consider anti-HIV Rx with zidovudine
200–300	every 3 mos	Nearing need for PCP prophylaxis, anti-HIV Rx
100–200	every 2–3 mos	PCP prophylaxis; consider altering anti-HIV Rx
<100	every 2 mos	Consider MAC and fungal prophylaxis, routine retinal exams for CMV

Hecht FM, et al (eds): HIV Infection, a Primary Care Approach. Boston, Massachusetts Medical Society, 1993.

Natural History

Studies of the natural history of HIV infection have usually focused on a portion of the disease process and not on the entire spectrum of disease. To interpret these studies, one must be familiar with the different portions of the process addressed by each study and understand how these relate to the complete spectrum of HIV disease. The studies described herein all refer to "AIDS" as defined in the August 1987 definition. That definition did not include a diagnosis of AIDS based on immune system testing alone (CD4+ count), as does the 1993 definition.

Starting points for natural history studies have been the date of seroconversion or the date when antibodies directed against HIV are first detected in a subject's serum, provided there are prior results showing the absence of these antibodies. After initial infection by HIV, the body's immune system responds with the formation of these antibodies, generally within 3 weeks, and >95% of the time within 3 months. Two types of studies have used this point as the beginning of the period of observation for natural history. The first type has gone back to previously obtained serum samples, identified specimens positive for anti-HIV antibodies, and then attempted to locate the individuals. Once located, the individuals are examined for prior manifestations of HIV infection and then enrolled in a prospective study. The San Francisco City Clinic Cohort Study (SFCCCS) is the prime example of this type. Due to their high risk of hepatitis B, homosexual men in San Francisco had been recruited in the late

```
Treponema pallidum  ------------------------------------------------------------>
     Streptococcus pneumoniae  --------------------------------------------------->
     Haemophilus influenzae  ----------------------------------------------------->
          Pulmonary tuberculosis --------------------------------------------------->
               Coccidioides immitis  --------------------------------------------->
               Oral/esophageal candidiasis  --------------------------------------->
               VZV (shingles)  ----------------------------------------------------->
                              Pneumocystis carinii  --------------------------->
                              Cryptococcus neoformans --------------->
                              Histoplasma capsulatum ------->
                              Mycobacterium kansasii --->
                              M. avium complex  ---------->
                                        Toxoplasma
                                        gondii ------------>
                                                  CMV ------>

1000         500                  200         100         50          0
```

CD4+ Count (cells/µl)

Relationship of CD4+ levels with opportunistic infections. The lower scale indicates the CD4+ count at the time of initial susceptibility to the indicated infections, such that pulmonary TB usually occurs earlier, at a higher CD4+ count, than PCP. The susceptibilities are lifetime (or until the CD4+ count recovers), as indicated by the extending arrows. (Shelhamer JH, et al: Respiratory disease in the immunosuppressed patient. Ann Intern Med 117:415–431, 1992.)

1970s for study of a vaccine against hepatitis B. Serum was obtained every 6 months as part of the vaccine study to evaluate the efficacy of the immunization against hepatitis. When it quickly became apparent that this same group represented the highest-risk group for HIV infection, the stored serum samples were tested for anti-HIV antibodies once such a test was available (mid-1980s). The date of seroconversion was then defined as that date midway between a last anti-HIV negative test and an initial positive test.

The second study type is that of the Multicenter AIDS Cohort Study (MACS). In this study, homosexual men in five cities around the United States were enrolled and followed prospectively for the development of AIDS. The initial enrollment took place before a test for anti-HIV antibodies was available, and thus both HIV-infected and noninfected individuals were enrolled. Once such an antibody test was available, the study group could be divided up into those infected prior to the time of enrollment and those not infected. For those infected prior to enrollment, no date of infection could be estimated. Those not previously infected would then be followed prospectively to identify those infected during follow-up. The date of infection was then taken as the midpoint between the last visit yielding a negative test for anti-HIV antibodies and the first visit yielding a positive test.

These two study types have thus far reported results describing the time from infection to the development of AIDS or the development of immune suppression severe enough to place one at imminent risk of AIDS. The SFCCCS identified 341 men infected with HIV during the years 1977–80. The median time to development of AIDS from the time of infection was 9.7 years. At 11 years, 54% of the group had a diagnosis of AIDS, and at 13 years, 65%. One quarter of the group remains free of symptoms, and 27% of these have a CD4+ count persisting above 500. In the MACS, 1,588 men were grouped according to initial CD4+ lymphocyte count and examined for development of a subsequent count <200 (which is the range within which the risk for developing an opportunistic infection, or AIDS, is high). Of the 483 men initially seen with a CD4+ count between 501 and 700, 1.3% were <200 at 12 months, 3.1% at 18 months, 5.5% at 24 months, 9.0% at 30 months, 14.4% at 36 months, and 20.2% at 42 months, in the last update published. MACS investigators have estimated that 9 to 17% of study subjects will be AIDS-free even at 20 years after seroconversion.

Additional studies have attempted to correlate laboratory tests with disease progression. CD4+ lymphocyte counts remain the most reliable and most accessible of these tests. CD4+ counts >500 have not been associated with rapid disease progression. One such study demonstrated that for men with CD4+ counts >550, a progression rate of 1.5 AIDS cases per 100 person-years could be expected. Of note, in these studies, much of the time had passed prior to the availability of specific anti-HIV therapy. Several therapies have been shown to prolong the time an individual remains free of AIDS.

Although these studies evaluated the natural history of HIV infection up to a diagnosis of AIDS, there is obviously a period of life after a diagnosis of AIDS and until death. That period of time is much easier to define and measure due to the clinical event that triggers an AIDS diagnosis and the ultimate end in death. It is also, however, the period most affected by medical interventions and improvements in management. Multiple studies have shown that the most important characteristics in determining prognosis following an AIDS diagnosis are the AIDS-defining event (PCP, KS, toxoplasmosis, etc.) and the year in which the diagnosis is made.

Diagnoses made in the early 1980s had a much worse prognosis than those made at the end of the decade. Median duration of survival following an AIDS diagnosis in 1993 would be 18–36 months based on current standards of care.

References: Lifson AR, et al: Progression and clinical outcome of infection due to human immunodeficiency virus. Clin Infect Dis 14:966–972, 1992.

Cooper GS, et al: The clinical prognosis of HIV-1 infection: A review of 32 follow-up studies. J Gen Intern Med 3:525–532, 1988.

Buchbinder S, et al: HIV disease progression and the impact of prophylactic therapies in the San Francisco City Clinic Cohort: A 13-year follow-up. Presented at the VII International Conference on AIDS, Vol. 2. Florence, Italy, June 16–21, 1991.

Tuberculosis in HIV-infected Patients

TB has emerged as one of the most important and difficult complications in HIV infection. It is important because unlike other infections associated with HIV, TB can readily be transmitted to persons with or without HIV infection. It is difficult because of the unusual ways in which TB can present during HIV infection and the associated development of drug-resistant TB in areas of the country with a high prevalence of HIV infection.

Compared to other AIDS-associated infections, TB occurs relatively early in the course of HIV infection. Thus the diagnosis of TB can allow for an HIV risk assessment and testing in order to facilitate earlier diagnosis of HIV infection. All individuals with TB should be offered HIV testing.

Manifestations of TB in Patients with HIV

- Depends upon stage of HIV
    Non-AIDS: more "typical" TB—cavitary, apical, pulmonary smear positive
    AIDS: more "atypical" TB—diffuse or focal, nonapical infiltrates; extrapulmonary
- Extrapulmonary sites
    Lymph nodes
    Bone marrow
    Urinary tract
    Blood (peripheral)
    CNS
- Tuberculin skin testing
    Anergy common, dependent upon stage of HIV
    5 mm significant positive

Recommendations for anti-TB therapy have been revised due to the emergence of multiple drug-resistant TB. The recommendations, as of May 1993, are shown in the following table:

Regimen Options for the Initial Treatment of TB in Children and Adults

TB without HIV infection

Option 1: Administer daily INH, RIF, and PZA for 8 weeks followed by 16 weeks of INH and RIF daily or 2–3 times/week* in areas where the INH resistance rate is not documented to be <4%. EMB or SM should be added to the initial regimen until susceptibility to INH and RIF is demonstrated. Continue treatment for at least 6 months and 3 months beyond culture conversion. Consult a TB medical expert if the patient is symptomatic or smear or culture positive after 3 months.

Option 2: Administer daily INH, RIF, PZA, and SM or EMB for 2 weeks followed by 2 times/week* administration of the same drugs for 6 weeks (by DOT), and subsequently, with 2 times/week administration of INH and RIF for 16 weeks (by DOT). Consult a TB medical expert if the patient is symptomatic or smear or culture positive after 3 months.

Option 3: Treat by DOT, 3 times/week* with INH, RIF, PZA, and EMB or SM for 6 months.† Consult a TB medical expert if the patient is symptomatic or smear or culture positive after 3 months.

TB with HIV infection

Options 1, 2, or 3 can be used, but treatment regimens should continue for a total of 9 months and at least 6 months beyond culture conversion.

---

*All regimens administered 2 or 3 times/week should be monitored by DOT (directly observed therapy) for the duration of therapy. INH = isoniazid; RIF = rifampin; PZA = pyrazinamide; EMB = ethambutol; SM = streptomycin.

†The strongest evidence from clinical trials is the effectiveness of all four drugs administered for the full 6 months. There is weaker evidence that SM can be discontinued after 4 months if the isolate is susceptible to all drugs. The evidence for stopping PZA before the end of 6 months is equivocal for the 3 times/week regimen, and there is no evidence on the effectiveness of this regimen with EMB for less than the full 6 months.

References: Centers for Disease Control: Initial therapy for tuberculosis in the era of multidrug resistance. MMWR 42(RR7):3, Table 1.

Barnes PF, et al: Tuberculosis in patients with human immunodeficiency virus infection. N Engl J Med 324:1644–1650, 1991.

HOMUNCULUS

The motor and sensory areas of the cerebral cortex are organized in a very precise, somatotopic fashion. Specific neurons in the motor strip (precentral gyrus) move specific muscles of the face, arm, and leg contralaterally, and similarly, specific neurons of the sensory strip (postcentral gyrus) receive sensory input from specific regions of the opposite face, arm, and leg. There is thus a representation of the body laid out upon the surface of the brain known as the homunculus.

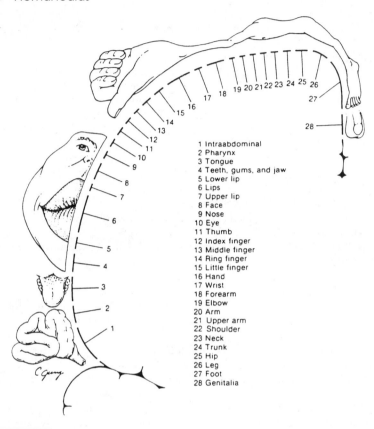

1 Intraabdominal
2 Pharynx
3 Tongue
4 Teeth, gums, and jaw
5 Lower lip
6 Lips
7 Upper lip
8 Face
9 Nose
10 Eye
11 Thumb
12 Index finger
13 Middle finger
14 Ring finger
15 Little finger
16 Hand
17 Wrist
18 Forearm
19 Elbow
20 Arm
21 Upper arm
22 Shoulder
23 Neck
24 Trunk
25 Hip
26 Leg
27 Foot
28 Genitalia

From: Penfield W, et al: The Cerebral Cortex of Man. New York, Macmillan, 1950, with permission.

It requires many neurons to perform the fine, detailed movements of the face and the hand, and similarly, sensation is quite accurate in the face and hand, so these areas are disproportionately well represented in the homunculus. In other words, the body map is distorted to reflect the relative neurologic importance of the different structures. The homunculus is a very ugly man.

An understanding of the homunculus organization of the brain has practical value for localizing neurologic lesions. Because neurons involved with motor and sensory functions of the leg are located on the very medial surface of the brain, between the hemispheres, most disease processes that affect the superficial cortex of the brain are unable to disturb leg function. Cortical lesions, such as strokes, will therefore produce deficits in the face and the arm, but not the leg. Fibers from the leg region do descend subcortically, deep within the brain, where they join the sensory and motor tracts in the spinal cord. Therefore, lesions deep within the brain, such as subcortical strokes and tumors, usually affect face, arm, and leg function. In other words, if the leg is affected, the lesion is subcortical.

Reference: Haerer A: DeJong's The Neurologic Examination, 5th ed. Philadelphia, J.B. Lippincott, 1992.

HYPERCALCEMIA, ACUTE

General Considerations and Treatment

The most common causes of hypercalcemia are cancer and primary hyperthyroidism. The two can be distinguished by measurement of serum PTH. Serum PTH is low in malignancy and high in hyperparathyroidism. Hypercalcemia that is symptomatic is usually caused by malignancy. Cancer induces hypercalcemia by several mechanisms.

1. Humeral hypercalcemia of malignancy is caused by secretion of a PTH-like protein. This is frequent in squamous cell carcinomas, especially those originating in the lung, head and neck, and esophagus.

2. Tumor cell secretion of osteolytic substances (IL-1, IL-6, and lymphotoxin) occurs in hematologic malignancies such as multiple myeloma.

3. Osteolytic bone metastases release calcium into the circulation in breast, renal, and other types of cancer.

4. Increased GI and renal tubular absorption of calcium infrequently plays a role in certain tumors.

Signs and Symptoms of Hypercalcemia

General: Fatigue, malaise, lassitude

CNS: Weakness, depressed DTRs, lethargy, confusion, personality changes or hallucinations, stupor progressing to coma

GI: Anorexia, nausea and vomiting, constipation, ileus, increased frequency of PUD and acute pancreatitis

GU: Polyuria; nephrolithiasis and nephrocalcinosis (in benign hypercalcemia only, because a long survival time is needed for renal stone formation), nephrogenic DI, renal insufficiency

Cardiovascular: Increased cardiac contractility and irritability, increased digoxin sensitivity, slowed conduction; at calcium levels >16 mg/dl, T-wave widening occurs, progressing to bundle branch block, complete heart block, and cardiac arrest

Other: Pruritus, arthralgias, band keratopathy

Treatment of Hypercalcemia

---

1. Vigorously hydrate with normal saline, at least 3 liters per day initially.
2. Stop all medications potentially contributing to the hypercalcemia. This includes calcium carbonate antacids (Tums), other calcium supplements, vitamins A and D, thiazide diuretics, and lithium. Rarely, estrogens, tamoxifen, or theophylline causes hypercalcemia.
3. Consider furosemide therapy once rehydration is complete.
4. Treat the underlying malignancy, or perform parathyroidectomy as indicated.

If the foregoing steps are not sufficient to bring the calcium to normal levels, there are several options for further treatment.

Treatment of Refractory Hypercalcemia

MEDICATION	DOSE	ADVANTAGES	DISADVANTAGES
Calcitonin	4–8 units/kg SC Q 6–12 hrs	Works quickly. Good for severe hypercalcemia. Safe, few side effects. Can be given at home.	Effects often short-lived due to tachyphylaxis.
Plicamycin (mithramycin)	25 μg/kg IVSS	Effective. Normocalcemia may last from a few days to a few weeks; suitable for intermittent outpatient administration.	Takes 48–72 hrs for maximum effect. Can be very toxic in large doses or in patients with renal or hepatic failure.
Biphosphonates Etidronate	7.5 mg/kg IV Q day × 3–7 days	Safe, effective. Pain relief and bone healing in some osseous metastases.	Expensive. Occasional nephrotoxicity. Onset of action 24–48 hrs.
Pamidronate	Several regimens		
Gallium nitrate	200 mg/m^2 continuous IV × 5 days	Effective. Modest antitumor activity in lymphomas and other malignancies.	Expensive, nephrotoxic. Works in 24–48 hrs.
Gluco-corticoids Hydro-cortisone	200–300 mg IV Q day x 3–5 days	Effective in hematologic malignancies.	Ineffective in most solid tumors except breast cancer. Takes 3–5 days.
Phosphate	1.5 gm IV over 6 hrs, then 1–3 gm/day PO in divided doses	IV: rapid action; for use only in life-threatening refractory hypercalcemia. Oral: good for chronic Rx once normocalcemic.	Risk of calcium-PO$_4$ complex deposition and fatal hypotension. Oral phosphates cause diarrhea.

Reference: Bilezikian JP: Management of acute hypercalcemia. N Engl J Med 326:1196–1203, 1992.

About 46 to 50% of calcium in the serum of normal persons is ionized (i.e., free calcium), with most of the remainder protein bound, principally to albumin and to a lesser extent to globulins. The normal range of total serum calcium is 8.7 to 10.1 mg/dl. With normal protein binding, values of the serum calcium above 10.1 mg/dl indicate hypercalcemia.

Causes of Hypercalcemia

1. Primary hyperparathyroidism (hypercalcemia, hypophosphatemia, increased serum alkaline phosphatase, and elevated level of PTH in the serum)
   Parathyroid adenoma (80% of hyperparathyroidism)
   Diffuse parathyroid hyperplasia (20% of cases)
      Spontaneous hyperplasia
      Familial hyperparathyroidism
      Hyperparathyroidism seen in MEN I and MEN IIa
   Parathyroid carcinoma (uncommon)
2. Secondary hyperparathyroidism
   Chronic renal failure
   Malignancies that produce PTH-like substances
3. Familial hypocalciuric hypercalcemia: Serum PTH levels are normal to low
4. Malignancies
   Metastatic malignancy to bone, causing direct osteolysis (e.g., carcinomas of breast, lung, kidney, and thyroid and acute leukemia)
   Multiple myeloma with osteolysis due to osteoclast-activating factor (OAF)
   Lymphoma with hypercalcemia due to OAFs or vitamin D derivatives
   Adult T-cell lymphoma caused by the retrovirus HTLV-I
   Squamous cell tumors, secreting PTH-related proteins
   Other malignancies, associated with other humoral substances
5. Vitamin D–related hypercalcemia
   Vitamin D intoxication
   Granulomatous diseases (sarcoidosis, tuberculosis, histoplasmosis, berylliosis)
6. Vitamin A intoxication
7. Milk alkali syndrome
8. Other endocrine disorders
   Hyperthyroidism, with increased bone turnover (hypercalcemia usually mild)
   Addison's disease
   Pheochromocytoma (rare)
   Acromegaly (rare)
   Pancreatic VIPoma
9. Drugs
   Thiazide diuretics
   Furosemide
   Aluminum intoxication, with decreased bone mineralization
   Calcium
   Lithium
10. Immobilization
   Paget's disease
   Other demineralizing diseases of bone

HYPERCOAGULABLE STATES

The occurrence of DVT in a young person, a family history of thrombosis, thrombosis at unusual sites, or recurrent thrombosis without precipitating factors should persuade the clinician to investigate the possibility of a hypercoagulable state. The disorder can be divided into hereditary and acquired states. The pathogenesis of the disorder and clinical approaches to the patient have been well reviewed by Schafer and are listed and described following.

The Hypercoagulable States

I. Hereditary disorders

Antithrombin III deficiency	Protein C, S deficiency
Plasminogen deficiency	Plasminogen activator deficiency
Dysfibrinogenemia	Homocysteinuria
Factor XII deficiency	

II. Acquired disorders

Lupus anticoagulant, antiphospholipid syndrome	Dysfibrinogenemia of liver disease
	Pregnancy
Malignancy	Hyperlipidemia
DM	Vasculitis
Drug induced	TTP
Heparin-induced thrombocytopenia	Prosthetic devices
Oral contraceptives	Valves, vascular grafts
Platelet disorders	Balloon pumps
Myeloproliferative disorders	Venous stasis
Paroxysmal nocturnal hemoglobinuria	Obesity
Hyperviscosity	Old age
Polycythemia	Postoperations
Leukemia	Prolonged bed rest
Nephrotic syndrome	Sickle-cell disease
Multiple myeloma	

These disorders are primarily marked by venous thrombotic disease: DVT, PE, and thrombosis in unusual sites. Antithrombin III deficiency is typical of these disorders. It is an autosomal-dominant disease with presentation with thrombosis at any time, but most often in the second or third decade. Most thrombotic events in this disorder are venous, but arterial thrombi have been recognized in the disorder. Some individuals are deficient in antithrombin III activity, but they lack any evidence of thrombosis. Factors that may dispose these patients to thrombosis are the typical risk factors for other adults: pregnancy, use of contraceptives, trauma, post-surgery, and in association with infections. Acquired antithrombin III deficiency has been observed in DIC, in severe liver disease (and post–liver transplantation), as a result of nephrotic syndrome, and in patients taking contraceptives. Symptomatic patients with this disorder may require lifelong anticoagulation Asymptomatic patients identified in family studies do not require anticoagulation, but may benefit from prophylaxis during periods of high risk for thrombosis.

The lupus anticoagulant and the related antiphospholipid syndrome are prototypic acquired disorders that result in an increased risk for arterial and venous thrombi. Although first described in SLE, the lupus anticoagulant is also found in adults without a known collagen vascular disease, in those with HIV infection, and in drug-induced lupus. The PTT is prolonged and does not correct with a one-to-one dilution with normal plasma. The PT is sometimes prolonged, and mild thrombocytopenia may also be present. The lupus anticoagulant may be confirmed by the Russel viper venom time. Some patients also have a positive test for anticardiolipin or other antiphospholipid antibodies. A significant group of patients with thrombotic disease have these antiphospholipid antibodies without the typical lupus anticoagulant.

Of particular note is the relationship between malignancy and thrombosis first described by Trousseau. Studies of patients with known malignancy demonstrate a high incidence (5–15%) of thromboembolic disease. In pancreatic carcinoma, the incidence is even higher. Certain patients may have migratory thrombophlebitis for months before their malignancy is recognized. How aggressively should we evaluate patients who present with DVT? A recent Italian study suggests that 3% of patients who do not have a typical risk factor for thrombosis will have cancer detected by routine tests at the time of presentation. During a 2-year follow-up of patients with idiopathic thrombosis, 7% were found to have cancer. About a third of that study's follow-up patients had a second thrombosis. Malignancy was identified in 17% of those patients. However, it is likely that the patients with DVT had very small neoplasms at first encounter. A diagnostic approach to locate such tumors, many of which were GI, breast, or lung carcinomas with a poor outlook, would have been prohibitively expensive. A prudent workup might include mammography in women, CEA and PSA determinations in men, and tests for fecal occult blood.

References: Schafer AI: The hypercoagulable states. Ann Intern Med 102:814, 1985.

Pradoni P, et al: Deep-vein thrombosis and the incidence of subsequent symptomatic cancer. N Engl J Med 327:1128–1133, 1992.

HYPERGLOBULINEMIA

Hyperglobulinemia exists when the serum globulin level is 3.8 g/dl or greater. The hyperglobulinemia may be due to an increase in a single Ig (monoclonal gammopathy) or to increased levels of multiple Igs (polyclonal hyperglobulinemia).

Causes of Hyperglobulinemia

Monoclonal gammopathies
1. Multiple myeloma: Monoclonal IgG, IgA, IgD (rare), or IgE (very rare) class.
2. Light chain gammopathy: Monoclonal light chain found in serum only if renal insufficiency present.
3. Macroglobulinemia: Monoclonal IgM
4. Primary amyloidosis
5. Heavy chain disease: An incomplete serum monoclonal Ig, usually in low concentration. Three types exist: alpha–heavy chain disease, gamma–heavy chain disease, and mu–heavy chain disease.
6. Lymphocytic lymphoma: A small number of patients have serum monoclonal Ig, usually IgM.
7. Chronic lymphocytic leukemia: IgM monoclonal serum protein is found in about 5% of patients.
8. Monoclonal gammopathy of undetermined significance (MGUS) (also called benign monoclonal gammopathy or essential monoclonal gammopathy): Common in elderly patients.
9. Cold agglutinin disease: Monoclonal cold-agglutinating IgM with associated chronic hemolytic anemia.
10. Cryoglobulinemia: Type I cryoglobulinemia has monoclonal IgG or IgM. Type II cryoglobulinemia is mixed with a monoclonal component, usually IgM, directed at polyclonal IgG.
11. Pyoderma gangrenosum: Monoclonal IgG, IgA, or IgM.
12. Papular mucinosis (i.e., lichen myxedematosus): Usually monoclonal IgG.

Table continued on next page.

Causes of Hyperglobulinemia (Cont.)

Polyclonal hyperglobulinemia
1. Chronic infections: HIV type 1 (HIV infection and AIDS), lymphogranuloma venereum, infective endocarditis, osteomyelitis, syphilis, chronic TB, leprosy, chronic invasive fungal infections (histoplasmosis), kala-azar, trypanosomiasis.
2. Granulomatous disorders: Sarcoidosis, Crohn's disease, granulomatous hepatitis.
3. Autoimmune disorders: SLE, rheumatoid arthritis, Sjögren's syndrome, Wegener's granulomatosis, immune vasculitis, autoimmune hepatitis, angioimmunoblastic lymphadenopathy.
4. Hepatic disorders: Chronic active hepatitis, cirrhosis.
5. Cryoglobulinemia: Type III (i.e., mixed polyclonal cryoglobulinemia).

HYPERKALEMIA

Hyperkalemia is defined as a serum K$^+$ level >5 mEq/L and is potentially lethal because of cardiac toxicity. In the evaluation of hyperkalemia, details pertaining to diet, medications, and a history of renal and endocrine disorders should be sought.

Etiology of Hyperkalemia

A. Spurious
Thrombocytosis	Mononucleosis
Hemolysis (leaky red cells)	Leukocytosis

B. Redistribution
Acidosis	Hyperkalemic periodic paralysis
DKA	Succinylcholine
Beta-blockers	Arginine
Digitalis overdose	Hyperglycemia

C. Potassium excess states
   Increased intake: oral or IV administration
   Tissue release: hemolysis, rhabdomyolysis, tumor lysis
   Renal failure: acute or chronic (GFR <20 ml/min)
   Aldosterone deficiency: Addison's disease
   - Hyporeninemic hypoaldosteronism
   - Hereditary adrenal enzyme defects
   - Drugs (decreased renin-angiotensin activity): ACE inhibitors, cyclosporine, NSAIDs, heparin (decreased aldosterone synthesis), spironolactone (aldosterone resistance)

   Tubular hyperkalemia without aldosterone deficiency:
   Obstructive uropathy, SLE, amyloidosis, sickle-cell nephropathy, renal transplant

Clinical and laboratory evaluation: Clinical manifestations include neuromuscular weakness, paraesthesia, and paralysis. It is important to rule out artifactual hyperkalemia secondary to elevation of WBCs, platelets, or hemolysis. Any serum K$^+$ of >6 mEq/L should be followed up with an ECG. The ECG abnormalities seen with hyperkalemia, in order of their appearance, include peaking of T waves, disappearance of P waves, prolongation of the PR interval, widening of the QRS complex, and ventricular fibrillation. Bladder catheterization should be done to rule out bladder neck obstruction. A renal ultrasound is useful to rule out hydronephrosis or the small, shrunken kidneys of ESRD.

Treatment: Hyperkalemia can be fatal if severe, due to the effects on cardiac conduction and rhythm. Various agents are used in the treatment. Calcium gluconate in doses of 10 to 30 ml of a 10% solution starts acting in 1 to 2 min, and the effect lasts for 10 to 20 min. Calcium antagonizes the action of K^+ on the cardiac conducting system. Calcium chloride can be used instead of gluconate in similar doses. Repeated doses will be effective only if hypocalcemia is present. $NaHCO_3$ in doses of 50-mEq ampules can be administered IV and can be repeated every 15 min if ECG changes persist. It can also be given mixed with 5% dextrose (2 amps in 1 L with 25–50 units of regular insulin/L) at the rate of 200 to 300 ml the first half-hour and then at a rate titrated by the falling serum K^+ level. Circulatory overload and hypernatremia are problems associated with $NaHCO_3$ therapy.

Insulin lowers the plasma K^+ by promoting K^+ entry into the cell by increasing the Na-K ATPase activity. Glucose alone given as 50 ml of 50% dextrose achieves this in nondiabetics by stimulating endogenous insulin release. Exogenous insulin may be unnecessary and often dangerous in nondiabetics, as it can cause hypoglycemia. In diabetics, 1 unit of regular insulin may be added to every 3 to 5 gm of glucose administered, and insulin alone may be sufficient if hyperglycemia is already present. This regimen quickly and predictably lowers the plasma K^+, especially in patients with renal failure. Kayexalate (sodium polystyrene sulfonate) is an Na-K^+ exchange resin that removes approximately 1 mEq of K^+/gm of resin administered orally and 0.5 mEq of K^+/gm by enema. The effect is seen in 1 to 2 hrs. The resin is usually dispensed in 20% sorbitol base to promote rapid GI transit and is repeated every 3 to 4 hrs until the serum K^+ is normal. Sodium retention and circulatory overload are problems of this therapy. Dialysis is needed when there is volume overload, severe azotemia or acidosis associated with hyperkalemia. Hemodialysis removes 20 to 30 mEq/hr; peritoneal dialysis removes 10 to 15 mEq/hr.

Chronic hyperkalemia as in the cases of chronic renal failure or hyperkalemic renal tubular acidosis can often be managed by dietary restriction of K^+ to 40 to 60 mEq/day. In patients with signs of fluid retention, loop diuretics may be used, and fludrocortisone acetate (Florinef) (0.1–0.4 mg daily) can be used in patients without evidence of Na^+ retention or HTN. Finally, Kayexalate (sodium polystyrene sulfonate) in doses of 15 to 60 gm QID can be used, as can $NaHCO_3$ tablets (650 mg TID).

HYPERMAGNESEMIA

Magnesium is an important intracellular cation, second in quantity only to potassium. It plays an important role in enzymatic activity and neurochemical transmission, and it serves as a cofactor in ATP metabolism. The usual serum concentration varies between 1.4 and 2.2 mEq/L but may rise with increased magnesium intake in the setting of renal failure. Magnesium acts as a direct muscle depressant and has effects on the cardiac conduction system similar to those of potassium.

Symptoms of magnesium toxicity begin at 4 mEq/L, with nausea, vomiting, and hypotension. As levels exceed 7 mEq/L, sedation and muscular hyporeflexia intervene, followed by coma and respiratory failure at levels above 12 mEq/L. For emergency management of these severe symptoms, IV infusion of 10 cc of 10% calcium gluconate will reverse the symptoms temporarily; peritoneal dialysis or hemodialysis will quickly lower serum levels.

HYPERNATREMIA

Hypernatremia is said to exist when the serum Na^+ concentration exceeds 145 mEq/L. It is seen in about 1% of elderly hospitalized patients.

Hypernatremia is a relative deficiency of total body water compared to total body Na^+. Thus it can result from an excessive loss of free water or an addition of solute. Accordingly, hypernatremia is classified as hypovolemic, normovolemic, or hypervolemic. Severe hypernatremia always requires a defective thirst mechanism or nonavailability of water.

Etiology of Hypernatremia

HYPOVOLEMIC	NORMOVOLEMIC	HYPERVOLEMIC
Diuretics	Diabetes insipidus	Excessive $NaHCO_3$ adminis-
Osmotic purgatives	Excessive cutaneous and pul-	tration
Excessive sweating	monary losses in hospital-	Hypertonic Na^+ dialysate
	ized patients	

Pathophysiology: The osmolality of body fluids is tightly maintained in a narrow range between 285 and 290 mOsm/kg H_2O. The plasma osmolality (Posm) can be estimated by the formula:

$$Posm = 2\,[Na^+\,(mEq/L)] + \frac{Glucose\,(mg/dl)}{18} + \frac{BUN\,(mg/dl)}{2.8}$$

Normally, the osmolality of extracellular and intracellular fluids is maintained in equilibrium by free permeability of cell membranes to water. Effective osmoles are those solutes that when administered would not freely penetrate cell membrane but would cause water shift from the cells. They include glucose, Na^+, mannitol, and glycerol. When Posm exceeds 300 mOsm/kg, the water thirst mechanism is stimulated. Hypovolemia and hypotension also stimulate the ADH and thirst mechanisms.

Hypovolemic hypernatremia results from loss of hypotonic fluids from the body such as by means of sweat, hypotonic urine loss from diuretics, or hypotonic stool losses. The degree of volume contraction and hypotension correlates best with the amount of salt loss. Administration of hypertonic $NaHCO_3$ solutions during cardiac arrest, and hypertonic saline in dialysate, can result in hypertonic hypernatremia. This causes rapid intracellular dehydration. On the other hand, loss of free water without any solute loss results in euvolemic hypernatremia because such electrolyte free water derives primarily from the cells. Hypotension does not occur until water loss is extreme. DI is a classic example of this kind of hypernatremia.

Clinical features: Neurological manifestations predominate in the clinical picture of hypernatremia and hyperosmolality. This is because of the cellular dehydration especially in the brain. The process leads to capillary and venous congestion, tearing of cerebral vessels, thrombosis of venous sinuses, and subcortical hemorrhages. Symptoms include irritability, muscular twitching, hyperreflexia, seizures, and coma. The morbidity and mortality of hypernatremia correlate with the rapidity of development, being worst in the acute forms. In adults, acute hypernatremia—a serum Na^+ >160 mEq/L—is associated with 75% mortality; in chronic hypernatremia of the same degree, the mortality is around 50%. However, these numbers indicate to some extent the seriousness of the underlying disorder.

Treatment: The primary aim of treatment is restoration of serum osmolality. Hypotonic hypernatremia should be corrected by administration of NS until hemodynamic stability is restored. After that point, hypernatremia should be corrected by administration of either D5W or 1/2 NS until the serum Na^+ is close to normal. Hypertonic hypernatremia is managed by the administration of D5W along with diuretics and by dialysis if the renal function is severely impaired. In normovolemic hypernatremia, the water loss is replaced by D5W. The free-water deficit is calculated as follows:

$$\frac{\text{Measured serum Na concentration}}{\text{Required serum Na concentration}} \times \text{TBW} = \text{ideal body water}$$

where TBW (total body water) is calculated as total body weight $\times 0.6$. This amount of fluid can generally be replaced in 48 hrs with a correction rate not faster than 2 mOsm/hr. It is believed that faster rates of correction are associated with seizures due to cerebral edema. Slower rates of correction prevent this by allowing idiogenic osmoles time to be dissipated.

Reference: Madsen PA, et al: Pathophysiological approach to patients presenting with hypernatremia. Am J Nephrol 5:229, 1985.

HYPEROSMOLALITY

Calculation of Water Deficits

Water disorders are osmolality disorders. Osmolality consists of the number of dissolved particles per unit of water. Although the type of osmotic particles varies between the inside of the cell and the extracellular compartment, intracellular and extracellular osmolalities are normally equal because of the free movement of water.

Na^+ salts are the principal extracellular osmoles. When the amount of Na^+ in the ECF increases, water is drawn out of cells, and cells shrink. Conversely, water enters cells and swells them when the amount of Na^+ in the ECF drops. We can look at the serum Na^+ concentration and draw conclusions about the presence of an osmolality (water) disorder. A low serum Na^+ (hyposmolality) is indicative of water excess; a high serum Na^+ (hyperosmolality) indicates a water deficit. Water deficit or excess (osmolality disorders) can coexist with Na^+ (volume disorders). The following formula estimates the plasma osmolality:

$$P_{osm} = 2 \times [P_{Na+}] + (\text{glucose}/18) + (\text{BUN}/2.8)$$

(When glucose and BUN are normal, P_{osm} approximates $2 \times P_{Na+}$.)

Clinically, patients with a pure water deficit (hyperosmolality) will have depression, confusion, coma, and seizures. A water deficit (hyperosmolality) can result from pure water loss, as seen with DI (though most adults with DI can maintain acceptable serum osmolality if they have access to and can drink free water). However, in internal medicine, the most common cause of a pure water deficit (hyperosmolality) is the inability of an elderly patient to obtain water because of bedfastness, dementia, or delirium. In elderly patients, water deficits are often accompanied by Na$^+$ (volume) deficits. That is, hypernatremia and hyperosmolality coexist with clinical evidence of volume depletion such as orthostatic hypotension. Pure Na$^+$ gain is a very infrequent cause of water deficit in adults.

Calculation of a water deficit is based on estimates of body water and the serum Na$^+$. In men, TBW accounts for about 60% of the body weight; in women, the proportion is 50%. Water deficit is normal body TBW minus present body water. Present total body water equals TBW × (current serum Na$^+$/normal serum Na$^+$). Assuming that normal body water is 60% of body weight and normal serum Na$^+$ is 140, the equation is:

$$\text{Water deficit [L]} = 0.6 \times \text{body weight [kg]} \times (1-140/\text{plasma Na}^+)$$

Water replacement should be slow so as not to cause cerebral edema or demyelination of the CNS. Most practitioners recommend that the serum Na$^+$ should not be brought down more quickly than 0.5 to 2 mEq/L per hr. When hypovolemia accompanies water deficit, saline (NS, $^1/_2$NS, $^1/_4$NS) infusions are necessary. Na$^+$ in the solution lowers the amount of free water in the infusion, and administration rates must be increased accordingly. It is important to include maintenance fluid requirements (skin and respiratory tract losses and obligate renal losses) in planning the hourly rate of infusion; otherwise, serum Na$^+$ will increase instead of decrease.

References: Feig PU, et al: The hypertonic state. N Engl J Med 297:1444–1454, 1977.
Gennari FJ: Serum osmolality: Uses and limitations. N Engl J Med 310:102–105, 1984.

HYPEROSMOLAR NONKETOTIC COMA

This condition is ten times less common than DKA. Although it may occur at any age, the median age at presentation is 60 to 70 years. It is much more common in patients with NIDDM. Two thirds of presenting patients do not have a previous history of DM.

Precipitating factors
1. Surgical stress
2. Hyperalimentation
3. Dialysis (either peritoneal or hemodialysis)
4. Drugs such as glucocorticoids, dilantin, and diazoxide
5. Chronic illnesses, particularly renal disease and CHF
6. Alcoholism
7. Stroke
8. Acute illnesses (cholecystitis, pancreatitis, pneumonia, MI)
9. Social isolation in elderly
10. Diuretics (aggravating factor)

Pathophysiology
1. Lack of insulin: There is, however, enough insulin to inhibit ketogenesis (typical of NIDDM).
2. Osmotic diuresis due to hyperglycemia and glycosuria
3. Decreased renal function is a common predisposing factor

Clinical presentation
1. Dehydration
2. Altered sensorium (confusion, stupor, or even coma) due to hyperosmolarity >350 mmol/kg may cause diagnostic problems

3. Convulsions
4. Other consequences—stroke, MI, peripheral gangrene, renal failure, and even death—may occur

Laboratory findings

1. Glucose >600 mg/dl (levels as high as 1,000 to 2,000 mg/dl common)
2. Slight or absent evidence of ketosis
3. Normal pH
4. Plasma osmolality >340 mOsm (osmolality = 2 × [Na + K] + glucose + BUN mmol/kg)
5. Evidence of prerenal azotemia with elevated BUN and creatinine
6. Serum sodium often elevated
7. Potassium either normal or elevated at presentation

Prognosis: There is a 50% mortality rate, especially in patients older than 50. These patients often have hypothermia, coma, and shock. About 50% of patients will have residual NIDDM after correction of hyperosmolar coma. Other complications related to management include hypoglycemia, cerebral edema, and hypokalemia.

Management: Rehydration is the main component of therapy. IV administration of 2 L of NS the first hour, then 1 L/hr in the second and third hours, followed by 250 to 500 ml/hr. When the vital signs are stabilized, fluids should be switched to 1/2 NS. As many as 10 L may be required for the first 24 hrs (watch for CHF and volume overload). In severe cases, monitoring CVP may be required to adjust fluid therapy. Insulin should be given at a low rate both to prevent a rapid drop in blood sugar and to avoid hypoglycemia. Plasma potassium levels should be followed very closely and will allow adjustment of potassium administration. Anticoagulation with heparin has been recommended by some, but is not widely used. Magnesium and phosphate levels should be monitored and replaced if necessary.

HYPERPIGMENTATION

Generalized brown pigmentation
Addison's disease
ACTH-producing pituitary tumors
MSH-producing pituitary tumors
Nelson's syndrome (high ACTH/MSH production after bilateral adrenalectomy in patients with Cushing's disease)
ACTH therapy
ACTH- and/or MSH-producing small cell carcinoma of lung
Pregnancy
Sun exposure and ultraviolet light
Hemochromatosis
Transfusional hemosiderosis
Porphyria cutanea tarda
Wilson's disease (hepatolenticular degeneration)
Malignant melanoma, with melanuria
Kwashiorkor and pellagra
Sprue
Arsenic poisoning
Busulfan therapy

Localized brown pigmentation
  Café au lait lesions of neurofibromatosis
  Addison's disease
  Acanthosis nigricans
  Albright's syndrome (polyostotic fibrous dysplasia)
  Xeroderma pigmentosa
  Estrogen therapy (increased pigmentation of nipples)
  Eczema, drug eruptions
  Urticaria pigmentosa
Generalized gray pigmentation
  Hemochromatosis (gray or brown appearance)
  Malignant melanoma with melanuria (gray or brown appearance)
  Argyria (silver intoxication) (gray-to-blue appearance)
  Bismuth intoxication (gray-to-blue appearance)
  Gold therapy
  Local application of mercury (gray or brown appearance)
Generalized blue appearance
  Cyanosis
  Methemoglobinemia
  Sulfhemoglobinemia
  Application of mercury
  Argyria
  Ochronosis
Yellow pigmentation
  Jaundice (particularly evident in conjunctivae, cartilages of ears, mucous membranes; due to hemolytic anemia, hepatocellular disease, or biliary obstruction)
  Carotenemia (evident in palms and soles, but not in conjunctivae or mucous membranes; observed in patients with myxedema or persons with ingestion of a large amount of carotenoid-containing foods)
  Quinacrine therapy (diffuse yellow color to skin)
  Picric acid exposure
  Rifampin therapy (transitory orange color of skin and mucous membranes)
  Sodium fluorescein (yellow appearance of skin for 1–2 days after IV injection for ophthalmologic studies)

HYPERSENSITIVITY REACTIONS

The four classic types of hypersensitivity reactions describe different mechanisms of immunologically mediated inflammation.

Types of Immunologically Mediated Inflammation

TYPE OF INFLAMMATION	RECOGNITION COMPONENT	SOLUABLE MEDIATOR	INFLAMMATORY RESPONSE	DISEASE EXAMPLE
Reaginic, allergic	IgE	Basophil and mast cell products (ECF)	Immediate flare and wheal, smooth muscle constriction	Atopy, anaphylaxis

Table continued on next page.

Types of Immunologically Mediated Inflammation (Cont.)

TYPE OF INFLAMMATION	RECOGNITION COMPONENT	SOLUBLE MEDIATOR	INFLAMMATORY RESPONSE	DISEASE EXAMPLE
Cytotoxic antibody	IgG, IgM	Complement	Lysis or phagocytosis of circulating antigens, acute inflammation in tissues	AIHA, thrombocytopenia associated with SLE
Immune complex	IgG, IgM	Complement, lipid mediators	Accumulation of PMNs and macrophages	RA, SLE
Delayed hypersensitivity	T lymphocytes	Cytokines	Mononulcear cell infiltrate	TB, sarcoidosis, polymyositis, granulomatosis, vasculitis

From Snyderman R: Mechanisms of inflammation and tissue destruction in the rheumatic diseases. In Wyngaarden JB, Smith LH (eds): Cecil Textbook of Medicine, 18th ed. Philadelphia, W.B. Saunders, 1988, p 1989, with permission.

HYPERTENSION

HTN can be classified according to the Joint National Committee on Detection, Evaluation, and Treatment of High Blood Pressure (1988) by the following categories, based on the average of two or more readings on two or more occasions:

RANGE, mm Hg	CATEGORY
Diastolic BP	
<85	Normal BP
85–89	High-normal BP
90–104	Mild HTN
105–114	Moderate HTN
>115	Severe HTN
Systolic BP (when diastolic BP is <90)	
<140	Normal BP
140–159	Borderline isolated systolic HTN
≥160	Isolated systolic HTN

Diagnosis

History
1. Known documentation and/or treatment of high BP, including side effects of medications
2. Family history of high BP and heart disease
3. Prior history of heart, kidney, cerebrovascular disease, or DM
4. Weight change; exercise; salt, fat, and alcohol intake

  5. Symptoms of secondary HTN: Secondary causes of HTN include pheochromocytoma, hyperthyroidism, hypothyroidism, Cushing's disease, aldosteronism, renal failure, renal artery stenosis.
  6. Psychosocial stressors

Physical examination
  1. Vital signs: Standing and seated BP in both arms, thigh BP, height, weight
  2. Optic fundus: Arteriolar narrowing, AV nicking, hemorrhages, exudates, papilledema
  3. Thyroid: Size and nodularity
  4. Heart: Point of maximum impulse (PMI), murmurs, gallops
  5. Abdomen: Bruits, enlarged kidneys
  6. Extremities: Equal peripheral pulses, edema
  7. Neurologic: Mental status changes, focal deficits

Laboratory tests
  1. Hemoglobin
  2. Potassium, calcium, creatinine, glucose, uric acid
  3. Cholesterol, triglycerides, HDL cholesterol
  4. UA
  5. ECG

Therapy (nonpharmacologic)
  1. Weight reduction
  2. Alcohol restriction (<1 oz of ethanol daily)
  3. Sodium restriction
  4. Tobacco cessation
  5. Exercise

Therapy (pharmacologic)

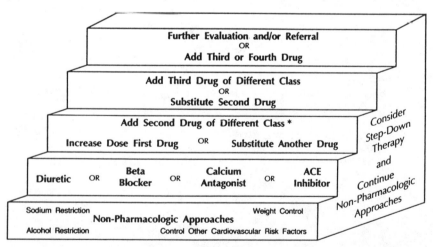

Individualized step-care therapy for hypertension. For some patients, nonpharmacologic therapy should be tried first. If BP goal is not achieved, then add pharmacologic therapy. Other patients may require pharmacologic therapy initially. In these instances, nonpharmacologic therapy may be a helpful adjunct. The asterisk indicates drugs such as diuretics, β-blockers, calcium antagonists, ACE inhibitors, α-blockers, centrally acting α₂-agonists, *Rauwolfia serpentina,* and vasodilators. (From 1988 Joint National Committee: The 1988 report of the Joint National Committee on Detection, Evaluation, and Treatment of High Blood Pressure. Arch Intern Med 148:1023–1038, 1988, with permission.)

Essential Hypertension

Of the more than 60 million in the United States who suffer from HTN, greater than 90% have essential type. HTN is defined as a systolic BP ≥140 mmHg and/or a diastolic BP ≥90 mmHg on three separate evaluations, measured with the proper-size cuff at an interval of at least 30 min since last ingestion of caffeine or use of nicotine.

Medical history should emphasize:

• **Family history:** HTN, cardiovascular disease, cerebrovascular disease, renal disease, endocrine disorders

• **Past medical history:** Previous HTN; HTN treatment responses; cardiac, cerebrovascular, renal, or endocrine diseases; peripheral vascular disease; hyperlipidemia; prescribed medications such as birth control pills, corticosteroids, NSAIDs, cyclosporine, diet pills

• **Social history:** Use of tobacco, alcohol, or stimulant drugs (including OTC nasal sprays and decongestants); recent stresses; dietary salt intake; activity level

• **Review of symptoms:** Symptoms of secondary HTN, recent change in weight, chest or abdominal pain, claudication symptoms, shortness of breath, swelling

• **Physical examination:** Best when directed at both attempting to detect a source for the HTN and documenting existing end organ damage and physical conditions that may prohibit the use of certain antihypertensive medications. BP readings should be taken both sitting and standing, and the pressure in both arms should be documented. Head and neck examination includes attention to the fundus (retinopathy helps establish duration of the hypertensive process), thyroid, and neck veins. Chest exam may give clues to underlying pulmonary problems (rales, wheezing, prolonged expiratory phase) as well as cardiac conditions such as valvular heart disease, LVH, CHF, and rate and rhythm disturbances. Examination of the abdomen may reveal kidney enlargement, bruits, or pulsatile masses suggestive of aneurysm. Vascular examination for carotid bruits or attenuated peripheral pulses is important, as is a baseline neurologic examination

• **Pertinent laboratory evaluation:** Should include hemoglobin, hematocrit, UA, BUN, creatinine, K^+, Ca^+, cholesterol, triglycerides, glucose (fasting), and ECG.

Treatment. Many studies have shown that effective treatment of HTN reduces the risk of mortality and morbidity from stroke, CHF, and hypertensive renal disease. The recently completed SHEP study (Systolic Hypertension in the Elderly Program) confirmed that reduction of isolated systolic HTN to levels under 160 mmHg in patients older than 65 years of age reduced the incidence of LVH by 54%, strokes by 36%, and CAD by 25%.

Once a decision has been made to initiate therapy for HTN, various nonpharmacologic and pharmacologic options exist. Weight loss, restriction of alcohol (no more than 2 oz of whiskey, 8 oz of wine, or 24 oz of beer daily), restriction of sodium

(4–6 g of salt daily), and regular aerobic exercise may be very effective in lowering BP. Recommendations regarding appropriate first-line drug therapy are constantly undergoing revision. Currently, several choices are available, including thiazide-type diuretics, beta-blockers, calcium channel blockers, ACE inhibitors, alpha-1 blockers, and central adrenergic inhibitors. If initial therapy is inadequate to maintain BP below 140/90 mm Hg, a step-care approach as diagrammed in the following figure may be utilized.

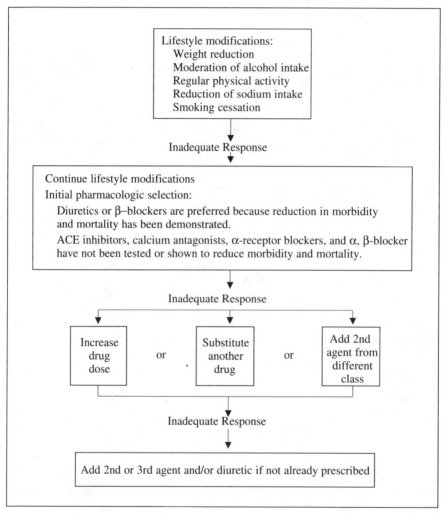

Treatment algorithm. Response means that the patient has achieved the goal BP or is making considerable progress toward this goal. (From The Joint Committee on Detection, Education, Evaluation and Treatment of High Blood Pressure. The Fifth Report of the Joint National Committee on Detection, Evaluation, and Treatment of High Blood Pressure. Arch Intern Med 153:154–183, 1993, with permission.)

Side Effects. Troublesome side effects may often be avoided by a judicious combination of medications at less than those medications' individual maximum doses. However, it is important to avoid beta-blockers in combination with central adrenergic inhibitors because the combination may cause a paradoxical rise in BP and marked bradycardia secondary to combined negative chronotropic effects. The following list may be helpful in choosing the right medication(s).

- **Blacks:** Do not in general respond well to beta-blockers or ACE inhibitors.
- **Elderly:** (>65 yrs): Often respond to smaller doses; orthostasis a problem with diuretics and vasodilators.
- **Pregnancy:** Bed rest and sodium restriction initially; methyldopa or hydralazine preferable (*avoid:* calcium channel blockers, which may decrease uterine contractions, and ACE inhibitors, which have been associated with increased fetal wasting in animal studies).
- **CHF:** Caution with negative inotropic or chronotropic agents (beta-blockers without intrinsic sympathomimetic activity, verapamil, diltiazem, clonidine).
- **Asthma, chronic bronchitis:** Beta-blockers may provoke bronchospasm.
- **Cerebrovascular disease:** Avoid overaggressive lowering of BP, especially with vasodilators.
- **Peripheral arterial disease:** Beta-blockers may aggravate claudication symptoms.
- **DM:** Beta-blockers may impair catecholamine-mediated response to hypoglycemia. ACE inhibitors and calcium channel blockers (except nifedipine) may decrease or retard the onset of proteinuria associated with diabetic nephropathy.
- **Hyperlipidemia:** Thiazide diuretics and beta-blockers may aggravate condition. Alpha-1 blockers and central adrenergic agonists may decrease lipid levels. ACE inhibitors and calcium channel blockers appear to have no effect.
- **Gout:** Avoid thiazide-type diuretics, which raise uric acid levels and may bring on acute attack.
- **Renal failure:** Need close monitoring with use of ACE inhibitors for deterioration of function and hyperkalemia.
- **Cardiovascular disease:** Avoid agents that may aggravate any associated hyperlipidemia. Recent studies demonstrate possible antiatherosclerotic effects of calcium channel blockers.

References: The Fifth Report of the Joint National Committee on Detection, Evaluation, and Treatment of High Blood Pressure. Arch Intern Med 153:154–183, 1993.

Mann SJ: Systolic hypertension in the elderly: Pathophysiology and management. Arch Intern Med 152:1977–1984, 1992.

Renovascular Hypertension

Renovascular HTN accounts for 0.5% of all cases of HTN and is the most common form of secondary HTN correctable with surgery. Stenotic lesions in the renal artery produce elevation of renin levels and secondarily elevate the angiotensin II and aldosterone levels, causing HTN by vasoconstriction and later by salt and water retention. Progressive occlusion of the renal artery leads to eventual loss of function in that kidney. Bilateral renal artery stenosis is now increasingly being recognized as a cause of chronic renal failure. Renovascular obstruction can be caused by intrinsic and extrinsic factors.

Etiology of Renovascular Hypertension

INTRINSIC LESIONS	EXTRINSIC LESIONS
Atherosclerosis	Retroperitoneal tumors
Fibromuscular dysplasia	Retroperitoneal fibrosis
Others: Emboli, vasculitis, renal cysts, trauma, "Page kidney"	

Atherosclerotic disease is seen in about 60% of cases of renovascular HTN, and fibromuscular dysplasia is seen in about one third of patients. There are several differences between the two forms of renal artery stenosis as follows.

Differences Between Atherosclerotic and Fibromuscular Stenosis

	FIBROMUSCULAR DYSPLASIA	ATHEROSCLEROSIS
Age at onset	<40	>45
Gender	80% female	Primarily males
Distribution of lesion	Distal main renal artery and intrarenal branches	Aortic orifice and proximal main renal artery
Extrarenal disease	Uncommon	Common
Progression	Uncommon	Common, may progress to complete occlusion
Prognosis	Better	Worse

Clinical Features: Renovascular HTN is suspected in patients with resistant HTN, abrupt onset of HTN before the age of 20 or after the age of 50 years, or sudden deterioration in BP control in a stable hypertensive and in those with high-pitched systolodiastolic bruit in the abdomen. Abdominal bruits are described in 50 to 70% of confirmed cases of renal artery stenosis. Acute renal failure developing in a patient with HTN upon treatment with an ACE inhibitor is a clue to the presence of underlying bilateral renal arterial disease.

Screening Tests: An abdominal ultrasound is useful in noting the renal size (a differential of >1.5 cm is consistent with renal artery stenosis in the smaller kidney). It can also exclude renal parenchymal disease and obstruction, which is a consideration in the differential diagnosis. A captopril screening test can be performed that consists of the administration of 25 to 50 mg of captopril after a washout of all anti-HTN agents for a week. The peripheral renin levels are obtained before and 1 hr after the administration, with the patient seated throughout the test. An increase in the renin levels by 4.7 ng/ml/hr is diagnostic of renal artery stenosis. This is a sensitive but not specific test for the diagnosis of renovascular disease. A captopril renogram using ^{131}I-Hippuran shows persistent cortical uptake with delayed excretion after captopril. A ^{99}Tc-DTPA renogram indirectly demonstrates decreases in the renal plasma flow and GFR that are improved with captopril. The captopril renogram provides indirect measure of renal blood flow and GFR, and a positive test indicates that a stenotic lesion is functionally significant. This test has largely replaced the rapid-sequence IVP once used as a screening test for renal artery stenosis. The sensitivity and specificity of the captopril renogram are not completely known.

The diagnosis is traditionally confirmed by selective renal angiography with differential renal vein renin measurements. If the lesions are typical, some physicians proceed with angioplasty without waiting for renal vein renin levels. A captopril renogram may be used in lieu of renal vein renin measurements to determine the functional significance of stenotic lesions.

Treatment: Percutaneous angioplasty of stenotic lesions is successful in >80% of cases, although restenosis is a major problem. Osteal lesions are corrected in only 20% of cases by this technique. Surgical revascularization is reserved for patients with angioplasty failures, osteal lesions, uncontrolled HTN (especially in the face of failing renal function) and aortic lesions.

Patients who are not surgical candidates for any reason should be considered for medical management. ACE inhibitors alone or in combination with diuretics are successful in controlling BP. ACE inhibitors are known to cause ARF in certain patient groups, including patients with bilateral renal artery stenosis, unilateral stenosis in a single or transplant kidney, or unilateral stenosis when the contralateral kidney has severe parenchymal disease. Serial estimations of renal lengths, measured every 3 to 6 months, is a sensitive index of renal mass and is important in the follow-up of patients on medical management.

Secondary Hypertension

Of all patients with HTN, only 5 to 10% present with a secondary, potentially reversible cause.

Causes of Secondary Hypertension

Renal disorders	Drug use
Volume overload with renal failure	Hormonal: contraceptives, anabolic steroids, glucocorticoids
Chronic renal failure: polycystic kidneys, glomerulonephritis	Nonhormonal: licorice, cocaine, amphetamines
Obstructive uropathy	
Primary abnormality in salt excretion	
Renovascular disease	Excess ethanol intake
Tumors	
	Ethanol or drug withdrawal
Endocrine disorders	
Adrenal: pheochromocytoma, Cushing's syndrome, primary hyperaldosteronism	Pregnancy
Pituitary: acromegaly, Cushing's syndrome	Aortic coarctation
Thyroid: hyperthyroidism, hypothyroidism	Neurologic disorders
Hyperparathyroidism	Increased ICP
	Quadriplegia
	Guillain-Barré syndrome
Pain or acute stress	
	Porphyria

From Nasir M, et al: Reversible hypertension in adults. Hosp Med (May):25, 1992, with permission.

Although rare, these diseases are important to recognize. Significant morbidity and even mortality may result from both the effects of severe HTN, as well as side effects of various therapeutic agents utilized to control it.

Clinical Findings Suggestive of Secondary Hypertension

HISTORY	PHYSICAL EXAMINATION
Age at onset <30 or >50 yr	Difference in BP in upper extremities
Absence of family history	Difference in BP and pulse in upper and
Poor control on 3-drug regimen	lower extremities
Uncontrolled BP after a period of good	Abdominal bruit
control	Abdominal mass
Palpitations, tremors, sweating, weight loss,	Peripheral cyanosis or gangrene
glucose intolerance	Peripheral edema
Ethanol intake >3 drinks/day	Needle marks
Use of cocaine, amphetamines, hormones	Perforated nasal septum
GU or renal disease	Thyroid enlargement
Deterioration in renal function induced by	Immature secondary sex characteristics
ACE inhibitors	Stigmata of Cushing's syndrome
Muscle pain (esp. after diuretic use)	

From Nasir M, et al: Reversible hypertension in adults. Hosp Med (May):26, 1992, with permission.

Useful Diagnostic Studies in the Diagnosis of Secondary HTN

Renal artery stenosis
 Captopril test: 60 min after ingestion of 25–50 mg captopril, a PRA (plasma renin activity) >12 ng/ml/hr plus an absolute increase in PRA >10 ng/ml/hr and a 150% increase in PRA (400% if the baseline was <3 ng/ml/hr) indicates the presence of renal artery stenosis.
Hyperaldosteronism
 Oral salt loading: After 3 days of oral salt loading (250–300 mEq/day), a urinary aldosterone excretion rate >14 μg/24 hr and/or a supine plasma aldosterone level >22 ng/dl (normal = 8.5 ng/dl) indicates hyperaldosteronism.
 IV (acute) salt loading: After 2 L NS IV over 4 hrs, a plasma aldosterone level >10 ng/dl indicates hyperaldosteronism.
Cushing's syndrome
 24-hr urinary free cortisol: A level >100 μg is abnormal.
 Low-dose dexamethasone suppression test: After 0.5 mg dexamethasone PO Q 6 hr for 2 days, a 24-hr urinary free cortisol <25 μg and a 24-hr urinary 17-hydroxycorticosteroid <4 mg is a normal response. An abnormal response indicates Cushing's syndrome and calls for a high-dose dexamethasone suppression test.
 High-dose dexamethasone suppression test: After 2 mg dexamethasone PO Q 6 hr for 2 days, a 24-hr urinary free cortisol level and a 24-hr urinary 17-hydroxycorticosteroid level ≤40% of baseline suggest a pituitary cause of Cushing's syndrome. If levels are >40% of baseline, a nonpituitary cause is likely.
Pheochromocytoma
 Resting plasma catecholamines (norepinephrine and epinephrine): A level >2,000 pg/ml is diagnostic; a level of 1,000 to 2,000 pg/ml is suspicious.
 24-hr urinary VMA: A level >10 mg indicates the presence of a pheochromocytoma.
 24-hr urinary metanephrines: A level >1.3 mg indicates the presence of a pheochromocytoma.

Clonidine suppression test: 3 hr after 0.3 mg clonidine PO, a normal response is a decrease of 500 pg/ml or more in plasma norepinephrine and epinephrine.

Glucagon stimulation test: After 1–2 mg glucagon IV, a positive response is at least a threefold increase in plasma catecholamines or a level >2,000 pg/ml.

Reference: Nasir M, et al: Reversible hypertension in adults. Hosp Med (May):26, 1992.

Treatment of Newly Detected Hypertension

The first principle in the approach to the patient with newly detected high BP is to ensure the BP is truly elevated before committing the patient to pharmacologic therapy. An expert committee comprising representatives of the World Health Organization and the International Society of Hypertension has recommended starting drug treatment only if the diastolic BP remains ≥95 mm Hg after 3 to 6 months in the face of nonpharmacologic therapies. Nonpharmacologic measures are effective in reducing BP. They include weight reduction, dietary Na^+ restriction, regular aerobic exercise, and moderation of alcohol intake to no more than two portions per day. At the same time it is important to consider the BP within the context of the patient's entire constellation of cardiovascular risk factors, including cigarette smoking, hyperlipidemia or dyslipidemia, LVH, obesity, DM, and sedentary lifestyle. Patients should be counseled on ways to modify all of their risk factors, not just BP.

Once the diagnosis of HTN not responsive to nonpharmacologic measures is established (systolic-diastolic HTN is present when the pressure exceeds 140/90 in adults under age 60 or 160/90 in adults over age 60, systolic HTN when the systolic BP exceeds 160 with the diastolic ≤90), drug therapy should be started. The one exception to this rule concerns the person who has borderline hypertension and no other risk factors. Studies have not shown that reducing BP in such persons reduces their already low cardiovascular risk.

When drug treatment is begun, it is safest to "start low and go slow." About 90% of hypertensives can be controlled on a one- or two- drug anti-HTN regimen. According to the U.S. Joint National Committee on Detection, Evaluation, and Treatment of High Blood Pressure, appropriate first-line choices include diuretics, beta-blockers, second-generation alpha-blockers, ACE inhibitors, and calcium channel blockers. Blacks and elderly patients respond particularly well to diuretics, less well to beta-blockers.

Concern that the lipid-raising effects of thiazides outweigh the benefits of using these agents to lower BP remains theoretical. In fact, two recently completed trials of the treatment of systolic HTN in the elderly have again proven that the use of a thiazide diuretic, in conjunction with a beta-blocker as a second agent when needed, reduces cardiovascular morbidity and mortality. The use of ACE inhibitors and calcium channel blockers as first-line agents may be acceptable under some circumstances but remains controversial. These agents undoubtedly reduce BP; however, their efficacy in reducing cardiovascular morbidity and mortality has never been proven. That fact, together with their high cost, should be taken into account in the design of a therapeutic regimen for a newly diagnosed hypertensive. To illustrate, the cost of 1 month of therapy using a two-drug regimen of generic hydrochlorothiazide (25 mg daily) plus generic propranolol (40 mg twice daily) is $11 compared to $47 for a one-month supply of captopril (still not available in a generic form) 25 mg every eight hours. With which of these two regimens is *your* self-pay patient likely to comply?

References: Kaplan NM: The appropriate goals of antihypertensive therapy: Neither too much nor too little. Ann Intern Med 116:686–690, 1992.

Mann SJ: Systolic hypertension in the elderly. Pathophysiology and management. Arch Intern Med 152:1977–1984, 1992.

National Heart, Lung, and Blood Institute. The fifth report of the Joint National Committee on the Detection, Evaluation, and Treatment of High Blood Pressure. NIH Pub. No. 93–1088. Bethesda, National Institutes of Health, 1993.

HYPERTENSIVE EMERGENCIES AND URGENCIES

Classifying a patient with elevated BP according to whether a hypertensive *emergency* or *urgency* exists is an excellent way to discipline oneself to tailor the intensity of treatment to the severity of the clinical situation. This is one setting in which failure to do so can have drastic consequences for the patient: undertreatment of the patient with a hypertensive emergency can lead to death or permanent organ dysfunction, and overtreatment of the patient with a hypertensive urgency can lead to both dangerous drops in BP and organ underperfusion. The Hx & PE distinguishes a hypertensive emergency from a hypertensive urgency. The actual BP numbers mean very little and can be misleading. Hypertensives can tolerate much higher elevations of BP than normotensives. The rule is to treat the patient, not the numbers.

A **hypertensive emergency** is a situation in which there is a severe elevation in BP accompanied by rapid or progressive CNS, myocardial, renal, or hematologic deterioration. **The goal of treatment is to lower the BP within 1 hour.** Signs and symptoms of a hypertensive emergency include CNS findings (confusion, disorientation, obtundation, headache, visual changes, nausea and vomiting from increased ICP, focal or generalized weakness, focal or generalized seizures, nystagmus, asymmetrical reflexes), eye ground changes (papilledema, exudates, hemorrhages), cardiac problems (angina, MI, pulmonary edema), acute renal insufficiency, and microangiopathic hemolytic anemia. Cerebral infarction, subarachnoid hemorrhage, intracerebral hemorrhage, and aortic dissection can occur. The diastolic BP should be lowered to 100 to 110 mm Hg within an hour. It should not be brought to normal levels. Sodium nitroprusside is the drug of choice, but because it may have adverse effects on the fetus, in eclampsia a reduced dose should be used or an alternative drug selected. Also, no reduction in blood pressure may be warranted if a cerebral infarct or bleed has occurred, because lowering BP may further threaten areas of cerebral ischemia. In such cases, immediate neurologic consultation is needed. See the Parenteral Drugs table for available drugs.

A **hypertensive urgency** is a situation in which there is severe elevation in BP but no evidence of end-organ damage or dysfunction. **The goal of treatment is to lower the BP slowly, over 6 to 24 (some say 48) hours.** The patient should be placed in a quiet, darkened area. If the BP comes down within 30 min, the patient can be started on a regular program of anti-HTN medication. If the pressure remains high, one of the drugs listed in the Oral Drugs table may be used.

Parenteral Drugs for Treatment of Hypertensive Emergencies

DRUG	DOSE	REACTION TIME (MIN)	ADVERSE REACTIONS
Vasodilators			
Sodium nitroprusside	0.5–10 μg/kg/min as IV infusion	Instant	Nausea, thiocyanate intoxication, methemoglobinemia
Nitroglycerin	5–100 μg/min as IV infusion	2–5	Headache, tachycardia, methemoglobinemia
Diazoxide	50–150 mg IV bolus, repeated, or 15–30 mg/min IV infusion	1–2	Hypotension, tachycardia, aggravation of angina pectoris
Hydralazine	10–20 mg IV bolus or 10–50 mg IM	10 20–30	Tachycardia, headache, aggravation of angina
Adrenergic inhibitors			
Phentolamine	5–15 mg IV bolus	1–2	Tachycardia, orthostatic hypotension
Trimethaphan	1–4 mg/min IV infusion	1–5	Paresis of bowel and bladder, orthostatic hypotension, blurred vision, dry mouth
Labetalol	20–80 mg IV bolus Q 10 min or 2 mg/min IV infusion	5–10	Bronchoconstriction, heart block
Methyldopa	250–500 mg IV infusion Q 6 hr	30–60	Drowsiness
Enalapril	0.625–1.25 mg Q 6 hr IV	15–60	Renal failure in bilateral renal artery stenosis, hypotension

Oral Drugs for Treatment of Hypertensive Emergencies and Urgencies

DRUG	DOSE	REACTION TIME (MIN)	ADVERSE REACTIONS
Nifedipine	10–20 mg PO; repeat after 30 min	15–30	Rapid, uncontrolled reduction may precipitate circulatory collapse in aortic stenosis.
Captopril	25 mg PO; repeat as required	15–30	Hypotension, renal failure in bilateral renal artery stenosis
Clonidine	0.1–0.2 mg PO; repeat Q 1 hr as required to a total dose of 0.6 mg	30–60	Hypotension, drowsiness, dry mouth
Labetalol	200–400 mg PO; repeat Q 2–3 hr	30 min–2 hr	Bronchoconstriction, heart block, orthostatic hypotension

From The Joint Committee on Detection, Education, Evaluation, and Treatment of High Blood Pressure. The fifth report of the Joint National Committee on Detection, Evaluation, and Treatment of High Blood Pressure. Arch Intern Med 153:154–183, 1993, with permission.

Caution should be used so as to avoid excessively rapid or aggressive lowering of the BP in the setting of an acute CVA because of the possibility of worsening the patient's condition due to interference with cerebral autoregulation. In this setting, short-acting agents such as nitroprusside or nicardipine are preferable. For pregnant patients, hydralazine or methyldopa is suggested.

References: Calhoun DA, et al: Treatment of hypertensive crisis. N Engl J Med 323:1177–1183, 1990.

Reuler JB, et al: Hypertensive emergencies and urgencies: Definition, recognition, and management. J Gen Intern Med 3:64–74, 1988.

HYPERTRIGLYCERIDEMIA

Hypertriglyceridemia represents an important risk factor for atherosclerosis. Age-related increases in plasma TG occur, and these increases are concurrent with a rise in VLDL. It is also related to premature atherosclerosis in specific disorders. Patients with severely elevated VLDL who have a family history of familial combined hyperlipidemia are at the same increased risk as those affected members of families with increased LDL, but those who come from families with pure monogenic familial hypertriglyceridemia do not seem to have increased risk. Increased VLDL may, however, increase the risk of premature atherosclerosis when associated with other risk factors for CAD such as DM, smoking, HTN, and renal failure on dialysis. There appears to be a progressive decline with age in the correlation of hyperlipidemia with acute MI. Hyperlipidemia is a more significant risk factor below age 50 and operates independently of other risk factors. After age 65, there is no evidence of correlation between hyperlipidemia and atherosclerosis.

Screening for hyperlipidemia should be done once between ages 20 and 30, especially in those who have a family history of premature atherosclerosis. In adults younger than 55, a cholesterol >240 mg/dl or a TG >250 mg/dl indicates further attention. If a secondary cause, such as uncontrolled DM, hypothyroidism, uremia, hypoproteinemia, obstructive liver disease, or dysproteinemia is identified, it should be treated. Medical regimens should be examined for the use of drugs such as oral contraceptives, estrogens, glucocorticoids, and some antihypertensives. If none of these are present, then dietary or genetic factors are responsible. TG >500 mg/dl usually indicates a genetic disorder, and the presence of xanthomas are virtually diagnostic. First-degree relatives of such patients should also be given medical attention.

All patients should be given careful and thorough dietary counseling to attain normal weight and decrease intake of saturated fat and cholesterol. Abstinence from alcohol is advisable. The maximum effect of diet is seen approximately 2 months after body weight has plateaued. If TG remains above 300 mg/dl after diet, 2 months of clofibrate may be prescribed. This can be used in combination with cholestyramine if cholesterol is also elevated.

HYPOCALCEMIA

Regulation of the extracellular Ca^+ level in humans is controlled primarily by interactions of PTH and calcitonin (polypeptide hormones) and vitamin D (a sterol hormone) in various target organs. Secreted in response to a decrease in serum Ca^+ level, PTH acts both on bone to increase Ca^+ resorption and on the kidney to decrease Ca^+ excretion and increase inorganic PO_4^- excretion. With vitamin D as a cofactor, PTH also increases intestinal absorption of dietary Ca^+. There are two bioequivalent forms of vitamin D: vitamin D_3, which is generated in the skin through solar irradiation of 7-dehydrocholesterol, and vitamin D_2 which is absorbed from the jejunum by a process involving chylomicron formation. Active metabolites of vitamins D_2 and D_3 are generated in the liver and kidney, the most potent being $1,25(OH)_2$ vitamin D_3 (calcitriol).

True hypocalcemia must be confirmed by correction for the serum albumin level. For every reduction of 1 gm/dl serum albumin, the serum Ca^+ level is reduced by 0.8 mg/dl. Classic symptoms and physical findings with hypocalcemia include:

- Trousseau's sign—carpopedal spasm
- Chvostek's sign—facial muscle spasm following tapping of the facial nerve
- Circumoral tingling
- Mental irritability
- Seizures
- Prolongation of the QT interval on electrocardiogram
- Lenticular cataracts
- Papilledema

Transient hypocalcemia may occur in the setting of sepsis, extensive burns, or transfusion with multiple units of whole citrated blood. Short-lived hypocalcemia may also occur with the use of heparin, protamine, or glucagon. Metabolic or respiratory alkalosis lowers serum Ca^+ concentration, in contrast to acidosis.

Etiologies and Treatment of Hypocalcemia

PTH absent
A. Hereditary or acquired
- Laboratory : $\downarrow Ca^+$, $\uparrow PO_4^-$, undetectable to normal PTH
- Emergency treatment: 10% calcium gluconate 10–20 cc IV over 10–15 min followed by IV infusion of 10 cc calcium gluconate 10% in 500 cc D5W over 6 hr, increasing by 5 cc every 6 hr to maintain serum Ca^+ in 7.5–9.0 mg/dl range
- Chronic treatment: 500–1,000 mg elemental Ca^+ PO BID or TID plus vit D_2 beginning with 8,000 U daily and increasing as needed to 50,000–100,000 U daily, or shorter-acting agent such as calcitriol $(1,25(OH)_2\ D_3)$ 0.25 μg PO daily (more expensive but less likely to cause prolonged vit D toxicity). Monitor serum Ca^+ levels monthly. Restrict PO_4^- with AlOH gel. Measure 24-hr urinary Ca^+ when serum Ca^+ level normalized, because hypercalciuria secondary to low or absent PTH levels may result in renal stones.
B. Hypomagnesemia
- Laboratory: $\downarrow Ca^+$, $\downarrow PO_4^-$, undetectable to normal PTH
- Emergency: 1–2 gm $MgSO_4$ (10% solution) IV over 15 min followed by 1 gm IM Q 4–6 hr as indicated by serum Mg^+ level (withhold if patellar reflexes absent).
- Chronic: Mg^{++} oxide tablets 600 mg, 1 or 2 tabs PO daily (diarrhea troublesome side effect)
PTH ineffective
A. Chronic renal failure
- Laboratory: $\downarrow Ca^+$, $\uparrow PO_4^-$, $\uparrow$ PTH, $\downarrow 1,25(OH)_2D$
- Treatment: Restrict dietary PO_4^-. AlOH antacids for PO_4^- binding. Elemental Ca^+ 1–3 gm PO daily. Calcitriol 0.25–1.0 μg daily.
B. Deficiency of active vit D ($\downarrow$ dietary intake or sunlight)
- Laboratory: $\downarrow Ca^+$, $\downarrow PO_4^-$, $\uparrow$ PTH, $\downarrow 1,25(OH)_2D$
- Treatment: Vit D 1,000–2,000 IU daily for several months, followed by 200–400 IU daily. Oral Ca^+ 1–3 gm daily.

Table continued on next page.

Etiologies and Treatment of Hypocalcemia (Cont.)

C. Defective metabolism
  1. Anticonvulsant therapy (phenytoin or phenobarbital)
    —Treatment: Change to alternative anticonvulsant, if possible, or vit D 2,000–4,000 IU daily plus 1–3 gm Ca^+ daily for several months, then changing to 50,000 IU vit D monthly.
  2. Vit D–dependent rickets, type I (relative end-organ resistance to vit D)
    —Treatment: Physiologic amounts of calcitriol
D. Vit D ineffective
  1. Intestinal malabsorption
    —Laboratory: $\downarrow Ca^+$, $\downarrow PO_4^-$, $\uparrow$ PTH, $\downarrow$ 1,25$(OH)_2$D
    —Treatment: Vit D 50,000–100,000 IU PO daily or vit D_2 in sesame oil 500,000 units IM every few months
  2. Vit D–dependent rickets, type II
    —Treatment: Same as type 1, but higher doses of vit D may be required.

Pseudohypoparathyroidism
  (Hereditary, with end-organ PTH resistance, plus skeletal and developmental defects)
  • Laboratory: $\downarrow Ca^+$ (most patients), $\uparrow PO_4^-$, $\uparrow$ PTH
  • Treatment: Same as hypoparathyroidism

PTH overwhelmed
A. Severe acute hyperphosphatemia (tumor lysis, acute renal failure, rhabdomyolysis)
  • Treatment: PO_4^-–binding antacids or dialysis; parenteral or oral Ca^+ replacement only if hypocalcemia severe and symptomatic. May lead to rebound hypercalcemia in recovery phase due to release of IM Ca^+ deposits.
B. Acute pancreatitis
C. Osteitis fibrosa (secondary to high bone cellularity after prolonged hyperparathyroidism, with severe hypocalcemia after parathyroidectomy)

Adapted from Potts JT: Diseases of the parathyroid gland and other hyper- and hypocalcemic disorders. In Wilson JD, et al (eds): Harrison's Principles of Internal Medicine, 12th ed. New York, McGraw-Hill, 1991, p 1915.

HYPOGLYCEMIA

Clinical hypoglycemia is defined as the documentation of a low plasma glucose concentration associated with symptoms and relief of symptoms by correction of the low blood sugar (Whipple's triad). In addition, the symptoms tend to be the same, to be repetitive, and to correlate very well with either fasting or food intake. *Fasting hypoglycemia* should be differentiated from *reactive* or *postprandial hypoglycemia* (which occurs following a glucose load or a meal). Whereas fasting hypoglycemia is often a manifestation of a major health problem that requires recognition and management, reactive or postprandial hypoglycemia is often secondary to a less severe condition. When hypoglycemia develops rapidly, often adrenergic symptoms predominate as follows:

nervousness	pallor	hunger
tremulousness	nausea	angina
sweating	flushing	anxiety
palpitations		

When hypoglycemia is severe enough, regardless of the rate of decrease of blood sugar, neuroglycopenic symptoms are usually the most predominant. The lower the blood sugar, the more severe are the neuroglycopenic manifestations:

headaches	difficulty awakening in the morning
blurred vision	senile dementia
paresthesia	organic personality syndrome
weakness	transient hemiplegia
tiredness	transient aphasia
confusion	seizures
dizziness	coma
amnesia	abnormal mentation
incoordination	behavioral changes

Causes of Fasting Hypoglycemia

1. Drugs
   a. Insulin (surreptitious use or overdose)
   b. Oral hypoglycemic agents: Consider drug interactions. Renal or hepatic failure are often predisposing factors.
   c. Salicylates, especially in children
   d. Ethanol (poststarvation)
   e. Beta-blockers impair recognition and recovery from hypoglycemia.
   f. Miscellaneous medications: Acetaminophen, disopyramide, pentamidine, propoxyphene, sulfa drugs
2. Endocrinopathies: Adrenal insufficiency, hypopituitarism (i.e., cortisol and growth hormone deficiency)
3. Liver diseases: Particularly hepatic failure due to acute fulminant hepatitis, secondary to CHF or cirrhosis
4. Chronic renal failure: Spontaneous hypoglycemia of uremia; consider drugs and malnutrition as potentiating mechanisms.
5. Insulinoma: Islet cell tumors, nesidioblastosis
6. Non–islet cell tumors: Due to secretion of insulin-like factors. Most common tumors are mesenchymal tumors, hepatomas, adrenocortical tumors, GI tumors, lymphomas, and leukemias; in leukemias, be aware of factitious hypoglycemia due to increased intracellular consumption of glucose by very high WBC count.
7. Autoimmune mechanisms: Presence of anti-insulin antibodies or insulin receptor antibodies.

Causes of Postprandial or Reactive Hypoglycemia

1. Alimentary hypoglycemia: Mostly in patients with history of gastric surgery; due to abnormally fast glucose absorption, which leads to hypersecretion of insulin; hypoglycemia occurs usually 1 hr after ingestion of the glucose load; symptoms of alimentary hypoglycemia may be severe; best managed with frequent, small meals.
2. Early DM: Controversial
3. Idiopathic reactive hypoglycemia: Symptoms seem to correlate better with the rapidity of fall of blood sugar rather than the absolute value of blood glucose; most

patients, however, turn out to have the "nondisease of nonhypoglycemia"; (no clear correlation between symptoms and plasma glucose levels).

4. Reactive clinical hypoglycemia may also occur as a result of hyperinsulinism due to an islet cell tumor or other endocrinopathies, such as adrenal insufficiency.

Evaluation

Fasting Hypoglycemia

After exclusion of obvious causes of fasting hypoglycemia (e.g., renal failure, hepatic disease, drugs, endocrinopathies), often the workup of fasting hypoglycemia is directed at confirming or excluding hyperinsulinism and, particularly, an insulinoma.

1. **Fasting insulin and glucose levels:** The patient should be evaluated in the hospital with a prolonged fast up to 72 hrs with frequent blood sugar measurement. When hypoglycemia occurs, plasma insulin, C peptide, cortisol, and growth hormone should be obtained. Nearly 60% of patients develop hypoglycemia within the first 24 hrs, up to 85% within 48 hrs, and up to 97 to 98% within 72 hours of fast. If hypoglycemia cannot be elicited by the fast test, dynamic studies should be performed. During prolonged fast, women, but not men, tend to decrease plasma glucose levels <60 mg/dl without significance. A high level of insulin during the fast in relationship to plasma glucose is virtually diagnostic of hyperinsulinism. Evidence of hyperinsulinism is provided by an insulin-glucose ratio higher than 0.3. A more discriminative ratio is the amended ratio of Turner (insulin × 100 ÷ glucose − 30). A ratio higher than 150% is clear-cut evidence of hyperinsulinism, and a ratio less than 50% basically excludes hyperinsulinism. Some obese patients with insulin resistance may have a ratio ranging between 50% and 150%.

2. **Proinsulin levels:** Proinsulin–insulin ratios are elevated in insulinomas (>30%).

3. **Dynamic tests:**

   a. Measurement of C peptide after insulin-induced hypoglycemia.

   b. Tolbutamide test should be done only in difficult cases, when previous maneuvers have failed to confirm the diagnosis of insulinoma with 100% certainty.

Differential Diagnosis of Hyperinsulinism

1. Insulinoma
2. Accidental or surreptitious administration of insulin (high total and free insulin; low C peptide)
3. Overdose with sulphonylureas (high total and free insulin levels, high C peptide)
4. Antiinsulin-antibody–mediated hypoglycemia (high insulin antibody titers, free insulin and C peptide levels)
5. Insulin-receptor-antibody–mediated hypoglycemia (high total free insulin levels and C peptide levels; presence in the serum of high titers of insulin receptor antibodies)

Thinking through these additional possible causes of hyperinsulinism may prevent an unnecessary surgery in a patient with hyperinsulinism due to causes other than insulinoma.

Imaging for insulinoma: The best procedure for visualization of a pancreatic islet cell tumor is the selective celiac arteriography, which can localize the tumor 80 to 90% of the time. Abdominal CT scan and ultrasound visualize a tumor in <50% of cases, and therefore their use has not been widely advocated. The percutaneous transhepatic route for selective sampling of the pancreatic venous drainage may help localize the tumor. About 90% of such tumors are benign, and therapy should consist of surgical removal of the tumor. The tumor is often difficult to find, particularly when it is located in the head of the pancreas.

Medical therapy:
1. In preparation for surgery
2. In malignant tumors
3. In patients in whom the tumor could not be located

Drugs:
1. Diazoxide
2. Phenytoin
3. Propranolol
4. Streptozocin
5. Fluorouracil

Reactive Hypoglycemia

The evaluation should include an oral glucose tolerance test, but clinicians should keep in mind that the glucose load is larger than that of a typical meal. Prior to the oral glucose tolerance test, the patient should be receiving a normal, adequate glucose intake for at least the preceding 3 days. Low blood sugar occurring 2 to 3 hrs after a meal occurs in nearly 10% of healthy adults.

HYPOKALEMIA

Diagnosis

Hypokalemia is said to exist when the serum K^+ level is below 3.5 mEq/L. The serum K^+ concentration is a general indicator of total body K^+. However, because only about 2% of total body K^+ exists in the ECF and 98% is in the cells, small changes in cellular K^+ can cause major changes in serum K^+.

The etiologies and diagnostic approaches to patients with hypokalemia are shown in the following figures. Hypokalemia results in clinical symptoms at levels below 2.5 mEq/L.

Clinical Manifestations of Hypokalemia

Cardiac
Predisposition to digoxin toxicity
Ventricular irritability
Abnormal ECG
T-wave flattening
U waves
ST segment depression
Cardiac necrosis

Renal
Polyuria (nephrogenic DI)
Polydipsia

Neuromuscular
Skeletal: weakness, cramps, tetany, paralysis, rhabdomyolysis
GI: constipation, ileus
Encephalopathy (liver disease)

Endocrine/metabolic
Carbohydrate intolerance
Decreased aldosterone levels

Diagnostic Approach to Hypokalemia in the Normotensive or Hypotensive Patient

Hypokalemia

- Artifactual
- Potassium depletion
  - **Extrarenal K losses**
    Urine K <20 mEg/day
    - Blood pH
      - Normal
        - Inadequate intake
        - Increased sweat loss
      - Metabolic acidosis
        - Diarrhea disorders
        - GI fistulas
        - Fasting/starvation
      - Variable
        - Villous adenoma
        - Laxative abuse
  - **Renal K losses**
    Urine K >20 mEg/day
    Normal/low blood pressure
    - Blood pH
      - Acidosis
        - Renal tubular acidosis
        - Carbonic anhydrase inhibitor
        - Diabetic ketoacidosis
        - Ureterosigmoidostomy
      - Alkalosis or normal
        - Urine chloride
          - Low
            (Cl < 10 mEq/day)
            - Vomiting
            - Nasogastric drainage
            - Diuretics
            - Posthypercapneic
          - High
            (Cl > 10 mEq/day)
            - Bartter's syndrome
            - Diuretics
            - Severe K depletion
            - Magnesium depletion
- Redistribution

Diagnostic Approach to Hypokalemia in the Hypertensive Patient

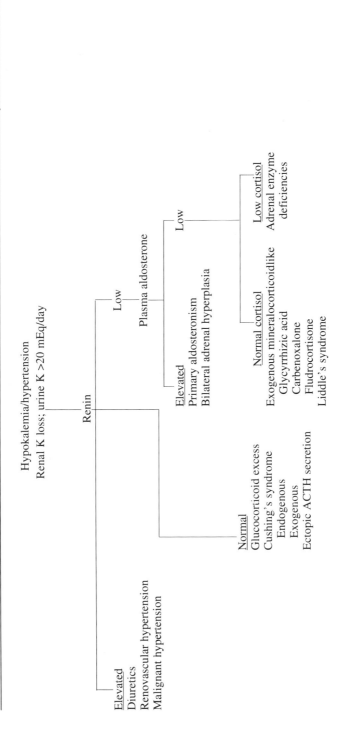

From Stephanz GB Jr, et al: Potassium disorders. In Tisher CC, et al (eds): Nephrology for the Houseofficer. Baltimore, Williams & Wilkins, 1989, pp 69–70, with permission.

Management

The first step is to ascertain whether hypokalemia is artifactual, redistributional, or real (depletional). Artifactual values are seen in leukemic patients with WBC counts over 100,000. Serum and urinary electrolytes, CBC, blood pH, serum renin, aldosterone, cortisol, and Mg levels are the laboratory tests often required in an investigation for hypokalemia.

Although serum K^+ cannot be taken as an index of total body K^+ stores, a few general guidelines can be applied to the correction of hypokalemia: A decrease of serum K^+ of 0.27 mEq/L (below 4 mEq/L) is approximately equal to 100 mEq/L of K^+ deficit. Therefore a serum K^+ level of 3 mEq/L reflects approximately 300 mEq/L of K^+ deficit, and serum K^+ of <2 mEq/L reflects deficits over 1,000 mEq/L. IV K^+ replacement should be used for patients with severe and dangerous hypokalemic situations such as neuroparalysis and digitalis toxicity. It should be noted that initially, K^+ replacement should be made in glucose-free solutions, for glucose can cause K^+ levels to drop. In less severe situations, oral therapy is preferred in supplements of 20 to 120 mEq/L per day. KCl is appropriate when there is concomitant Cl^- depletion. Oral tablets are often associated with GI ulceration. In general, K^+ can be given IV in rates up to 10 mEq/hr through a peripheral vein, but when K^+ has to be infused at higher rates, it should be done through a central vein with ECG monitoring. Doses of 40 mEq/hr can then be given. The best guide to replacement remains frequent serum K^+ measurements. It should be remembered that overzealous K^+ replacement can result in hyperkalemia and that concomitant hypomagnesemia renders correction of hypokalemia difficult.

Etiologies

Hypokalemia exists when the serum potassium concentration is less than 3.5 mEq/L. Hypokalemia may result from diminution in both intracellular and extracellular potassium or from a shift of potassium from the extracellular to the intracellular compartment. Hypokalemia results in muscular weakness, diminished deep tendon reflexes, decreased bowel sounds progressive to ileus, and ECG changes such as decreased T-wave voltage, depression of the ST segment, and increased prominence of U waves.

Causes of Hypokalemia

Shift of potassium to the intracellular compartment
Acute alkalosis
Following correction of metabolic acidosis (e.g., diabetic acidosis)
Hypokalemic periodic paralysis
Insulin administration
Administration of beta-2-agonists
Conditions of catecholamine excess
   Cardiac surgery
   Myocardial infarction
   Delirium tremens
Barbiturate intoxication
Vitamin B_{12} therapy
Thyrotoxicosis (rare)

Table continued on next page.

Causes of Hyperkalemia (Cont.)

Inadequate potassium intake (uncommon because of
renal conservation of potassium)
Starvation
Postoperative state without replenishment

Gastrointestinal potassium loss
Diarrhea
Laxative abuse
Villous adenoma of rectum
Vomiting
Fistulas

Renal potassium loss (renal cause of hypokalemia should be sought
if the urinary loss of potassium exceeds 20 mEq/day)
Osmotic diuresis
Magnesium depletion
Acute leukemia
Antimicrobial agents (such as carbenicillin, gentamicin, amphotericin B)
Cisplatin administration
Renal conditions with metabolic acidosis
Distal renal tubular acidosis
Proximal renal tubular acidosis
Ureterosigmoidostomy
Administration of acetazolamide
Conditions with metabolic alkalosis
Cushing's syndrome
Exogenous corticosteroid administration
Primary aldosteronism
Licorice usage
Renovascular hypertension
Malignant hypertension
Renin-producing renal tumor
Diuretics (thiazides, furosemide)
Liddle's syndrome
Bartter's syndrome

HYPOMAGNESEMIA

Low serum Mg^{++} is very common in the elderly and is often caused by poor oral intake or the high frequency of diuretic use. Mg^{++} plays a key role in antagonizing the effects of Ca^{++} in the cardiovascular and nervous systems and is essential for the function of many enzymes. Evaluation should proceed with a 24-hr urine collection for Mg^{++}. If, despite hypomagnesemia, urinary excretion of Mg^{++} is high (>2 mmol/day), urinary Mg^{++} wasting may be implicated. If low (<0.5 mm/day), then low Mg^{++} intake may be implicated.

Manifestations of Hypomagnesemia

- Cardiovascular: refractory dysrhythmias, hypotension or hypertension, increased sensitivity to digoxin effects
- Neuromuscular: tetany, weakness, tremor, spasticity
- CNS: agitation, delirium, seizures, depression
- Metabolic: hypokalemia (renal K^+ wasting), hypocalcemia

Hard water has more Mg^{++}, and the drinking of hard water is associated with less cardiovascular disease and less sudden death. Thiazides may cause more wasting of Mg^{++} than loop diuretics do. Cisplatinum and aminoglycosides produce hypermagnesiuria leading to low serum Mg^{++}.

Treatment: Potassium-sparing diuretics also spare Mg^{++}. Oral repletion with Mg^{++} oxide is better absorbed than are the Mg^{++}-containing antacid preparations, but diarrhea is common. Parenteral replacement with Mg^{++} sulfate or chloride is reserved for those who are symptomatic or have serum Mg^{++} ≤ 0.5 mmol/L. The initial dose should be 600 to 900 mg of elemental Mg^{++} over 3 hr. For refractory ventricular arrhythmias, it can be given over 20 min. Some authors have recommended up to 2 gm of $MgSO_4$ over 1 min followed by 5 gm over the next 6 hr for torsades de pointes or digoxin-induced arrhythmias.

Salem M, et al: Hypomagnesemia in critical illness. Crit Care Clin 7:225–252, 1991.

HYPONATREMIA

Hyponatremia is defined as a serum Na^+ level of <135 mEq/L. It is the commonest electrolyte disorder and occurs in about 2.5% of hospitalized patients. Total body Na^+ content is dependent on the balance between Na^+ intake and Na^+ excretion. Normally, this does not vary by more than 2 to 5%, and serum Na^+ is normally held in the normal range despite wide fluctuations in Na^+ intake thanks to the ability of the kidneys to modify renal Na^+ excretion over a wide range.

The principal determinant of serum Na^+ level is total body water rather than total body Na^+. Alterations in total body Na^+ alter the ECF volume rather than the serum Na^+ concentration, and changes in serum Na^+ usually reflect changes in total body water. An increase in plasma osmolarity by 2% usually stimulates ADH secretion, and a decrease in the ECF volume by 10% also stimulates ADH secretion. Often, volume-mediated changes in ADH secretion override the osmotic regulation of ADH.

Classification and differential diagnosis: Hyponatremia is classified into three types depending on serum osmolality: isosmolar, hyperosmolar, and hyposmolar hyponatremia.

Pseudohyponatremia results from accumulation of large quantities of glucose or

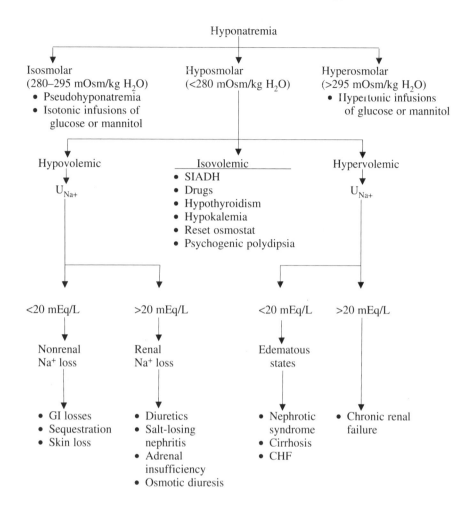

protein, which displace a fraction of the salt-containing water from plasma and replace it with salt-free solids. The osmolality remains normal because each liter of plasma has a smaller Na^+ and water portion but the concentration of salt in the water portion is normal. In hyperglycemia, osmotic withdrawal of water from the cells decreases the plasma Na^+. For every 100 mg/dl increase in serum glucose concentration, serum Na^+ concentration decreases by 0.6 mEq/l.

Hyposmolar hyponatremia can be associated with hypovolemia, isovolemia, or hypervolemia. Hypovolemic hyponatremia can be differentiated into renal and nonrenal conditions depending on the urinary Na^+ excretion. Diuretic administration is the most frequent cause of hypovolemic hyponatremia. Thiazide diuretics inhibit urinary dilution, but unlike loop diuretics, they do not inhibit urinary concentration and hence cause more severe hyponatremia. Salt-losing renal conditions such as polycystic kidney disease, pyelonephritis, and other interstitial diseases are associated with hyponatremia. Euvolemic hyponatremia is often due to SIADH and is discussed elsewhere. Hypervolemic hypernatremia is often due to expansion of ECF and edematous states. In chronic renal failure, hyponatremia results from decreased GFR, which diminishes the delivery of solute to the distal diluting segment.

Clinical features: Most patients with hyponatremia are asymptomatic. The severity of the symptoms depends on the degree and the rate of development of hyponatremia. Early symptoms are GI (nausea and vomiting) but soon are replaced by neurological features (agitation, lethargy, hyperreflexia, seizures, and coma). Severe symptoms are associated with serum Na^+ levels <120 mEq/L.

Treatment: Treatment of euvolemic hyponatremia is discussed elsewhere (see SIADH). Hypovolemic hyponatremia requires correction of the underlying etiologic factors such as discontinuation of diuretics and specific treatment for GI fluid losses. Volume reexpansion with NS is necessary to correct the Na^+ deficit. The Na^+ deficit is calculated by subtracting current total body Na^+ (current TBW $\times$ current serum Na^+) from normal total body Na^+ (normal TBW $\times$ normal serum Na^+). One third of this deficit is replaced in the first 6 hrs and the rest in 24 to 48 hrs. Concomitant K^+ deficit should also be replaced.

Hypervolemic hyponatremia is treated by salt and water restriction. Severe symptomatic hyponatremia needs careful correction in the intensive care unit. Salt and water diuresis is initiated with furosemide (1.0 mg/kg body weight), and urinary Na^+ and K^+ losses are replaced hourly with 3% NS and KCl until the serum Na^+ level is approximately 125 mEq/L. Sodium should be corrected no faster than 1.5 to 2.0 mEq/L/hr and not more than 25 mEq/L over the first 48 hrs. Overzealous correction can result in a neurological complication termed central pontine myelinosis (CPM). Patients with liver disease and hypoxia are more likely to develop CPM.

Reference: Anderson RJ: Hospital associated hyponatremia. Kidney Int 29:1237–1247, 1986.

HYPOPHOSPHATEMIA

The serum phosphorus concentration in adults varies between 2.5 and 4.5 mg/dl. Values are somewhat higher in children, presumably because of the need for phosphorus in growth.

Causes of Hypophosphatemia

1. Hyperparathyroidism: Serum calcium and alkaline phosphatase values are elevated while serum phosphorus is mildly to moderately decreased due to renal loss.
2. Vitamin D deficiency: Patients develop rickets or osteomalacia.
3. Familial hypophosphatemic, vitamin-D-resistant rickets
4. Fanconi syndrome: Impaired renal proximal tubular function results in excessive phosphaturia, glycosuria, excessive aminoaciduria, hyperuricosuria, and metabolic acidosis.
5. Hypomagnesemia: Excessive loss of phosphorus through the renal tubules.
6. Increased carbohydrate metabolism
7. Recovery phase of DKA: Osmotic renal loss of phosphorus followed by shift of phosphorus to intracellular compartment during treatment with insulin; severe hypophosphatemia (i.e., serum phosphorus <1.0 mg/dl) may be encountered.
8. Extracellular fluid expansion: Mild hypophosphatemia due to decreased renal tubular reabsorption of phosphate
9. Acute respiratory or metabolic alkalosis
10. Hemodialysis: Insufficient phosphate in the dialysis solution.
11. Hyperalimentation: Excessive phosphate utilization in restoring good nutritional state.

Table continued on next page.

Causes of Hypophosphatemia (Cont.)

12. Recovery phase from malnutrition: Severe hypophosphatemia may occur as patient's nutritional state is restored.
13. Phosphate-binding antacids: Prevent absorption of dietary phosphate (e.g., aluminum hydroxide).
14. Alcohol withdrawal: Hypophosphatemia may be severe in alcoholic patients during withdrawal (with values of the serum phosphorus <1.0 mg/dL); reasons for phosphate depletion are poor dietary intake, diarrhea, magnesium deficiency, and excessive loss of phosphate in the urine.

Consequences of Phosphate Depletion

1. Erythrocyte abnormalities
   a. Depletion of 2,3-DPG in RBCs, thereby increasing affinity of hemoglobin for oxygen and decreasing oxygen delivery to the tissues
   b. Depletion of erythrocyte ATP such that at serum phosphorus levels <0.5 mg/dL, hemolysis may occur because of lack of energy to maintain the red cell membrane
2. Platelet dysfunction: Depletion of ADP and ATP in platelets
3. Leukocyte dysfunction: Low content of ATP in leukocytes impairs chemotaxis and phagocytosis
4. Muscle weakness
5. Rhabdomyolysis: With severe hypophosphatemia, deficiency of muscle ATP results in rhabdomyolysis
6. CHF: A cardiomyopathy related to phosphate depletion
7. Neurologic dysfunction
   a. Peripheral neuropathy
   b. Metabolic encephalopathy

HYPOXEMIA

Hypoxemia is defined as deficient oxygenation of the blood. The five basic pathophysiologic mechanisms that can cause hypoxemia are:

1. Decreased inspired oxygen (P_IO_2)
2. Hypoventilation
3. Diffusion abnormality
4. Ventilation/perfusion (V/Q) abnormality—mismatching of ventilation and perfusion—the most common cause of hypoxemia
5. Shunt—perfusion of nonventilated alveoli

Differentiation of the Causes of Hypoxemia

MECHANISM	P_aO_2	P_aCO_2	A-aO$_2$ GRADIENT	RESPONSE TO 100% O$_2$
↓ P_IO_2	↓	→ or ↓	→	N/A
Hypoventilation	↓	↑	→	N/A
Diffusion abnormality	↓	→ or ↓	↑	Yes
V/Q mismatch	↓	→ or ↓	↑	Yes
Shunt	↓	→ or ↓	↑	No

From Goodnight-White S, et al: Pulmonary secrets. In Zollo AJ (ed): Medical Secrets. Philadelphia, Hanley & Belfus, 1991, p 302, with permission.

Treatment of Hypoxemia

MECHANISM	EXAMPLES	TREATMENT
Hypoventilation (normal A–a gradient)	Overdose (opioid, phenobarbitol), neuromuscular disease (myasthenia gravis, Guillain-Barré)	Increase ventilation (will also benefit from supplemental oxygen)
V/Q mismatch (increased A–a gradient)	Pneumonia, asthma, COPD, CHF	Supplemental oxygen
Shunt (increased A–a gradient)	ARDS (noncardiac pulmonary edema), cardiac pulmonary edema, atelectasis	Treat underlying abnormality, administer PEEP
Diffusion block (increased A–a gradient)	Interstitial fibrosis	Supplemental oxygen
Decreased F_IO_2/P_IO_2 (normal A–a gradient)	Improper gas mixture/altitude	Supplemental oxygen

Alveolar-arterial oxygenation gradient ($P_{(A-a)}O_2$): The $P_{(A-a)}O_2$ can be useful in differentiating the causes of hypoxemia as previously noted. However, it is used primarily as a mechanism to objectively quantitate the degree of derangement in oxygenation. The $P_{(A-a)}O_2$ is the difference between the PO_2 in the alveolar air (P_AO_2) and the oxygen in arterial blood (P_aO_2): $A–aO_2 = P_AO_2 – P_aO_2$. The $P_{(A-a)}O_2$ is normally 10 to 15 mm Hg and increases gradually with age (age $\times$ 0.04).

$$P_AO_2 = P_IO_2 – (P_aCO_2/RQ)$$

P_aCO_2 measured by ABG
RQ (respiratory quotient) assumed to be 0.8

where P_IO_2 (inspired O_2) = F_IO_2 ($P_{atm} – P_{H2O}$)

F_IO_2 is the fraction of inspired O_2(21% room air)
P_{atm} is atmospheric pressure (760 at sea level)
P_{H2O} is vapor pressure of H_2O (assumed 47 mm Hg)

Therefore, on room air, at sea level, with a P_aCO_2 of 40 mm Hg:

$$P_IO_2 = 0.21 (760 – 47) – 40/0.8$$
$$150 – 50 = 100$$

The $P_{(A-a)}O_2$ would be $100 – P_aO_2$ (measured by ABG).

Criteria for O_2 therapy: In acute hypoxemia, the goal of O_2 therapy is to raise the P_aO_2 so that it is no longer on the steep portion of the oxyhemoglobin dissociation curve. The following table demonstrates various oxygen delivery systems available for use in the patient with acute hypoxemia.

Which Oxygen Delivery System Should You Use?

SYSTEM	FEATURES
Nasal prongs	Depends on respiratory frequency and depth of respiration F_1O_2 is about $20 + 4 \times$ oxygen flow in L/min Oxygen flow is 1–6 L/min Delivers a low F_1O_2 when precise concentration is unimportant Patient can converse and eat normally
Standard (non-Venturi) mask	Delivers an F_1O_2 of 35%, depending on oxygen flow (6–10 L/min) and patient's minute ventilation Delivers an intermediate F_1O_2 when precise concentration is unimportant Produces discomfort and restrictions on eating
Partial rebreathing reservoir mask	Delivers a high F_1O_2 of 40%–90% High oxygen flow (8–15 L/min) flushes the reservoir bag to maintain high oxygen concentration and to avoid CO_2 buildup
Nonbreathing reservoir mask	Delivers an F_1O_2 of about 90% High oxygen flow (8–10 L/min) fills reservoir bag to give inspiration, through a one-way valve, of mostly oxygen
Venturi mask	Delivers a specific low F_1O_2 to the oxygen-sensitive patient Specific masks are used, depending on the pairing of concentration and flow, as follows: F_1O_2 — Flow 24% — 2 L/min 28% — 4 L/min 31% — 6 L/min 35% — 8 L/min 40% — 10 L/min Fixed oxygen flow pulls air into the mask to deliver specific F_1O_2 and to wash out CO_2 produced by patient Inhalation of a constant F_1O_2 regardless of respiratory rate or depth of respiration Uncomfortable for prolonged use; eating is affected Does not provide proper humidification

From Carlton TJ, et al: A guide for judicious use of oxygen in critical illness. J Crit Care 7:1744–1761, 1992, with permission.

Criteria for continuous low-flow O_2 therapy: The role of continuous low-flow O_2 therapy was largely established by the Nocturnal Oxygen Therapy trial in the United States and the Medical Research Council in Great Britain. This therapy is indicated for any of the following conditions:

1. A patient at rest and on an optimal medical regimen, whose P_aO_2 is <55 mm Hg
2. A patient at rest and on an optimal medical regimen, whose P_aO_2 is >55 mm Hg and <60 mm Hg, if there is evidence of hypoxic end-organ damage manifested by one or more of the following:
   cor pulmonale
   secondary pulmonary hypertension
   secondary erythrocytosis
   impaired mentation

3. A patient whose P_aO_2 drops below 55 mm Hg on exercise and who has evidence of significant improvement in one or both of the following:
   exercise duration
   exercise performance
4. A patient whose P_aO_2 falls below 55 mm Hg during sleep and who has evidence of one or more of the following:
   hypoxic organ dysfunction
   disturbed sleep pattern
   significant cardiac dysrhythmia

References: Nocturnal Therapy Trial Group: Continuous or nocturnal oxygen therapy in hypoxemic chronic obstructive lung disease. Ann Intern Med 93:391–398, 1980.

Medical Research Council Working Party: Long term domiciliary oxygen therapy in hypoxemic cor pulmonale complicating chronic bronchitis and emphysema. Lancet 681–686, 1981.

I

IDIOPATHIC (IMMUNE) THROMBOCYTOPENIC PURPURA

ITP, an autoimmune disorder, results in the production of antibodies that react with major platelet glycoproteins IIb/IIIa and Ib. Platelet destruction occurs via macrophage recognition of the bound antibody and phagocytosis in the spleen and other reticuloendothelial tissues. Thrombocytopenia, even when compensated by an increased marrow production of megakaryocytes, may be severe and life threatening. Patients present with purpura, petechiae, bleeding oral ulcers, hematuria, or GI hemorrhage. Intracranial hemorrhage, the dreaded complication of ITP, is relatively uncommon. However, treatment is aimed at avoiding all significant bleeding. In the past, ITP—like other autoimmune disorders—was more frequently observed in young women but is now increasingly seen in both young men and women in association with HIV infection or IV cocaine use.

A thorough Hx & PE of the thrombocytopenic patient is imperative because of the variety of disorders associated with immune destruction of platelets. As previously noted, the sexual history should be taken, and high-risk behaviors for HIV should be discovered. A careful review of the patient's prescription and over-the-counter drug use is important. Quinine is a cause of ITP that may be overlooked if the physician forgets to ask for details about a patient's drinking habits. Quinine, present in tonic or taken as a relief for leg cramps, has been recognized as a cause of ITP and more recently as a cause of hemolytic uremic syndrome. Lymphoproliferative disorders such as Hodgkin's disease, non-Hodgkin's lymphoma, and CLL are also associated with thrombocytopenia. Collagen vascular diseases such as lupus may have mild thrombocytopenia (sometimes in association with a lupus anticoagulant) or full-blown ITP. Other disorders such as Graves' disease and myasthenia gravis also may be associated with thrombocytopenia. In addition, infections are associated with significant thrombocytopenia. DIC usually causes a low platelet count, as does thrombotic thrombocytopenic purpura (TTP).

In the physical exam, careful attention should be paid to the presence of lymphadenopathy or splenomegaly. Such findings suggest the presence of a lymphoproliferative disorder or chronic infection such as brucella or TB. In the initial laboratory evaluation, it is important that the practitioner personally review the peripheral blood film to look for fragmentation of RBCs (DIC or TTP) and to evaluate platelet morphology and numbers. In ITP, platelet destruction results in a population of young, large platelets. Patients who have a low platelet count but no clinical bleeding may have spurious thrombocytopenia caused by agglutination of platelets in the presence of EDTA. Clumps of platelets are found on the peripheral blood film and a normal count is obtained when blood is anticoagulated with citrate.

Hematologists are occasionally referred patients who seem to have mild thrombocytopenia with a family history of thrombocytopenia. If large platelets are seen along with obvious Döhle bodies in the granulocytes, then May-Hegglin syndrome may be present. This disorder seldom results in clinical bleeding, but its recognition helps to avoid unnecessary bone marrow examination or splenectomy.

Treatment of patients with a platelet count less than 20,000 and bleeding should begin by observation in the hospital while prednisone (1.0 mg/kg) is begun. Platelet transfusions are not useful because they are rapidly consumed and so are used only in desperate situations. Patients who are either refractory to steroids, who relapse once off steroids, or who develop complications of steroid treatment (hyperglycemia, HTN) should be considered for splenectomy. Prior to splenectomy, immunization against pneumococcal infection by means of a polyvalent vaccine should be given. Infusion of IV gamma globulin can result in dramatic but transient (2–3 weeks) improvement of the platelet count. This treatment is costly and is usually given either when a procedure is necessary or prior to splenectomy. Some patients who are refractory to steroids, splenectomy, or other forms of treatment are managed with IV gamma globulin chronically. Danazol has been found to be effective in patients who have been splenectomized. It is frequently used before splenectomy when delay or avoidance of splenectomy is desirable.

Patients who have HIV infection present with ITP early in the course of their illness. These patients respond to steroids and splenectomy in the same way that non-HIV-infected patients do. To date there has been no evidence for acceleration of the progression to AIDS by either brief treatment with corticosteroids or splenectomy. Still, there are reports of successful alternative therapies for ITP in HIV infection. These include low-dose corticosteroids, splenic irradiation, and administration of Rh antibody to Rh(+) individuals. The management of ITP during pregnancy is a complex issue, and the reader is referred to an excellent recent review.

References: Karpatkin S: Autoimmune thrombocytopenic purpura. Semin Hematol 22:260–288, 1985.

McCrae KR, et al: Pregnancy-associated thrombocytopenia: Pathogenesis and management. Blood 80:2697–2714, 1992.

IMMUNIZATIONS IN THE ADULT

Immunizations Recommended for Adults 18 Years of Age and Older

IMMUNOBIOLOGIC	MAJOR INDICATIONS	DOSE SCHEDULE	MAJOR PRECAUTIONS
Influenza vaccine	Adults with high-risk conditions, residents of nursing homes or other chronic care facilities, medical care personnel, healthy persons aged 65 or older	Annual vaccination with current vaccine; either whole- or split-virus vaccine may be used IM	History of anaphylactic hypersensitivity to egg ingestion
Pneumococcal polysaccharide vaccine (23-valent)	Adults at increased risk of pneumococcal disease and its complications because of underlying health conditions; healthy older adults, especially those 65 or older	One 0.5-ml dose IM or SC	Vaccine safety in pregnant women has not been evaluated; revaccination may be recommended for some high-risk persons

Table continued on next page.

Immunizations Recommended for Adults 18 Years of Age and Older (Cont.)

IMMUNOBIOLOGIC	MAJOR INDICATIONS	DOSE SCHEDULE	MAJOR PRECAUTIONS
Hepatitis B vaccine	Adults who are at increased risk of occupational, environmental, social, or familial exposure to hepatitis B; certain travelers to foreign countries	Two 1-ml doses IM 4 weeks apart; 3rd dose 5 months after 2nd; booster doses not routinely recommended	Pregnancy should not be considered contraindication if woman is otherwise eligible
Tetanus-diphtheria toxoid (Td)	All adults at mid-decade ages; susceptible travelers to foreign countries	Two 0.5-ml doses IM 4 weeks apart; 3rd dose 6–12 months after 2nd; 0.5-ml booster every 10 years	History of neurologic or hypersensitivity reaction following previous dose
Measles vaccine	Adults born after 1956 without verification of live measles vaccine on or after 1st birthday, of clinician-diagnosed measles, or of laboratory evidence of immunity; susceptible travelers to foreign countries	One 0.5-ml dose SC	Pregnancy; history of anaphylactic reaction following egg ingestion or receipt of neomycin; immunosuppression
Mumps vaccine	Adults born after 1956 without verification of clinician-diagnosed mumps, without laboratory evidence of immunity, or without proof of vaccination on or after 1st birthday; susceptible travelers to foreign countries	One 0.5-dose SC; no booster	Pregnancy; history of anaphylactic reaction following egg ingestion or receipt of neomycin; immunosuppression
Rubella vaccine	Adults without verification of live vaccine on or after 1st birthday or without laboratory evidence of immunity; susceptible travelers to foreign countries	One 0.5-ml dose SC; no booster	Pregnancy; history of anaphylactic reaction following receipt of neomycin; immunosuppression

Modified from Myers JP: Immunizations in adults. Infect Med (May/Jun):83, 1989.

IMMUNODEFICIENCY

Infections in Immunocompromised Hosts

Infections in the Immunocompromised Host

IMMUNE DEFECT/ORGANISM	SITE OF INFECTION
I. Cell-mediated immune defects (e.g., Hodgkin's lymphoma, transplant recipients, steroid recipients, AIDS)	
A. Viruses	
1. Herpes zoster	Cutaneous
2. Herpes simplex	Mucocutaneous
3. JC virus	Progressive multifocal leukoencephalopathy
4. Cytomegalovirus	Disseminated disease, pneumonia, enteritis, retinitis
B. Bacteria	
1. *Listeria monocytogenes*	Meningitis, bacteremia
2. *Salmonella* sp.	Enteritis, bacteremia
3. *Nocardia asteroides*	Pulmonary, cerebral abscess
4. *Mycobacterium tuberculosis*	Pulmonary, disseminated disease
5. Nontuberculosis mycobacteria (*M. kansasii, M. chelonei, M. fortuitum, M. avium-intracellulare*)	Disseminated disease
6. *Legionella* sp.	Pulmonary
C. Fungi	
1. *Cryptococcus neoformans*	Meningitis, pulmonary, disseminated
2. *Histoplasma capsulatum*	Disseminated, pulmonary
3. *Coccidioides immitis*	Meningitis, disseminated, pulmonary
4. *Candida* sp.	Mucocutaneous
D. Parasites	
1. *Strongyloides stercoralis*	GI, hyperinfection syndrome
2. *Cryptosporidium*	GI
3. *Pneumocystis carinii*	Pulmonary
II. Humoral immunodeficiency	
A. Hypogammaglobulinemia (congenital or acquired)	
1. *Streptococcus pneumoniae*	Pneumonia, bacteremia
2. *Haemophilus influenzae*	Pneumonia, bacteremia
3. *Pseudomonas aeruginosa*	Pneumonia, bacteremia
4. *Neisseria meningitidis*	Meningitis, bacteremia
5. Enteroviruses	Severe disseminated infections
6. *Pneumocystis carinii*	Pulmonary
B. Selective IgA deficiency	
1. *Giardia lamblia*	GI
2. Respiratory pathogens	Respiratory tract infections
C. Selective IgG deficiency	
1. *Streptococcus pneumoniae*	Pulmonary, bacteremia
2. *Haemophilus influenza*	Pulmonary, bacteremia
3. *Pseudomonas aeruginosa*	Pulmonary, bacteremia
III. Neutrophil disorders	
A. Neutropenia (leukemia, aplastic anemia, secondary to cytotoxic chemotherapy):	
1. Coagulase-neg. staphylococci	Bacteremia
2. *Staphylococcus aureus*	Bacteremia, focal infections
3. *Pseudomonas aeruginosa*	Cutaneous, bacteremia, pneumonia

Table continued on next page.

Infections in the Immunocompromised Host (Cont.)

IMMUNE DEFECT/ORGANISM	SITE OF INFECTION
4. Enterobacteriaceae	Cutaneous, bacteremia, pneumonia
5. *Candida* sp.	Fungemia, focal infections
6. *Aspergillus* sp.	Pneumonia, CNS, cutaneous
7. Zygomycetes	Pneumonia, CNS, cutaneous

B. Intracellular killing defects
    1. Defective oxidative metabolism (chronic granulomatous disease)

a. *Staphylococcus aureus*	Cutaneous, focal, pulmonary
b. Enterobacteriaceae	Cutaneous, focal, pulmonary
c. *Pseudomonas aeruginosa*	Cutaneous, focal, pulmonary
d. *Nocardia asteroides*	Pulmonary, CNS
e. *Aspergillus* sp.	Pulmonary, cutaneous

C. Myeloperoxidase deficiency
    1. *Candida* sp.
D. Defective chemotaxis (Chédiak-Higashi, Job syndromes):
    1. *Staphylococcus aureus*
    2. *Haemophilus influenzae*
    3. Beta-hemolytic streptococci
E. Defects in leukocyte adhesion molecules
    1. *Staphylococcus aureus*
    2. *Pseudomonas aeruginosa*

IV. Complement defects
  A. C3 deficiency
    1. *Streptococcus pneumoniae*
    2. *Haemophilus influenzae*
    3. *Neisseria* sp.
  B. C5 to C8 deficiency

1. *Neisseria* sp.	Disseminated

  C. Properdin deficiency

1. *Neisseria meningitidis*	Disseminated

V. Splenectomy/hyposplenism (surgical asplenia, sickle cell)

A. *Streptococcus pneumoniae*	Pneumonia, bacteremia
B. *Neisseria* sp.	Pneumonia, bacteremia
C. *Babesia microti*	Disseminated

IMPOTENCE

Erection requires parasympathetic activity and arterial filling of the corpora cavernosa. The orgasm is mediated by the alpha-adrenergic system. Although the prevalence of impotence is high, it remains underestimated in most surveys and is not a part of normal aging. Healthy community-dwelling men aged 75 to 79 have sexual intercourse twice a month on average. Even in men over 80, sexual interest is present although to a somewhat decreased degree, and it requires increased stimulation to attain and maintain erection.

The most common etiologies include vascular insufficiency, diabetic or nondiabetic neuropathies, and a combination of vascular and neurologic mechanisms. Reversible etiologies include drug effects, hypogonadism, and hyperprolactinemia. If these remediable causes are not present, treatment can include:

1. *Self-injection of phentolamine, papaverine, or prostaglandin E into corpora cavernosa:* This is less effective in cases of vascular etiology and more effective in neurogenic cases. Chronic use of phentolamine or papaverine may result in fibrosis.

2. *Penile prostheses:* These are safe and effective for those who have failed the workup and self-injection. (Vacuum devices are also potentially useful.)

Fear and anxiety are the worst enemies of sexual performance, and oftentimes a frank discussion that allays fears is the best therapy, especially post-MI.

Drugs That Can Produce Impotence

- Digoxin (increases estradiol)
- Antihypertensives: methyldopa, clonidine, reserpine, beta-blockers (↓ libido)
- Diuretics: thiazide diuretics, spironolactone
- Phenothiazines (↑ prolactin and ↓ testosterone)
- Tricyclic antidepressants
- Benzodiazepines
- Cimetidine (? other H_2 blockers)
- Estrogens
- Ketoconazole
- Corticosteroids

Weiss JW, et al: Sexual dysfunction in elderly men. Clin Geriatr Med 6:185–196, 1990.

INCREASED INTRACRANIAL PRESSURE

ICP rises when one of the substances inside the skull increases (the brain, the blood flowing in the blood vessels, or the spinal fluid). The most common causes of increased ICP are as follows.

1. A **mass lesion,** such as a brain tumor, abscess, intracerebral hemorrhage, or subdural hematoma. Such mass takes up space and must displace brain, blood, or spinal fluid.
2. **Edema** can occur around a mass such as a tumor, or it can occur diffusely such as after global hypoxia or a head injury. Edema arises from three main sources:
   a. *Vasogenic edema:* Breakdown of the blood-brain barrier causes fluid to leak out of the vascular compartment and into brain tissue. This commonly occurs around brain tumors or abscesses.
   b. *Cytotoxic edema:* When cells die, they lyse open and spill their intracellular fluids. This is most common after ischemic cell death, such as from a stroke.
   c. *Interstitial edema:* CSF is forced out into the brain parenchyma, such as from hydrocephalus.

The most sensitive sign of increased intracranial pressure is altered mental status, which begins to present before any changes in cranial nerves, motor, sensory, or cerebellar testing. Other findings may include projectile vomiting and headache, which may worsen with maneuvers that increase intracranial pressure, such as bending over or Valsalva.

The increased pressure may cause herniation when the medial, midline structures of the brain (such as the uncus and hippocampal gyrus) are pressed downward against the hard sheath of the tentorium. The earliest consistent sign of such uncal herniation is the unilaterally dilated pupil, which occurs when the third nerve, at the top of the brain stem, becomes compressed. Parasympathetic fibers surrounding the third nerve are damaged immediately, leading to dilatation of the pupil. Once the pupil dilates, CNS deterioration is often rapid. The cerebral peduncle of the midbrain, containing the pyramidal tract, is pushed against the opposite tentorial edge (producing Kernohan's notch), resulting in hemiparesis ipsilateral to the mass. The patient thus has a dilated pupil and a hemiparesis on the same side as the expanding mass.

Treatment for increased intracranial pressure must effect a reduction in the volume of one of the three components of the intracranial compartment as follows.

1. **The brain:** Brain edema can be treated by hyperosmolar agents. Mannitol or glycerol are most commonly used, but diuretics such as furosemide may also be effective. These agents are most useful for vasogenic edema (such as brain tumors) but have less efficacy for cytotoxic edema (such as strokes). Steroids may also benefit the vasogenic edema of tumors but are not indicated for intracerebral hemorrhages or infarctions.

2. **The blood within blood vessels:** Vasoconstriction reduces ICP, which can best be accomplished by intubation and hyperventilation. However, equilibrium returns quickly, so this is a temporizing measure until definitive therapy can be applied.

3. **Spinal fluid:** Emergency placement of an intraventricular shunt by the neurosurgeons can drain off spinal fluid and allow the tissues to collapse, making some space for the mass. Removal of spinal fluid by lumbar puncture should not be attempted in the setting of a mass lesion.

Other measures to reduce ICP involve common sense approaches such as keeping the patient's head elevated and maintaining relative dehydration.

Reference: Hayek DA, et al: Physiologic concerns during brain resuscitation. In Civetta JM, et al (eds): Critical Care, 2nd ed. Philadelphia, J.B. Lippincott, 1992, pp 1449–1466.

INFECTIOUS ARTHRITIS

The search for an infectious cause of chronic arthritis is one of the oldest quests in medicine. Clinicians were so convinced that a chronic indolent infection was responsible for RA that they often recommended complete dental extraction, tonsillectomy, and cholecystectomy. Nonetheless, direct involvement of infectious agents as a source of articular inflammation is well-known. Direct bacterial infection of the joint (septic arthritis) can result in articular destruction and ankylosis if not aggressively treated. Most commonly, bacteria arrive in the joint as a result of hematogenous spread from another site of infection or from IV drug use. In addition, direct infection of the joint from puncture wounds or, more rarely, from direct progression from adjacent osteomyelitis can occur. Surgery, trauma, or damage to the joint predisposes to seeding the infectious agent. Thus patients with a chronic destructive arthropathy (such as RA), a total joint replacement, or even an old injury are at highest risk for developing septic arthritis. Finally, one should not forget that recent intraarticular injection, too, can track organisms into the joint.

Bacterial: Some strains of bacteria seem to be arthrogenic. About 70% of nongonococcal bacterial infections result from *Staphylococcus* and *Streptococcus* (*pyogenes, pneumoniae,* and *viridans*). Gram-negative bacilli such as *Escherichia coli, Salmonella,* and *Pseudomonas* develop occasionally. The last is more common in patients with sickle-cell anemia. *Haemophilus influenzae* is more common in children.

The clinical features of septic arthritis include acute onset of intense pain, swelling, and redness. Elevated temperature is common, although chills occur less frequently. The knee is the most commonly involved joint. Polyarticular involvement in nongonococcal arthritis is rare (<10%) and is usually associated with an underlying systemic illness. Occasionally, synovial tissue is required to identify an organism, particularly in mycobacterial or fungal infections. Up to 50% of patients with established nongonococcal bacterial arthritis may have a positive blood culture. Most patients have an elevated WBC count.

Synovial fluid evaluation is the key to diagnosis. Culture is mandatory, and best results are obtained when fluid is inoculated onto media at the bedside. Cell count, together with Gram and AFB stains, can provide initial insights. In infected joints, synovial fluid glucose is usually below corresponding serum levels, although low levels can be seen in noninfectious inflammatory arthropathies as well. Glucose levels less than half of serum levels suggest a tuberculous etiology.

Treatment revolves primarily around the sensitivity of the microbe. Splinting the joint in addition to providing necessary analgesia is important. Once the intense inflammation subsides, slow and progressive mobilization should be initiated. Decompression of the joint with serial aspirations allows adequate drainage and monitoring (synovial fluid WBC counts and culture). If aspiration is difficult, access incomplete, or lack of treatment response documented, then open or arthroscopic drainage should be undertaken.

Gonococcal: Gonococcal arthritis remains a common cause of acute bacterial arthritis and in some series accounts for up to 50% of cases. The clinical features are less distinctive than in nongonococcal septic arthropathy. A tenosynovitis is present in the majority of patients and may not be associated with the swollen and painful joints. Small papules, particularly in distal extremities, can often provide a diagnostic clue. Gonococcus is cultured from the infected joint in less than 50% of cases. Often, either a clinical history of active infection or a positive culture of the urethra, cervix, throat, or rectum suggests the diagnosis.

Viral: Hepatitis B infection can also produce an active inflammatory arthropathy, believed to be caused by immune complex production rather than by direct joint infection. Articular symptoms generally occur in the prodromal phase of illness, before patients become icteric. The small joints of the hands are the most commonly involved areas. Symptoms usually resolve as icterus develops. Patients with chronic hepatitis B antigenemia can develop symptoms later in the illness. From a rheumatic disease standpoint, the latter can sometimes appear as a syndrome of polyarteritis nodosa, of glomerulonephritis, or of cryoglobulinemia.

The arthropathy associated with the rubella virus occurs with mild infection and can even occur after vaccination. Rash, low-grade fever, and posterior cervical adenopathy are often present. The incidence of arthritis increases with the age at which the vaccination is given or the infection acquired. It occurs much less commonly in men than in women. Joint symptoms usually occur early in the course of the illness and may be the presenting complaint. Symptoms usually are quick to resolve but rarely may develop into a chronic polyarthropathy (3–4% of cases).

Musculoskeletal complaints are uncommon in mumps. Men who encounter the infection in their 20s are perhaps the most likely to develop arthritis. Their joint symptoms antedate the glandular swelling by 7 to 21 days. Three distinct syndromes are described. The first is simple arthralgia or arthritis. Occasionally, a monarticular arthritis, particularly of the large, weight-bearing joints, can be present. Finally, a migratory polyarthropathy (the most common) can be present. There is a high association of such arthropathy with the development of orchitis in adult men.

Recently, data have shown that parvovirus infection can be associated with articular inflammation. Specifically, P19, the virus responsible for erythema infectiosum (fifth disease, or slapped-cheek syndrome in children) can produce a symmetric polyarthropathy involving the knees, the small joints of the hands, and the wrists. As with rubella, women are more commonly affected. Joint symptoms commonly persist for months, but documentary evidence of viral culpability for a chronic arthropathy is lacking.

Spirochetal: Spirochete infection can lead to arthritis. Lyme arthritis is well-known and covered separately. Syphilis rarely causes joint symptoms alone, although musculoskeletal pains are common. Secondary syphilis may present with polyarthralgias or frank arthritis. Tenosynovitis is often present, and destructive sacroiliitis may also occur. It is more common in men aged 20 to 45 and is usually associated with lymphadenopathy, rash, and mucocutaneous lesions. Bone pain secondary to periosteitis can be present. Tertiary syphilis usually presents as a Charcot's joint.

Reference: Goldenberg DL, Reed JI. Bacterial arthritis. N Engl J Med 312:764–771, 1988.

INFLAMMATORY BOWEL DISEASE

Two major categories of IBD are Crohn's disease and chronic ulcerative colitis.

Comparison of the Pathologic and Clinical Features
of Ulcerative Colitis and Crohn's Disease

FEATURE	CUC	CROHN'S
Pathology		
Discontinuous involvement	0	++
Transmural inflammation	0/+*	+++
Deep fissures and fistulas	0	++
Confluent linear ulcers	0	++
Crypt abscesses	+++	+
Focal granulomas	0	+
Clinical		
Rectal bleeding	+++	+
Malaise, fever	+	+++
Abdominal pain	+	+++
Abdominal mass	0	++
Fistulas	0	+++
Endoscopic		
Diffuse, continuous involvement	+++	0/+
Friable mucosa	+++	0/+
Rectal involvement	+++	+
Cobblestoning	0	+++
Linear ulcers	0	++

*In toxic megacolon.

From Bass NM, et al: Gastrointestinal diseases. In Andreoli TE, et al (eds): Cecil Essentials of Medicine, 2nd ed. Philadelphia, W.B. Saunders, 1990, p 292, with permission.

Chronic ulcerative colitis involves inflammation of the epithelial layer of rectum and distal colon. It is four times more common in whites and more common in females. There are three recognized categories:

- Mild   60% of cases   Seldom progresses proximally
  No extracolonic symptoms
  Fewer than 5 stools per day

- Moderate   25%   Systemic symptoms (fever/fatigue)
  Greater than five stools per day

- Severe   15%   Severe systemic symptoms
  Recurrent hospitalizations

The earliest symptoms are usually constipation and passage of mucus or blood with bowel movements, with progression to diarrhea, and systemic symptoms may occur slowly over several months or years. Long-term complications include the following.

Complications of Ulcerative Colitis

COMPLICATION	INCIDENCE (%)
I. Colonic	
Toxic megacolon	1–3
Perforation	3
Stricture	10
Severe hemorrhage	4
Carcinoma	2.5–3.0
II. Extracolonic*	
Skin lesions	
Erythema nodosum	3
Pyoderma gangrenosum	0.5
Aphthous mouth ulcers	10
Iritis, episcleritis	5–10
Arthritis	5–10
Liver lesions	
Fatty infiltration	40
Pericholangitis (portal triaditis)	5–10[+]
Cirrhosis (postnecrotic)	3
Sclerosing cholangitis	<1
Bile duct carcinoma	0.5

*Extracolonic complications in Crohn's disease are similar in prevalence to those in ulcerative colitis.

[+]Based on clinical and laboratory abnormalities; a higher incidence (30–50%) is found on liver biopsy.

From Gray, G: Inflammatory bowel disease. In Rubenstein E, et al (eds): Scientific American Medicine. New York, Scientific American, 1991, p 4(IV):8, with permission.

Treatment involves antidiarrheal agents, sulfasalazine, and topical and systemic corticosteroids. Sulfasalazine is most effective in maintaining remissions, usually starting at a dose of 500 mg BID and increasing over 2 to 4 days to 500 to 1,500 mg QID. Side effects include nausea, epigastric discomfort, oligospermia, and folate deficiency, which may require folic acid supplementation at a dose of 1 mg/day. For more severe symptoms, prednisone may be initiated at a dosage of 40 to 80 mg daily and continued for approximately 4 weeks, slowly tapering the dose after that time. If symptoms are severe enough to necessitate hospitalization, IV fluids, NG suction, and parenteral corticosteroids must be utilized. Proctocolectomy may be indicated if there is an inadequate clinical response after 96 hrs of such treatment.

Crohn's disease involves inflammation of all layers of bowel but most often involves the terminal ileum, cecum, and/or ascending colon. The usual presentation is one of gradual progression of abdominal pain and nonbloody diarrhea and anorexia. Symptoms may be present for several years before the diagnosis is established. The most common complications are rectal fissures, rectocutaneous fistulas, perirectal abscesses, and enteroenteric fistulas. Sigmoidoscopy may be normal in up to 50% of patients; when positive, it often demonstrates granularity and linear ulceration. Characteristic changes on barium enema include segmental involvement of two or more areas with normal-appearing areas in between, as well as thumbprinting of the mucosa and the presence of rectocutaneous and entero-enteric fistulae. Therapy is similar to that for ulcerative colitis. Prednisone at doses of 40 to 60 mg daily may be required for up to 12 weeks to bring severe symptoms under control, followed by a gradual taper. In milder and less urgent cases, standard doses of sulfasalazine may achieve remission after 3 to 4 months and provide relief of local symptoms. Metronidazole is also effective in Crohn's disease at a dose of 250 mg TID, but long-term use (2–4 months) is associated with the development of peripheral neuropathy.

Surgical therapy varies for these two diseases. In ulcerative colitis, proctocolectomy with ileostomy is preferred in order to prevent fulminant recurrences. Indications include severe colitis persisting for 2 to 4 weeks in spite of intensive therapy, persistence of toxic megacolon in spite of intensive therapy for 96 hours, a high suspicion of cancer due to severe dysplasia or stricture, and severe extracolonic symptoms. Approximately 25% of ulcerative colitis patients require surgery in the first 5 years of their disease. In contrast, greater than 60% of patients with Crohn's disease undergo surgery in the first 5 years of their illness, usually for intraabdominal fistulas or strictures. Furthermore, unlike ulcerative colitis, there is a high postoperative recurrence rate of 20 to 80% within the 5 years following surgery.

Mortality rates for the two diseases vary greatly. The rate for Crohn's disease is only 5% within the first 5 years compared to a 10 to 25% mortality rate for severe ulcerative colitis and a 1% rate for mild disease.

INFLUENZA

Influenza is an epidemic illness caused by two types of influenza viruses (A and B) that occurs annually December through April. Although patients and physicians frequently think of influenza as the flu or a common cold, it is a potentially lethal disease. Each year, influenza accounts for approximately 40,000 deaths during the epidemic from pneumonia and influenza. Influenza takes its greatest toll in those over 65 years of age and those with chronic underlying illness such as cardiac and pulmonary disease.

Influenza frequently begins with the *sudden* onset of fever (usually greater than 38.5°C), sore throat, and myalgia. Many patients can exactly time the onset of the illness and find the myalgia to be the most uncomfortable symptom. Patients frequently have a nonproductive cough.

For most people, influenza resolves in 3 to 5 days. Even after the acute illness has passed, patients may be left with a prolonged postviral asthenia characterized by fatigue. In some patients, complications may occur, including primary viral pneumonia, secondary bacterial pneumonia (most often with *Streptococcus pneumoniae, Staphylococcus aureus,* and *Haemophilus influenzae*), Reye's syndrome, encephalitis, myocarditis, pericarditis, and Guillain-Barré syndrome. Both viral and secondary bacterial pneumonia may lead to respiratory failure and death.

The symptoms, but not the complications, of influenza A can be reduced through the early use of amantadine. If given within 24 hours of the onset of symptoms, amantadine can reduce such symptoms' duration and severity. The dose of amantadine is 200 mg/day, but 100 mg/day is given to elderly patients and patients with renal failure. The side effects of amantadine include confusion, delirium, and impaired thinking.

Influenza can be prevented through immunization. Each year a new vaccine is formulated that contains antigen to the three viral strains most likely to circulate during the upcoming epidemic. The vaccine should be repeated annually and is best given before the epidemic begins. Vaccination can begin as soon as the vaccine is available in September and can continue throughout the epidemic. It takes 2 weeks to develop immunity. The vaccine is approximately 80% effective in preventing the complications of influenza in the elderly and over 90% effective in preventing disease in young patients. Side effects include a mild, flulike illness that occurs in 10% of vaccinees in addition to a sore arm. Allergy to eggs is the only contraindication. Guillain-Barré syndrome occurred following the administration of swine influenza vaccine in 1976 but has not been reported since then.

INSOMNIA

Insomnia is defined as abnormal sleep patterns resulting in adverse consequences during waking hours. Approximately one third of all patients complain of insomnia in any particular year, of either increased sleep latency or increased wakening. Causes of insomnia include:

- *Physical disorders:* periodic movements during sleep, restless legs, gastroesophageal reflux, sleep apnea, fibromyalgia, arthritis, chronic pain, cardiac problems
- *Substances:* caffeine, nicotine, alcohol, hypnotics, tranquilizers, prescription medications, substances of abuse
- *Circadian rhythm problems:* shift work, jet lag, delayed sleep phase syndrome, advanced sleep phase syndrome
- *Psychological factors:* stress, psychopathology, nightmares, inactivity, reinforcement for insomnia
- *Poor sleep environment:* noise, ambient temperature, light, sleeping surface, bed partner
- *Poor sleep habits:* extended time in bed, naps, irregular schedule, bed as a cue for arousal

Several studies have shown a greater degree of depression and anxiety in insomniacs, often associated with decreased job performance, impaired interpersonal relationships, chronic fatigue, and irritability. Transient insomnia may be either situational or related to phase shift. Chronic insomnia (lasting longer than 3 weeks) is more common in the elderly and appears to be related to an impairment in normal circadian rhythm. Several medications that may be responsible for sleep disturbance are:

Methyldopa	Propranolol
Theophylline	Thyroid hormone
Cimetidine	Phenytoin
Levodopa	OTC nasal decongestants
Quinidine	

Nonpharmacologic Therapy for Insomnia

- Avoidance of naps
- Avoidance of heavy exercise in the evenings
- Proper bedroom temperature

Table continued on next page.

- Use of the bed only for sleeping
- Avoidance of stimulants such as caffeine and nicotine
- Leaving the bed after a 10- to 20-min period of wakefulness

Pharmacologic Therapy for Insomnia

AGENT	SIDE EFFECTS
Alcohol	Decreased REM sleep
Diphenhydramine, hydroxyzine	Urinary retention
Benzodiazepines	Tolerance, psychologic dependence, antero-grade amnesia (impaired information acquisition and recall), rebound insomnia
Chloral hydrate	Low toxic-to-effective dose ratio
Antidepressants	Orthostasis, ? cardiac conduction defects

In the choice of a benzodiazepine, intermediate-acting agents such as temazepam or lorazepam (half-life 8–15 hrs) are preferable to longer-acting agents (e.g., flurazepam with a half-life of greater than 100 hrs). Although they are excellent sedating agents, antidepressants such as amitriptyline and doxepin should be used with caution in the elderly, for whom desipramine or nortriptyline may be preferable because they cause fewer anticholinergic side effects. Barbiturates should be avoided due to the high rate of addiction associated with their use as well as the risks of lethal overdose.

Nocturnal polysomnography studies in a sleep laboratory may be indicated for the following reasons:

1. Failure to respond to traditional sleep hygiene and sedative-hypnotic therapies.

2. Unacceptable side effects arising from careful, supervised use of sedative-hypnotic medications, resulting in an apparent lack of suitable treatment alternatives.

3. Suspicion of, but inability to confirm, primary sleep disorders such as sleep apnea and periodic leg movements (nocturnal myoclonus).

4. Desire for diagnostic or therapeutic consultation in complicated or refractory cases or when multiple etiologies are suspected.

References: Moran MG, et al: Sleep disorders in the medically ill patient. J Clin Psychiatry 53:6(Suppl):33, 1992.

Bootzin RR, et al: Nonpharmacologic treatments of insomnia. J Clin Psychiatry 53:6(Suppl):37, 1992.

INTRAVENOUS DRUG USE

Associated Medical Conditions

Intravenous drug use (IVDU) is a twentieth-century phenomenon, initially described in the 1920s. It was not until the 1930s, however, that reports describing complications of IVDU appeared in the medical literature. The initial complications described were transmission of malaria through the sharing of needles among addicts along the eastern seaboard. As drug dealers began to cut heroin with quinine, this complication was minimized. During the 1960s to 1970s, HBV infection became a major complication of IVDU. Although this continues, vaccination against HBV could eliminate it as a problem. Today, HIV occupies center stage in the medical complications of IVDU. During the mid-to-late 1980s, HIV widely penetrated most IVDU communities, resulting in high rates of HIV infection. As a result, heterosexual transmission of HIV to the sexual partners of users is increasingly common, as is perinatal transmission to the children of such couples.

Infections remain the primary complication of IVDU, with HIV representing only a small portion of these. There are three sources for infectious agents. The first is the external environment such as the drug itself or the paraphernalia used for preparation or injection. As a second source, other addicts can act as such when needles and other equipment are shared. The third source consists of addicts themselves with intact or altered skin defenses and flora.

Drug preparation techniques often vary with locality and may include dilution with varying degrees of clean or unclean water. Clusters of candidemia have been described resulting from dilution of drugs with contaminated lemon juice. Some drugs, such as heroin, require heat to go into solution, rendering the solution relatively sterile. Other drugs (cocaine) are readily soluble. Cleansing of the skin may minimize infection by skin flora, but the not-uncommon practice of quickly wiping the injection site with saliva raises the possibility of other infectious etiologies.

The route of administration can alter the complications found. IV injection is more frequently associated with bacteremia, whereas intraarterial injection is associated with embolic events. SC injection commonly causes abscess formation with skin flora and clostridial species sometimes resulting in tetanus or botulism.

Skin and soft tissue infections constitute the vast majority of complications in all series, with acknowledgment of underreporting due to self-treatment by addicts. The degree of involvement can range from mild cellulitis to abscess to frank ulceration. Close observation and surgical consultation are necessary in all but the most mild cases. Staph and strep species are the most common etiologic organisms. If a history of wiping with saliva is obtained, consideration of anaerobes is important. The physical exam of abscesses in IVDU is unreliable in anatomical areas such as the neck and groin. Deep, dissecting involvement can be well hidden. Mycotic aneurysms and osteomyelitis occur with regularity in such complicated processes.

Infectious endocarditis is the most well-known complication of IVDU and must be considered in the febrile user with no other apparent source. There is a continual high-grade bacteremia, which can be diagnosed with routine bacterial blood cultures.

Because of the high prevalence of TB in the IVDU community, PPD skin testing should be a routine part of the health examination in these individuals. With varying degrees of immunocompetence, results should be recorded in millimeters of induration, not as merely negative or positive. Proper interpretation of the PPD also requires knowledge of the IVDU's HIV status.

Reference: Levine DP, et al (eds): Infections in Intravenous Drug Abusers. New York, Oxford University Press, 1991.

J

JAUNDICE

Differential Diagnosis

Bilirubin is a waste product of hemoglobin metabolism. A normal serum bilirubin concentration (0.3–1.0 mg/dl) represents a balance between the rate of heme production and the hepatic clearance of bilirubin. Jaundice—the accumulation of excess bilirubin in the skin—occurs when bilirubin exceeds clearance, as in hemolytic states, or when elimination is impaired owing to a liver abnormality. Jaundice presents as an orange-yellow color of the skin and is usually seen when serum bilirubin levels are greater than 2.5 mg/dl.

Unconjugated bilirubin, which is insoluble in water and cannot be easily excreted from the body, is taken up by the liver and converted to a conjugated, water-soluble form by attachment to glucuronic acid. This conjugated bilirubin is then excreted in the bile. If the conjugated level of bilirubin becomes greater than 2 mg/dl, it will be excreted in the urine and the urine will turn black. Hyperbilirubinemia can be classified into the following groups: prehepatic (i.e., increased bilirubin production such as in hemolysis), intrahepatic (i.e., a defect in uptake, transport, or conjugation of bilirubin), and posthepatic (i.e., a defect in biliary excretion as would occur in obstructive jaundice).

Causes of Jaundice

| | INTRAHEPATIC | | |
PREHEPATIC	Congenital	Acquired	POSTHEPATIC
Hemolysis (drugs, autoimmune, hemoglobinopathies)	Gilbert syndrome	Viral hepatitis	Common bile duct stone
Dyserythropoiesis	Dubin-Johnson syndrome	Alcohol	Benign bile duct strictures
Transfusion	Crigler-Najjar syndrome	Drugs	Pancreatic cancer
Hematoma resorption	Rotor's syndrome	Sepsis	Pancreatitis
		Heart failure	Bile duct cancer
		Parenteral nutrition	Ampullary cancer
		Malignancy	Choledochal cyst
		Primary biliary cirrhosis	Sclerosing cholangitis

Evaluation

The first step in the evaluation of jaundice is a thorough Hx & PE that looks for clues that will aid in the differential, such as a history of drug abuse (supportive of

351

hepatitis), signs of cirrhosis, or a palpable gallbladder (suggestive of extrahepatic obstruction). The initial laboratory assessment of the jaundiced patient includes CBC, UA, AST, ALT, alkaline phosphatase, total and direct bilirubin, albumin, PT, and stool examination for occult blood. If the patient is anemic, if the urine is negative for bilirubin, and if the patient has a primary unconjugated hyperbilirubinemia, a high reticulocyte count, and fragmented RBCs, then one should suspect hemolysis as the cause. The workup of jaundice after the initial tests is described in the following table.

Clinical Approach to Jaundice

TEST RESULTS	LIKELY MECHANISM	ETIOLOGY

Mostly conjugated bilirubin
  Alk phos >3x normal
  ALT <500
	Likely obstruction; obtain
	  CT scan, ultrasound, or
	  ERCP
		Infiltrating tumor, biliary or
		  pancreatic cancer

Mixed bilirubin
  ALT >500
  Hepatomagaly
  Alk phos <3 × normal
	Likely a hepatocellular
	  disorder; obtain hepati-
	  tis serologies
		Viral hepatitis, drug-related
		  hepatitis, ischemic hepati-
		  tis

Unconjugated
  Normal ALT
	Likely hemolysis or inher-
	  ited defect
		Hemolysis, Gilbert or Crigler-
		  Najjar syndrome

It must be noted that if the AST and ALT are less than 50 IU and the alkaline phosphatase is greater than three times normal, one needs to distinguish between intrahepatic cholestasis and extrahepatic cholestasis. An ultrasound should be obtained to look for dilated bile ducts; if ducts are not dilated, viral serologies should be done. In that situation, alcoholic hepatitis is also a consideration.

K

KAPOSI'S SARCOMA

KS, along with PCP, was one of the sentinel events that alerted health authorities in 1980 to a new syndrome of immunodeficiency, soon known as AIDS. The reasons for the high prevalence of KS in AIDS remain unknown, as does the pathogenesis of KS. Also unknown are the reasons both for the predilection of KS for homosexual men with HIV as opposed to all other risk groups and for the steadily decreasing incidence of KS in all HIV risk groups over the past 5 years.

KS in HIV-infected patients is most often seen as cutaneous or oropharyngeal nodules. These nodules usually range from 0.5 to 2.0 cm in diameter, although multiple nodules may coalesce and form a larger plaque. The nodules are most often raised and readily palpable, as well as painless and nonpruritic, and they have no evidence of inflammation or exudate. Rarely, lesions may become friable or verrucous-like and may weep or bleed with trauma. The lesions are usually blue or violet-to-purple in color; in darker-skinned individuals, they may appear almost black. Any area of the body may be involved, although the head, neck, and oral cavity are very common. Multiple sites may be involved at initial presentation, highlighting the need for a complete physical examination during the initial evaluation of even an outwardly healthy appearing HIV-infected patient.

Because other infectious processes that are associated with HIV may present similarly, biopsy of suspicious areas should be considered. Both disseminated fungal infections, particularly histoplasmosis, and bacillary angiomatosis may be indistinguishable from KS, yet are fully treatable with proper therapy.

Therapy against KS is hampered by our lack of understanding of its pathogenesis. Therapy is indicated primarily for control of local complications such as edema, for cosmetically disfiguring lesions, or for visceral (particularly pulmonary) involvement. Local therapy such as radiation, cryotherapy with liquid nitrogen, or intralesional injection of vinblastine can yield very good results for limited disease. No single regimen of systemic chemotherapy has yielded totally satisfactory results, so several options consisting of both single-agent and combination chemotherapy exist. Differentiation between limited and extensive disease can assist the clinician in

Kaposi's Sarcoma Assessment in AIDS

LIMITED DISEASE	EXTENSIVE DISEASE
No previous OI	Previous OI
No ''B'' symptoms	''B'' symptoms
No edema	Edema of face or extremities
CD4+ T lymphocytes >200	CD4+ T lymphocytes <200
KS lesions <25	KS lesions >25
Slow-appearing KS <10/month	Rapidly progressive KS >10/month
No pulmonary KS lesions	Pulmonary involvement with KS
Tolerant of zidovudine	Intolerant of zidovudine
Serum p24 <35 pg/ml	Serum p24 >35 pg/ml

From Kahn J, et al: AIDS-associated Kaposi's sarcoma. In Volberding P, et al (eds): AIDS Clinical Review, 1992. New York, Marcel Dekker, 1992, p 268, with permission.

353

prescribing a particular course of therapy. One such system to classify patients, which is utilized by San Francisco General Hospital, is presented here.

The decision to utilize systemic chemotherapy should be made on an individual basis until better data are available to indicate such use more definitively. Consideration needs to be given to the ways therapy may interfere with other life-supporting or life-improving interventions such as antiretroviral therapy or PCP prophylaxis.

L

LAMBERT-EATON MYASTHENIC SYNDROME

Lambert-Eaton myasthenic syndrome (LEMS) is an autoimmune disease affecting the neuromuscular junction, caused by antibodies that attack the L-type calcium channel on the presynaptic neuron. The motor nerve synapsing on the muscle fiber cannot be depolarized adequately and so does not release enough of its neurotransmitter, acetylcholine. As a result, the contraction of the muscle is weak.

Clinically, this syndrome is often extremely difficult to differentiate from myasthenia gravis (MG), because patients usually present identically, with proximal weakness in the limbs, which fatigues with repetitive testing.

Clues to Differentiating LEMS from MG

1. The eyes are never involved in LEMS. MG frequently causes ptosis or diplopia.

2. Clinically, repetitive testing in LEMS sometimes leads to incremental strengthening rather than decremental weakening. With repeated use, a muscle may actually increase in strength in LEMS, whereas it usually fatigues and weakens in MG. Although the phenomenon is often difficult to appreciate at the bedside, electrical studies show it easily; therefore nerve conduction studies with repetitive stimulation are essential tests for LEMS. (Pathophysiologically, the reason for this phenomenon is probably because repetitive firing and depolarization of the nerve, leading to repetitive inflow of calcium through the damaged calcium channel, gradually result in accumulation of enough intracellular calcium to cause release of more and more neurotransmitter.)

3. LEMS frequently causes autonomic dysfunction, especially dry mouth and dry eyes.

4. LEMS usually does not respond to cholinesterase inhibitors, such as pyridostigmine.

Most cases of LEMS are associated with small-cell carcinoma of the lung, and LEMS is one of the best examples of a paraneoplastic syndrome, or remote effect of cancer (the antibody causing the disease is produced by the lung tumor). Patients with LEMS require evaluation for an underlying malignancy.

The best therapy is treatment of the underlying neoplasm. Some medications, such as guanethidine, can enhance neurotransmitter release and thus provide some improvement. Plasmapheresis to decrease levels of the circulating antibody can also offer some relief, as can steroids and other immune suppressants.

Brooke MH: A Clinician's View of Neuromuscular Diseases, 2nd ed. Baltimore, Williams & Wilkins, 1986.

LEUKEMIA

Acute: French-American-British (FAB) Classification

Acute myeloblastic leukemia (AML)

M1: *AML without maturation.* The bone marrow is almost totally infiltrated with myeloblasts. At least 90% of the nonerythroid cells must be blasts, with at least 3% of the blast cells showing myeloid histochemical markers (positive for peroxidase or Sudan black). A few granules, Auer rods, or both are seen; one or more distinct nucleoli are evident, but no further maturation.

M2: *AML with maturation.* From 30 to 89% of the nonerythroid cells of the bone marrow are blast cells, some showing positive histochemical stains for myeloblasts. At least 10% of nonerythroid cells are more mature myeloid cells (promyelocytes to segmented neutrophils), and less than 20% of the cells are monocytic. Myelocytes, metamyelocytes, and mature granulocytes are seen. Eosinophilia may predominate in some cases.

M3: *Promyelocytic leukemia.* The predominant nonerythroid cell in the bone marrow is the promyelocyte, with reniform (kidney-shaped) nuclei and bundles of Auer rods; also some have closely packed bright pink or purple granules. DIC is very common in this type of leukemia.

M4: *Myelomonocytic leukemia.* Myeloblasts constitute 30% or greater of the nonerythroid marrow cells, the percentage of monocytic cells is at least 20%, and the percentage of myeloid cells (myeloblasts and all more mature forms including segmented neutrophils) is 30 to 80%. An eosinophilic variant is also recognized.

M5: *Monocytic leukemia.* At least 80% of the nonerythroid cells in the marrow are of monocytic lineage, with less than 10% granulocytes. Two forms exist:

M5a: *Monoblastic leukemia* (poorly differentiated). At least 80% of the monocytic lineage cells are monoblasts.

M5b: *Monocytic leukemia* (differentiated). At least 20% or greater of the monocytic cells are more mature than monoblasts (i.e., promonocytes and monocytes). Monocytoid cells have a fluoride-sensitive esterase reaction cytochemically.

M6: *Erythroleukemia.* About 30% of the nonerythroid cells are myeloblasts. Numerous bizarre erythroblasts are found in the bone marrow.

M7: *Megakaryoblastic leukemia.* The bone marrow contains at least 30% blast cells. Megakaryocytic lineage of blast cells is identified by electron microscopy or platelet-specific monoclonal antibodies. Myelofibrosis, or increased marrow reticulin, is usually a prominent feature recognized by bone marrow biopsy. Cytoplasmic budding is also a feature.

Acute lymphoblastic leukemia (ALL)

L1: *Lymphoblastic leukemia with small lymphoblasts:* the most common form in children, 85% of all cases of ALL.

L2: *Lymphoblastic leukemia with medium-size lymphoblasts:* the most common form in adults, approximately 14% of all cases of ALL.

L3: *Lymphoblastic leukemia with lymphoblasts that have deep-blue cytoplasm and often cytoplasmic vacuoles:* the form of ALL seen in Burkitt's cell leukemia and in patients with AIDS. Frequently associated with very high values for the serum uric acid and serum LDH.

Reference: Bennett JM, et al: Proposed revised criteria for the classification of acute myeloid leukemia. Ann Intern Med 103:620–625, 1985.

Acute Myelogenous Leukemia

Acute leukemia in adults is mainly AML, a proliferation of primitive cells with monocytic or granulocytic characteristics. Only 10% of adult leukemia is lymphoid in origin. AML can arise de novo or evolve from a myeloproliferative or myelodysplastic disorder. CML uniformly advances to AML, with about 20% transforming into blast crises each year after diagnosis.

Secondary leukemia is an unfortunate consequence of the success of therapy for Hodgkin's disease, multiple myeloma, and other malignancies for which alkylating agents and/or radiation are utilized. These leukemias are often preceded by a period of myelodysplasia and are associated with characteristic abnormalities of chromosomes 5 and 7. Usually the response to therapy is poor, and death constitutes a tragic punctuation of a "cure" for the original malignancy. The success of antithymocyte globulin (ATG) therapy for aplastic anemia has also been marred in some patients by myelodysplasia and leukemia after several years of follow-up in remission.

AML in adults presents with bleeding, fever, and anemia. Some patients do not have a markedly elevated WBC count, although myeloblasts are easily recognized upon examination of the peripheral blood. Occasional patients present with atypical abdominal pain, splenomegaly, pericarditis, or gum and skin involvement (often in monocytic leukemias). Marked leukocytosis (blast counts of 60,000–100,000) marks the most dramatic presentation. Because the myeloblast is large, poorly deformable, and sticky, the small vessels of the circulation are choked by leukemic cells. This hyperleukostasis syndrome is manifested by altered mental status, pulmonary infiltrates, abnormal bleeding into tissues, and vasoocclusive events such as priapism and stroke. Perivascular cuffing by abnormal cells leads to breakdown of hemostasis and death due to CNS hemorrhage. Emergent leukapheresis and institution of cytoreductive chemotherapy may be lifesaving. Laboratory artifacts associated with very high WBC counts include hypoxemia, hypoglycemia, and hyperkalemia.

Some important general measures are avoidance of aspirin, IM injections, and manipulation of the rectum. Establishment of a central venous access catheter is often helpful, and blood bank support should emphasize the use of single-donor platelet units.

The classification of AML has been codified by the FAB group, and its essential elements are shown in the table on the preceding page. This scheme is morphologic and depends on specific staining patterns as well as analysis of a significant number of bone marrow cells by a trained hematologist. Currently, marrow cells are routinely cultured for cytogenetic evaluation, and determination of surface markers is made by flow cytometry. These maneuvers have resulted in the recognition of distinct cytogenetic abnormalities associated with many of the FAB morphologic subgroups, which are summarized in the second table. The markers facilitate recognition of biphenotypic disease (blasts that have simultaneous expression of myeloid and lymphoid disease) or biclonal disease (in which patients have two distinct clones—one myeloid, the other lymphoid). Problems arise in the classification of erythroid leukemias and myelodysplastic states. M7, or megakaryocytic leukemia, is a relatively new diagnostic entity resembling acute myelofibrosis. The identification of this form of leukemia is possible because of the availability of antibodies that recognize vWF and platelet-specific glycoproteins.

Cytogenetics in AML

CYTOGENETIC ABNORMALITY	LEUKEMIA TYPE	PROGNOSIS
Trisomy 8	M2	Average
t(8;21)	M2 with splenomegaly, chloromas, Auer rods	Good
t(15;17)	M3, many promyelocytes, DIC	Average
inv 16	FAB M4 with abnormal eosinophils	Good
t(9;11)	M5, monocytic leukemia	Average
t(6;9)	M2 with increased basophils	Average
t(4;11)	Biphenotypic leukemia lymphoid and monocytic phenotype	Poor
5q–,7q–,5–,7–	Therapy-related leukemia	Poor

Acute promyelocytic leukemia (M3) is an interesting disease because of the early recognition of a frequent translocation (15:17) in this disorder. The retinoic acid receptor on chromosome 17 is split by the translocation. Retinoic acids and their receptors are important agents in cellular differentiation and morphogenesis. When patients with promyelocytic leukemia receive transretinoic acid, their promyelocytes appear to differentiate into more mature neutrophils. Therapeutic trials are under way with retinoic acid to establish the place of this differentiation agent in modern chemotherapy of acute promyelocytic leukemia. Clinically, the recognition of M3 by the FAB subgroups is also important because of its association with DIC. The DIC in this disorder responds to heparin or in some instances to intensive support with platelets, fresh frozen plasma, and cryoprecipitate.

Another common cytogenetic abnormality is the 8:21 translocation in M2. Although some centers report that these patients have excellent results with chemotherapy alone, there is some controversy about the role of bone marrow transplantation. Allogeneic transplantation should be considered for most patients who are in first remission, are young, and have siblings who may be suitable donors. Although the potential for a fatal outcome is a significant factor with this procedure, the long-term outlook is very good because of the low relapse rate for leukemia posttransplant.

What is the outlook for a young person (i.e., less than 45 years of age) with AML? With conventional DAT chemotherapy, long-term disease-free survival is possible for 20 to 25% of those in first remission. For HLA-identical sibling-donor-marrow transplants, the rate is 40 to 60%. Unfortunately, the two regimens are difficult to compare due to the selection bias of institutions in which either chemotherapy or bone marrow transplantation, but not both, predominate.

References: Mastrianni DM, et al: Acute myelogenous leukemia: Current treatment and future directions. Am J Med 92:286–295, 1992.

Bennet JM, et al: Proposed revised criteria for the classification of acute myeloid leukemia: A report of the French-American-British Cooperative Group. Ann Intern Med 103:620–625, 1985.

Chronic Lymphocytic Leukemia

CLL is a neoplasm of mature lymphocytes. The disease is marked by the accumulation of lymphocytes in the bone marrow, blood, lymph nodes, and spleen. CLL may be a manifestation of the absence of the normal demise of cells via programmed cell death or apoptosis. Immune dysfunction may be manifested by autoimmune hemolytic anemia, ITP, and susceptibility to recrudescence of herpes zoster. The typical patient is elderly, and the peripheral blood film shows increased numbers of mature-appearing lymphocytes as well as disrupted lymphs or basket cells. Nucleoli are infrequently observed. The diagnostic criteria for CLL are set forth in the table that follows.

Certain closely related disorders may be confused with CLL: Prolymphocytic leukemia is marked by cells with a single distinct nucleolus and splenomegaly. Hairy-cell leukemia has lymphocytes with characteristic spiny projections and bone marrow fibrosis. Indolent non-Hodgkin's lymphomas may have a leukemic phase, with mature but clefted or folded nuclei. The immunologic phenotype of CLL is helpful in distinguishing CLL from other disorders of lymphocytes; for example, the CLL cell expresses surface Ig weakly and a T-cell activation antigen, CD5, strongly.

Diagnostic Criteria for CLL

To make a diagnosis of CLL, criterion 1 should be satisfied along with either criterion 2 or 3. If criterion 1 is not satisfied, criteria 2 *and* 3 must be present.
1. Sustained lymphocyte count $\geq 10 \times 10^9$/L. Morphology should be typical.
2. Bone marrow involvement (>30% lymphocytes)
3. B-cell immunophenotypes (typically weak expression of membrane Ig, CD5 expression and rosette formation with mouse erythrocytes)

Patients can be staged according to the systems devised by Rai or Binet (see tables). Later stages are associated with a poorer prognosis. Patients who have only lymphocytosis without significant lymphadenopathy, splenomegaly, thrombocytopenia, or anemia enjoy a better outlook. Their life expectancy may be determined by other disorders prevalent in the elderly. The course of CLL in some individuals is marked by transformation into a more malignant, large-cell lymphoma that responds poorly to therapy. This transformation, or Richter's syndrome, can be suspected when there is fever, or new lymphadenopathy, or retroperitoneal disease.

Rai Staging System for Chronic Lymphocytic Leukemia

STAGE	CLINICAL FEATURES	SURVIVAL* (MO)
0	Lymphocytosis in blood and bone marrow only	> 120
I	Lymphocytosis and enlarged lymph nodes	95
II	Lymphocytosis plus hepatomegaly, or splenomegaly, or both	2
III	Lymphocytosis and anemia (hemoglobin <100 gm/L)	30
IV	Lymphocytosis and thrombocytopenia (platelets <100 × 10^9/L)	30

*Weighted median survival was derived from eight different series that involved a total of 952 patients.

Binet Staging System for Chronic Lymphocytic Leukemia

STAGE	CLINICAL FEATURES	SURVIVAL* (MO)
A	Hemoglobin ≥100 gm/L, platelets ≥100 × 10^9, and <3 areas[+] involved	>120
B	Hemoglobin ≥100 gm/L, platelets ≥100 × 10^9, and ≥3 areas involved	61
C	Hemoglobin <100 gm/L or platelets <100 × 10^9 or both (independently of the areas involved)	32

*Weighted median survival was derived from eight different series that involved a total of 1,117 patients.

[+]The 3 areas are the cervical, axillary, and inguinal lymph nodes (whether unilateral or bilateral); the spleen; and the liver.

From International Workshop on Chronic Lymphocytic Leukemia: Chronic lymphocytic leukemia: Recommendations for diagnosis, staging, and response. Ann Intern Med 110:236–238, 1989, with permission.

Advanced or symptomatic disease may be amenable to therapy with chlorambucil and prednisone. Recently, new antimetabolites such as fludarabine have been shown to be effective agents. Fludarabine may work by inducing apoptosis in CLL cells. Fludarabine is immunosuppressive, and a number of patients have presented months after completion of therapy with unusual infections such as listeriosis, *Pneumocystis carinii*, and fungi. Although some patients are severely hypogammaglobulinemic, prophylactic use of IV gamma globulin does not seem to be cost-effective therapy.

Reference: Keating MJ: Chemotherapy of chronic lymphocytic leukemia. In Cheson, BD (ed): Chronic Lymphocytic Leukemia: Scientific Advances and Clinical Developments. New York, Marcel Dekker, 1990, pp 297–336.

Complications of CLL

Anemia, mechanisms of:

1. Myelophthisic: due to marrow infiltration with lymphocytes
2. Autoimmune hemolytic: warm antibody type, 8% of patients with CLL, direct Coombs' reaction positive
3. Hemolytic: due to cold agglutinins, IgM antibody mediated; occurs rarely
4. Hypersplenism
5. Anemia of chronic disorders
6. Pure erythroid aplasia; rarely occurs
7. Related to cytotoxic chemotherapy

Neutropenia, mechanisms of:

1. Myelophthisic: due to marrow infiltration with lymphocytes; leads to severe neutropenia in late CLL
2. Immune destruction of neutrophils: difficult to prove clinically
3. Hypersplenism
4. Chemotherapy

Thrombocytopenia (15% of CLL patients), mechanisms of:

1. Myelophthisic: due to marrow infiltration with lymphocytes
2. Immune destruction of platelets; occurs occasionally
3. Hypersplenism: degree of thrombocytopenia approximates extent of splenomegaly
4. Chemotherapy

Infections, predisposing causes:

1. Neutropenia: leads to infections with gram-negative organisms, *Candida,* and *Aspergillus*
2. Immunoglobulin deficiency: occurs in >50% of patients with CLL; leads to infections with pneumococci and other encapsulated organisms
3. Poor antibody response to specific antigens: causes poor response to immunizations, as well as increased viral and bacterial infections
4. T-lymphocyte dysfunction: sometimes associated with impaired delayed-type hypersensitivity
5. Chemotherapy related: fludarabine plus prednisone predisposes to *Listeria monocytogenes* infections

Monoclonal immunoglobulins:

1. IgM serum paraprotein in about 5% of CLL
2. Rarely IgG or IgD serum paraprotein or light chain paraprotein in urine

Lymphadenopathy causing obstruction:

1. Lymphedema of lower extremities
2. Obstruction of ureters, leading to renal insufficiency
3. Obstruction of bronchus, resulting in atelectasis and pneumonia

Increased frequency of second malignancies (10–20% of patients):

1. Multiple myeloma
2. Carcinomas of colon and rectum
3. Carcinoma of lung'
4. Carcinoma of skin
5. Malignant melanoma

Transformation of CLL to other lymphoid malignancies:

1. Richter transformation of CLL to diffuse large-cell lymphoma
2. Prolymphocytic leukemia (5–10% of patients with CLL)
3. Acute lymphoblastic leukemia (ALL)

Chronic Myelogenous Leukemia

CML is a clonal myeloproliferative disorder that involves stem cells and is characterized by a proliferation of granulocytes. The chronic phase lasts 3 to 7 years and leads to an acute blastic transformation with a survival of 3 to 6 months. CML is associated with the Philadelphia (Ph) chromosome, a shortened chromosome 22, which results from a translocation between chromosomes 22 and 9. As a result of the translocation, *abl* proto-oncogene on 9 is inserted into the breakpoint cluster region (*bcr*) of 22. A new gene is created, which can be identified by Southern blot analysis. Detection of the Ph chromosome in cells aspirated from the bone marrow offers a precise diagnosis of CML in most patients. Occasional patients are Ph chromosome negative but still show the *abl/bcr* fusion gene on Southern analysis.

CML may be discovered in patients referred for evaluation of an elevated WBC count, splenomegaly, or unexplained fever and weight loss. The peripheral blood usually shows an increased granulocyte count, which may include promyelocytes, myelocytes, and metamyelocytes as well as a small number of blasts. Unlike the leukocytosis associated with infections and inflammation, CML is marked by an increased number of basophils and eosinophils, some of which are atypical. Atypical platelet morphology may also be present. In secondary leukocytosis, promyelocytes and myelocytes are typically absent, and metamyelocytes are less common. The bone marrow in CML shows marked myeloid hyperplasia. Occasionally, CML presents with significant fibrosis and, in the absence of the means to detect the Ph chromosome, cannot be distinguished clinically from myelofibrosis. Thrombocytosis and erythrocytosis also can accompany CML.

CML is a disease of distinct phases. In the chronic phase, treatment with hydroxyurea can control the blood counts, delay splenomegaly, and reduce any hypermetabolic symptoms (fever, night sweats). The onset of painful splenomegaly, basophilia, marrow fibrosis, bone pain, or refractoriness to hydroxyurea heralds the blast transformation of CML. Most of the time this represents a progression to AML, but 30% of patients have blasts that are lymphoid. More rarely the transformation is to megakaryocytic leukemia or erythroleukemia. Patients with the features of ALL may enjoy a good (but brief) response to typical ALL therapy. Once the blast phase is established, however, the outlook is poor. Most patients respond briefly to chemotherapy and succumb to their illness within 3 to 6 months.

In the chronic phase, patients below age 50 to 55 should be evaluated for allogeneic bone marrow transplantation. Older patients, or younger patients without suitable marrow donors, can be treated with hydroxyurea. Matched, unrelated donor transplants remain investigational. Interferon-α is an effective, albeit expensive, form of therapy that results in cytogenetic remission in 25% of patients treated. In those patients whose Ph chromosomes have disappeared, there is the possibility that blast transformation may be delayed. It may not be well tolerated by older individuals. Leukapheresis is used in patients who develop the leukostasis syndrome and in pregnant women.

Reference: Kantarjian HM, et al: Chronic myelogenous leukemia: A concise update. Blood 82:691–703, 1993.

Hairy-Cell Leukemia

HCL, or leukemic reticuloendotheliosis, is an uncommon neoplasm of B-lymphoid cells that are intermediate in differentiation between the B-lymphocytes of CLL and multiple myeloma. When first described by Bertha Bouroncle, this disorder was called leukemic reticuloendotheliosis, reflecting the notion that the cell of interest might be a monocyte. HCL is clinically manifested by splenomegaly, bone marrow involvement, and atypical lymphs surrounded by a reticulin web. Adenopathy is typically absent. The peripheral blood picture is usually that of pancytopenia, monocytopenia, and circulating lymphocytes demonstrating generous cytoplasm with hairy projections and bean-shaped nuclei with lacy reticulum. The cells have an acid phosphatase that is tartrate resistant and a characteristic immunophenotype that consists of B-cell markers, CD11 and CD25—the receptor for IL-2. Unlike CLL, typical HCL cells do not have the T-cell antigen CD5.

If HCL is uncommon, why is it so interesting? This disorder has fascinating presentations and complications and is amenable to therapy. Recognition of HCL requires diagnostic acumen and can lead to successful therapy. The diagnostic challenge consists of the difficulty in obtaining the cells of interest from the bone marrow. Efforts to aspirate the marrow frequently result in a dry tap. The fibrosis and splenomegaly of HCL may lead to confusion of it with myelofibrosis. In fact, in some series of myelofibrosis, HCL was found retrospectively to be the true diagnosis in a significant number of cases. HCL may have aplastic presentations and there are examples of HCL with lytic lesions or aseptic necrosis of the femoral head. About 10% of HCL patients have no splenomegaly at presentation. HCL is also associated with a predilection for atypical mycobacterial infections and fungal disease. Vasculitis and paraproteinemia have also been observed in HCL.

In the past, the mainstay of treatment for HCL was splenectomy. Because HCL is often an indolent disorder, splenectomy was often beneficial, resulting in improved peripheral counts. The discovery that interferon-α was an effective form of therapy inaugurated the modern era of therapy for HCL, but interferon-α is expensive and associated with flulike symptoms and a high relapse rate off-therapy. Complete remissions of HCL have been achieved with 2-deoxycoformycin but at the cost of severe immune suppression. Recently, remarkable success in the treatment of HCL was achieved with 2-chlorodeoxyadenosine (2-CdA).

Reference: Golomb HM, et al: Hairy cell leukemia: A clinical review based on 71 cases. Ann Intern Med 89:677, 1978.

LEUKEMOID REACTION

A leukemoid reaction is defined as a peripheral leukocyte count greater than 25,000 to 30,000 cells/mm³ (although some authors use the more stringent definition of 50,000 cells/mm³). In the most common type of leukemoid reaction, the WBC count is elevated because of an increased number of myeloid cells in the peripheral blood. The blood smear shows a left shift, with bands, metamyelocytes, myelocytes, and even promyelocytes or blasts in severe cases. If infection is the cause of the leukocytosis, neutrophils may show toxic granulations, Döhle bodies, or cytoplasmic vacuoles. A myeloid leukemoid reaction with blasts, myelocytes, and promyelocytes may be confused with CML, but the two can usually be distinguished by the leukocyte alkaline phosphatase (LAP) blood test and/or a bone marrow karyotype.

Leukemoid Reaction Versus CML

TEST	LEUKEMOID REACTION	CML
LAP score	High or normal	Low
Philadelphia chromosome in bone marrow	Absent	Present

Blasts and mature neutrophils in the peripheral blood without any intermediate neutrophil precursors (leukemic hiatus) suggest acute leukemia rather than a leukemoid reaction. However, this pattern can sometimes also occur with TB, alcoholic hepatitis, or recovery from agranulocytosis. Leukemoid reactions involving lymphoid cells also occur, most often in young patients with pertussis or infectious mononucleosis.

Causes of Leukemoid Reaction

A. Primary
- Hereditary neutrophilia, chronic idiopathic neutrophilia
- Leukocyte adhesion factor deficiency
- Down's syndrome, congenital anomalies

B. Secondary
1. Acute infection
   - Bacterial: staphylococcal pneumonia, meningococcal meningitis, pertussis, *Salmonella* sepsis, *Shigella* dysentery, pneumococcal endocarditis, diphtheria, bubonic plague
   - Disseminated TB
   - Viral: infectious mononucleosis (EBV and CMV), infectious hepatitis, mumps
2. Neoplasms
   - Lung cancer, other solid tumors
   - Hodgkin's disease, multiple myeloma, myelofibrosis
   - Many types of cancer metastatic to bone marrow
3. Intoxications
   - Drug reactions, mercury poisoning
   - Severe burns, eclampsia
4. Severe blood loss
   - Hemorrhage, hemolysis

Table continued on next page.

Causes of Leukemoid Reaction (Cont.)

5. Miscellaneous
   - DKA
   - RA, ulcerative colitis
   - Recovery from agranulocytosis
   - Alcoholic hepatitis

Reference: Athens JW: Variations of leukocytes in disease. In Lee GR, et al (eds): Wintrobe's Clinical Hematology, 9th ed. Malvern, PA, Lea and Febiger, 1993, pp 1579–1581.

LEUKOPENIA

Leukopenia results when there is decreased production or increased destruction of WBCs. A low peripheral WBC count may be caused by a decreased number of polymorphonuclear leukocytes (neutropenia), a decreased number of lymphocytes (lymphocytopenia), or both. Neutropenia and lymphocytopenia are defined as having absolute values below 1,500 cells/mm^3 in the adult. The following conditions may result in leukopenia.

Causes of Leukopenia

A. Congenital
   - Benign familial leukopenia, chronic benign neutropenia of infancy and childhood
   - Cyclic neutropenia, chronic idiopathic neutropenia
   - Kostmann's syndrome (infantile agranulocytosis)
   - Shwachman-Diamond-Oski syndrome, Chédiak-Higashi syndrome
   - Immunodeficiency disorders: DiGeorge syndrome, severe combined immunodeficiency, reticular dysgenesis
B. Acquired
   1. Infections
      - Bacterial: typhoid, paratyphoid, brucellosis, tularemia (rarely), *Staphylococcus aureus*
      - Viral: influenza, measles, infectious hepatitis, chicken pox, rubella, Colorado tick fever, dengue, yellow fever, sandfly fever, AIDS
      - Rickettsial: rickettsial pox, typhus, Rocky Mountain spotted fever
      - Protozoal: malaria, kala-azar, relapsing fever
      - All types of overwhelming infections, such as miliary TB and sepsis (especially in debilitated adults or newborns)
   2. Physical agents, chemicals, and drugs
      - Ionizing radiation, benzene
      - Chemotherapy: alkylating agents, antimetabolites, anthracyclines
      - Drugs: colchicine, aminopyrine, phenothiazines, sulfonamides, antithyroid drugs, nonsteroidal antiinflammatory drugs, anticonvulsants, antihistamines, meprobamate, semisynthetic penicillins, chloramphenicol, many others
   3. Decreased or ineffective production of leukocytes
      - Pernicious anemia, folate deficiency, malnutrition/debilitated states (e.g., alcoholism)
      - Aplastic anemia, chronic hypochromic anemia, myelodysplastic syndromes

Table continued on next page.

Causes of Leukopenia (Cont.)

---

4. Myelophthisis in bone marrow
   • Myelofibrosis, leukemia, metastatic cancer
5. Increased utilization, physical destruction, or sequestration
   • Liver cirrhosis with splenomegaly, other hypersplenic states, Gaucher's disease, uremia, hemodialysis
6. Immune-mediated destruction or suppression
   • SLE, Felty's syndrome, thymoma
   • Anaphylactoid shock, acute immunologic reactions

From Athens, JW: Neutropenia. In Lee GR, et al (eds): Wintrobe's Clinical Hematology, 9th ed. Malvern, PA, Lea and Febiger, 1993, p 1590, with permission.

To determine the absolute neutrophil or lymphocyte count, the WBC count is multiplied by the percentage of mature neutrophils and bands, or the percentage of lymphocytes, and then divided by 100. The danger of serious infection rises sharply if the absolute neutrophil count drops below 500 cells/mm^3. Severely neutropenic patients may show few clinical signs of infection because of the lack of inflammatory cells. When such patients become febrile, they should be hospitalized and managed aggressively with IV antibiotics. Therapy should be continued until the patient is afebrile and the absolute neutrophil count is above 500. The use of colony-stimulating factors such as G-CSF (granulocyte colony-stimulating factor) or GM-CSF (granulocyte-monocyte colony-stimulating factor) may be considered in cases of prolonged neutropenia.

LOW BACK PAIN

LBP is an extremely common complaint. In a frustratingly high number of cases, a definite etiology cannot be established. However, by means of a standard approach to Hx & PE, it is possible to make a presumptive diagnosis and determine which patients need further investigation (imaging) and referral because of the possibility of serious disease. Only a minority of patients with back pain need diagnostic imaging, including plain radiographs.

LBP can be caused by musculoligamentous injuries; degenerative changes in discs and facet joints; nerve root irritation from a herniated nucleus pulposus; spinal stenosis; anatomic abnormalities of the spine such as scoliosis; systemic disease such as neoplasm, spinal osteomyelitis, or ankylosing spondylitis; and diseases of the internal organs and vessels such as pyelonephritis and dissecting aortic aneurysm.

The history should include questions about the pain itself (mode of onset, duration, point of maximal intensity, radiation, worsening factors, easing factors), specific activities the pain makes it impossible to do, occupation, previous attacks, and prior back surgery and other past medical history. It is also important to elicit generalized symptoms such as fever and weight loss, because these suggest that osteomyelitis or neoplasm involving the spine may be the etiology of the pain. (However, vertebral osteomyelitis and epidural metastasis account for <2% of cases of LBP.)

The examination should include inspection of the posture and the shape and curvature of the back. Having the patient repeatedly flex and extend the spine helps localize pain. Two passive stretch tests should be performed: the straight-leg-raising test for sciatic nerve irritation and the femoral stretch test for irritation of the femoral nerve (L-2, L-3, L-4 nerve root). L-5 conduction should be tested by examining ankle dorsiflexion, great toe extension, and hip abductor strength. S-1 conduction should be tested by examining plantar flexion, the ankle reflex, and gluteus maximus strength. (The great majority of persons with a herniated nucleus pulposus have abnormal L-5 or S-1 conduction tests.) Saddle sensation (S-3, S-4, S-5) should be tested. (Saddle anesthesia plus decreased anal sphincter tone suggest cauda equina syndrome.) Finally, Babinski's reflexes should be elicited. (An upgoing toe indicates an upper motor neuron lesion.)

It has been suggested that the Hx & PE of a patient with LBP should be conducted so that three questions can be answered after the evaluation:

1. Is a serious systemic disease (cancer, spinal infection, osteoporotic compression fracture, ankylosing spondylitis) causing the pain?
2. Is there neurologic compromise (disc herniation, spinal stenosis, cauda equina syndrome) that might require surgical evaluation?
3. Is there social or psychological distress amplifying or prolonging the pain?

In the great majority of patients presenting with LBP, the answers to the first two questions are no. Imaging studies and referral are needed when the answer is maybe or yes.

References: Deyo RA, et al: What can the history and physical examination tell us about low back pain? JAMA 268:760–765, 1992.

Hall H: A simple approach to back pain management. Patient Care (Dec 15):77–98, 1992.

LUNG CANCER

Lung cancer is the leading cause of cancer death in the United States, accounting for 35% of male deaths and 21% of female deaths. About 80 to 90% of the mortality is directly related to smoking. However, of people who smoke, only 1 of 11 develop lung cancer, supporting the theory that genetic predisposition may be an important factor. It is known that women develop lung cancer at a younger age with a smaller pack-year history. There is a 35 to 53% increase in lung cancer for nonsmokers who live with smokers, and wives of smokers have a two to three times increased risk of developing lung cancer. Another risk factor is radon exposure, with 25% of cancer in nonsmokers and 5% in smokers attributed to this substance. Investigations into effects of diet have been done and are inconclusive, but it is possible that vitamin A, selenium, and vitamin E confer a protective effect.

The most common cell types in smokers are squamous and adenocarcinoma, each accounting for about 35 to 40% of cases. Other cell types are small cell (about 25% of cases) and large cell. In nonsmokers, adenocarcinoma accounts for 55 to 70% of cases.

Large-scale screening with CXRs and/or sputum cytologies has not been shown to have an impact on survival and is not cost-effective, but current recommendations by the National Cancer Institute recommend yearly CXRs for those at risk. Obviously, this is much more important for smokers.

Tumor-associated genes for lung cancer as well as cancer suppression appear to be on chromosome 3, although 11 and 18 are also implicated. The effect of these markers continues to intrigue investigators.

The staging of lung cancer is by an American joint committee TMN system and correlates well with survival. However, other prognostic factors in lung cancer include systemic signs such as fever, weight loss, and performance status.

Treatment of lung cancer is curative only in the very early stages of non-small-cell lung cancer, when surgery is possible. For small-cell lung cancer, impressive responses have been achieved with chemotherapy, but long-term survivors remain few. For localized but unresectable stages of non-small-cell lung cancer, radiation therapy is often palliative, and a few long-term survivals are seen. Radiation therapy is most useful in controlling symptoms of bone and brain metastases.

Agents Implicated in the Development of Lung Cancer

CARCINOGEN	EXPOSURE SOURCE	ASSOCIATED LESIONS
Arsenic	Pesticides, smelters	Keratoses of palms and soles
Asbestos	Miners, millers, fitters, shippers	Pulmonary asbestosis, asbestos bodies in sputum
Bis-chloromethyl ether	Plastics, chemical workers	None
Chromate	Smelters	Perforated nasal septum
Hematite	Miners	None
Isopropyl oils	Chemical workers	None
Nickel (carbonyl)	Miners, refiners, shippers	Nasal polyps, chronic dermatitis
Radioisotopes	Miners (uranium), fluorspar, iron ore	None
Radon	Homes	None
Soot, tars, oils	Oil refiners, asphalt workers, coke oven workers	Chromic dermatitis, photosensitivity, warts

LUNG NODULES

Solitary Pulmonary Nodule

A pulmonary nodule can be described as a rounded lesion on CXR measuring less than 3 cm. Although no single characterisic or group of characteristics can definitely predict the nature of a solitary nodule, the following chart, differential diagnosis, and algorithm may be helpful.

Differentiation of Benign and Malignant Solitary Pulmonary Nodules

FACTORS	BENIGN	MALIGNANT
Clinical		
Age	<40 yrs (except with hamartoma)	>45 yrs
Sex	Female	Male
Symptoms	Absent	Present
Past history	Lives in area of high granuloma incidence, exposure to TB, mineral oil medication	Diagnosis of primary lesion elsewhere
Skin tests	Positive, usually with specific infectious organisms	Negative or positive
Roentgenographic		
Size	Small (<2 cm in diameter)	Large (>2 cm in diameter)
Location	No predilection (except for TB [upper lobes])	Predominantly upper lobes (except for lung metastases)

Table continued on next page.

Differentiation of Benign and Malignant Solitary Pulmonary Nodules (Cont.)

FACTORS	BENIGN	MALIGNANT
Definition and contour	Margins well defined and smooth	Margins ill defined, lobulated, umbilicated
Calcification	Almost pathognomonic of a benign lesion, particularly if of a laminated, multiple punctate, or popcorn variety	Very rare, may be eccentric (scar carcinoma)
Satellite lesions	More common	Less common
Serial studies with no change over 2 yrs	Almost diagnostic of a benign lesion	Most unlikely
Doubling time	<30 or >490 days	30–490 days

From Fraser RG, et al: Diagnosis of Diseases of the Chest, 3rd ed. Philadelphia, W. B. Saunders, 1989, p 1390, with permission.

Categories of Solitary Pulmonary Nodules

Malignant neoplasms
  Primary lung neoplasms
    Bronchogenic carcinoma—common*
    Bronchial adenoma—uncommon
    Alveolar cell carcinoma—uncommon
    Sarcoma—rare†
    Localized pulmonary lymphoma—rare*
  Solitary metastasis from extrathoracic source
    Carcinoma from GI tract, kidney, breast, etc.—relatively common (3 to 5% of SPNs)
    Sarcoma, melanoma, etc.—uncommon as solitary lesions; usually present as multiple nodules
Benign lesions
  Infectious granuloma—common‡
    Tuberculoma
    Histoplasma
    Coccidioma
    Miscellaneous types
  Benign neoplasma
    Hamartoma
    Dermoid—teratoma
    Tumorlith
    Miscellaneous lesions
  Cysts
    Bronchial
    Infections, e.g., echinococcal, dog worm
  Inflammatory
    Rheumatoid nodule
    Wegener's granuloma
    Organizing pneumonia
    Pulmonary infarct
    Foreign body
  Vascular
    AV malformation
    Varix
  Miscellaneous

*Approximately 90% of malignancies occur in cigarette smokers.
†Except in AIDS.
‡Incidence closely correlated with geographic epidemiology.
From Neff TA, et al: Asymptomatic solitary pulmonary nodule. In Schwarz MI (ed): Pulmonary Grand Rounds. Toronto, B. C. Decker, 1990, p 295, with permission.

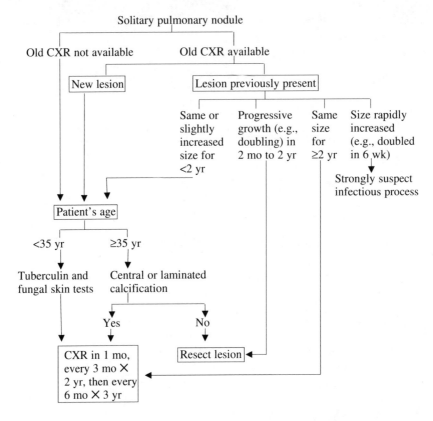

Guidelines for approaching the solitary pulmonary nodule. (From Casciato DA, Lowitz BB: Manual of Clinical Oncology, 2nd ed. Boston. Little, Brown, 1988, p 120, with permission.)

Multiple Pulmonary Nodules

Types of Multiple Pulmonary Nodules

CATEGORY	ETIOLOGY	CAVITATION
Developmental	Pulmonary AV fistula	No
Infectious	Pyemic abscesses	Common, thick walls
	Pseudomonas pseudomallei	Common
	Coccidioides immitis	Common, thick or thin walls
	Histoplasma capsulatum	No
	Paragonimus westermani	Common
Immunologic	Wegener's granulomatosis	Common, thick irregular walls
	Rheumatoid necrobiotic nodules	Common, thick smooth walls

Table continued on next page.

Types of Multiple Pulmonary Nodules (Cont.)

CATEGORY	ETIOLOGY	CAVITATION
Neoplastic	Papilloma	Frequent
	Hematogenous metastasis	Rare, 4%, usually in upper lobes
	Non-Hodgkin's lymphoma	Rare
	Multiple myeloma (plasmacy-toma)	No
	Bronchopulmonary amyloidosis	Sometimes
Traumatic	Multiple pulmonary hematomas	No
Idiopathic	Sarcoidosis	No

Reference: Pare JA, et al: Synopsis of Diseases of the Chest. Philadelphia, W. B. Saunders, 1983, pp 778–783.

LYME DISEASE

Lyme disease is a multisystem disorder caused by the spirochete *Borrelia burgdorferi*. Originally described in 1976 after an unusual outbreak of childhood arthritis in Lyme, Connecticut, it is currently recognized as the most common vector-borne disease in the United States. The disease is now well recognized to have worldwide distribution. In Europe, the manifestations are slightly different and the condition is referred to as Bannworth syndrome or acrodermatitis. The distribution and timing of the illness reflect the spirochete's life cycle, its primary tick vector, and the tick's reservoir host.

In Europe, three species of spirochetes are known to produce disease, whereas in the United States, only *B. burgdorferi* has been implicated in producing disease. The natural host of *B. burgdorferi* is the ixodid tick. In the Northeastern United States, the disease is transmitted mostly by the nymphal stage of *Ixodid dammini*. The white-footed mouse is the primary reservoir host of the larval and nymphal stages of the tick. The uninfected larval tick acquires the spirochete by feeding on an infected mouse. By the next spring, the larva molts and an infected nymph develops. It may feed on the mouse (thus completing the cycle) or on humans. The seasonality of Lyme disease is explained, because the nymphs are active late in spring and early summer, which is the time that most cases of Lyme are reported. The nymph eventually molts to become an adult, which feeds once more (preferred host: the white-tailed deer), mates, and lays uninfected eggs (no vertical transmission); then the cycle begins again. In California, the cycle is more complicated. It is likely that there are several hosts and two different ixodid ticks required. This complex interaction is probably responsible for the relatively low rate of Lyme transmission in the Western United States.

Clinical manifestations: The classic manifestations of Lyme disease follow an established pattern. Although the tick may bite where it lands (usually on the lower limbs), it may migrate to the groin or axilla. Erythema chronicum migrans, the pathognomonic skin lesion of early Lyme disease, begins as a red macule at the site of the tick bite and expands. *B. burgdorferi* can often be isolated in the advancing edge. Subsequently, a flulike syndrome of generalized achiness, fatigue, and even arthralgia can present within the first 2 to 4 weeks. Two to 6 weeks after the onset of the rash, cardiac manifestations can occur. These often present as conduction abnormalities but cardiomyopathy has been documented. Probably less than 10% of patients develop cardiac manifestations. A sizable minority (20%) may subsequently develop neurologic manifestations. Cranial nerve palsies are the most common manifestations, but chronic neuropathy and rarely demyelinating conditions are seen.

The majority of untreated patients develop arthritis. Occasionally, arthritis can be the initial manifestation in patients who do not develop a rash or other earlier event. Knees are the most commonly involved joints, and popliteal cysts can be present. Occasionally, patients have arthralgia and chronic fatigue but do not develop frank synovitis.

The diagnosis can be quite difficult and is based primarily on the complete clinical picture. It is definitively established when the organism is isolated in culture, but this is rarely possible. Laboratory data can be quite helpful in detecting exposure to *B. burgdorferi* (antibody studies by ELISA).

Chronic manifestations of untreated Lyme include persistent arthritis, most commonly in the knees. Patients with DR4 or DR2 may have a higher predisposition to develop a chronic arthritis. This phenotype may also be a marker for poor response to treatment. Occasionally, there are chronic neurologic manifestations, including an encephalopathy and peripheral neuropathies.

Treatment: Treatment has improved significantly. Studies have shown that simple removal of the tick is probably sufficient to prevent early disease. Prophylactic treatment at the time of the tick bite has not been shown to be helpful. Early in the disease at the time of erythema chronicum migrans, amoxicillin or doxycycline can be quite successful. Once systemic manifestations have occurred, aggressive treatment probably should be pursued. Lumbar puncture should be undertaken in patients who develop headaches, Bell's palsy, or facial or peripheral paresthesias. If meningeal irritation appears present, IV antibiotics are required. A 4-week course of doxycycline is generally effective in individuals with Lyme arthritis. IV penicillin and ceftriaxone are also effective.

Reference: Steere AC: Current understanding of Lyme disease. Hosp Pract Apr:37–44, 1993.

LYMPHADENOPATHY

Benign Causes

Enlargement of lymph nodes requires investigation when there are one or more new nodes that are ≥ 1 cm in diameter and that are not known to have arisen from a previously recognized source.

Differential Diagnosis of Benign Lymphadenopathy

I. **Infectious diseases**
  A. Viral infections: infectious hepatitis, infectious mononucleosis (CMV, EBV), AIDS, rubella, varicella zoster, vaccinia
  B. Bacterial infections: staphylococci, *Salmonella, Brucella, Francisella tularensis, Listeria monocytogenes, Yersinia pestis, Haemophilus ducreyi,* cat-scratch disease
  C. Fungal infections: coccidioidomycosis, histoplasmosis
  D. Chlamydial infections: lymphogranuloma venereum, trachoma
  E. Mycobacterial infections: TB, leprosy
  F. Parasitic infections: trypanosomiasis, microfilariasis, toxoplasmosis
  G. Spirochetal diseases: syphilis, yaws, endemic syphilis (bejel), leptospirosis
II. **Immunologic diseases**
  A. Rheumatoid arthritis
  B. Systemic lupus erythematosus
  C. Dermatomyositis
  D. Serum sickness
  E. Drug reactions: phenytoin, hydralazine, allopurinol
  G. Angioimmunoblastic lymphadenopathy
III. **Endocrine diseases:** hyperthyroidism, adrenal insufficiency, hypopituitarism
IV. **Lipid storage diseases:** Gaucher's and Niemann-Pick diseases
V. **Miscellaneous diseases and diseases of unknown cause**
  A. Giant follicular lymph node hyperplasia
  B. Sinus histiocytosis
  C. Dermatopathic lymphadenitis
  D. Sarcoidosis
  E. Amyloidosis
  F. Mucocutaneous lymph node syndrome (Kawasaki's syndrome)
  G. Lymphomatoid granulomatosis
  H. Multifocal Langerhan's cell (eosinophilic) granulomatosis

Modified from Haynes BF: Enlargement of lymph nodes and spleen. In Braunwald E, et al (eds): Harrison's Principles of Internal Medicine, 11th ed. New York, McGraw-Hill, 1987, Table 55–1, p 274, with permission.

LYMPHOCYTES, ATYPICAL

Atypical, or reactive, lymphocytes are cells that have been stimulated and are actively synthesizing DNA. These lymphocytes are called atypical because their morphologic appearance deviates considerably from that of normal lymphocytes. Atypical lymphocytes are larger than normal lymphocytes, may have nuclei that are kidney bean shaped or convoluted, commonly have abundant cytoplasm (sometimes with vacuoles), and may exhibit cytoplasmic pseudopods and dark-blue staining of the periphery of the cytoplasm. In contrast, malignant lymphocytes have less nuclear chromatin clumping, may exhibit prominent nucleoli, and usually have very little cytoplasm. The lymphocyte population in disorders with reactive lymphocytosis (atypical lymphocytes) is generally quite heterogeneous morphologically, whereas in malignant lymphoid disorders involving the blood, there is much greater homogeneity in the appearance of the lymphoid cell population.

Disorders with Substantial Numbers of Atypical Lymphocytes

Infectious mononucleosis	CMV infection
HIV type I infection	Rubella
Reaction to phenytoin	Herpes simplex virus type II
or mephenytoin	Toxoplasmosis

Disorders with Small Numbers of Atypical Lymphocytes

Viral hepatitis	PAS hypersensitivity
Adenovirus infection	Other viral infections

Infectious mononucleosis is an infection of B lymphocytes by the EBV. Usually more than 50% of the leukocytes of the blood are lymphocytes with 20 to 80% atypical. Most of the atypical cells are T lymphocytes.

In patients with CMV infection, after the first few days, usually 20% or more of the lymphocytes are atypical. In an immunocompetent host, acute CMV infection causes a clinical picture quite similar to infectious mononucleosis, except that pharyngitis and palatal petechiae are infrequent and lymphadenopathy is less extensive.

In rubella, similar to EBV infection, there are enlarged posterior cervical lymph nodes and atypical lymphocytes. The rash of rubella distinguishes the two illnesses.

Early after contracting the virus, persons with HIV type I may experience an illness characterized by fever, malaise, enlarged lymph nodes, and atypical lymphocytes in the blood. These findings ordinarily disappear after a short time, and the patient remains asymptomatic for months or years.

On rare occasions, hypersensitivity to phenytoin or mephenytoin leads to an EBV-like illness with fever, malaise, generalized lymphadenopathy, splenomegaly, variable abnormalities in liver function tests, and numerous atypical lymphocytes in the blood. Withdrawal of the drug results in gradual disappearance of the features of the illness.

LYMPHOMA

Hodgkin's Lymphoma

This treatable lymphoma was recognized by Thomas Hodgkin, a physician at Guy's Hospital in London in 1832. The significant enlargement of the lymph nodes persuaded Hodgkin that this was a disease that could be differentiated clinically from TB, although Hodgkin did not have the benefit of a microscope. [Quick quiz in the history of medicine: Thomas Hodgkin was a member of the trio of famous physicians known as the Three Great Men of Guy's. Who were the other two? Answer is given in footnote.]

The very tissues that Hodgkin examined that formed the basis of his report have been resectioned and evaluated by more modern pathologists, and because of the remarkable preservation of the samples, Hodgkin's disease was confirmed in several. In one case there was underlying TB, which Hodgkin also recognized. The typical cell in Hodgkin's disease is the Reed-Sternberg cell, which may exist in the presence of reactive lymphocytes, plasma cells, eosinophils, and granulocytes. In the nodular sclerosing type, the Reed-Sternberg cell and its companions are swathed by bands of fibrosis. The presence of reactive lymphocytes suggests lymphocyte predominance.

Recently a type of large-cell lymphoma called T-cell-rich B-cell lymphoma has been recognized, which is often misdiagnosed as Hodgkin's disease. This disorder has large cells surrounded by a polyclonal reaction of T cells. The large cells, which account for only 10% of the cells, demonstrate B-cell immunologic markers and do not possess the Ki-1 antigen typically present on Reed-Sternberg cells. Patients typically respond better to non-Hodgkin's lymphoma treatment regimens such as CHOP. Diagnostic confusion also occurs between lymphocyte-depleted Hodgkin's disease and peripheral T-cell lymphomas. These confusions reflect the ever-increasing need for expert pathologists and determination of the presence of surface markers in Hodgkin's and non-Hodgkin's lymphomas.

Hodgkin's disease may present as a painless, enlarging lymph node or may be asymptomatic and discovered as a mediastinal mass on routine CXR. Hodgkin's may be diagnosed as the consequence of an evaluation for FUO. Patients may have fever and other B symptoms such as weight loss and night sweats. Pruritus and ichthyosis are skin manifestations of Hodgkin's disease. Some patients describe unusual pain when drinking alcohol in the site of an involved lymph node or chest mass. Hodgkin's disease is also manifested by autoimmune disease. Patients may present with ITP during active Hodgkin's disease, or ITP may develop in the patient during remission. Autoimmune hemolytic anemia, glomerulonephritis and nephrotic syndrome, and arthritis are features of Hodgkin's disease. Hodgkin's disease patients are susceptible to unusual infections and, when splenectomized for staging purposes, prone to postsplenectomy pneumococcal sepsis. Some patients with Hodgkin's disease have a striking eosinophilia, and rare cases of eosinophilic meningitis have been described as well.

The staging of Hodgkin's disease is also a critical issue. Patients should have an adequate biopsy of a lymph node or mediastinal mass. In addition to routine blood counts and chemistry, a determination of LFTs and an ESR should be obtained. CT scans of the chest and abdomen and lymphangiograms are also routinely obtained. A bone marrow examination is also a necessary part of the evaluation. If indicated, a liver biopsy should be obtained. If the bone marrow is unremarkable and limited disease is present, then most physicians consider a staging laparotomy to determine the pathological stage. The general rule is that results of the laparotomy should change the therapy. If radiotherapy is to be combined with chemotherapy, there is no need for laparotomy. Laparotomy followed by mantle radiotherapy remains a good approach to the treatment of limited disease. The need for staging laparotomy is controversial in certain circumstances and might be avoided in patients with B symptoms or large mediastinal masses, who should receive combined modality treatment or chemotherapy. Negative laparotomies are frequent in patients with clinical stage IA, lymphocyte-predominant disease, and disease limited to the submandibular space.

Because the results of therapy in Hodgkin's disease are so good, there are a significant number of long-term survivors cured of their disease. In these patients, the late consequences of mantle radiation and chemotherapy can be sources of major morbidity and even mortality. Primary care physicians should be aware of these late complications (see table) and should take steps to recognize them when they occur.

Late Effects of Therapy and Prolonged Survival in Hodgkin's Disease

A. Hematologic	
Myelodysplastic syndrome	Acute myelogenous leukemia
Non-Hodgkin's lymphoma	
B. Neurologic	
Chronic progressive myelopathy	Peripheral neuropathy
(reversible form with Lhermitte's sign,	Brachial plexopathy
paresthesias, weakness, incontinence,	Lumbosacral plexopathy
paraplegia)	Cranial neuropathy

Table continued on next page.

Late Effects of Therapy and Prolonged Survival in Hodgkin's Disease (Cont.)

C. Endocrine	
Hypothyroidism	Infertility
D. Cardiovascular	
Accelerated CAD	Arrhythmias, conduction system disease
Cardiomyopathy	
Pericarditis	
E. Pulmonary	
Radiation pneumonitis	Fibrosis
Spontaneous pneumothorax	
F. Skeletal system	
Scoliosis	Avascular necrosis of the femoral or
Osteoporosis	humoral head
G. Solid tumors	
H. Infection/immunity	
Meningitis	Pneumonia
Postsplenectomy sepsis	

Answer to quick quiz: Thomas Addison and William Bright.
Reference: Urba WJ, et al: Hodgkin's disease. N Engl J Med 327:678–687, 1992.

Non-Hodgkin's Lymphoma

Classification

The non-Hodgkin's lymphomas constitute a diverse group of disorders in respect to both histologic features and clinical manifestations. Currently, the most useful classification is that of the Working Formulation, which in 1982 defined three broad groups of non-Hodgkin's lymphoma:

1. *Low grade:* low aggressiveness of the malignancy, favorable prognosis
2. *Intermediate grade*
3. *High grade:* usually a highly malignant, aggressive disorder with a poor prognosis when untreated

Classification of Non-Hodgkin's Lymphoma

WORKING FORMULATION TERMINOLOGY	RAPPAPORT TERMINOLOGY	% OF CASES
Low-grade lymphoma		
Small lymphocytic	Diffuse well-differentiated lymphoma (DWDL)	4
Follicular small cleaved	Nodular poorly differentiated lymphoma (NPDL)	25
Follicular mixed	Nodular mixed lymphoma (NML)	9
Intermediate-grade lymphoma		
Follicular large cell	Nodular histiocytic lymphoma (NHL)	4
Diffuse small cleaved	Diffuse poorly differentiated lymphocytic lymphoma (DPDL)	8
Diffuse mixed	Diffuse mixed lymphoma (DML)	8
Diffuse large cell	Diffuse histiocytic lymphoma (DHL)	22
High-grade lymphoma		
Immunoblastic	Diffuse histiocytic lymphoma (DHL)	9
Lymphoblastic	Lymphoblastic lymphoma (LBL)	5
Small noncleaved	Diffuse undifferentiated lymphoma (DUL)	6

The ten-year survival of patients with non-Hodgkin's lymphoma is:

Low grade	45%
Intermediate grade	26%
High grade	23%

Intermediate-grade and high-grade lymphomas are potentially curable in some patients, whereas low-grade lymphomas are rarely curable, but patients with low-grade lymphomas may have extended survival because of lack of aggressiveness of the malignancy.

The aforementioned non-Hodgkin's lymphomas are usually of B-cell lymphoid lineage except that

- 1 to 2% of small lymphocytic lymphomas are T cell.
- Diffuse, small-cleaved cell lymphomas are occasionally T cell.
- Diffuse mixed and diffuse large-cell lymphomas may be either B cell or T cell, with B-cell somewhat exceeding T-cell lineage in frequency.
- Lymphoblastic lymphomas are of T-cell lineage.

Lymphoblastic lymphomas are subdivided into convoluted-cell and non-convoluted-cell types. Small noncleaved-cell lymphomas are divided into Burkitt's cell lymphoma and non-Burkitt's lymphoma.

There are several non-Hodgkin's lymphomas in addition to those shown in the table:

- Mycosis fungoides (CD4 T-cell lymphoma)
- Adult T-cell lymphoma (a lymphoma of CD4 lymphocytes due to the HTLV-I retrovirus)
- True histiocytic lymphoma
- Malignant histiocytosis (histiocytic medullary reticulosis)
- Lymphomatoid granulomatosis (poorly defined illness presenting as prelymphoma or actual lymphoma)

References: Simon R, et al: The non-Hodgkin lymphoma pathologic classification project. Ann Intern Med 109:939–945, 1988.

The Non-Hodgkin Lymphoma Pathologic Classification Project: National Cancer Institute sponsored study of classifications of non-Hodgkin's lymphomas: Summary and description of a working formulation for clinical usage. Cancer 49:2112–2135, 1982.

MALABSORPTION

Clinically, malabsorption is generally recognized as malabsorption of dietary fat. Based on the normal physiology of digestion and absorption, fat malabsorption can be divided into three categories: intraluminal maldigestion, mucosal malabsorption, and postmucosal malabsorption related to lymphatic obstruction.

The following tables and approach to the patient with malabsorption are based on these broad categories.

Causes of Malabsorption

I. Intraluminal maldigestion
    Chronic liver disease and bile duct obstruction
    Bacterial overgrowth
    Pancreatic exocrine insufficiency
II. Mucosal malabsorption
    Drugs (colchicine, neomycin, para-aminosalicylic acid)
    Infectious diseases (*Giardia, Isospora, Strongyloides, Mycobacterium avium-intracellulare*)
    Immune diseases (systemic mastocytosis, eosinophilic gastroenteritis)
    Tropical sprue
    Celiac sprue
    Whipple's disease
    Abetalipoproteinemia
III. Postmucosal obstruction
    Intestinal lymphangiectasia (congenital, posttraumatic, lymphoma, carcinoma, Whipple's disease)
IV. Mixed causes of steatorrhea
    Short bowel syndrome
    Metabolic diseases (thyrotoxicosis, adrenal insufficiency, protein-calorie malnutrition)

The following two tables characterize signs and symptoms commonly seen in patients with malabsorption, mechanisms for these problems, and laboratory tests that may help delineate the exact type of malabsorptive process and its location. In general, the clinical history may lead to a suspicion of one of the three major classes of malabsorptive disease. If mucosal disease is suspected, then a D-xylose absorption test combined with small bowel biopsy are likely to be of high yield. A 72-hr stool fat collection is imperative to document the presence or absence of malabsorption but is not specific as to the cause. If impaired intraluminal digestion is suspected, then tests aimed at detecting bacterial overgrowth or pancreatic disease should be performed. If lymphatic obstruction is suspected, then small bowel biopsy may be of high yield in detecting the abnormality.

Correlation of Clinical Manifestations, Pathophysiology, and Laboratory Findings in Malabsorptive Processes

SIGNS AND SYMPTOMS	PATHOPHYSIOLOGIC MECHANISM	LABORATORY ABNORMALITIES
Gastrointestinal		
Diarrhea	Malabsorption of fat, cholesterol, and protein	Stool weights >200 g
	Increased secretion due to crypt hyperplasia, inflammatory mediators, bile and fatty acids	Stool weight ↓ to normal with fast
		Stool osmotic gap >100 mOsm/kg H_2O [Na] <60 mmol/L
Weight loss	Nutrient malabsorption, anorexia in mucosal diseases	↑ stool fat, ↓ serum proteins
Flatulence, borborygmus, abdominal distention, foul-smelling stools	Bacterial fermentation of malabsorbed carbohydrates and proteins	↑ flatus production
Bulky, greasy stools	Fat malabsorption	↑ stool fat, low serum carotene
Abdominal pain	If severe, due to chronic pancreatitis	
	If mild, distention of bowel and inflammation	
Hematopoietic		
Anemia	Fe, pyridoxine, folate, and B_{12} deficiency	Microcytic, macrocytic, or dimorphic anemia
Hemorrhagic diathesis	Vitamin K deficiency	Prolonged PT
Musculoskeletal		
Bone pain (osteopenic bone disease)	Ca, vitamin D, and protein malabsorption	Hypocalcemia, hypophosphatemia, ↑ serum alkaline phosphatase
Tetany	Ca, Mg, vitamin D malabsorption	Above, plus hypomagnesemia
Endocrine		
Amenorrhea, infertility, impotence	Malabsorption with protein-caloric malnutrition	Low serum proteins; may have abnormalities in gonadotropin secretion
Secondary hyperparathyroidism	Probably vitamin D and Ca deficiency	↑ alkaline phosphatase, increased serum PTH
Skin and mucous membranes		
Cheilosis, glossitis, stomatitis	Iron, riboflavin, niacin, folate, and B_{12} deficiency	Low serum Fe, folate B_{12}
Purpura	Vitamin K deficiency	Prolonged PT
Follicular hyperkeratosis	Vitamin A deficiency	Low serum carotene
Scaly dermatitis or acrodermatitis	Zinc and EFA deficiency	Low serum or urinary Zn
Hyperpigmented dermatitis	Niacin deficiency	
Edema and/or ascites	Protein malabsorption	Low serum albumin
Nervous system		
Xerophthalmia and night blindness	Vitamin A deficiency	↓ serum carotene
Peripheral neuropathy	Vitamin B, thiamine deficiency	↓ serum B_{12}

From Trier JS: Intestinal malabsorption: Differentiation of cause. Hosp Pract 23:195, 1988, with permission.

Comparison of Laboratory Results in the Three Types of Malabsorption

TEST	MUCOSAL DISEASE	IMPAIRED LUMINAL DIGESTION		LYMPHATIC OBSTRUCTION
		Pancreatic Disease	Bacterial Overgrowth	
Stool fat	↑↑	↑↑↑	↑	↑↑
Intestinal biopsy	Abnormal	Normal	Mildly abnormal	Usually abnormal
Screening (blood) tests of malabsorption				
PT	May be ↓	May be ↓	May be ↓	May be ↓
Serum carotene	↓	↓	May be ↓	↓
Serum cholesterol	↓	↓	↓	↓
Serum albumin	↓	Normal	May be ↓	↓
Serum Fe	↓	Normal	Normal	Normal
Serum folate	↓	Normal	Normal	Normal
Serum B_{12}	Normal	Normal	May be ↓	Normal
Specific malabsorption tests				
^{14}C-triolein breath test	↓	↓	↓	↓
D-Xylose absorption	↓	Normal	May be ↓	Normal
Schilling test	Normal	↓	↓	Normal
Breath tests (H_2, ^{14}C-xylose, or ^{14}C-cholylglycine)	Normal or abnormal	Normal	Abnormal	Normal
Bentiromide test	Normal or ↓	Normal or ↓	?	Normal

From Trier JS: Intestinal malabsorption: Differentiation of cause. Hosp Pract 23:195, 1988, with permission.

MALARIA

Chemoprophylaxis for Malaria*

ORGANISMS AND ANTIMALARIAL AGENT	DOSE
Plasmodium vivax, P. ovale, P. malariae, and chloroquine-susceptible P. falciparum:	
Chloroquine phosphate (Aralen)	300 mg of base (500 mg of chloroquine phosphate) per week

Table continued on next page.

Chemoprophylaxis for Malaria* (Cont.)

ORGANISMS AND ANTIMALARIAL AGENT	DOSE
Chloroquine-resistant *P. falciparum:*	
Mefloquine (Lariam)	228 mg base (250 mg salt) orally once/ week beginning 1 week before travel and continuing for 4 weeks after departure from malarious areas
Doxycycline (Vibramycin)†	100 mg/day
Proguanil (Paludrine)	200 mg/day orally
Pyrimethamine-sulfadoxine (Fansidar)	1 tablet (25 mg of pyrimethamine + 500 mg of sulfadoxine) per week
Late relapse caused by *P. vivax* or *P. ovale:*	
Primaquine phosphate	15 mg of base (26.3 mg of salt) per day for 14 days with the last 2 weeks of chloroquine chemoprophylaxis

*Chemoprophylaxis should begin 1 week before departure. This permits monitoring for tolerance of the drug(s) and any required changes in the regimen. Chemoprophylaxis should be continued for 4 to 6 weeks after leaving the endemic area to protect against symptomatic parasitemia from infections acquired shortly before departure (6 weeks for chloroquine; 4 weeks for doxycycline, proguanil, and pyrimethamine-sulfadoxine). Doxycycline plus chloroquine has been used more extensively in Southeast Asia, whereas the proguanil-plus-chloroquine combination has been used more extensively in East Africa. Pyrimethamine-sulfadoxine plus chloroquine has been used in both Southeast Asia and Africa but has been associated with serious reactions.

†A number of investigators now suggest using doxycycline without chloroquine for chemoprophylaxis of chloroquine-resistant *P. falciparum.*

Modified from Herwaldt BL, et al: Antimalarial agents: Specific chemoprophylaxis regimens. Antimicrob Agents Chemother 32:953–956, 1988.

Clinical and Laboratory Differentiation of Malarial Types

CHARACTERISTICS	P. FALCIPARUM	P. VIVAX	P. OVALE	P. MALARIAE
Incubation period (days):				
Range	8–25	8–27	9–17	15–40
Mean	12	14	15	
Erythrocyte cycle (hrs)	48	48	48	72
Duration of malarial attack (wks)	Up to 2	2–4	2–4	4–8
Persistent extraerythrocytic stages	No	Yes	Yes	No
Parasitemia (/mm^3):				
Average	50,000–500,000	20,000	9,000	6,000
Maximum	Up to 2,500,000	50,000	30,000	20,000
Multiple infection of RBC	Usual	Rare	Rare	Rare
Duration of untreated infection (yrs)	0.5–2.0	1.5–4.0	1.5–4.0	1–30
Forms in circulation	Rings and gametocytes	All	All	All
Gametocyte shape	Crescent	Oval	Oval	Oval
Age of infected RBCs	All ages	Younger	Younger	Older

Modified from Brown HW, et al: Basic Clinical Parasitology, 5th ed. Norwalk, CT, Appleton-Century-Crofts, 1983, p 80.

Treatment of Malaria

ORGANISM(S) AND DRUG	TREATMENT
Plasmodium vivax, P. ovale, P. malariae,* and chloroquine-susceptible *P. falciparum:	
Chloroquine regimens	
PO	600 mg of base (10 mg of base/kg; 1,000 mg of chloroquine phosphate) initially, followed by an additional 300 mg of base (5 mg of base/kg) in 6 hrs and again on days 2 and 3
IM	2.5 mg of base/kg every 4 hrs or 3.5 mg of base/kg every 6 hrs (total dose not to exceed 25 mg of base/kg)
IV	10 mg of base/kg over 4 hrs, followed by 5 mg of base/kg every 12 hrs (given by infusion over ≥1 hr) until the patient is alert (total dose not to exceed 25 mg of base/kg)
P. vivax, P. ovale, P. malariae,* and chloroquine-resistant *P. falciparum:	
Quinidine regimens*	
IV quinidine gluconate for adults	24 mg of quinidine gluconate/kg (15 mg of base/kg) over 4 hrs, followed by 12 mg of quinidine gluconate/kg (7.5 mg of base/kg) over 2–4 hrs every 8 hrs
Pyrimethamine-sulfadoxine regimen	3 tablets (75 mg of pyrimethamine and 1,500 mg of sulfadoxine) in a single
PO	dose
Mefloquine regimens for mild to moderate *P. falciparum* or *P. vivax:*	
Oral mefloquine alone	1,000 or 1,500 mg of base as a single dose (25 mg of base/kg)
Oral mefloquine plus pyrimethamine-sulfadoxine	750 mg of mefloquine base plus 3 pyrimethamine-sulfadoxine tablets (75 mg of pyrimethamine plus 1,500 mg of sulfadoxine)
To prevent relapses of *P. vivax* and *P. ovale* after leaving endemic areas:	
Primaquine	15 mg base (26.3 mg salt) orally, once/day for 14 days or 45 mg base (70 mg salt) orally once/week for 8 weeks

*Oral doses are as with IV quinidine, using quinidine sulfate capsules (248 mg of base per 300 mg of quinidine sulfate).

Modified from Krogstad DJ, et al: Antimalarial agents: Specific treatment regimens. Antimicrob Agents Chemother 32:957–961, 1988, p 958.

MAMMOGRAPHY

Breast cancer currently affects one out of every eight women in the United States. The chance of curing a patient with breast cancer is best at the very earliest stages of cancer development, before the malignant cells have had an opportunity to disseminate. Randomized trials have shown that screening mammography can reduce breast cancer mortality by 20 to 30% by increasing the rate of detection of early breast cancers. Mammography can be used to screen asymptomatic women, to evaluate palpable breast lesions, or to follow up the contralateral breast in a patient who has had a mastectomy for breast cancer.

Characteristics of mammographic lesions suspicious for malignancy include:

- Spiculated, irregular, crablike densities
- Clusters of 5 or more microcalcifications within a 1-cm area
- Distortion of normal breast architecture without a benign explanation (such as a scar from a previous biopsy)

Because the quality of a mammogram depends highly on proper breast compression, imaging, and interpretation, it is essential that mammograms be performed by trained personnel and read by highly experienced radiographers. However, even in the best of situations, it is not always possible to determine if a mammographic abnormality represents a benign or malignant lesion. Adjunctive tests such as ultrasound or MRI may help to determine if a lesion is solid or infiltrative. If available, serial mammograms can be examined to assess whether changes are progressive over time. Questionable findings should be reviewed by a second trained mammographic radiologist before proceeding to biopsy.

For lesions that are suspicious for malignancy on mammogram, either fine-needle aspiration or surgical biopsy can be performed. Nonpalpable lesions seen on mammograms are localized by guide wire prior to biopsy. Mammography of the excised specimen will confirm that the mammographic abnormality has been removed.

It is important to remember that approximately 10 to 15% of breast cancers are not detectable by mammography, even if a mass is palpable. *A normal mammogram should not prevent a physician from obtaining a biopsy if the patient has a clinically suspicious lesion.*

The American Cancer Society advises that women should obtain screening mammography as follows:

Age	Recommendation
35–40	Obtain baseline mammogram
40–49	Screening mammogram every 1–2 yrs
50+	Annual mammogram

Women with increased risk factors for breast cancer should be tested more frequently. These include a mother or sister with breast cancer, a personal history of breast cancer, or a history of mantle irradiation for Hodgkin's disease (see also Cancer: Screening Recommendations). With modern mammographic techniques, the radiation dosage per mammogram is well under 1 rad, leading to an estimated 0.1% lifetime risk of radiogenic breast cancer for women who begin their screening at age 35. It is predicted that 93,000 breast cancers would be detected over the same period in a cohort following the same screening schedule.

References: Paulus DD, et al: Mammography and early breast cancer detection. Oncol Case Rep Rev 7:1–10, 1992.

France AC, et al: Controlling breast cancer in older women: The physician's role. Tex Med 88:68–70, 1992.

MARANTIC ENDOCARDITIS

Marantic endocarditis, also known as nonbacterial thrombotic endocarditis (NBTE), results from deposition of sterile fibrin thrombi on heart valves, without valve destruction. This type of endocarditis is most common in patients with mucinous adenocarcinomas of the lung, pancreas, stomach, and ovary. Marantic endocarditis has also been reported in nonmalignant states such as SLE, chronic rheumatic heart disease, various infections, and bone marrow transplants.

Clinical manifestations in marantic endocarditis arise because of embolization of valvular vegetations. Marantic endocarditis should be suspected in a cancer patient with any one of the following conditions:

- Arterial emboli to visceral organs
- Peripheral arterial insufficiency
- Acute multifocal neurologic disease
- Cerebrovascular accidents

Because the clinical signs of NBTE are subtle and nonspecific, a high index of suspicion is required to make the diagnosis before death. Heart murmurs and the other stigmata of bacterial endocarditis are typically absent. Vegetations are usually too small to be visualized by traditional 2-D echocardiography. Transesophageal and Doppler echocardiography may be helpful.

Treatment involves the use of anticoagulants or antiplatelet drugs. If removal of the underlying malignancy is possible, the condition may resolve. Otherwise, the prognosis is very poor.

Reference: Blanchard DG, et al: Nonbacterial thrombotic endocarditis: Assessment by transesophageal echocardiography. Chest 102:954–956, 1992.

MEDIASTINAL MASSES

Differential Diagnosis

The differential diagnosis of mediastinal masses should be guided by their location in the anterosuperior, middle, and posterior mediastinum.

Differential Diagnosis of Mediastinal Masses

1. Anterosuperior mediastinum
- Thymic tumor or cyst
- Germ cell neoplasm: teratoma, seminoma, nonseminomatous germ cell tumor, choriocarcinoma, endodermal sinus tumor
- Thyroid enlargement: goiter or carcinoma
- Malignant lymphadenopathy: lymphoma, leukemia, carcinoma
- Other lymphadenopathy: Castleman's disease, granulomatous disease, angioimmunoblastic lymphadenopathy
- Parathyroid tumor
- Mesenchymal neoplasm: lipoma, fibroma, hemangioma, lymphangioma
- Vascular disease: aortic aneurysm

2. Middle mediastinum
- Malignant lymphadenopathy: lymphoma, leukemia, carcinoma
- Infectious lymphadenopathy: fungus, TB, mononucleosis
- Primary tracheal neoplasms
- Other lymphadenopathy: Castleman's disease, granulomatous mediastinitis, amyloidosis
- Bronchogenic cyst
- Anterior cardiophrenic masses: pleuropericardial cysts, foramen of Morgagni hernia, pericardial fat pad or fat necrosis, enlarged diaphragmatic lymph nodes
- Vascular dilatation or aneurysm: pulmonary artery, azygos or hemiazygos veins, aorta

Table continued on next page.

Differential Diagnosis of Mediastinal Masses (Cont.)

3. **Posterior mediastinum**
   - Neurogenic tumor
   - Periaortic, periesophageal, paraspinal, or retrocrural adenopathy
   - Lateral meningocele
   - Intrathoracic goiter
   - Foregut cysts: bronchogenic, neurenteric, or gastroenteric cysts
   - Lymphangioma (cystic hygroma)
   - Esophageal lesions: carcinoma, diverticula, megaesophagus, hiatal hernia, varices
   - Hernia through the foramen of Bochdalek
   - Thoracic spine diseases: neoplasm, paraspinal abscess due to infectious spondylitis, traumatic paraspinal hematoma
   - Extramedullary hematopoiesis
   - Pancreatic pseudocyst
   - Mediastinal lipomatosis

The most common causes of mediastinal masses are:

1. *Adults:* neurogenic tumors, malignant lymphoma, thymoma, metastatic carcinoma, germ cell tumors, cysts
2. *Children:* neurogenic tumors, malignant lymphoma, teratomas, benign thyroid enlargement, foregut cysts

---

References: Kawashima A, et al: CT and MR evaluation of posterior mediastinal masses. Crit Rev Diagn Imag 33:311–367, 1992.

Weisbrod GL, et al: Mediastinal masses: Diagnosis with noninvasive techniques. Semin Thorac Cardiovasc Surg 4:3–22, 1992.

MENINGITIS

Aseptic Meningitis

Many conditions may present with a picture of acute meningitis. Although the vast majority of these diagnoses are infectious in nature, a minority respond to specific antiinfectious therapy. Many of these belong in the category of aseptic meningitis syndrome in that Gram stain and bacterial culture of CSF are negative. This is not to imply, however, that aseptic is equivalent to noninfectious.

Conditions Presenting as Acute Meningitis

Infectious diseases
Bacteria and spirochetes
    Streptococcus pneumoniae
    Neisseria meningitidis
    Haemophilus influenzae
    Streptococcus (particularly group B)
    Listeria monocytogenes
    Treponema pallidum

    Leptospires
    Staphylococcus aureus
    Pseudomonas aeruginosa
    Enteric gram-negative bacilli
    Staphylococcus epidermidis
    Propionibacterium acnes

Viruses
    Echovirus
    Coxsackievirus types A and B
    Enterovirus
    Mumps virus
    Herpes simplex virus types 1 and 2
    Epstein-Barr virus
    Human immunodeficiency virus

    Herpes zoster virus
    CMV
    California encephalitis virus
    St. Louis encephalitis virus
    Colorado tick fever virus
    Lymphocytic choriomeningitis virus
    Poliovirus

Parasites
    Naegleria
    Angiostrongylus

    Strongyloides stercoralis (hyperinfection syndrome)

Infections resembling acute meningitis
    Rickettsiosis and ehrlichiosis
    Brain abscess
    Epidural or subdural abscess

    Tuberculosis, cryptococcosis, and other forms of chronic meningitis
    Viral and other causes of encephalitis

Noninfectious causes of acute meningitis syndrome
    Mollaret's meningitis
    Drug-induced meningitis
    Epidermoid cyst of the meninges

From McGee ZA, et al: Acute meningitis. In Mandell GL, et al (eds): Principles and Practice of Infectious Diseases, 3rd ed. New York, Churchill Livingstone, 1990, p 743, with permission.

When most people speak of aseptic meningitis, they are referring to viral meningitis. From the foregoing table it is clear that a large number of viruses cause meningitis, but 80 to 90% of those with an eventual specific viral diagnosis are caused by echovirus, coxsackievirus types A and B, and enterovirus.

In viral meningitis, the specific neurologic symptoms usually begin within the first or second day following the more nonspecific systemic symptoms of fevers, sore throat, and myalgias. There is a sudden onset of headache, stiff neck, and photophobia. The presence of altered mental status represents a more diffuse encephalitis. Patients are generally younger than age 40 and present during the later summer and the fall months. A specific diagnosis requires submission of specimens of pharyngeal washings and stool, because CSF usually will not yield the organism.

CSF findings usually include the following:

- WBC   50–500 per mm^3
- WBC diff: lymphocytic (neutrophils may predominate in the first 12–24 hrs)
- Glucose   >50 mg/dl
- Protein   normal–150 mg/dl

These CSF findings should not be used as the sole evidence to exclude the possibility of bacterial meningitis nor to withhold antibiotics, for there is considerable overlap between these findings and those of bacterial etiologies. However, bacterial etiologies usually result in a higher CSF WBC count (250–1,000), neutrophilic predominance (>80%), lower glucose (<40 mg/dl), and higher protein (>100 mg/dl). A prudent course is to administer empiric antibiotic therapy while awaiting laboratory confirmation of negative cultures. Patients clinically improve within 48 hrs of presentation and often can be released at this time. Care must be taken to consider parameningeal processes as a source of the CSF abnormalities.

Bacterial Meningitis

The most common etiologies of bacterial meningitis are shown in the table.

Bacterial Causes of Meningitis

	NEONATES (≤1 MO) (%)	CHILDREN (1 MO–15 YRS) (%)	ADULTS (>15 YRS) (%)
S. pneumoniae	0–5	10–20	30–50
N. meningitis	0–1	25–40	10–35
H. influenzae	0–3	40–60	1–3
Streptococci	20–40 *	2–4	5
Staphylococci	5	1–2	5–15
Listeria	2–10	1–2	5
Gram-negative bacilli	50–60 †	1–2	1–10

*Almost all isolates from neonatal meningitis are group B streptococci.

†Of all cases of neonatal meningitis, *E. coli* accounts for about 40% and *Klebsiella-Enterobacter* for about 8%.

From Swartz MN: Bacterial meningitis. In Wyngaarden JB, et al (eds): Cecil Textbook of Medicine, 18th ed. Philadelphia, W. B. Saunders, 1988, p 1604, with permission.

In some cases, the clinical setting may give diagnostic clues to the etiologic agent. Meningitis due to *Streptococcus pneumoniae* is often associated with a focus of infection elsewhere. Acute otitis media or pneumonia is present in about half the cases of pneumococcal meningitis. Meningococcal meningitis may occur in outbreaks, among close contacts. Staphylococcal meningitis is most common following neurosurgical interventions and trauma with penetrating injuries. Of note is the dramatic decrease in serious illness due to *Haemophilus influenzae* type b as a result of immunization programs. As the immunized cohort advances in age, the above table will undoubtedly show a remarkable shift in the most common etiologies for children under 15 years of age.

Symptoms generally have an acute onset, with fever, headache, stiff neck, and vomiting followed by rapid progression to impaired cognition, with confusion, lethargy, and loss of consciousness.

Examination of CSF is the diagnostic procedure of choice and needs to be done expeditiously. In presentations that raise the possibility of an intracranial mass lesion, antibiotics may be administered while an imaging procedure is obtained, because cultures of the CSF should continue to yield the causative organism for up to an hour after antibiotic infusion. Antibiotics should not be withheld due to slow progression of the diagnostic evaluation, nor should CSF examination be approached less urgently because antibiotics have been given.

Clues to Specific Etiologies

Data Suggesting Specific Etiologic Agents for Meningitis

CLUES	MICROORGANISMS
Epidemiologic clues	
Age	
Neonates	*E. coli,* group B streptococci, *Listeria,* HSV 2
Infants <2 months	Group B streptococci, *Listeria, E. coli*
Children <10 years	Viruses, *H. influenzae,* pneumococci, meningococci
Young adults	Viruses, meningococci
Adults	Pneumococci, meningococci
Elderly	Pneumococci, gram-negative bacilli, *Listeria*
Epidemiology	
Summer and fall	Coxsackievirus or echovirus, leptospires
Hospital acquired	Gram-negative bacilli, staphylococci, *Candida*
Sibling with meningitis	Meningococci, *H. influenzae*
Swimming in fresh water	Amoebas
Handling hamsters or mice	Lymphocytic choriomeningitis
Contact with water frequented by rodents or domestic animals	Leptospires
Exposure to TB	*M. tuberculosis*
Prior meningitis	Pneumococci
Associated infection	
Upper respiratory infection	Viruses, *H. influenzae,* pneumococci, meningococci
Pneumonia	Pneumococci, meningococci
Sinusitis	Pneumococci, *H. influenzae,* anaerobic bacteria
Otitis	Pneumococci, *H. influenzae,* anaerobic bacteria
Cellulitis	Streptococci, staphylococci
Brain abscess	Anaerobes
Trauma	
Closed skull fracture	Pneumococci, gram-negative bacilli
Open skull fracture or craniotomy	Gram-negative bacilli, staphylococci
CSF otorrhea and rhinorrhea	Pneumococci, gram-negative bacilli, staphylococci, *H. influenzae*
Underlying condition	
Diabetes mellitus	Pneumococci, gram-negative bacilli, staphylococci, *Cryptococcus,* agents of mucormycosis
Alcoholism	Pneumococci
Leukemia, lymphoma	Pneumococci, gram-negative bacilli, *Cryptococcus, M. tuberculosis*
Steroid therapy	*Cryptococcus, M. tuberculosis*
AIDS	HIV, *Cryptococcus, M. tuberculosis*
Sickle-cell disease	Pneumococci
Cancer	*Listeria*

Modified from McGee ZA, et al: Acute meningitis. In Mandell GL, et al (eds): Principles and Practice of Infectious Diseases, 3rd ed. New York, Churchill Livingstone, 1990, p 750.

MENOPAUSE

Menopause is that period of time in a woman's life when there has been neither ovulation nor menstrual function for 6 months or more. It usually occurs between the ages of 48 and 55, but occurrence at a younger age is not unusual. The majority of women develop symptoms secondary to hypoestrogenism. Due to the longer life expectancy in the United States nowadays, most women live approximately one-third of their life after menopause.

By the time of menopause only a few thousand of the ovarian follicles with which a woman is born remain, and the follicles that remain are less sensitive to the stimulatory effects of FSH and LH, and they therefore secrete less estrogen. Initially, the length of the menstrual cycle shortens due to a reduced follicular phase, and the menses become scant. Then the cycle lengthens, finally disappearing entirely. During the years before climacteric, FSH increases due to the failure of the primordial follicles, but LH is usually normal. In addition, ovarian estradiol production is reduced markedly, and plasma levels decrease significantly from a mean of 160 to 13 pg/mL. In postmenopausal women, the main estrogen is estrone, and the adrenal glands contribute 70% of the androstenedione production, which is converted peripherally to estrone. Postmenopausal testosterone is either unchanged or greater than that of the premenopausal state, accounting for the changes in hair growth that may be seen. However, levels may not always be helpful in identifying menopause due to the wide variations in hormone production.

About 80% of menopausal women experience hot flashes for more than one year. These can occur before menopause because they are due to falling levels of estrogens rather than estrogens' total absence. Often a prodrome of 4 to 5 minutes occurs, with a sensation of pressure, headache, or palpitations. This is followed by a sensation of heat, which begins in the head, neck, and upper body, and then profuse diaphoresis. Weakness, fatigue, faintness, and vertigo may ensue. This may last from a few seconds to as long as 45 minutes. In some women, hot flashes during the night may cause enough sleep disturbance to produce cognitive and affective dysfunction. The hot flash is due to a sudden downward regulation of the thermoregulatory center in the anterior hypothalamus. Estrogen sensitivity alters hypothalamic sensitivity, resulting in greater pulsatile GnRH release and instability in the thermoregulatory center.

Results of estrogen deficiency include atrophy of the reproductive and genitourinary tracts, which leads to changes in the vaginal mucosa, with excessive dryness and dyspareunia. Urethral dryness causes dysuria, frequency, and urgency. Postmenopausal osteoporosis is also a major problem, leading to 100,000 radial fractures and 200,000 hip and vertebral fractures per year. About 25% of women over the age of 60 years and 50% of women over the age of 75 years will have vertebral fractures. With estrogen deficiency, the bone mass decreases, and bones become more brittle and more easily fractured. It is also known that the incidence of atherosclerotic heart disease increases significantly after menopause.

Estrogen therapy reverses or improves the subjective and objective changes that occur in menopause. It prevents osteoporosis, abolishes hot flashes, minimizes urethral and vaginal dryness, and decreases the incidence of atherosclerotic cardiovascular disease. Contraindications to estrogen therapy are breast or endometrial cancer, predisposition to thrombosis or history of stroke, liver disease, and hyperlipidemia. Careful thought must also be given when prescribing for patients who have

seizures, HTN, fibrocystic breast disease, CAD, migraine headaches, thrombophlebitis, endometriosis, or gallbladder disease. Usually a combination of estrogen and
progesterone is used to prevent the long-term complications of unopposed estrogen
therapy.

MENSTRUAL DISORDERS

Amenorrhea is defined as the absence of menses for at least 6 months. Primary
amenorrhea is considered at age 14 if no secondary sexual characteristics have
developed, or at age 16 if menarche has not occurred. **Oligomenorrhea** refers to
reduced frequency of menses, usually occurring only three to four times a year. The
following list covers the most important diagnoses to consider in the evaluation of
amenorrhea/oligomenorrhea.

1. **Lesions of the CNS:** organic brain disease (tumors, toxins, infectious
diseases), hypothalamic defects or dysfunction (nutritional, exercise associated,
stress induced, polycystic ovary syndrome, obesity, medication or drug induced),
pituitary disturbances, psychogenic causes (acute emotional disturbances, anorexia
nervosa, pseudocyesis)

2. **Intermediary factors:** nutritional, chronic illness, endocrinologic disorders
(thyroid or adrenal dysfunction, hyperprolactinemia, DM), renal or hepatic disease

3. **Gonadal factors:** congenital defects (gonadal dysgenesis, hermaphroditism),
premature menopause, insensitive ovary syndrome, tumors

4. **End-organ causes:** hysterectomy, Asherman's syndrome, cervical stenosis

5. **Physiologic causes:** menopause, pregnancy, lactation

A thorough history must include attention to a previous history of menstrual
change when the patient has been under stress: use of any drugs; a history of
abdominal pain or distension; and the phase of reproductive life. The physical
examination should include attention to body habitus, the distribution and amount of
body hair, stage of breast development, presence of nipple discharge, appearance of
external genitalia (properly developed labia minora, clitoris size), appearance of the
distal genital tract (possible causes of obstruction to menstrual flow), degree of
maturation of vaginal mucosa, and the possibility of intrauterine or extrauterine
pregnancy.

Laboratory evaluation should include serum pregnancy test; serum prolactin
level; serum LH, and TSH, FSH levels, and thyroid function studies. FSH levels >40
mIU/ml suggest ovarian failure and should be followed by chromosomal analysis
in women <30 years of age. Polycystic ovary syndrome may be suspected if the
LH:FSH ratio is elevated with slight increases in the levels of testosterone and
dihydroepiandrosterone sulfate (DHEA-S). Very low levels of LH and FSH suggest the presence of a hypothalamic or pituitary neoplasm. In patients with signs
of androgen excess, testing of serum testosterone levels (ovarian androgen production) and DHEA-S level (adrenal androgen production) should be performed.
Levels <200 ng/dl testosterone and <7.0 µg/ml DHEA-S rule out adrenal or ovarian
tumors. DHEA-S levels of 5.0–7.0 µg/ml suggest adult-onset congenital adrenal
hyperplasia.

When initial testing is unrevealing, and after pregnancy has been ruled out, a
progesterone withdrawal test may be administered with 50 to 100 mg progesterone
in oil IM or with medroxyprogesterone acetate 10 mg orally daily for 5 consecutive

days. Withdrawal bleeding within a few days indicates a high estrogen status, and endometrial biopsy may be indicated for further evaluation. Treatment includes either oral contraceptives if appropriate or cyclic administration of a progestational agent to protect the endometrium, coupled with estrogen support if the patient is at risk for osteoporosis secondary to hypoestrogenization.

Dysfunctional uterine bleeding refers to an excessive length, amount, or frequency of menstrual flow. The three steps comprising the evaluation are to:

1. Confirm that bleeding is actually coming from the uterus.

2. Decide whether the patient is ovulatory or anovulatory: Ovulatory bleeding may be suspected with dysmenorrhea or premenstrual complaints of emotional lability or fluid retention, and clues to anovulatory bleeding include infrequent and often heavy menses at intervals of 6 to 12 weeks.

3. Decide whether or not an organic lesion is present by means of complete physical examination attentive to all organ systems (including endometrial biopsy for patients older than 35 years of age), Pap smear, CBC, coagulation studies, thyroid function studies and TSH, liver and renal function studies, dexamethasone suppression test, serum glucose, and pregnancy test.

The following diagram outlines the major causes of altered menstrual patterns in females.

Management of **acute vaginal hemorrhage** involves routine stabilization of vital signs and careful physical examination directed toward establishing the etiology of the bleeding episode. Sometimes emergency surgery may be indicated. However, often

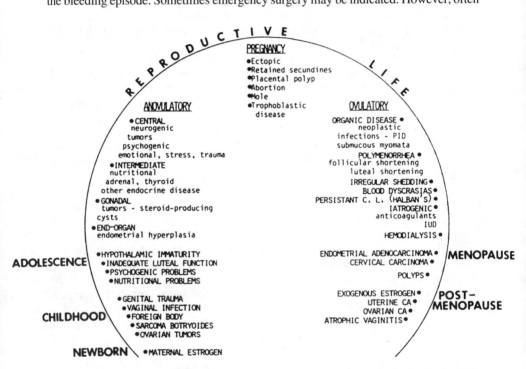

Etiologic causes of abnormal bleeding throughout female life. CA = cancer; Persistent C. L. = corpus luteum. (From Wentz AC: Abnormal uterine bleeding. In Jones HW, et al (eds): Novak's Textbook of Gynecology, 11th ed. Baltimore, Williams & Wilkins, 1988, p 380, Fig. 14.1, with permission.)

hormonal therapy effectively arrests bleeding within 24 to 36 hrs (e.g., progesterone in oil 100–200 mg IM repeated in 2–4 hrs, followed by oral progesterone 10–30 mg/day for 7–10 days). Long-term therapeutic options to prevent recurrent hemorrhage are the same as those discussed for management of amenorrhea.

Reference: Wentz AC: Amenorrhea: Evaluation and treatment. In Jones HW, et al (eds): Novak's Textbook of Gynecology, 11th ed. Baltimore, Williams & Wilkins, 1988, p 352.

MENTAL STATUS EVALUATION

The Mini-Mental State Examination (MMSE) by Folstein takes 10 min to administer and is quite sensitive to moderate impairment but relatively insensitive to mild impairment (especially in those with higher education). False positives (low scores in those without cognitive impairment) are seen in illiterate persons and those with very little formal education. Patients must be examined at their best, in the absence of sedation, and while not acutely ill.

Mini-Mental State Examination

			Score		Total
1.	**Orientation**				
	What is the	day	_____ 1		
		date	_____ 1		
		month	_____ 1		
		year	_____ 1		
		season	_____ 1	_____ 5
	What is the	city	_____ 1		
		state	_____ 1		
		county	_____ 1		
		building	_____ 1		
		floor	_____ 1	_____ 5
2.	**Registration**				
	Name 3 objects and take 1 second to say each. Then ask the patient to repeat all 3 objects. (Give 1 point for each correct answer. Repeat until patient can get all 3 objects.)				_____ 3
3.	**Attention and calculation**				
	Serial 7s: Ask the patient to count backward by 7s from 100. (Stop after 5 answers. Give 1 point for each correct answer.) Alternate: Spell *world* backward. (Give 1 point for each correctly placed letter.)				_____ 5
4.	**Recall**				
	After 2 minutes, ask for the 3 objects' names in question 2. (Give 1 point for each correct answer.)				_____ 3
5.	**Language**				
	Point to a pencil and a watch. Ask the patient to name each as you point. (Give 1 point for each correct answer.)				_____ 2
	Ask the patient to repeat the following phrase: No *if's, and's,* or *but's.* (Give 1 point for each correct answer.)				_____ 1
	Ask the patient to perform the following three-stage command: Take this piece of paper in your left hand, fold it in half, and lay it on the table. (Give 1 point for each correct step.)				_____ 3

Table continued on next page.

Mini-Mental State Examination (Cont.)

Ask the patient to read and carry out the following written command: Close your eyes. (Give 1 point for each correct response.)	_____	1
Ask the patient to write a sentence. It must contain a noun and a verb and make sense. Ignore spelling errors. (Give 1 point for each correct answer.)	_____	1
Ask the patient to draw 2 interlocking pentagons. There must be 5 sides to each pentagon and 4 interlocking sides. Example: (Give 1 point for each correct answer.)	_____	1
TOTAL	_____	30

From Yoshikawa T, et al: Ambulatory Geriatric Care. St. Louis, Mosby-Year Book, 1993, p 114, with permission.

Using a cutoff score of 23 or below to indicate dementia, when compared with the gold standard of a full psychiatric interview, the MMSE has a sensitivity of 87%, a specificity of 82%, a false-positive rate of 39%, and a false-negative rate of 4.7%. A somewhat shorter version may have the same sensitivity and specificity as tested on white persons of unclear educational status.

Persons with a low score merit an evaluation for reversible dementias or sources of excess morbity (see dementias), including depression.

Reference: Folstein MF, et al: "Mini-mental state." 1. Practical method for grading the cognitive state of patients for the clinician. J Psych Res 12:189–198, 1975.

MIGRAINE HEADACHES

Migraine headaches are one of the commonest reasons for consulting a physician.

Characteristics of Migraine Headaches

1. More common in women than men by a ratio of at least 3:1
2. Onset prior to age 25
3. Family history in 50% of patients
4. Headaches are paroxysmal, occurring once or twice per month on average.
5. Often associated with trigger factors

Typical Triggering Factors for Migraine Headaches

1. Foods, especially those rich in tyramine, such as cheese and chocolate
2. Alcohol
3. Psychological stress
4. Sleep, or sometimes sleep deprivation
5. Hormonal changes, especially menstruation

Characteristics of migraine headaches include:

1. Approximately 20% of patients have an aura preceding their headache, usually of zigzag, scintillating, visual scotomas and lights. Occasionally, the aura is a vague mood change or a focal neurologic deficit such as weakness or numbness in a limb.

2. The headache itself generally appears 10–30 min after the aura. The headache is hemicranial in one-third of patients and involves the entire head in two-thirds.

3. Headaches last 4–12 hrs but seldom persist overnight.

4. Although headaches may be pulsatile, many are not.

5. Accompanying symptoms include anorexia, nausea, vomiting, photophobia, and hypersensitivity to sound. Patients generally withdraw to a dark, quiet room.

6. Resolution of the migraine headache may leave the patient tired, unable to concentrate, or moody.

A clinical pearl: If a patient can eat during a headache, it is probably not migraine.

Acute Therapy for Migraine Headaches

1. Ergotamines, such as Cafergot, 1–3 mg PO or sublingually at the time of the aura or as soon as the pain begins
2. Inhalation of pure oxygen to promote vasoconstriction and minimize painful vasodilatation
3. NSAIDs, especially aspirin
4. Serotonin analogs
   a. Dihydroergotamine (DHE), 1 mg parenterally
   b. Sumatriptan (given parenterally via an autoinjector; this has become the treatment of choice for acute migraine)

Prophylactic Therapy for Migraines

1. Propranolol: Most other beta-blockers are not as effective as propranolol.
2. Amitriptyline: Most other tricyclics are not as effective as amitriptyline.
3. Calcium channel blockers
4. Cyproheptadine (Periactin)
5. Methysergide (Sansert): This is an excellent preventative medication, but because of the small risk of fibrosis, it is used only rarely.

Reference: Saper JR, et al: Handbook of Headache Management. A Practical Guide to Diagnosis and Treatment of Head, Neck and Facial Pain. Baltimore, Williams & Wilkins, 1993.

MITRAL REGURGITATION

Differential Diagnosis

Differential Diagnosis of Mitral Regurgitation

1. Rheumatic heart disease
2. Ischemic heart disease
3. Mitral valve prolapse
4. Infective endocarditis
5. Mitral annular dilatation
6. Mitral annular calcification
7. Congenital valve deformities
   a. Parachute mitral valve
   b. Endocardial cushion defects
   c. Endocardial fibroelastosis
   d. Transposition of the great arteries
8. Cardiac trauma
9. Prosthetic mitral valve malfunction

One or two decades ago, rheumatic heart disease was by far the commonest cause of mitral regurgitation. The steady decrease in the incidence of rheumatic heart disease in industrialized countries has markedly reduced the incidence of mitral regurgitation from this cause. Thus, in the United States today, the most common cause is MVP rather than rheumatic heart disease.

On gross examination, a myxomatous mitral valve shows characteristic bulky mitral valve leaflets, thickened chordae tendineae, and ruptured chordae resulting in regurgitation.

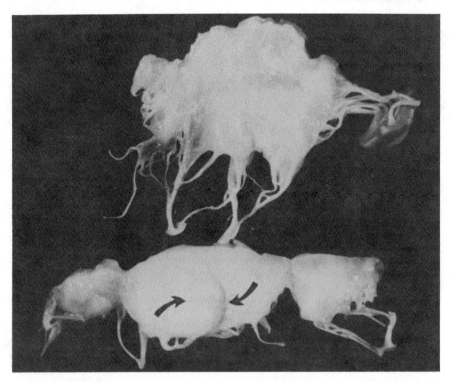

A resected floppy mitral valve from a 60-year-old man. Note the gelatinous appearance of the leaflets. The central scallop of the mural leaflet (arrows) shows a doming deformity. Some tendinous cords are ruptured in the vicinity of the dome. (From Turri M, et al: Surgical pathology of disease of the mitral valve, with special reference to lesions promoting valvular incompetence. Int J Cardiol 22:213, 1989, with permission.)

MITRAL VALVE PROLAPSE

MVP is one of the most prevalent cardiac valvular abnormalities, affecting 5 to 10% of the population. Barlow was first in demonstrating that mid-systolic clicks and late systolic murmurs—the auscultatory hallmark of the MVP syndrome—are frequently associated with MVP and often with mitral regurgitation and are intracardiac in origin.

Historical Findings

The large majority of subjects with MVP are asymptomatic. Nonspecific symptoms include chest pain, fatigability, palpitations, postural orthostasis, and neuropsychiatric symptoms. Chest pain may be typical of angina pectoris but is more often atypical. Some patients with MVP have associated cardiovascular and skeletal anomalies. Ostium secundum ASD is the most commonly associated cardiovascular anomaly. In 54 patients with ostium secundum ASD, 20 (37%) had angiographically proven MVP and 11 (20%) had auscultatory findings of MVP (a late systolic or pansystolic murmur or one or more mid-systolic clicks).

Moreover, about 5% of all patients have an ostium secundum ASD. Other commonly associated findings are thoracic skeletal anomalies such as pectus excavatum, straight back, and scoliosis. Thus, patients with MVP may present with signs and symptoms related to these associated anomalies rather than to the incidental finding of the prolapse.

Physical Findings

The distinctive physical findings on ausculation of subjects with MVP are one or more mid-systolic clicks and a late systolic murmur. In MVP, clicks are nonejection clicks; that is, they occur *after* the onset of the carotid upstroke. (This is in contrast to the ejection click of aortic stenosis.) The murmur of MVP typically occurs in late systole and corresponds to the late systolic occurrence of MVP. However, as MVP advances in severity and becomes associated with increasing mitral regurgitation, the murmur tends to occupy a greater portion of ventricular systole. In severe cases, with moderate to severe mitral valve regurgitation, the murmur is both pansystolic and indistinguishable from the murmur of mitral regurgitation due to other etiologies such as rheumatic heart disease or ischemic heart disease.

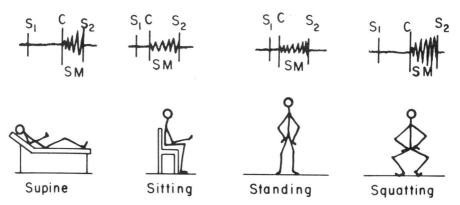

Postural changes affecting the auscultatory signs of mitral prolapse. On sitting and standing, the systolic click moves closer to S_1, and the murmur is prolonged. On squatting, the click moves toward S_2, and the murmur becomes shorter. These auscultatory variations are related to changes in left ventricular volume and shape. (Adapted from Devereux RB, et al: Mitral valve prolapse. Circulation 54:3–14, 1976, with permission.)

Since patients with a large number of valvular abnormalities can present with a systolic murmur, it is essential to recognize the unique response of the systolic click and late systolic murmur of MVP to various physical or pharmacologic maneuvers. It is this unique response to physical maneuvers that constitutes the basis for the concept of **dynamic auscultation,** the art of recognizing valvular abnormalities by evaluating the patient's response to various maneuvers.

The results of dynamic auscultation in MVP can best be understood in the context of the effect of alterations in LV volume on the degree and duration of prolapse of the mitral valve. As shown in the figure, a change from a supine to a sitting or standing position results in a reduction in venous return to the heart, thus causing a reduction in LV volume. In prolapse, any reduction in LV systolic volume increases the duration and severity of MVP into the left atrium by decreasing the tension exerted by the chordae tendineae on the mitral valve leaflets. Thus, a change from supine to sitting or standing results in a longer systolic murmur and earlier occurrence of the systolic click(s). The same result can be obtained by administration of inotropic drugs such as isoproterenol or by administration of an afterload-reducing drug such as amyl nitrite.

Conversely, as the LV systolic volume increases, there is greater tension exerted by the chordae tendineae on the mitral valve leaflets, thus preventing them from prolapsing into the left atrium. Thus, any increase in LV systolic volume decreases the duration and severity of MVP. Thus, during squatting, or upon assuming a sitting

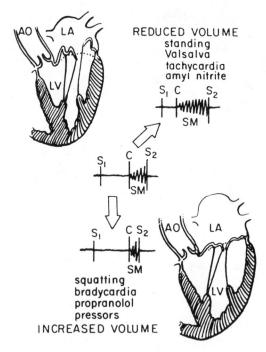

The effect of interventions on the timing of ausculatory events is related to changes in left ventricular volume and shape. Maneuvers which reduce ventricular volume enhance leaflet redundancy, hasten prolapse, and move click and murmur earlier in systole. An increase in left ventricular dimensions has the opposite effect. The loudness of ausculatory events is governed independently by left ventricular systolic pressure. (From Devereux RB, et al: Mitral valve prolapse. Circulation 54:3–14, 1976, 5, p 8, with permission.)

or supine position from a standing position, venous return to the heart increases LV volume and thereby decreases the duration and intensity of prolapse. In MVP, squatting delays the systolic click(s) and shortens the systolic murmur. The same result can be obtained by elevating legs while in the supine position, by administration of vasoconstrictors resulting in an increase in LV systolic volume, or with negative inotropic drugs.

References: Salomon J, et al: Thoracic skeletal abnormalities in idiopathic mitral valve prolapse. Am J Cardiol 36:32–36, 1975.

Betriu A, et al: Prolapse of the posterior leaflet of the mitral valve associated with secundum atrial septal defect. Am J Cardiol 35:363–369, 1975.

MONONUCLEOSIS

Although infectious mononucleosis is most often associated with EBV infection, it is also caused by other agents such as CMV, toxoplasmosis, and HIV. The infectious mononucleosis caused by the EBV is a self-limited disease that is accompanied by fever, sore throat, and adenopathy. Patients may also experience malaise, headache, loss of appetite, myalgias, and arthralgias. In addition to lymphadenopathy, splenomegaly and hepatomegaly may be observed. A rash and sometimes jaundice occurs. An absolute lymphocytosis with an increased percentage of atypical lymphocytes is also present. Diagnosis is confirmed by a positive heterophile antibody titer of at least 1:56.

Complications of mononucleosis include autoimmune hemolytic anemia, thrombocytopenia, and granulocytopenia. Aplastic anemia has been encountered, but this may be an indication of underlying immune deficiency. In immunosuppressed individuals, the hemophagocytic syndrome has been observed with EBV infection. The bone marrow contains numerous histiocytes that chew up platelets, RBCs, and WBCs. Other herpesvirus infections, brucellosis, and typhoid can also cause hemophagocytosis. Splenic rupture is a rare complication of the splenomegaly seen in this disorder. Neurologic complications include encephalitis, Guillain-Barré syndrome, and Bell's palsy. Hepatitis and massive hepatic necrosis have also been observed.

In patients with acquired or congenital immune deficiency, EBV infection may be prolonged and associated with immunoproliferative disorders. Persistent infectious mononucleosis has been observed rarely in previously well individuals. Such patients have chronic fatigue, reactive adenopathy, polyneuropathy, and evidence for cellular and humoral immune dysfunction.

Therapy in the uncomplicated patient is largely supportive. The pharyngitis can be complicated by bacterial infection. When beta-hemolytic streptococcus is present, penicillin prophylaxis is warranted. However, neither ampicillin nor amoxicillin should be used because of their association with rash in patients who have mononucleosis. Corticosteroids are not advisable in uncomplicated cases but have a role in the treatment of the autoimmune manifestations of EBV infection.

Reference: Straus SE, et al: Epstein-Barr virus infections: Biology, pathogenesis, and management. Ann Intern Med 118:45–58, 1993.

MULTIPLE ENDOCRINE NEOPLASIA SYNDROMES

The MEN syndromes are familial disorders with autosomal dominant inheritance. Affected members present with benign or malignant tumors of specific endocrine organs. The neoplasms tend to be multiple, with diffuse glandular involvement. Serious sequelae can be prevented by early recognition, careful clinical screening, and appropriate intervention. Three syndromes are currently recognized, as follows:

The MEN Syndromes

---

1. **MEN Type 1** (Wermer's syndrome, also called MEN I; defect on chromosome 11q13)
   a. Hyperparathyroidism
      - Most common feature of MEN 1 (80% of patients)
      - Complications: hypercalcemia, renal stones, skeletal fractures, peptic ulcer disease
      - Early diagnosis: serum PTH, ionized calcium
      - Treatment: total parathyroidectomy with autotransplantation to forearm
   b. Pituitary adenomas
      - Prevalence 70–80%
      - Tumors produce prolactin, GH, or ACTH or are nonsecretory
      - Complications are related to mass effect and hormone that is produced
      - Diagnosis: serum hormone screening, CT or MRI of pituitary
      - Treatment: surgical resection, radiotherapy, or medical treatment (bromocriptine)
   c. Pancreatic tumors
      - In 75% of affected patients; most tumors are functional.
      - These cause the most important life-threatening complications of MEN 1.
      - Diagnosis (general): CT/MRI, arteriography, serum hormone levels
         i. Gastrinoma (Zollinger-Ellison syndrome)
            —Complications: GI hemorrhage, diarrhea, malignant transformation
            —Diagnosis: serum gastrin level, secretin test
            —Treatment: omeprazole or H_2 blockers, pancreatic surgery (pancreaticoduo-denectomy in families with high incidence of malignancy)
         ii. Insulinoma
            —Complications: severe persistent hypoglycemia
            —Diagnosis: fasting hypoglycemia with increased insulin and C-peptide
            —Treatment: subtotal pancreatectomy
         iii. Other endocrine pancreatic tumors
            —Glucagonoma, VIPoma, pancreatic polypeptide-producing tumor
            —Treatment: surgical resection
   d. Duodenal microadenomas
      - Multiple, mainly gastrin secreting
   e. Carcinoid tumors
      - Thymus, bronchus
2. **MEN Type 2a** (Sipple's syndrome, also called MEN II; defect on chromosome 10p11)
   a. Medullary thyroid carcinoma
      - Earliest tumor to appear in MEN 2a patient
      - Complications: lethal if untreated
      - Diagnosis: serum calcitonin, pentagastrin, or calcium infusion tests
      - Treatment: total thyroidectomy
   b. Pheochromocytoma
      - Onset years after medullary thyroid carcinoma
      - Complications: sweating, tachycardia, episodic HTN (may be severe)
      - Diagnosis: CT/MRI, urinary epinephrine excretion
      - Treatment: bilateral adrenalectomy (recurrence is high for unilateral resection)

Table continued on next page.

The MEN Syndromes (Cont.)

---

c. Hyperparathyroidism
  - Last tumor to appear
  - Rare if thyroidectomy performed early in life for medullary thyroid carcinoma; may be related to constant calcitonin exposure
3. **MEN Type 2b** (mucosal neuroma syndrome, also called MEN III)
  a. Medullary thyroid carcinoma and pheochromocytoma; no hyperparathyroidism
  b. Oral mucosal neuromas at an early age, before other tumors
  c. Other physical characteristics: marfanoid habitus, characteristic facies (large lips, flat nasal bridge), retinal changes

---

DNA screening is currently being developed to identify family members at risk for these genetic syndromes.

Reference: Bone HG III: Diagnosis of the multiglandular endocrine neoplasias. Clin Chem 36:711–718, 1990.

MULTIPLE MYELOMA

Plasma cell dyscrasias are now frequently recognized early as a result of the investigation of mild anemia or an increased globulin determination on routine blood chemistry. Multiple myeloma (MM) consists of the malignant proliferation of a clone of plasma cells. The disorder is more common in blacks and the elderly. Differentiating it from benign monoclonal gammopathy is an important task of the internist. Now that indolent or localized forms of myeloma have been recognized, it is important to identify those patients who may benefit from less aggressive therapy or in fact may be observed without therapy. In some instances, the ß-2 microglobulin level is a useful adjunct. When it is above 3.0 or 4.0 mg/L, then MM is more likely.

A solitary plasmacytoma may be discovered in bone or in soft tissue such as the nasal sinuses or lung parenchyma. Of interest are the findings that only one-half of such patients have a monoclonal protein in the serum or urine and that, when present, the amount is usually small. Solitary plasmacytomas of the bone are not associated with either other lytic bone lesions, renal failure, hypercalcemia, or bone marrow plasmacytosis. About 15% of patients with MM have an indolent disease at presentation. A recent follow-up study suggests that such patients can be observed without treatment for an average of 26 months. If no lytic lesions were present, if the paraprotein were less than 3.0 gm/dl, and if the urine protein were less than 500 mg/dL, then the median time to progression of disease was 61 months. Treatment for these patients was offered either when the paraprotein increased to 5.0 g/dl (IgG) or when there was an unequivocal increase in the size or number of lytic lesions. Similarly, frank complications of myeloma such as pathologic fractures, hypercalcemia, and azotemia also constituted criteria for progression and the need to treat.

In the patient with overt MM, elevated LDH, azotemia, and hypercalcemia have been identified as indicators of a poor prognosis. Although most patients do well when treated with melphalan and prednisone, those with poor prognostic indicators may do better with more aggressive treatment by such regimens as VAD (dexamethasone along with a 4-day continuous infusion of doxorubicin and vincristine). Probably the most potent agent in the VAD protocol is high-dose dexamethasone, and some patients do well on this form of oral therapy alone. Those who achieve a response to chemotherapy may benefit from maintenance with interferon. Trials of allogenic and autologous bone marrow transplantation are also under way. Though these trials offer hope for improved therapy in the younger patient with aggressive disease, the cost and morbidity of bone marrow transplantation may be significant factors in application to older individuals.

New understanding of the biology of MM may have an impact on management of this disorder. IL-6 is produced by marrow stromal cells, may act as a paracrine growth factor, is elevated in MM, is an osteoclast-activating factor, and may be the cause of anemia in MM. The increase in IL-6 production may also explain the typical absence of thrombocytopenia in MM, for IL-6 appears to support megakaryocytopoiesis. Interventions such as blockade of the action of IL-6 may offer a new approach to the treatment of this disorder.

Reference: Dimopoulos MA, et al: Risk of disease progression in asymptomatic multiple myeloma. Am J Med 4:57–61, 1993.

MULTIPLE SCLEROSIS

MS is an inflammatory disease, probably of autoimmune etiology, which damages the proteolipid myelin sheath that coats nerves in the brain and spinal cord. When the myelin is destroyed, nerve membranes may no longer be capable of depolarization and cannot conduct action potentials or transmit information. In this fashion, demyelination causes dysfunction exactly as though the nerve itself had been destroyed.

Common Symptoms of Multiple Sclerosis

1. Weakness	45%
2. Optic neuritis	40%
3. Numbness	35%
4. Cerebellar ataxia and tremor	30%
5. Diplopia and brain stem symptoms	25%
6. Sphincter changes	20%

Variability is the hallmark of MS, as can be seen by the large number of symptoms it can produce. The pattern also varies greatly, ranging from abrupt onset of symptoms to gradual progression of disability. This variability is vexing in attempts to diagnose MS, but clinical criteria do allow for an accurate diagnosis.

Schumacher Criteria for Clinical Diagnosis of MS

1. Two separate CNS symptoms
2. Two separate attacks or occurrences of symptoms
3. Objective deficits on the neurologic examination
4. White matter symptoms
5. Age between 10 and 50 years
6. No other disease present

The first two features of the Schumacher criteria are generally taken as the *sine qua non* of MS, namely, two separate lesions at two separate times.

Diagnostic aid can come from the MRI, which shows multiple scattered abnormalities in the white matter of the brain and spinal cord. The CSF also usually contains elevated levels of IgG, often clumped together in distinctive oligoclonal bands.

Diseases that mimic MS include vasculitis affecting the CNS and spinocerebellar degenerations, but the commonest condition in the differential diagnosis is hysteria.

Variability is characteristic of the clinical course of MS. Thirty years after the diagnosis, as many as one-third of patients may remain normal, with no persistent deficit, another third may have some degree of disability (although still be able to lead a functional life), and the final third may become disabled—in a wheelchair or bedridden. MS is not fatal, but death may occur from complications such as falls, aspiration, and sepsis.

There is no treatment that is known to alter the natural history of MS, but steroid therapy can provide at least temporary relief. Most regimens utilize high-dose pulse methylprednisolone (Solu-Medrol), 1 gm per day for 3 to 7 days, often followed by a brief taper of oral prednisone. Other immune suppressant agents, such as cyclophosphamide, azathioprine, plasmapheresis, or IV immunoglobulin, remain in the therapeutic arsenal, but scientific data on their effectiveness are not yet compelling. Beta-interferon may be of value in slowing progression of the disease.

Reference: Rolak LA: Multiple sclerosis. Curr Neurol 9:109–148, 1989.

MYASTHENIA GRAVIS

MG is an autoimmune disease caused by circulating antibodies directed against the acetylcholine receptor at the neuromuscular junction. It is the commonest disease affecting the neuromuscular junction. Its hallmark is fatigability, defined as the weakening of muscles with use, followed by recovery with rest. Because muscles recover with rest, a pattern of variability or fluctuation is typical. Patients thus report weakness that waxes and wanes and fluctuates throughout the day.

The weakness is generally symmetric and proximal, involving especially muscles of the eyelids, eyes, face, tongue, jaw, and neck. Ptosis and double vision are common early symptoms of MG.

The diagnosis of MG can be confirmed through the use of three primary tests.

1. **Tensilon (edrophonium):** This is administered as a 10-mg IV push. This is an acetylcholine esterase inhibitor, which rapidly reverses muscular weakness. Symptoms return back to baseline in just a few minutes, as the medication is cleared.

2. **Electromyography:** The nerve is stimulated repeatedly and the electrical potential recorded from the muscle. With repetitive stimulation, muscle contraction becomes weaker and weaker, and this decrease can be recorded on the EMG.

3. **Acetylcholine receptor antibodies:** The circulating antibodies against the acetylcholine receptor can be measured directly.

Treatment for myasthenia involves the following.

1. **Mestinon (pyridostigmine):** This acetylcholinesterase inhibitor has a duration of 3 to 4 hrs and is commonly given as 60 mg PO Q 4 hrs. It often provides significant symptomatic relief, but, of course, has no influence on the underlying autoimmune pathogenesis of the disease.

2. **Steroids:** Use of steroids represents an attempt to produce immune suppression. Prednisone in doses of 20 to 100 mg given usually every other day often provides excellent relief.

3. **Immune suppression:** More intense immune suppression than can be obtained with steroids is often accomplished using cyclophosphamide, azathioprine, or cyclosporine.

4. **Plasmapheresis:** As an acute therapy, removal of circulating antibodies by plasmapheresis often provides significant benefit. The benefit is not long lasting, however, and within a few weeks symptoms may return, necessitating the use of chronic immune suppressants as an accompaniment to plasmapheresis. Infusions of IV immunoglobulin may produce similar acute benefits.

5. **Thymectomy:** The procedure often leads to improvement, although there remains controversy regarding which patients are benefited most from thymectomy. It is becoming increasingly common and is routine for most patients at many centers. Although the thymus has some immunologic connections, the mechanism of improvement in MG following thymectomy remains mysterious.

Myasthenic crisis occurs when respiratory muscles become sufficiently involved to impair breathing. Management of myasthenic crisis involves:

1. Intubation of the patient or preparations to at least support respirations
2. Admission to an intensive care unit
3. Discontinuation of acetylcholinesterase medications such as Mestinon
4. Initiation of a long-acting immune suppressant, such as steroids
5. Implementation of acute therapy, such as plasmapheresis or IV immunoglobulin
6. Possible restart of acetylcholinesterase medications once it is clear the patient is not experiencing cholinergic side effects.

Reference: Verma P, et al: Treatment of acquired autoimmune myasthenia gravis: A topic review. Can J Neurol Sci 19:360–375, 1992.

MYCOBACTERIA, NONTUBERCULOUS

Nontuberculous Mycobacteria

MICROORGANISM	PREDISPOSING FACTORS	DISEASE
I. Photochromogens (Runyon Group I)		
M. kansasii	Middle-aged white males with underlying chronic pulmonary disease	Apical, cavitary pulmonary infection
	Urban children	Cervical lymphadenitis
	Patients with impaired cellular immunity (AIDS, transplant recipients)	Disseminated disease, misc. infections involving skin or musculoskeletal structures
M. marinum	Almost always associated with aquatic activities (e.g. aquariums, unchlorinated swimming pools)	Local granuloma or sporotrichoid lesions, synovitis, arthritis, bursitis, osteomyelitis

Table continued on next page.

Nontuberculous Mycobacteria (Cont.)

MICROORGANISM	PREDISPOSING FACTORS	DISEASE
II. Scotochromogens (Runyon Group II)		
M. scrofulaceum	Children aged 1–5 yrs	Cervical lymphadenitis
M. szulgai	Middle-aged men	Cavitary pulmonary infection, rarely tenosynovitis, bursitis, osteomyelitis or cutaneous infection
III. Nonchromogens (Runyon Group III)		
M. avium-intracellulare complex:		
Ssp. *avium*	AIDS	Disseminated and focal infections
Ssp. *intracellulare*	Middle-aged white men with underlying lung disease Middle-aged women without preexisting factors	Chronic pulmonary infection, frequently with thin-walled cavities
Ssp. *paratuberculosis*	Cattle	Johne's disease
M. xenopi	Middle-aged men with preexisting pulmonary disease, alcoholism, diabetes or malignancy	Chronic pulmonary infection
M. asiaticum	? Chronic pulmonary disease	Chronic pulmonary infection
M. ulcerans	Endemic disease in Zaire, Uganda, Nigeria, Ghana, Cameroon, Malaysia, New Guinea, Guyana, Mexico, and Australia	Indolent cutaneous ulcers
M. haemophilum	Transplant recipients, AIDS, lymphoma	Multiple nodular or ulcerative skin lesions
M. malmoense	Middle-aged men with preexisting chronic pulmonary disease (e.g., pneumoconiosis)	Chronic pulmonary infection, lymphadenitis
IV. Rapid growers (Runyon Group IV)		
M. fortuitum	Frequently none Immunosuppression	Progressive pulmonary infection Abscesses, ulcers, sinus tracts, and bone infections
M. abscessus	Frequently none	Progressive pulmonary infection with bilateral, apical infiltrates
	Immunosuppression (e.g., transplant recipients)	Abscesses, ulcers, sinus tracts, and bone infections

Reference: Woods GL, et al: Mycobacteria other than *Mycobacterium tuberculosis*: Review of microbiologic and clinical aspects. Rev Infect Dis 9:275–294, 1987.

MYELODYSPLASTIC SYNDROMES

Classification

The myelodysplastic syndromes are disorders of the differentiation of hematopoietic cells that result in cytopenias and have a potential for transformation into acute leukemia. The entities embraced by the term *myelodysplasia* are shown in the following table as classified by the French-American-British (FAB) scheme. These disorders, although they are thrown together, probably represent the result of several different pathophysiologic processes. It is likely that these disorders are the result of somatic mutations in stem cells, with clonal expansion and evolution as further genetic mishaps occur. About half of patients with myelodysplasia have cytogenetic abnormalities.

FAB Classification of Myelodysplasia

Refractory anemia
Refractory anemia with ringed sideroblasts
Refractory anemia with excess blasts (RAEB): blasts make up 5–20% of marrow cells
Refractory anemia with excess blasts in transformation (RAEB-T): blasts make up 20–30% of marrow cells
Chronic myelomonocytic leukemia (CMML): Often confused with CML, but Ph chromosome and the *abl/bcr* gene fusion are absent and there are both an excess of monocytes and significant splenomegaly.

The clinical features of myelodysplasia are manifestations of anemia, thrombocytopenia, or neutropenia. Refractory anemia is observed and marked by macrocytic RBCs, dyserythropoietic-marrow erythroid cells, and ringed sideroblasts. Anemia may be significant and require frequent blood transfusions, which eventually result in iron overload. Some patients with prolonged courses require chelation therapy to minimize the effects of iron deposition on the heart, liver, and pancreas. Splenomegaly is a feature of CMML and is observed less frequently in other myelodysplastic disorders.

Abnormal lobation of the neutrophils is a hallmark of myelodysplasia. Characteristic bilobed pince-nez granulocytes or pseudo-Pelger-Huët cells are seen. Unilobed mature granulocytes or Stodtmeister cells may also be observed. Neutropenia, if severe or accompanied by dysfunctional cells, increases the susceptibility for infection. Abnormal megakaryocytic differentiation is present in varying degrees and may result in bleeding due to significant thrombocytopenia.

The bone marrow in myelodysplasia is usually cellular, with dyserythropoiesis, abnormal development of myeloid, and megakaryocytic cells. The number of myeloblasts is increased significantly in RAEB and portends a particularly poor prognosis. Management of most patients consists basically of supportive therapy. Young patients who have suitable donors may do well with allogeneic bone marrow transplantation. Attempts to improve counts with colony-stimulating factors and erythropoietin have met with only modest success. To date, none of these modalities has made a significant impact on thrombocytopenic patients. Once these patients transform into acute leukemia, their response rate to standard chemotherapeutic regimens is low.

Reference: List AF, et al: The myelodysplastic syndromes: Biology and implications for management. J Clin Oncol 8: 1424–1441, 1990.

MYOCARDIAL INFARCTION

Antiarrhythmic Drug Therapy Post-MI

Several studies have consistently reported that the frequency and complexity of ventricular arrhythmias after acute MI are associated with a greater risk of death. Moreover, LVEF is the most powerful predictor of short- and long-term clinical outcome post-MI. The most definitive clinical study that systematically examined the relative contributions of LV function and of ventricular arrhythmias to prognosis in the post-MI period is the Multicenter Post-Infarction Research Group Study.[1] This was a prospective study of 766 patients recovering from acute MI followed for an average of 22 months post-MI. Most patients underwent 24-hr ambulatory ECG monitoring and had an assessment of LV systolic function by radionuclide ventriculography prior to hospital discharge. Both the LVEF and the frequency and complexity of ventricular arrhythmias were independently predictive of 2-yr survival. Two-year mortality post-MI increased 3.5-fold in patients with an LVEF <30% and increased 2-fold in those with >3 ventricular premature beats (VPBs). This study was the first clinical study to demonstrate the independence of the associations between ventricular arrhythmias or EF, and survival post-MI.

Based on these results, the following hypothesis was tested: Does drug therapy aimed at reducing or abolishing ventricular arrhythmias decrease post-MI mortality? In the Cardiac Arrhythmia Prevention Trial (CAPS)[2]—a prospective, randomized, double-blind, placebo-controlled clinical trial—it was first shown that three antiarrhythmic drugs—encainide, flecainide, and moricizine, can be titrated to achieve a significant (≥70%) reduction of VPB frequency and >90% suppression of runs of VPBs.

Most recently, a prospective, randomized, placebo-controlled clinical trial—the Cardiac Arrhythmia Suppression Trial (CAST)—was designed to determine whether antiarrhythmic drug therapy with encainide, flecainide, or moricizine, titrated to achieve a drastic suppression of VPBs in patients recovering from acute MI, decreases mortality. Preliminary results of that trial indicated a surprising **3.5-fold excess mortality** due to arrhythmias and shock in patients who received flecainide or encainide.[3] More recently, moricizine was also reported to cause a slightly greater mortality.[3] In view of these results, we do not recommend the routine administration of antiarrhythmic drugs in all patients post-MI. Patients with frequent VPBs (defined as ≥10 VPB/min) or with nonsustained VT post-MI, particularly those with a depressed EF, should undergo further diagnostic workup such as electrophysiologic testing to determine whether antiarrhythmic drugs are recommended.

References: 1. Bigger JT, et al: The relationships among ventricular arrhythmias, left ventricular dysfunction, and mortality in the two years after myocardial infarction. Circulation 69:250–258, 1984.

2. The CAPS Investigators: Effects of encainide, flecainide, imipramine and moricizine on ventricular arrhythmias during the year after acute myocardial infarction: The CAPS. Am J Cardiol 61:501–509, 1988.

3. Echt DS: Mortality and morbidity in patients receiving encainide, flecainide or placebo. The CAST. N Engl J Med 324:781–788, 1991.

Beta-Adrenergic Receptor Blockers Post-MI

It was shown in the early 1970s that administration of beta-blockers reduces myocardial ischemia and infarct size in experimentally induced MI. Based on those experimental observations, over 30 clinical trials have been conducted in more than 25,000 patients worldwide to test the hypothesis that oral beta-blockers reduce mortality and reinfarction.

Historically, the first published, large-scale, prospective, randomized, double-blind, placebo-controlled clinical trial was reported by the Norwegian Multicenter Study Group in 1981.[1] A total of 1,884 patients received the nonselective beta-blocker timolol (10 mg twice daily) or placebo 5 to 28 days after MI and were followed for 12 to 33 months. Timolol resulted in a 45% reduction of sudden death rate and a 28% reduction of reinfarction rate during follow-up.

This was followed 5 months later by the reported results of a Swedish clinical trial of metoprolol.[2] The cardioselective beta-blocker metoprolol was given as a 15-mg intravenous dose followed by oral administration of 100 mg twice daily for 90 days and was associated with a 36% reduction of total mortality (from 8.9% to 5.7%, $p<0.03$).

Results of the first and largest U.S. clinical trial of oral beta-blockers post-MI—the Beta-Blocker Heart Attack Trial (BHAT)—were published soon thereafter.[3] In this prospective, randomized, double-blind, placebo-controlled clinical trial, 3,837 patients with acute MI who were aged 30 to 69 years were randomized to receive the noncardioselective beta-blocker propranolol 180 or 240 mg daily over a mean 25-month follow-up period. This clinical trial was terminated because of the significant reduction in mortality among propranolol-treated patients. Total mortality decreased from 9.8% to 7.2% (26%). Similarly, sudden cardiac death decreased significantly, from 4.6 to 3.3% (28%).

References: 1. Norwegian Multicenter Study Group. Timolol-induced reduction in mortality and reinfarction in patients surviving acute myocardial infarction. N Engl J Med 304:801–807, 1981.

2. Hjalmarson A, et al: Effect on mortality of metoprolol in acute myocardial infarction. Lancet 1:823–827, 1981.

3. BHAT Research Group: A randomized trial of propranolol in patients with acute myocardial infarction. 1. Mortality results. JAMA 247:1707–1714, 1982.

Calcium Channel Blockers Post-MI

The role of calcium channel blockers has been carefully evaluated in a large number of clinical trials. It is important to recognize that the three prototype calcium antagonists (nifedipine, diltiazem, and verapamil), which share an inhibitory effect on the calcium channel of vascular smooth muscle cells, are structurally different and have different pharmacologic properties. Thus, it is important to evaluate the roles of these three drugs separately in patients with acute MI.

1. **Nifedipine:** Extensive clinical trials evaluating the role of nifedipine in acute MI have provided substantial evidence to support the following recommendation[1]: the acute administration of nifedipine in evolving MI in an attempt to limit infarct size, reduce reinfarction, or improve survival is *contraindicated.* No clinical trial has demonstrated clinically favorable effects of nifedipine post-MI.

2. **Diltiazem:** In patients recovering from acute non-Q-wave MI *without pulmonary congestion* (or with an LVEF >40%), diltiazem has two favorable effects: it reduces reinfarction during hospitalization by about 50%, and it decreases recurrent fatal or nonfatal cardiac events, i.e., death or reinfarction at 2 years after hospital discharge. It is important to *avoid* the use of diltiazem in patients recovering from acute MI with pulmonary congestion or with a depressed LV function (LVEF <40%). In such patients, the use of diltiazem may *increase* the risk of recurrent fatal or nonfatal cardiac events. Based on the available evidence, it is now recommended to use diltiazem in patients recovering from acute non-Q-wave MI for 1 year.[2]

3. **Verapamil:** Verapamil has been shown to reduce death or reinfarction in acute MI. However, since it may cause conduction abnormalities in patients with acute MI or may worsen heart failure symptoms, it is recommended that verapamil be used in patients recovering from a non-Q-wave MI only if there is a contraindication to the use of diltiazem.

References: 1. Habib G, et al: Calcium channel blockers in the treatment of acute myocardial infarction. In ER Bates (ed): Thrombolysis and Adjunctive Therapy for Acute Myocardial Infarction. New York, Marcel Dekker, 1993.

2. ACC/AHA Task Force Report: Guidelines for the early management of patients with acute myocardial infarction: A report of the American College of Cardiology/American Heart Association Task Force on assessment of diagnosis and therapeutic cardiovascular procedures. J Am Coll Cardiol 16:249–292, 1990.

Diagnosis by Cardiac Enzymes

The diagnosis of acute MI has been traditionally based on the finding of at least two of the three diagnostic hallmarks of myocardial necrosis: chest pain suggestive of ischemic origin, classical ECG findings, and enzymatic changes. It is now well established that the single most sensitive and specific diagnostic finding for acute MI is elevation of the cardiac enzyme creatine kinase (CK) and of its myocardial isoenzyme MB-CK. Acute MI commonly results in an elevation of other enzymes such as AST and LDH. However, although these enzymes are still routinely obtained in many hospitals, the diagnosis of acute MI should not usually rely on such measurements.

A distinct exception to this rule is the patient presenting with a history of chest pain suggestive of acute MI 2 to 5 days before initial evaluation, who is found by ECG to have an evolving infarction. In such patients, CK enzymes may be normal, and an elevated total LDH enzyme, an elevated cardiac isoenzyme LDH1, or an elevated ratio of LDH1/LDH2 may be one of the few clues for a diagnosis of acute MI. LDH has five isoenzymes, which are numbered LDH1 to LDH5 in the order of the rapidity of their migration toward the anode of an electrophoretic field. The heart contains principally LDH1, whereas liver and skeletal muscle contain primarily LDH4 and LDH5. An elevated LDH1/LDH2 ratio of >1.0 is the most commonly used cutoff, above which acute MI is diagnosed. Another helpful test to diagnose acute MI in patients presenting a few days after the onset of symptoms is cardiac imaging with a calcium-avid radionuclide (technetium pyrophosphate).

More important for the diagnosis of acute MI than an elevation of CK and MB-CK are the serial changes in CK enzyme levels in the first 24 to 48 hrs after onset of MI. It is important to document a rise in CK enzyme levels followed by a gradual decline in the first 24 to 48 hs. Generally, CK enzyme levels start rising at 6 to 8 hrs, reach a peak level at 16 to 18 hrs, and normalize at 24 to 48 hrs. Other clinical conditions such as stroke, acute pericarditis, and rhabdomyolysis that result in elevation of CK levels are not characterized by similar temporal changes in CK levels and can thus be differentiated from acute MI.

Predicting Outcome and Risk Stratification

In the patient recovering from acute MI, the following factors have been consistently shown to be independently predictive of long-term survival following discharge:

1. Exercise-induced myocardial ischemia
2. Left ventricular ejection fraction
3. Ventricular ectopy (frequency and complexity)

The large majority of patients hospitalized with acute MI have uncomplicated infarction, meaning the absence of any one or more of the following potentially life-threatening complications:

1. Post–myocardial infarction ischemia
2. Congestive heart failure
3. Malignant ventricular arrhythmias such as sustained or nonsustained V tach or V fib.

Patients with an uncomplicated MI are routinely subjected to a predischarge diagnostic workup to evaluate their risk of recurrent cardiac events after hospital discharge. Because exercise-induced ischemia, LVEF, and malignant ventricular arrhythmias are independently predictive of prognosis after hospital discharge, it is recommended that performance of the following diagnostic tests occur before hospital discharge to risk stratify the patients with uncomplicated MI:

1. Exercise testing
2. Assessment of LVEF
3. Quantitation of cardiac arrhythmias by ambulatory ECG monitoring

By far the best test to risk stratify patients recovering from an uncomplicated MI is a treadmill exercise ECG test using a modified (or submaximal) Bruce protocol. A landmark study that clearly established the prognostic value of exercise ECG testing after recovery from ECG was reported by Theroux in 1979.[1] In that study, 210 patients, aged 28 to 70 years who sustained an acute MI uncomplicated by post-MI angina in the 4 days preceding hospital discharge or overt CHF (pulmonary rales, sinus tachycardia, or S_3) underwent a submaximal treadmill test 1 day before discharge. They were then followed for a period of 1 year for death, recurrent infarction, or need for CABG. One-year mortality was 2.1% (3/146) in patients without ST-segment changes during exercise compared to 27% (17/64) of those with ST-segment depression. Sudden death occurred in 1 of 146 (0.7%) patients with no exercise-induced ST-segment changes and in 10 of 64 (16%) with exercise-induced ST-segment depression.

In addition to exercise-induced myocardial ischemia, assessment of LV systolic function and of the frequency and complexity of ventricular arrhythmias can provide valuable clues to the overall assessment of the risk of death or recurrent cardiac events after hospital discharge.

The independent prognostic value of LVEF and of ventricular arrhythmias was best demonstrated in the Multicenter Post-Infarction Research Program.[2] Finally, it is important to recognize that even an initial 12-lead ECG can help predict the risk of complications during initial hospitalization for MI. In a study of 469 patients admitted to the hospital with a suspected acute MI, life-threatening complications (such as V fib, sustained V tach, or heart block) were 23 times more likely, and death during initial hospitalization was 17 times more likely, in patients with an abnormal admission ECG compared to patients with a normal admission ECG.

References: 1. Theroux P, et al: Prognostic value of exercise testing soon after myocardial infarction. N Engl J Med 301:341–345, 1979.

2. Bigger JT, et al: The relationships among ventricular arrhythmias, left ventricular dysfunction, and mortality in the 2 years after myocardial infarction. Circulation 69:250–258, 1984.

3. Brush JE, et al: Use of the initial electrocardiogram to predict hospital complications of acute myocardial infarction. N Engl J Med 312:1137–1141, 1985.

Prevention

CAD accounts for approximately one of every three deaths in the United States. Primary prevention, through the modification of risk factors rather than treatment of already existing disease, has the greatest potential for impacting this mortality. Many studies have looked at the impact of such changes, and the following tables list risk factors and summarize various interventions. The estimated achievable decrease in risk of MI and the efficacy of current strategies to modify risk factors are also outlined. Remember that regression of established atherosclerotic plaques is possible with reduction of risk factors.

CAD Risk Factors

I. Nonmodifiable
- Age (most powerful)
- Menopause
- Sex (male)
- Family history

II. Modifiable
- Cigarette smoking
- Hypercholesterolemia
- HTN (esp. systolic)
- DM, glucose intolerance
- Weight gain
- Central obesity
- ECG evidence of LVH
- Lack of physical activity (relative risk increases with age)
- Lack of postmenopausal estrogen
- Stress (some types)
- Ethanol use (U-shaped curve) (lowest risk at 1 or 2 drinks/ day)
- Dietary
  Diet high in saturated fatty acids
  Diet low in monounsaturated fatty acids
  Diet low in (ω-3) fish oil
  High % of total calories from fat
  Low dietary fiber
- Dyslipidemia
  Total-to-HDL cholesterol ratio (women with total chol = 240 often *not* at ↑ risk because of high HDL)
  LDL-to-HDL cholesterol ratio
  Total cholesterol predictive power ↓ after age 50

Effectiveness of MI Risk Factor Reduction

INTERVENTION	ESTIMATED MEAN REDUCTION IN MI RISK	EFFICACY OF CURRENT STRATEGIES
Smoking cessation	50–70% lower risk in former compared with current smokers, within 5 years of cessation	Fair
Reduction in serum cholesterol	2–3% decline in risk for each 1% reduction in serum cholesterol. Reductions in total cholesterol average 10% with diet therapy and often exceed 20% with drug therapy.	Fair to good
Treatment of hypertension	2–3% decline for each 1 mm Hg decline in diastolic BP. Reductions in diastolic BP average 5–6 mm Hg with combination diet/drug therapy, although decreases of 20 mm Hg are frequently achieved in clinical practice.	Good
Exercise	45% lower risk for active versus sedentary lifestyle	Fair
Maintenance of ideal body weight	35–55% lower risk for patients with ideal body weight versus those who are obese (>20% above ideal body weight)	Poor
Maintenance of normoglycemia in diabetics	(Data currently insufficient to provide estimates)	Fair to poor
Postmenopausal estrogen replacement therapy	44% lower risk in users compared to nonusers (although data not available for combined estrogen-progesterone therapy)	Data not available
Mild to moderate alcohol consumption	24–45% lower risk compared to nondrinkers	Data not available
Prophylactic low-dose aspirin	33% lower risk in users compared to nonusers	Data not available

Modified from Manson JE, et al: The primary prevention of myocardial infarction. N Engl J Med 326(21):1406–1416, 1992, Table 1 on p 1407, with permission.

Exercise and Risk Reduction

Benefits of regular exercise
    Difficult to isolate exercise as separate factor
    Health-seeking individuals exercise, but also do other "healthy" things
    Exercise will ↑ HDL cholesterol, ↓ VLDL cholesterol
    Exercise will ↓ systolic and diastolic BP by 10–15 mm Hg
    Exercise improves glucose tolerance
    Exercise may ↓ obesity
    Exercise reduces stress and ↓ activity of sympathetic nervous system
Contraindications to exercise
    Uncontrolled arrhythmias   Uncontrolled HTN
    Uncontrolled CHF   Unstable angina
    Initial days post-MI
Risks of exercise
    ↑ Angina   Myocardial infarction
    Arrhythmias   Sudden death
    Musculoskeletal problems

Recommendations for Exercise

- Exercise for 30 min 3 times a week (or more), or perform 60 min of movement per day.
- Check with physician before starting program
  1. Antecedent cardiac symptoms from history
  2. Physical exam
  3. Lab: glucose, cholesterol/lipid profile, CBC, UA
  4. ECG and graded exercise stress test (for age >35)

Reference: Frohich ED (ed): Preventive aspects of coronary heart disease. Cardiovasc Clin 20:3, 1990.

Prognosis of an Unrecognized MI

In the Framingham Heart Study—a large prospective cohort study of participants initially free of cardiovascular disease followed for over 30 years—the prevalence of unrecognized MI was about 25%. Unrecognized MI includes silent MI (MI without any symptoms) and clinically unsuspected MI (MI with atypical clinical presentation not recognized at the time as likely due to MI). Typically, patients with unrecognized MI are found at a routine biannual evaluation to have new pathologic Q waves on a routine 12-lead ECG.

It is generally recognized that the natural history of unrecognized MI is similar to that of recognized infarcts. In both men and women in the Framingham Heart Study, the 10-year survival in patients with unrecognized MI was even slightly worse than that of clinically recognized infarction. It is thus recommended to evaluate patients with a clinically unrecognized MI the same way as evaluation is routinely performed for recognized infarction, by including a treadmill exercise stress test for risk stratification and an assessment of LV function. As in patients with a clinically recognized MI, cardiac catheterization is recommended if the stress test is indicative of ischemia, particularly if ischemia is evident at an early exercise threshold (the first 5 min of a standard Bruce exercise protocol).

Q-Wave Versus Non-Q-Wave MI

Historically, the terms *transmural* and *subendocardial* were used to refer to MI with and without pathologic Q waves. The assumption behind the use of this terminology was that the presence of ECG Q waves indicates that the MI involves the full thickness of the myocardium, a so-called transmural infarction. The terminology also assumes that the absence of a pathologic Q wave indicates that only part of the myocardial thickness, namely, the subendocardial area, is involved. Autopsy studies have consistently shown that such assumptions are erroneous. In fact, only 60% of Q-wave infarcts are strictly transmural, and a similar percentage of non-Q-wave infarcts are subendocardial. The expressions *transmural* versus *subendocardial* were thus abandoned in favor of the ECG descriptive terms *Q-wave* and *non-Q-wave MI*, respectively.

It soon became recognized that patients recovering from a non-Q-wave MI have a different prognosis compared to patients with Q-wave MI. Clinical outcome variables in Q-wave versus non-Q-wave MI are illustrated in the following table. In

25 reported studies, short-term (i.e., hospital) mortality was 10.2% in patients recovering from a non-Q-wave infarct compared to a twofold greater, 19.9% hospital mortality in patients with Q-wave MI. However, when long-term follow-up (6 to 96 months) was undertaken, pooled data from 22 clinical studies showed a slightly greater mortality *after* hospital discharge of 31.2% in patients with a non-Q-wave infarct compared to 26.3% in patients with a Q-wave infarct. This prognostic paradox, that is, the contrast between the better clinical prognosis during initial hospitalization and the worse long-term clinical outcome, perplexed clinicians and researchers for many years.

Clinical Outcome Variables in Q-Wave versus Non-Q-Wave MI:
Results of Pooled Data

ENDPOINT OF STUDY	DURATION OF FOLLOW-UP	QMI (% DEATH OR REINFARCTION	NQMI (% DEATH OR REINFARCTION)	*p* VALUE
Short-term mortality (25 studies)	5–30 days	11,400 (19.9)	3,751 (10.2)	<0.0001
Long-term mortality (22 studies)	6–96 mos	7,641 (26.3)	3,346 (31.2)	<0.001
Reinfarction (14 studies)	Up to 44 mos	4,095 (5.7)	1,201 (15.7)	<0.001
Peak CK level (12 studies)		(1,167)	(538)	<0.001

Adapted from Gibson RS: Non-Q wave myocardial infarction: Diagnosis, prognosis and management. Curr Prob Cardiol 13:1–72, 1988, pp 29–33.

The prognostic paradox of non-Q-wave MI is now clearly explained by the greater propensity of patients with a non-Q-wave MI to develop reinfarction during initial hospitalization.[1] This important observation, subsequently confirmed by several investigators, supports the concept that a non-Q-wave MI results from spontaneous early reperfusion of an infarcted area. Further support for the concept was provided by the following findings.

1. Non-Q-wave MIs are smaller than Q-wave MIs.
2. The residual ischemic area is larger in non-Q-wave MI.
3. The risk of reinfarction is substantially greater during initial hospitalization as well as after hospital discharge.
4. Reinfarction occurs in the same anatomic area as the initial infarction in the majority of patients with a non-Q-wave MI.

The Diltiazem Reinfarction Study, reported in 1986, has conclusively demonstrated that the higher reinfarction rate of patients with a non-Q-wave MI can be effectively reduced by as much as 45% by the calcium antagonist diltiazem.[3] Thus, diltiazem is generally recommended for 1 year in patients recovering from a non-Q-wave MI. An alternative drug that has also been shown to reduce reinfarction in these patients is verapamil, which, like diltiazem (but unlike nifedipine), is a heart-rate-lowering calcium antagonist.[4]

References: 1. Marmour A, et al: Factors presaging early recurrent myocardial infarction ("extension"). Am J Cardiol 13:603–610, 1981.

2. Habib GB, et al: Calcium channel blockers in the treatment of acute myocardial infarction. In Bates ER (ed): Thrombolysis and Adjunctive Therapy for Acute Myocardial Infarction: New York, Marcel Dekker, 1992, pp 167–189.

3. Gibson RS, et al: Diltiazem and reinfarction in patients with non-Q-wave myocardial infarction: results of a double-blind, randomized, multicenter trial. N Engl J Med 315:423–429, 1986.

4. Danish Study Group on Verapamil in Myocardial Infarction: Effect of verapamil on mortality and major events after acute myocardial infarction (Danish Verapamil Infarction Trial II, DAVIT-II). Am J Cardiol 66:779–785, 1990.

Right Ventricular Infarction

Although about 35 to 40% of all patients with acute inferior wall MI have objective evidence of RV involvement (by echocardiography or radionuclide ventriculography), only 10% present with the clinical syndrome of acute RV infarction. The classic clinical triad of acute RV infarction consists of:

1. Hypotension
2. Elevated jugular venous pressure
3. Clear lungs

The diagnosis of RV infarction should be suspected in any patient with acute inferior wall MI presenting with this classic triad. However, it is important to recognize that the same triad can occur in patients with acute cardiac tamponade or acute exacerbation of chronic pulmonary disease. Thus, in such patients, the clinical suspicion of acute RV infarction should be confirmed with one of two tests: a right-sided ECG or a radionuclide ventriculogram. The presence of ≥ 1 mm ST segment elevation in the right-sided chest lead RV3 or RV4 (i.e., the right-sided chest leads that are the mirror-images of V3 and V4, respectively) is the most specific ECG finding for acute RV infarction, with >90% of patients having radionuclide evidence of a depressed RV systolic function. On the other hand, documentation of RV systolic dysfunction by echocardiography or by radionuclide ventriculography in a patient with acute inferior wall MI is a very reliable finding for acute RV infarction.

The major implication of an early diagnosis of acute RV infarction is the planning of a rational therapeutic approach. Despite their elevated jugular venous pressure, patients with acute RV infarction generally have a low LVEDP and a low cardiac output due to decreased venous return to the LV. Thus, the first line of therapy should target an increase in intravascular blood volume by means of IV fluids. However, IV fluid therapy alone rarely normalizes LVEDP in these patients, and thus dopamine is often necessary to improve pump function. It is important to recognize in this context that the optimal LVEDP in patients with acute MI and a noncompliant left ventricle is 15 to 17 mm Hg, rather than the usual, normal range of 8 to 12 mm Hg. Thus, IV fluids and dopamine therapy should be titrated to obtain an optimal LVEDP of 15 to 17 mm Hg in these patients in order to achieve optimal cardiac output.

Thrombolytic Drug Therapy

The role of thrombolytic therapy in the treatment of acute MI became the focus of increasing attention after early observations by Dewood in 1980 that total coronary occlusion was observed in 110 of 126, or 87%, of all patients with acute MI evaluated within 4 hrs of the onset of symptoms.[1] Since then, many clinical trials have consistently demonstrated that thrombolytic therapy reduces infarct size, improves LV function, and improves both the short- and long-term clinical outcomes of patients with MI. Although there remains substantial controversy about which of the currently commercially available thrombolytic drugs is most effective, there is a clear consensus in the medical community that the beneficial effect of thrombolytic therapy outweighs any other therapeutic intervention in these patients.

One of the most crucial factors affecting benefit from thrombolytic therapy is the timing of initiation of therapy. The critical role of timing has been most clearly shown in the GISSI trial—a prospective, randomized, controlled clinical trial of IV streptokinase versus placebo in 11,712 patients admitted to one of 176 coronary care units in Italy within 12 hrs of onset of symptoms of acute MI. At 21 days, overall hospital mortality was 10.7% in streptokinase recipients compared to 13% in controls—an 18% reduction in mortality.[2] Moreover, at 12 months, mortality was 17.2% in the streptokinase group compared to 19.0% in the control group—a statistically and clinically significant 9.5% reduction in 1-year mortality.[3] The reduction in hospital mortality was 51% in patients treated within 1 hr, 26% in those treated within 3 hrs, 20% in those treated within 3 to 6 hrs, and only a statistically insignificant 13% among those treated 6 to 9 hrs after onset. Patients treated 9–12 hrs after symptom onset experienced no reduction in mortality. Thus, the greatest reduction in mortality is achieved in patients who receive thrombolytic therapy in the first few hours of symptom onset. The crucial importance of timing in the administration of thrombolytic therapy is commonly illustrated by the statement "Time is muscle."

References: 1. Dewood MA, et al: Prevalence of total coronary occlusion during the early hours of transmural myocardial infarction. N Engl J Med 303:897–902, 1980.

2. GISSI: Effectiveness of intravenous thrombolytic treatment in acute myocardial infarction. Lancet 1:397–401, 1986.

3. GISSI: Effectiveness of intravenous thrombolytic treatment in acute myocardial infarction. Lancet 2:871–874, 1987.

MYOPATHY

The conditions known to produce weakness and muscle pain are legion. History can provide important clues to understanding the source and etiology of a patient's weakness. The pattern of muscles involved can provide important information. Associated symptoms such as spasm and twitching, fatigue, low-grade fever, alcohol consumption, and medication lists are all important as well. Physical examination of gait together with a careful musculature exam, particularly with repetitive testing, can lead to better understanding of muscle weakness. Muscle bulk with atrophy implies neurologic disease. Conversely, hypertrophy or pseudohypertrophy occurs in many muscular dystrophies. Severe weakness with little atrophy occurs commonly in patients with polymyositis, myasthenia gravis, periodic paralysis, steroid myopathy, Addison's disease, and hypothyroidism.

Probably the most well accepted muscle strength grading system comes from the Medical Research Council of Great Britain:

0	No motion (complete paralysis)
1	Minimal contraction
2	Active movement in the same plane as gravity
3	Weak muscular motion against gravity
4	Active movement against gravity and resistance
5	Normal strength

Polymyositis

Polymyositis is a systemic inflammatory disorder leading to breakdown of skeletal muscle. **Dermatomyositis,** a variant of polymyositis, is characterized by muscle inflammation associated with a characteristic skin rash. It can occur idiopathically or as part of an established systemic rheumatic disease, most commonly, scleroderma, SLE, or one of the inflammatory vasculopathies. There is an association between polymyositis/dermatomyositis and malignancy. Between 10 and 20% of patients with these conditions may have an underlying malignancy. In as many as 70% of patients, the inflammatory component may precede the development of malignancy by as much as 1 to 2 years. Careful follow-up studies reveal that **HIV-associated myositis** exists as a separate and distinct entity from a myopathy secondary to antiviral medication.

The incidence of disease appears to approach five cases per million population. Adult-onset disease generally begins between the fifth and sixth decades, and women are affected by a greater than 2:1 ratio. Worldwide, the Japanese are the least affected adult population, whereas African-Americans seem to suffer the highest incidence.

Both HLA B8 and DR3 have been associated with active myopathy. These antigens are commonly found together in patients with polymyositis. In addition, patients with this linkage have a higher incidence of circulating anti-Jo-1 antibody. These genetic factors in conjunction with the disease's pathologic changes have led investigators to conclude muscle damage is based on cell-mediated, antigen-specific cytotoxicity. The presence of circulating autoantibodies also suggests an immune pathogenesis. These antibodies are not found in other autoimmune conditions, are generally directed at cytoplasmic antigens (specifically, transfer ribonucleic acid), and, when present, can provide prognostic information. Finally, the recognized association with other autoimmune conditions (in addition to those previously noted, Hashimoto's thyroiditis, primary biliary cirrhosis, and primary vitiligo) also implies an autoimmune pathogenesis.

Viruses and altered muscle energetics have been proposed as playing roles in the production of inflammatory myopathy. In addition to frank necrosis, certain metabolic derangements may be contributing to muscle dysfunction and weakness. It seems likely, however, that inflammatory myopathies are the result of an immune response against certain environmental agents in the susceptible host.

The unifying clinical feature in these conditions is weakness. Onset is rarely explosive. More commonly, fatigue associated with leg and arm weakness is generally noted. Muscle pain and tenderness may also be present. Common complaints such as inability to rise from the commode or a low chair may be heard. Some patients have trouble putting dishes away overhead or in combing their hair. Stiffness, arthralgia, fever, and weight loss attest to the systemic nature of the disease. The rash of dermatomyositis commonly precedes the myopathy and may progress along an independent course. Raynaud's is more commonly associated with dermatomyositis than polymyositis.

Examination shows proximal weakness. Neck flexors should be carefully examined, as they are commonly involved. Distal weakness is uncommon unless disease is severe or long standing. Lack of ocular muscle involvement in polymyositis/dermatomyositis can be a helpful distinguishing feature.

In dermatomyositis, the classic rash is lilac in color (heliotrope) and is present over the eyelids. Violaceous scaly discolorations over the knuckles are known as Gottron's papules. Similar discoloration and scaling can occur at the elbows and knees. Cutaneous vasculitis, livedo reticularis, and digital infarcts are also not infrequent cutaneous manifestations.

Laboratory data provide important information. There are a few reports of inflammatory myopathy with a normal CPK, but these are truly the exception. Other muscle enzymes such as aldolase, AST and ALT are also elevated. EMG/NCV show increased insertional activity, bizarre high-frequency discharge, and polyphasic motor unit potentials of low amplitude. These findings are compatible with, but not diagnostic of, polymyositis/dermatomyositis.

Pathological evidence of muscle necrosis is present in patients with polymyositis/dermatomyositis. Regeneration fibers may also be seen, and normal fibers can be interspersed; these are inflammatory changes that include lymphocyte, plasma cell, and histiocytic infiltration. Interstitial edema is often present.

Treatment consists of hyperphysiologic doses of glucocorticoids. Methotrexate has been used successfully both as treatment for refractory cases and as a steroid-sparing agent.

Other Myopathies

Some specific infectious conditions can lead to myopathy. Trichinosis, less common today, is suggested by weakness in association with eosinophilia. Plain x-ray can sometimes reveal calcified cysts. Toxoplasmosis can cause a muscular weakness, but this usually occurs with liver disease and encephalopathy. Viral infections such as echovirus, adenovirus, and herpetic viruses such as EBV can be associated with muscular weakness.

Inflammatory myopathy is one of the most common rheumatic complications of HIV infection. Dermatomyositis can also be seen in HIV-infected patients although less frequently. The incidence of inflammatory myopathy in HIV patients is somewhat higher than in the general population. Myopathy has been reported to be the initial manifestation of infection and thus is clearly independent of treatment. Biopsy reveals the classical inflammation indistinguishable from idiopathic polymyositis. Several studies have been unsuccessful despite vigorous attempts to isolate virus from biopsy specimens. Other infections have also been reported and should be considered. Treatment carries the risk of further immunosuppression, but when faced with debilitating weakness and classical history of EMG/NCV findings, some investigators report success with oral glucocorticoids.

Inclusion body myositis affects mainly the pelvicrural muscles, but lower limb muscles can also be involved. Males are more frequently affected than females, and upper limbs are more involved than lower. Injury to the muscle is felt to be T cell mediated. A diagnosis must usually await muscle biopsy and demonstration of the classical intranuclear and intracytoplasmic inclusions. Patients do not seem to respond to glucocorticoids, and the condition is uniformly fatal.

Rhabdomyolysis occurs with rapid destruction of striated muscle fibers. Myoglobin from the destroyed fibers enters the blood and ultimately appears in the urine.

The myoglobinuria can lead to progressive renal failure. The most common causes include crush injuries or infarction of the muscles and, occasionally, aggressive polymyositis. Although alcoholic polymyopathy can sometimes present in this fashion, severe muscle necrosis in the alcoholic patient more commonly results from compression injury after prolonged unconsciousness.

The **muscular dystrophies** can be suggested on the basis of the pattern of muscle involvement. Polyneuropathies occur in the distal muscles of the limbs, whereas dystrophies affect mainly the girdle muscles in the proximal limb and oculopharyngeal muscles. In general, these are progressive, hereditary, degenerative diseases of skeletal muscles. There is preservation of cutaneous reflexes and often an obvious familial incidence. Duchenne muscular dystrophy is commonly encountered in children and does not present in adults. Becker's muscular dystrophy can sometimes occur in young adults, with weakness the presenting feature and CPK levels markedly elevated. Becker's and Duchenne muscular dystrophies are felt to be related through the gene product known as dystrophin. In Duchenne dystrophy, this compound is absent, whereas in Becker's dystrophy, it is present in normal amounts but is nonfunctional.

Central core myopathy is an example of a congenital myopathy that occasionally does not present until the middle years. A unique feature of this disease is dense amorphous mass in the central portion of type 1 muscle fiber. **Mitochondrial myopathy** is another congenital myopathy that can sometimes present in adulthood. These diseases are associated with the presence of large and overtly abundant mitochondria in many muscle fibers.

Finally, **metabolic diseases** are known to produce muscle dysfunction. Thyroid disease can cause a significant myopathy. Myasthenia gravis is associated with diffuse toxic goiter and hypothyroidism. Muscle hypertrophy and slow contraction occur in myxedema. Long-standing use of glucocorticoids can also produce a myopathy. Rarely is there any associated elevation of circulating CPK levels. Primary aldosteronism including adrenal adenoma leads to muscular weakness. Generalized weakness is likewise a characteristic of Addison's disease. Hypoparathyroidism can cause muscular problems and weakness as well. Glycogen storage diseases such as acid maltase deficiency and McArdle's disease may need to be considered in the differential diagnosis.

Reference: Cronin ME, et al: Idiopathic inflammatory myopathies. Rheum Dis Clin North Am 16(3):655–666, 1990.

MYXEDEMA COMA

Myxedema coma is the extreme expression of severe hypothyroidism. It is most often seen in hospitalized, elderly women with long-standing hypothyroidism. Despite vigorous and intensive therapy, the mortality rate is nearly 60%.

Clinical Features

1. All typical signs of severe hypothyroidism usually present
2. Depressed ventilatory response to hypercapnia, impaired ventilation (depression of respiratory drive), diaphragmatic muscle dysfunction

3. Impaired LV function, hypotension, collapse and shock in extreme cases
4. Paralytic ileus (to be differentiated from mechanical obstruction)
5. Gastric atony (severe)
6. Hyponatremia (secondary to impaired water diuresis—may be responsible for mental confusion and coma)
7. CNS manifestations: lethargy, seizures (25%), and, in extreme cases, coma
8. Hypothermia (75% of patients) may be profound (less than 80°F); profound hypothermia is often associated with a worse prognosis.
9. Hypoglycemia

Precipitating Factors

1. Administration of large amounts of IV fluids
2. Use of sedatives and hypnotic drugs in hypothyroid patients
3. Exposure to cold
4. Infection (lungs, urinary tract)

Thyroid Function Tests

TSH levels may be spuriously lowered by coexistent illness or dopamine infusion. An elevated TSH is indicative of primary hypothyroidism. A normal or low TSH suggests pituitary-hypothalamic disease. If so, cortisol-level measurement and assessment of pituitary adrenal reserve are crucial for survival.

Therapy

Management of Myxedema Coma

PROBLEM	SPECIFIC THERAPY
Hypercapnia, hypoxemia	Ventilatory support (up to 2–3 weeks)
Hyponatremia	Diuretics (if severe, infuse small amounts of hypertonic saline)
Hypothermia	Ordinary (avoid electric) blankets
	Increased room temperature
Hypotension	Hydrocortisone, pressor agents
Thyroid hormone deficiency	Levothyroxine (T_4) bolus (500 μg)
	Followed by 50–100 μg L-T_4 IV daily
	OR
	T_3 IV (higher risk of cardiac events)
	OR
	Combination of T_4 and T_3 IV until improvement
Possible coexistent adrenal insufficiency	Glucocorticoids
Precipitating illness	Antibiotics for infection, other specific treatment as needed

N

NAUSEA

Nausea is a nonspecific symptom associated with many conditions. It is perhaps most useful to consider it as an early form of vomiting, to which it may progress if the underlying cause is serious and/or significant. Thus, many of the same conditions that cause one also cause the other, and the mechanisms are similar.

The CNS center for nausea and vomiting is located in the lateral reticular formation of the medulla and receives signals from:

1. The GI tract via vagal and sympathetic afferent nerves
2. The midbrain receptors of intracranial pressure
3. The labyrinthine apparatus
4. Higher CNS structures such as the limbic system reacting to psychic stimuli
5. The chemoreceptor trigger zone (CTZ)

The CTZ is a distinct medullary center situated in the floor of the fourth ventricle, where it is in contact with both CSF and blood. Noxious materials activate the CTZ, which is abundant in neuroreceptors stimulated by histamine, dopamine, and acetylcholine. Stimuli are delivered to the CTZ, and efferent signals are sent via phrenic nerves to the diaphragm, spinal nerves to the abdominal musculature, and visceral nerves to the stomach and esophagus. The autonomic nervous system signs of nausea include salivation, tachycardia, diaphoresis, and pallor. Somatic efferent nerves coordinate the muscles of respiration, which are responsible for retching and contribute to the sensation of nausea.

Causes of Nausea

I. CNS
  A. Increased intracranial pressure
    1. Brain tumors, primary or metastatic
    2. Cerebral hemorrhage
    3. Meningitis
    4. Encephalitis
    5. High-altitude sickness
    6. Migraine headaches
    7. Acute hydrocephalus
  B. Labyrinthine dysfunction
    1. Meniere's disease
    2. Toxic labyrinthitis

II. Hypotension
  A. Acute MI (especially inferior wall MI)
  B. Septic shock

III. Toxic
  A. CO poisoning
  B. Chemotherapy
  C. Toxic chemical exposure
  D. Food poisoning
  E. Digitalis or theophylline toxicity
  F. Antibiotic (sulfa, tetracycline, erythromycin) side effects

IV. Anatomic/functional
  A. Early outlet obstruction
  B. Diabetic gastroparesis
  C. Functional bowel obstruction due to:
    1. Overuse of analgesics
    2. Constipation

Table continued on next page.

Causes of Nausea (Cont.)

V. Metabolic
    A. DKA   C. Renal failure/uremia
    B. Hyponatremia   D. Adrenal crisis

VI. Infectious
    A. Gastroenteritis   C. Hepatitis
    B. Tabetic crisis

VII. Miscellaneous
    A. Hereditary angioedema   B. Early pregnancy

Treatment of nausea is often symptomatic, since the mechanisms are similar for all causes. Drugs such as the phenothiazines, dopamine antagonists that block dopamine receptors at the CTZ, are the most commonly used drugs. Butyrophenones and substituted benzamides such as metoclopramide are more potent dopamine receptor blockers. Antihistamines such as diphenhydramine act by blocking labyrinthine impulses. Some drugs, such as metoclopramide, also act by increasing lower esophageal sphincter tone, by promoting gastric emptying, and by accelerating small bowel transit, thus minimizing gastric stasis and reflux. This is often useful in diabetic gastroparesis and other motility disorders. Cannabinoids are believed to suppress nausea by inhibiting efferent pathways from the CTZ.

Of course, if the etiology can be identified, the nausea may resolve with treatment of the primary problem. Thus infectious causes of gastroenteritis and meningitis should be treated, overuse of analgesics should be avoided, and the toxicities of any drugs being used should be considered in approaches to this problem.

NEEDLESTICK INJURIES

Needlestick injuries and the risk of subsequent infection with HIV or HBV are a concern of all health care workers. The risk of contracting HBV after a needlestick is much greater than the risk of contracting HIV. According to estimates by the CDC, each year 12,000 health care workers whose jobs entail exposure to blood become infected with HBV. Of these, 250 die: 170 to 200 from cirrhosis, 40 to 50 from liver cancer, and 12 to 15 from fulminant hepatitis.

The risk of contracting HIV infection from a needlestick injury is only now becoming quantified. As of 1988, 5% of the AIDS cases reported to the CDC were health care workers. However, 95% of these persons also reported engaging in high-risk behavior. Data on the incidence of HIV infection after needlestick injuries are now available from three large studies. In all three, seroconversion occurred in fewer than 0.5% of persons. In contrast, the risk of infection with HBV after a needlestick injury is about 12%.

Despite their frequency (one study found 0.75 needlestick injuries/person-year in an internal medicine training program), needlestick injuries are largely preventable, as has been shown by several before-after studies of educational programs in hospitals. Needles should never be recapped. All sharps should be disposed of promptly in appropriately labeled puncture-resistant containers. Needles should never be left on bedside stands, on beds, or plunged into mattresses after use.

A safe and effective vaccine is available against HBV. Vaccination is recommended for all health care workers regularly exposed to blood or body fluids. By mandates of the U.S. Departments of Labor and of Health and Human Services, HBV vaccine has been supplied free to health workers since 1988.

A worker should report promptly to the employee health clinic after a needlestick injury. All such clinics have protocols to manage needlestick injuries. The HBV and HIV status of the injured person should be determined immediately after the needlestick, and seronegative persons should be retested at 6 weeks, 12 weeks, and 6 months. Medical evaluation should be sought for any acute febrile illness occurring within 12 weeks of exposure. During the follow-up period (especially the first 12 weeks), the exposed worker should follow U.S. Public Health Service recommendations regarding prevention of transmission of HIV (refrain from donating blood, use appropriate protection during sexual intercourse, etc.). The role of zidovudine after needlestick injuries is not clear.

References: Centers for Disease Control: Guidelines for the prevention of transmission of human immunodeficiency virus and hepatitis B virus to health care and public safety workers. MMWR 38:1–32, 1989.

Owens DK, et al: Occupational exposure to human immunodeficiency virus and hepatitis B virus: A comparative analysis of risk. Am J Med 92:503–512, 1992.

Centers for Disease Control: Protection against viral hepatitis. Recommendations of the Immunization Practices Advisory Committee (ACIP). MMWR 39:19–25, 1990.

NEPHROLITHIASIS

Renal calculi are abnormal concretions occurring in the kidneys and consist of an organic matrix and a crystalline component. They are usually present in the renal pelvis or calyx but can migrate to the ureter or the bladder. The term *nephrolithiasis* indicates renal stones; *nephrocalcinosis* indicates calcification of the renal parenchyma. Renal stones are seen in 1 to 5% of the general population. Calcium stones are the most frequent and constitute 80 to 95% of all renal stones.

Classification of Kidney Stones

TYPES OF STONES	% INCIDENCE	PREDISPOSING FACTORS
Calcium salts	70	—
Calcium oxalate	67	Hypercalciuria, hyperoxaluria, hyperuri-
Calcium oxalate and hydroxyapatite	—	cosuria
Brushite and hydroxyapatite	3	Renal tubular acidosis, alkaline urine
Struvite	20	Alkaline urine due to urea-splitting or-
		ganisms
Uric Acid	5	Gout, hyperuricosuria, acidic urine
Cystine	2	Triamterene

Pathophysiology: Urinary supersaturation with certain salts is the primary event in the stone formation. This could be due to low urinary volume, high excretory rate of these ions, abnormalities of urinary pH, or deficiency of inhibitors of renal stone formation such as citrate, magnesium, and glycoproteins. The addition of urinary debris initiates nucleation, which leads to crystal growth and eventual stone formation.

Clinical features: Quite often, renal stones are asymptomatic but sometimes they present with hematuria from erosion into a renal pelvis or flank pain due to the dislodging of a stone. Other manifestations are urinary tract obstruction, urinary infection, nephrocalcinosis, and renal failure.

Diagnosis: In the workup of renal stones, details of diet and drug ingestion and family medical history should be obtained. UA will show hematuria and/or pyuria. If crystalluria is present, it gives a clue to the type of renal stone. Plain abdominal x-ray reveals the urinary stones in 85% of cases. Uric acid stones are radiolucent. Renal ultrasound can be used to document presence of stones and hydronephrosis. An IVP is used to determine whether a suspected radio-opaque object is located in the urinary tract. The chemical nature of the stone is established by crystallographic stone analysis. Urinary excretion of various salts should be determined to delineate the metabolic abnormalities predisposing to renal stone formation. Normal excretion of some of these salts is indicated in the table.

Urinary Excretion Rates of Salts

	UPPER LIMITS OF NORMAL	
SUBSTANCE	Men	Women
Calcium, mg/24 hr	300	250
Calcium, mg/kg/24 hr	4	4
Calcium, mg/mg creatinine	0.14	0.14
Oxalate, mg/24 hr	50	50
Uric acid, mg/24 hr	800	750

In patients with calcium stones, hypercalciuria is seen in 50% of cases. Hypercalciuria is idiopathic in 40% of cases and is secondary to other conditions in the remaining cases.

Major Metabolic Causes of Hypercalciuria

Primary hyperparathyroidism	Excess vitamin D and calcium intake
Sarcoidosis	Immobilization
Distal renal tubular acidosis	Milk-alkali syndrome

Idiopathic hypercalciuria is often due to intestinal hyperabsorption (absorptive hypercalciuria), which suppresses the serum PTH. In other cases, the abnormality is decreased renal tubular reabsorption (renal hypercalciuria) and is associated with normal PTH. Calcium phosphate stones occur in patients with persistently alkaline urine such as those with infections, distal RTA, and chronic alkali ingestion. Hyperoxaluria predisposes to calcium oxalate stone formation. Idiopathic hyperoxaluria is uncommon and is treated with pyridoxine and phosphates. The secondary causes of hyperoxaluria are listed in the table.

Secondary Causes of Hyperoxaluria

GI disorders
    Bacterial overgrowth, jejunoileal bypass, ileal resection
    Chronic pancreatitis, biliary disorders
    Inflammatory bowel disease
Other causes
    Dietary excesses of oxalate, ascorbic acid ingestion
    Pyridoxine deficiency, ethylene glycol intoxication
    Methoxyflurane

Struvite (magnesium ammonium phosphate) stones develop in the presence of urinary infections by urea-splitting organisms such as *Proteus, E. coli, Klebsiella,* and *Pseudomonas* species. In 50% of cases, struvite stones develop on another form of stone such as calcium or uric acid stones. Struvite stones grow rapidly in the presence of alkaline urine to form staghorn calculi and may cause urinary obstruction. Uric acid stones develop in persistently acidic urine, especially in patients with dehydration. Chemotherapy for malignant disorders as well as myeloproliferative syndromes are the other predisposing factors for uric acid stones. Cystine stones develop in patients with cystinuria, which is a rare, inherited tubular defect. These stones develop in acidic urine.

Management: About 80% of the stones are passed spontaneously. The treatment is often symptomatic in the acute phase. This includes pain relief, hydration, and treatment of concomitant infection if present. If there is urinary tract obstruction, the stone should be disimpacted by extracorporeal shock-wave lithotripsy or be surgically removed. Patients with metabolic disorders predisposing to stones need long-term therapy. In patients with calcium stones, dietary restriction of calcium may be considered, but if hyperoxaluria is present, calcium intake should not be restricted because this increases oxalate absorption. Restriction of dietary oxalate and Na^+ is helpful in patients with hyperoxaluria and hypercalciuria, respectively. Thiazides (25–50 mg BID) are helpful in decreasing calcium and oxalate excretion. Cellulose phosphate and neutral sodium phosphate bind to intestinal calcium and hence are useful in hypercalciuria. Struvite stones are managed by antimicrobial therapy, lithotripsy, and acidification of urine. Uric acid stones require alkalinization of urine ($NaHCO_3$ 1–3 mEq/kg/day), as well as avoidance of purine rich foods and allopurinol (if the uric acid is high). Cystine stones, too, are treated with alkalinization of urine, dietary restriction of methionine, and D-penicillamine (in cases with cystinuria >1 gm/day). In all forms of stone disease, urine output should be maintained at around 2 to 3 L/day.

Reference: Coe FL, et al: Pathophysiology of kidney stones and strategies for treatment. Hosp Pract 23:145, 1988.

NEPHROTIC SYNDROME

Nephrotic syndrome is generally defined as a symptom complex resulting from various etiologies and characterized by heavy proteinuria (usually >3.5 gm/day), generalized edema, and lipiduria with hyperlipidemia. Since all the other features are a consequence of marked proteinuria, some authorities restrict the definition of nephrosis to heavy proteinuria alone.

Common Causes of Nephrotic Syndrome

GLOMERULAR DISEASES	OTHERS
Primary	
Minimal change disease	CHF
Membranous nephritis	Drugs: NSAIDs, gold, phenytoin, penicil-
Membranoproliferative	lamine, captopril
Focal glomerulosclerosis	Hypothyroidism
Acute proliferative (rare)	Constrictive pericarditis

Table continued on next page.

Common Causes of Nephrotic Syndrome (Cont.)

GLOMERULAR DISEASES	OTHERS
Secondary	
DM	Dysproteinemias: amyloidosis, light chain
SLE	deposit disease
Endocarditis	Sarcoidosis
Hepatitis B	Serum sickness
HIV nephropathy	Massive obesity
Heroin abuse	Ulcerative colitis
Mixed cryoglobulinemia	Preeclampsia
Hereditary: Alport's syndrome	Neoplasia: Hodgkin's and non-Hodgkin's
Vascular: renal vein thrombosis,	lymphoma, carcinomas
rejection glomerulopathy	

Complications of Nephrotic Syndrome

1. Edema and ascites
2. Hypovolemia with acute prerenal and/or parenchymal renal disease: The nephrotic syndrome is a state of decreased effective arterial blood volume that can lead to various degrees of renal hypoperfusion. In severe cases, the renal hypoperfusion can lead to renal failure.
3. Protein malnutrition can occur because of massive protein losses in excess of dietary replacement.
4. Hyperlipidemia, which raises the risk of CAD and ASCVD.
5. Increased susceptibility to bacterial infection, which occurs most frequently in the lungs, meninges (meningitis), and peritoneum: Common organisms include *Streptococcus* species (including *S. pneumoniae*), *Haemophilus influenzae,* and *Klebsiella* species.
6. Proximal tubular dysfunction, which may lead to Fanconi's syndrome with urinary wasting of glucose, phosphate, amino acids, uric acid, K^+, and HCO_3^-.
7. Hypercoagulable state manifested by increased incidence of venous thrombosis, particularly in the renal vein: The precise mechanism is not clear, but it appears to be partially due to urinary loss of factors that normally inhibit clotting.

Management: Management of some of the common problems associated with all forms of nephrotic syndrome is discussed here. Edema is usually treated with thiazide or loop diuretics and salt and water restriction. However, overzealous diuresis can result in hypotension and renal failure. A protein-restricted diet (0.5–0.6 g/kg/d) along with ACE inhibitors often decreases protein loss. When the protein loss exceeds 10 gm/day, additional protein should be supplemented in the diet. Chronic urinary losses of vitamin D metabolites result in osteomalacia and often require replacement therapy with vitamin D. Hyperlipidemia is usually managed with both dietary reduction of saturated fat and regular exercise. Drug therapy with lovastatin and other lipid-lowering agents is generally reserved for patients with resistant hyperlipidemia. All patients with long-standing nephrotic syndrome should be vaccinated with the pneumococcal vaccine, as they are at risk for development of bacterial infections. Thromboembolism occurs in 20% of patients with nephrosis due to a multifactorial hypercoagulable state. Renal vein thrombosis occurs in 2 to 60% of cases of nephrotic syndrome but is an important source of pulmonary embolism. Long-term prophylactic anticoagulation is reserved for those at high risk of thrombosis or with prior thromboembolism.

The differential characteristics and response to treatment of various primary glomerulopathies leading to nephrotic syndrome are represented in the table that follows.

Summary of Primary Renal Diseases that Present as Idiopathic Nephrotic Syndrome

	MINIMAL CHANGE NEPHROTIC SYNDROME (MCNS)	FOCAL GLOMERULO-SCLEROSIS	MEMBRANOUS NEPHROPATHY	MEMBRANOPROLIFERATIVE GLOMERULONEPHRITIS (MPGN)	
				Type I	Type II
Frequency*					
Children	75%	10%	<5%	10%	10%
Adults	15%	15%	50%	10%	10%
Clinical manifestations					
Age	2–6, some adults	2–6, some adults	40–50	5–15	5–15
Sex	2:1 male	1.3:1 male	2:1 male	Male-female	
Nephrotic syndrome	100%	90%	80%	60%	
Asymptomatic proteinuria	0	10%	20%	40%	
Hematuria	20%	60–80%	60%	80%	
Hypertension	10%	20% early	Infrequent	35%	
Rate of progression	Does not progress	10 years	50% in 10–20 years	10–20 years	5–15 years
Associated conditions	Allergy, Hodgkin's disease	None	Renal vein thrombosis, cancer, SLE	None	Partial lipodystrophy
Laboratory findings	Manifestations of nephrotic syndrome	Manifestations of nephrotic syndrome	Manifestations of nephrotic syndrome	Low C1, C4, C3–C9	Normal C1, C4, low C3–C9, C3 nephritic factor
Immunogenetics	HLA-B8, B12 (3.5)†	Not established	HLA-DRw3 (12–32)†	Not established	
Renal pathology					
Light microscopy	Normal	Focal sclerotic lesions	Thickened GBM, spikes	Thickened GBM, proliferation, lobulation	
Immunofluorescence	Negative	IgM, C3 in lesions	Fine granular IgG, C3	Granular IgG, C3	C3 only
Electron microscopy	Foot process fusion	Foot process fusion	Subepithelial deposits	Mesangial and subendothelial deposits	Dense deposits
Response to steroids	90%	15–20%	May be slow progression	Not established	

* Approximate frequency. GBM = glomerular basement membrane. About 10% of adult nephrotic syndrome (NS) is due to various diseases that usually present with acute glomerulonephritis (GN).

† Relative risk.

From Couser WG: Glomerular disorders. In Wyngaarden JB, et al (eds): Cecil Textbook of Medicine, 19th ed. Philadelphia, W.B. Saunders, 1992, p 560, with permission.

Minimal change disease carries excellent prognosis in children and very good prognosis in adults: over 90% respond to steroids. Cyclophosphamide or chlorambucil induces remissions in steroid-resistant cases. Prognosis is generally poor in nephrotic patients with progressive renal failure as in focal sclerosis, membranous nephropathy, and membranoproliferative nephritis. About 40% of patients with focal sclerosis experience a remission when treated with prednisone (2 mg/kg per day for 8 weeks followed by a 4-week taper). Cyclosporine induces remission in about 30% of steroid-resistant adults with focal sclerosis. Steroid treatment in membranous nephropathy is often rewarding in the short-term preservation of renal function, but there is no difference in the long-term prognosis between treated and untreated patients. More than 50% of patients with membranoproliferative nephritis progress to renal failure, and the benefits of treatment on long-term renal function are questionable. It is claimed that prolonged alternate-day steroid therapy in children and antiplatelet agents in adults are beneficial but this remains to be proved.

Cameron JS: The nephrotic syndrome and its complications. Am J Kidney Dis 10:157, 1987.

NEPHROTOXINS

Renal injury resulting directly or indirectly from exposure to exogenous chemical toxins is referred to as toxic nephropathy. Drug-related renal injury is the most common cause of toxic nephropathy. In the majority of instances, the resulting renal damage is prominent in the tubules and interstitium, although some nephrotoxins such as gold and nonsteroidal analgesics cause severe glomerular injury. (NSAIDs and analgesics as nephrotoxins are discussed separately. This section deals with the other nephrotoxins.)

Prominent or Common Nephrotoxins

Anticonvulsants: paramethadione, phenytoin, trimethadone
Antihypertensive drugs: angiotensin-converting enzyme inhibitors
Antimicrobials: acyclovir, aminoglycosides, amphotericin B, cephalosporins, ethambutol, isoniazid, para-aminosalicylic acid, penicillins, pentamidine, rifampin, sulfonamides, tetracyclines
Antineoplastic agents: cisplatin, methotrexate, mitomycin C, nitrosoureas, radiation
Endogenous compounds: Bence Jones proteins, calcium, hemoglobin, myoglobin, oxalate, uric acid
Halogenated alkanes, hydrocarbons, and solvents: carbon tetrachloride, ethylene glycol, paraquat, toluene
Iodinated radiographic contrast media
Metals: arsenic, bismuth, cadmium, copper, gold, lead, lithium, mercury
Miscellaneous compounds: acetaminophen, allopurinol, amphetamines, azathioprine, cimetidine, cyclosporine, heroin, methoxyflurane, methysergide, D-penicillamine, phenacetin, phenindione, silicon
Nonsteroidal anti-inflammatory drugs
Sulfonamide diuretics: acetazolamide, chlorthalidone, furosemide, thiazides

---

From McKinney TD: Tubulointerstitial diseases and toxic nephropathies. In Wyngaarden JB, et al (eds): Cecil Textbook of Medicine, 19th ed. Philadelphia, W.B. Saunders, 1992, p 572, with permission.

Aminoglycosides

Aminoglycosides are the most common nephrotoxins among the antibiotics. The drugs accumulate in the kidney, causing various renal effects that include ARF and tubular functional abnormalities such as potassium and magnesium wasting. ARF, the most significant tubulotoxic result of aminoglycosides, occurs in up to 10% of patients receiving these agents and results from acute tubular necrosis (ATN). Aminoglycoside toxicity accounts for as many as 10 to 15% of cases of ARF in the United States. The ARF is mostly nonoliguric, occurs a few days after the drug has been started, and is often reflected by mild elevations of serum creatinine that return to normal in another few days. However, some patients develop oliguria and severe azotemia necessitating dialysis. Risk factors for development of nephrotoxicity include dose and duration of aminoglycoside therapy, volume depletion, K^+ depletion, preexisting renal and hepatic failure, concomitant administration of cephalosporins, and advanced age. Streptomycin is the least nephrotoxic, and neomycin the most nephrotoxic of this group; tobramycin and gentamicin are intermediate in toxicity. Management consists of discontinuation of the aminoglycoside and, if no suitable alternative is available, continuation at lower doses. Management of ARF is similar to that caused by other conditions, and the prognosis is most often excellent.

Amphotericin B

Amphotericin causes nephrotoxicity in most patients receiving a cumulative dose of more than 2 g. The initial effects are reversible upon discontinuation of the drug and consist of distal tubular defects such as distal tubular acidosis, nephrogenic DI, and renal K^+ leak. Serious toxicity includes ARF, is often progressive and irreversible, and results from renal vasoconstriction and direct tubular toxicity. The predisposing factors include volume depletion and underlying renal failure. Management consists of either discontinuation of the drug when renal failure occurs or decreasing the frequency of dosing to alternate days.

Other Antibacterial Agents

Tetracyclines cause increase in urea synthesis and elevate BUN without causing elevation of serum creatinine. This could be a major problem in patients with underlying renal insufficiency. Tetracyclines are thus contraindicated in the presence of renal insufficiency except for doxycycline and minocycline, which require slight dosage adjustment. Outdated tetracyclines cause Fanconi's syndrome. Demeclocycline causes nephrogenic DI and is used in the management of SIADH. However, it may cause renal failure when used to treat hyponatremia in patients with cirrhosis. Cephalosporins rarely cause ARF, but when used in combination with aminoglycosides, they are more nephrotoxic than either agent used alone.

Radiographic Contrast Agents

Radiographic contrast agents cause ARF in as many as 2 to 13% of patients exposed to them and are a common cause of ATN. Predisposing factors include underlying renal failure, DM, dehydration, old age, and probably multiple myeloma.

DM with preexisting renal insufficiency constitutes the most common risk factor (75% incidence of ATN), although diabetics with normal renal function seem to carry no increased risk. Pathogenetic factors incriminated include renal vasoconstriction, tubular obstruction by precipitated proteins, and tubulotoxicity. Elevations in serum creatinine are noted in 1 to 2 days, they plateau in 7 to 10 days, and thereafter recovery occurs over a variable period of time.

More severe forms of renal failure often needing dialysis are seen in patients with more severe underlying renal disease. Avoidance of dehydration, minimizing the dose of the contrast agent, and use of hypertonic mannitol in high-risk patients (25–50 gm in 1 hr) immediately following the contrast administration often prevent renal toxicity. Nonionic agents are not less nephrotoxic than conventional contrast agents.

Miscellaneous Nephrotoxins

A number of antineoplastic agents are nephrotoxic. These include cisplatin (ATN, renal Mg^+ and K^+ wasting), methotrexate (ARF due to tubular precipitation), nitrosureas (proteinuria, tubular abnormalities), and mitomycin C (hemolytic uremic syndrome).

In addition, several metals such as gold (membranous nephropathy), mercury (ATN, proteinuria), and lead (interstitial nephritis) are nephrotoxic. D-Penicillamine causes proteinuria and azotemia; ACE inhibitors cause azotemia in patients with bilateral renal artery stenosis, CHF, cirrhosis, hypovolemia, and, rarely, proteinuria. Pentamidine causes ARF in 25% of cases, and a similar toxicity is seen with foscarnet, used in the treatment of CMV retinitis.

Reference: Berns AS: Nephrotoxicity of contrast media. Kidney Int 36:730, 1989.

NEUROGENIC BLADDER

Dysfunction of the lower urinary tract can be a difficult problem for patients. Discomfort and embarrassment can lead to social isolation or reliance on various pads and diapers that are uncomfortable stop-gap measures. The physiological accomplishment of the seemingly mundane task of bladder emptying requires a complex integrated system: The detrusor muscle (bladder) is innervated by parasympathetic fibers via nerves of the sacral plexus. The internal sphincter (smooth muscle) is innervated by sympathetic fibers via hypogastric nerves, while the external sphincter (striated muscle) is supplied by the pudendal nerve. Finally, the entire process of micturition must be orchestrated by the CNS micturition center.

In the simplest terms, bladder and lower urinary tract functions can be divided into two segments—that of bladder filling and urine storage and that of bladder emptying. Accumulation and storage of urine should occur painlessly but with the appropriate sensibility at fullness. There should be no involuntary bladder contractions, and the bladder outlet should be closed at rest or with increased levels of intra-abdominal pressure. Initiation of voluntary emptying of the urinary bladder requires a coordinated contraction of the detrusor and release of smooth muscle and striated sphincters. In men there must be additional coordination, with closure of the internal sphincter and relaxation of the external sphincter at orgasm, to prevent retrograde ejaculation. Neurologic dysfunction of the urinary tract can generally be traced to problems in one of these spheres.

CNS impairment commonly is associated with voiding problems. Patients with dementia and Parkinson's disease often have difficulty with incontinence. Central deficits are one of the many ways multiple sclerosis can adversely affect bladder control. Without awareness of fullness, there are detrusor hyperactivity and contraction, resulting in overflow incontinence.

Spinal cord lesions, depending on their location, have an effect on the urinary tract. Upper cord lesions lead to the so-called spastic bladder. These lesions interrupt central inhibition of bladder contraction leaving detrusor reflex contractions intact. Likewise, the bulbocavernosus reflex (contraction of the bulbocavernosus muscle after stimulation of the glans penis or clitoris) remains intact. Because these lesions abolish voluntary external sphincter control, involuntary voiding results with bladder spasm. Cystometrogram (CMG) shows uninhibited contraction of the detrusor in response to small volumes. Lesions below T12 leave the detrusor atonic. Overflow incontinence occurs with a loss of both perineal sensation and the bulbocavernosus and anal reflexes. In this case, a CMG shows low pressure and no emptying contractions.

The impact of peripheral nerve lesions depends somewhat on their location. For example, the bulbocavernosus reflex is generally a good indication that the second and fourth sacral nerves are intact. Dyssynergy can sometimes develop between the detrusor and external sphincter muscles. Urinary frequency can be an especially troubling symptom. Although it can be psychologic, this symptom is commonly present in patients with low-volume bladder distention or detrusor hyperactivity. Failure to completely empty because of atonia can lead to urinary frequency. Nocturia implies nonpsychogenic urinary frequency. Urinary hesitancy and straining suggest difficulty in emptying. Radical pelvic surgery can lead to pelvic plexis injury and neurologic dysfunction. Loss of parasympathetic fibers leads to unrestricted sympathetic stimulation and hyperreflexia with loss of normal relaxation and voiding dysfunction.

With neurologic voiding abnormalities, symptoms may be related to other organs innervated by the same somatic and autonomic nerves. Altered genital and perineal sensation or changes in sexual function may be present. Abdominal pain, cramping, incontinence, or constipation can occur. Patients most commonly have an atonic bladder as motor impulses to the bladder are interrupted.

DM is perhaps one of the most common diseases leading to voiding dysfunction. Initially, the autonomic neuropathy leads to reduced bladder sensation followed by bladder decompensation with resultant hypotonia. Patients may experience sudden voiding if there is an involuntary bladder contraction. Urgency is usually associated with involuntary bladder contraction.

Nonneurologic problems can lead to bladder dysfunction and symptoms of urinary leakage. When it occurs only in association with increased intra-abdominal pressure, stress incontinence syndrome is suggested. Enlargement of the prostate gland can lead to obstruction and, ultimately, bladder dysfunction.

Treatment depends on the level of dysfunction. If flaccid paralysis is present, bethanecol can produce bladder tone and contractions. Bladder relaxation is required if a CNS lesion has produced a spastic bladder. Both propantheline and oxybutynin can be effective. When nerve root impingement is playing a role in urologic dysfunction, laminectomy can sometimes help if no permanent damage is present. Bladder suspensions or prostatectomy can provide significant relief when appropriate. Commonly, self-catheterization may be required. In selected patients, implanted nerve stimulation can sometimes be helpful.

Reference: Adams RD, et al: Principles of Neurology, 4th ed., New York, McGraw-Hill, 1989, pp 422–444.

NITRATE TOLERANCE

Organic nitrates are a mainstay in the treatment of angina pectoris and CHF. That humans developed tolerance to nitrates was first noted in munitions workers and reported in 1946, but it was not until the late 1970s and the 1980s that the clinical relevance of nitrate tolerance became apparent. It is now known that dosage strategies designed to provide therapeutic blood levels throughout the 24-hr day produce nitrate tolerance within a week. That is, hemodynamic, exercise tolerance, and antianginal effects become attenuated if blood levels are maintained at therapeutic levels—so attenuated in some cases that the drug is no better than placebo. Tolerance occurs regardless of the route of administration.

Fortunately, tolerance is rapidly reversible and easily prevented. With as short a period as an 8-hr nitrate-free interval each day, nitrate tolerance will not occur. This nitrate-free interval can be achieved by using a TID (e.g., 0900, 1300, 1700, no bedtime dose) schedule in a patient taking oral isosorbide dinitrate or by having the patient remove transdermal nitrates (paste or patch) at bedtime. The nitrate-free interval can be arranged for the daytime in patients whose angina is more frequent at night than during the daytime. Other antianginal therapy may be needed during the nitrate-free interval.

References: Parker JO: Nitrate tolerance. Am J Cardiol 60:44H–48H, 1987.
Packer M, et al: Prevention and reversal of nitrate tolerance in patients with congestive heart failure. N Engl J Med 317:799–804, 1987.

NOBEL PRIZE WINNERS IN AMERICAN MEDICINE

1930: Karl Landsteiner
1933: Thomas H. Morgan
1934: George R. Minot, William P. Murphy, George H. Whipple
1936: Otto Loewi
1937: Albert Szent-Gyorgyi
1943: Edward A. Doisy
1944: Joseph Erlanger, Herbert S. Gasser
1946: Hermann J. Muller
1947: Carl F. Cori, Gerty T. Cori
1950: Philip S. Hench, Edward C. Kendall
1951: Max Theiler
1952: Selman A. Waksman
1953: Fritz A. Lipmann
1954: John F. Enders, Frederick C. Robbins, Thomas H. Weller
1956: Andre F. Cournand, Dickinson W. Richards Jr.
1958: George W. Beadle, Edward L. Tatum, Joshua Lederberg

1959: Arthur Kornberg, Severo Ochoa
1961: Georg von Bekesy
1962: James D. Watson
1964: Konrad E. Bloch
1966: Charles B. Huggins, Francis Peyton Rous
1967: Halden Keffer Hartline, George Wald
1968: Robert W. Holley, H. Gobind Khorana, Marshall W. Nirenberg
1969: Max Delbruck, Alfred D. Hershey, Salvador Luria
1970: Julius Axelrod
1971: Earl W. Sutherland Jr.
1972: Gerald M. Edelman
1974: Albert Claude, George Emil Palade
1975: David Baltimore, Howard Temin, Renato Dulbecco
1976: Baruch S. Blumberg, Daniel Carleton Gajdusek
1977: Rosalyn S. Yalow, Roger C.L. Guillemin, Andrew V. Schally
1978: Daniel Nathans, Hamilton O. Smith
1979: Allan M. Cormack
1980: Baruj Benacerraf, George Snell
1981: Roger W. Sperry, David H. Hubel, Tosten N. Wiesel
1983: Barbara McClintock
1985: Michael S. Brown, Joseph L. Goldstein
1986: Rita Levi-Montalcini, Stanley Cohen
1988: Gertrude B. Elion, George H. Hitchings
1989: J. Michael Bishop, Harold E. Varmus
1990: Joseph E. Murray, E. Donnall Thomas
1992: Edmond Fischer, Edwin Krebs

NONSTEROIDAL ANTI-INFLAMMATORY DRUGS

Rational Use of NSAIDs

Many rheumatic diseases are associated with acute and intense inflammation. Thus, great strides in treatment and in pain control were made with the discovery and institution of NSAIDs. Although they do not change the long-term course of disease, they do have an analgesic effect and reduce ongoing inflammation. The analgesic effect is achievable at a lower dose than required to achieve a reduction in inflammation. Other properties include suppression of fever, reduced platelet aggregation, and promotion of the closure of a patent ductus arteriosus.

Although no single mechanism completely explains all aspects of NSAID actions, prostaglandin inhibition remains the currently favored hypothesis. Inflammation leads to the production of thromboxane A_2, prostacyclin, and prostaglandin E_2. The latter two compounds are the primary mediators of the vasodilatory phase of the inflammatory response and are believed to account for many of the clinical signs of inflammation. NSAIDs are thought to inhibit production of these mediators by inhibiting cyclo-oxygenase, a key enzyme in the pathway. Aspirin inhibits this enzyme irreversibly, whereas nonacetylated salicylates and other NSAIDs accomplish this in a reversible fashion.

Classification schemes exist and are based primarily on the NSAIDs' chemical structure. Most, but not all, are organic acids and are mostly protein bound in circulation. Their efficacy when compared to placebo is well documented, especially in patients with active RA and osteoarthritis. Comparisons between NSAIDs

Nonsteroidal Anti-inflammatory Drugs

GENERIC NAME	TRADE NAME (PARTIAL LISTING)	TABLET SIZE (MG)	STARTING DOSAGE (MG)	MAXIMUM DAILY DOSE (MG)
Salicylates				
Aspirin[a]	Aspirin	325	650–1300 q4–6h	[b]
	Encaprin	500	1000 q6–8h	[b]
	ZORprin	800	1600 q12h	[b]
Choline salicylate	Arthropan liquid	1 tsp = 870	—	[b]
Choline magnesium trisalicylate[a]	Trilisate	500, 750, 1000 1 tsp = 500	1000–1250 bid	[b]
Magnesium salicylate[a]	Mobidin	600	600–1200 tid–qid	[b]
	Magan	545	545–1090 tid–qid	[b]
Salsalate	Disalcid	500	1000 bid–1500 tid	[b]
Nonsalicylates				
Diclofenac sodium	Voltaren	25, 50, 75	50–75 bid	200
Diflunisal	Dolobid	250, 500	250 bid	1500
Etodolac	Lodine	200, 300	400 bid–tid	1200
Fenoprofen calcium	Nalfon	200, 300, 600	300–600 qid	3200
Flurbiprofen	Ansaid	50, 100	50–100 tid	300
Ibuprofen	Motrin, Rufen	400, 600, 800	400 qid	3200
Indomethacin	Indocin	25, 50, 75	25 tid–qid	200
	Indocin SR	75	75 qd	200
	Indocin suppositories	50	50 bid	200
Ketoprofen	Orudis	50, 75	75 tid	300
Meclofenamate sodium	Meclomen	50, 100	50 tid–qid	400
Naproxen[a]	Naprosyn	250, 375, 500	250–500 bid	1250
Naproxen sodium	Anaprox	275	275 q6–8h	1375
Phenylbutazone	Butazolidin	100	100 tid	600
Piroxicam	Feldene	10, 20	20 qd	20
Sulindac	Clinoril	150, 200	150–200 bid	400
Tolmetin sodium	Tolectin	200, 400, 600	400 tid	1600

[a] Available as a suspension.
[b] Determined by measurement of serum salicylic level.
From Woodley M, et al (eds): Manual of Medical Therapeutics, 27th ed. Boston, Little, Brown, 1992, p 447, with permission.

generally have shown less dramatic differences in efficacy. Striking variability in efficacy and dose response among patients with the same disease is well described. Thus, if the initial dose is not effective, relief can often be obtained by increasing the dose within the therapeutic range. Some authors have hypothesized that if a patient does not respond to an NSAID in a given class, efficacy might be more likely by changing to a compound from another chemical class. This practice, although intellectually reasonable, has not been studied carefully.

Although the benefits of a specific NSAID cannot be predicted, some prescribing patterns have been successful. Indomethacin has proven efficacy in acute crystalline arthropathies, and for many it remains the drug of choice. Many authorities also see its use in the B27-related spondyloarthropathies. Some experts maintain that phenylbutazone is the most efficacious medication for many of the articular manifestations of HIV-related arthritis.

Adding a second NSAID to an ineffective regimen seems to add toxicity rather than benefit. Just as benefit can be variable between NSAIDs, toxicity can also be quite variable. Idiosyncratic adverse effects occur with NSAIDs just as with all medications. Some unwarranted effects actually occur by the same mechanism as the beneficial effects (i.e., prostaglandin inhibition). In general, these effects are dose related.

In addition to NSAID-induced gastroduodenopathy and nephropathy (discussed later), NSAIDs have many other adverse effects. Another prostaglandin-mediated function adversely affected by NSAIDs is renal blood flow. In patients who require renal prostaglandins (e.g., patients with CHF) to maintain GFR, there can be a substantial increase in sodium retention, leading to worsening edema, poorer BP control, and general reduction in renal function. Reduced efficacy of diuretics and other antihypertensive medications is documented. NSAID use increases the risk of hyperkalemia as well. Acute interstitial nephritis has also been documented with NSAID use. The latter is felt to be idiosyncratic rather than related to prostaglandin inhibition.

Other idiosyncratic side effects include rashes and photosensitivity, urticaria, and exacerbations of asthma in patients with aspirin sensitivity. Bone marrow suppression is best described with phenylbutazone but has been reported with other NSAIDs. As with gastric ulceration, women over age 60 may be at highest risk for bone marrow supression. Finally, CNS effects range from headache to psychosis. Aseptic meningitis has been reported in patients with SLE who take NSAIDs. As with all medications these risks must be balanced against the benefits.

Reference: Borda IT, et al (eds): NSAIDs. A Profile of Adverse Effects. Philadelphia, Hanley & Belfus, 1992.

Gastroduodenopathy

NSAIDs are well-known to cause gastric ulceration. Prostaglandins have been shown to promote gastric mucus secretion and reduce acid production. By inhibiting the production of these mediators, NSAIDs increase the risk of gastric injury. Although there may be some direct local effect, the route of medication administration (i.e., by suppository or even parenterally) does not substantially change the risk of these effects. Symptoms such as dyspepsia or indigestion often, but not invariably, accompany gastric ulceration. Occult blood loss may be the only suggestion of developing toxicity. Risk for toxicity increases with age, debility, and concomitant use of glucocorticoids. H_2 blockers and sucralfate are often helpful with symptoms of dyspepsia, although their efficacy in preventing ulceration has not been convincingly demonstrated. Conversely, the prostaglandin analog misoprostol has been less efficacious in reducing symptoms of indigestion and heartburn despite its demonstrated ability to reduce gastric erosions and ulceration. Other GI adverse effects include hepatic toxicity, pancreatitis, stomatitis, and diarrhea.

Patients at increased risk of NSAID-induced gastroduodenopathy include those with:

1. Increasing age (especially age >60 years)
2. Previous history of PUD (especially ulcer-related bleeding or perforation)
3. Concomitant steroid or anticoagulant therapy
4. A requirement for higher doses or longer duration of therapy
5. *Helicobacter pylori* infection (proposed)
6. Alcohol and/or tobacco use (although not well proven)

Reference: Loeb DS, et al: Management of gastroduodenopathy associated with use of nonsteroidal anti-inflammatory drugs. Mayo Clin Proc 67:354–364, 1992.

Nephrotoxicity

NSAIDs are being recognized as an important cause of acute renal failure. Aspirin and NSAIDs cause inhibition of vasodilatory prostaglandins in the kidney and thus cause renal ischemia. The toxic renal effects of these agents include ischemic ARF, acute interstitial nephritis, papillary necrosis, hyporeninemic hypoaldosteronism, edema, proteinuria, and nephrotic syndrome. These complications and other electrolyte disorders associated with the use of NSAIDs are listed in the following table.

Renal and Electrolyte Complications of NSAIDs

1. Renal failure
   a. Hemodynamic: Major risk factors are sodium depletion and low "effective" arterial blood volume.
   b. Acute interstitial nephritis with or without nephrotic syndrome
   c. Glomerulonephritis associated with diffuse vasculitis
   d. Papillary necrosis with chronic interstitial nephritis
2. Sodium and fluid retention
3. Hyperkalemia, metabolic acidosis: Occurs more often in patients with renal insufficiency, sodium depletion, or other factors predisposing to hyperkalemia.

From McKinney TD: Tubulointerstitial diseases and toxic nephropathies. In Wyngaarden JB, et al (eds): Cecil Textbook of Medicine, 19th ed. Philadelphia, W.B. Saunders, 1992, p 573, with permission.

Mechanism of nephrotoxicity: Many of the renal effects of NSAIDs are very predictable if the role of renal prostaglandins is understood. The vasodilatory prostaglandins (PGE_2, PGI_2) cause renal vasodilatation and preserve the renal blood flow in states of Na^+ depletion and diminished effective arterial blood flow. In these states, the angiotensin and catecholamines are elevated and help in maintenance of systemic BP. Elevated levels of angiotensin II decrease renal perfusion, which is normally balanced by the vasodilatory effects of prostaglandins. NSAIDs block prostaglandin synthesis, thereby disrupting the balance between angiotensin II and prostaglandins and hence resulting in severe decrement of GFR. The renal prostaglandins also cause natriuresis and diuresis, and they stimulate rennin release. A more chronic variety of renal failure associated with heavy proteinuria and interstitial nephritis on renal biopsy is seen with several types of NSAIDs and is also slowly reversible upon cessation of these agents.

Risk factors for nephrotoxicity: Various conditions associated with decreased effective arterial blood volume such as cirrhosis with ascites, nephrotic syndrome, CHF, renal insufficiency, diuretic use, renovascular disease, and DM are the important predisposing factors for nephrotoxicity from NSAIDs.

Clinical features: Patients who have diminished effective arterial blood volume develop a hemodynamically mediated ARF, which is associated with low fractional excretion of Na^+ and oliguria resembling prerenal azotemia. Urine sediment is unremarkable, and renal biopsy shows acute tubular necrosis. A different syndrome, consisting of acute interstitial nephritis (AIN) and heavy proteinuria, has been described with the use of several NSAIDs, especially fenoprofen. Heavy proteinuria in the nephrotic range results from a lesion in the glomeruli similar to the so-called minimal change lesion. In addition, AIN with microscopic pyuria and hematuria often accompanies this syndrome. Skin rash, eosinophilia, and eosinophiluria are uncommon. The disorder usually resolves within several days of discontinuing the drug. Corticosteroids are believed to hasten recovery in resistant and severe cases. Unlike the hemodynamically mediated ARF, this syndrome is seen only after exposure to the drug for several weeks to months.

Renal retention of salt and water is perhaps the most common renal side effect of NSAIDs. It is particularly prominent in patients with HTN and CHF. Hyperkalemia and metabolic acidosis due to hyporeninemic hypoaldosteronism are seen especially in patients with renal insufficiency, those with volume depletion, and those on K^+-sparing diuretics.

Analgesic nephropathy: Chronic exposure to excessive amounts of certain analgesics results in chronic interstitial nephritis and chronic renal failure. In the United States, 2 to 10% of all cases of ESRD are caused by analgesic nephropathy, which in Australia accounts for at least 25% of ESRD cases. The most common offending agents are phenacetin and acetaminophen, although several analgesics, in sufficient quantities, are known to cause this entity. In general, a cumulative ingestion of 3 kg of any of the aforementioned drugs in a 2 to 3-year period would result in analgesic nephropathy.

Most patients abusing analgesics do not admit to doing so. The diagnosis is suspected on the basis of circumstantial evidence and medical history. Analgesic abuse is four to six times more common in females and occasionally is familial. Anemia is a prominent feature and may be due to chronic GI blood loss. Bone disease is particularly prominent. UA shows pyuria, hematuria (often gross with papillary necrosis), and modest proteinuria. Sometimes patients develop focal sclerosis, which is associated with heavy proteinuria. Renal tubular defects with renal salt wasting, nephrogenic DI, and renal tubular acidosis are seen. IVP often reveals caliceal defects and sloughed papilla (ring sign). Demonstration of papillary necrosis in patients without DM, sickle-cell disease, or urinary obstruction with infection gives a clue to analgesic nephropathy.

Therapy: Prevention by way of avoidance of these agents is of utmost importance. Patient education and counseling are indicated. The reversible elements in the course of the disease, such as urinary obstruction from sloughed papilla, HTN, and volume depletion, should be recognized and promptly treated.

Reference: Dunn MJ, et al: Renal effects of NSAIDS. Am J Med 81(Suppl 2B):1, 1986.

NORMAL-PRESSURE HYDROCEPHALUS

This uncommon but important, treatable cause of dementia manifests with the classic clinical triad of gait disturbance, dementia, and bladder and/or bowel incontinence. It is often a sequela of subarachnoid hemorrhage, meningitis, and other conditions that lead to scarring of the basal meninges leading to decreased resorption of CSF.

A clue to the diagnosis is that the lateral ventricles are larger on CT scan or MRI than the degree of cortical atrophy. This is in contrast to hydrocephalus ex vacuo, in which the ventricles enlarge to fill the space of atrophied cortex, which occurs in many other types of dementia (such as Alzheimer's disease).

In NPH, because of pressure on the floor of the fourth ventricle, incontinence is seen *early* in the progression of the disease. This is the opposite of most other dementing conditions, in which incontinence is a late finding. The gait abnormalities present as lower leg spasticity and magnetic gait.

The treatment consists of ventriculoperitoneal shunting. There is a correlation between the presence of all three parts of the triad and the response to treatment. There is also a correlation between NPH of short duration and improvement. Usually, with treatment, incontinence reverses, but dementia does not (although it remains stable). A trial lumbar puncture with removal of 30 to 40 ml of CSF results in improvement among those likely to respond well to shunting.

Reference: Turner DA, et al: Normal pressure hydrocephalus and dementia—evaluation and treatment. Clin Geriatr Med 4:815–830, 1988.

OBESITY

Obesity is common (10–12% of the U.S. population) and is associated with HTN, hypercholesterolemia, NIDDM, and certain malignancies (e.g., colon, rectal, and prostate cancer in men; carcinoma of the gallbladder, biliary tract, breast, ovaries, uterus, and endometrium in women). It is defined as an increase of 20% above ideal weight and a body mass index >30.

Pathogenesis

1. Excessive lipid deposition: increased food intake, increased appetite due to hypothalamic abnormality (i.e., decreased satiety peptides such as corticotropin-releasing factor or increased neuropeptide Y)
2. Diminished lipid mobilization
3. Decreased lipid utilization possibly due to defective thermogenesis

Causes of Human Obesity

1. Hypothalamic abnormalities (1–2% of all cases of obesity): trauma, adenoma of the third ventricle, an inflammatory process, chordoma, lipoma, craniopharyngioma, aneurysm of the internal carotid, neuroma of the right optic nerve (Patients with hypothalamic obesity rarely weigh >140 kg.)
2. Hyperphagia and excessive food intake
3. Diminished metabolic rate and energy expenditure
4. Genetic predisposition

Management of Obesity

The failure rate of most dietary programs is approximately 90%.

1. **Reduction of caloric intake:** The most appropriate diet for the obese patient is a balanced diet (approximately 1,000–1,200 calories per day with frequent feedings) to achieve a gradual weight reduction. Low-calorie diets and total starvation have been associated with many complications, including anemia, metabolic acidosis, potassium depletion, hyperuricemia, gouty arthritis, LFT abnormalities, hypotension, and, sometimes, unexplained sudden death. Very-low-calorie diets may cause loss of lean mass and changes in body composition.

2. **Exercise:** By itself exercise is not an efficient means of losing weight (100 calories burned in 20 min of walking). However, it clearly contributes to the feeling of well-being in obese subjects undergoing an integrated program of weight loss.

3. **Behavioral modification:** modification in lifestyle, techniques directed at changing the patient's attitude toward the weight problem, relationship modification and nutrition techniques. The importance of behavior modification is to help sustain the weight loss.

4. **Medications:** The most important ones are the class IV appetite-suppressing medications—the catecholamine congeners, which include diethylpropion (Tenuate), fenfluramine (Pondimin), mazindol (Mazanor), and phentermine (Ionamin^R). Investigational drugs are aimed at increasing the thermogenic expenditure.

ONCOGENES

Role in Human Malignancies

The term *oncogene* is used to describe a gene associated with the development of a malignancy. Oncogenes were first detected in animal tumor viruses, which had acquired them during the course of infection of mammalian cells in the remote past. It is believed that oncogenes arise from mutations in normal genes that regulate essential cellular functions. The conversion of a gene to an oncogene is either caused by a spontaneous error during cell replication or induced by damage from radiation, chemicals, or viral agents. Usually, a series of mutations to multiple genes is required to transform a healthy cell into a malignant cell. Thus, several different oncogenes may be associated with the development of a particular type of cancer.

Three categories of oncogenes have been associated with human malignancy:

1. **Proto-oncogenes:** This class of genes is essential to cellular growth, transcription, or signaling pathways. When intact, their functions are tightly regulated by complex physiologic controls. Mutations to these genes result in loss of regulation, leading to unrestricted or constitutive proliferation of cells. Alteration to one chromosomal copy of the gene is sufficient for the neoplastic effect (dominant oncogene) (e.g., c-*myc, ras*).

2. **Tumor suppressor genes (anti-oncogenes):** These genes normally function as cell regulators, turning off proliferation and other active processes when growth is no longer needed. Inactivation of a gene in this class leads to inability to shut down cell growth. Damage to both chromosomal copies of the gene is generally necessary for the neoplastic effect (recessive oncogene) (e.g., *Rb* [retinoblastoma gene], *p53*).

3. **Cell death genes:** This class of genes controls the normal programmed death of cells (apoptosis). A mutation causes cells to live when they should have died, leading to excessive accumulation of cells (e.g., *bcl-2*).

In familial cancer, there is a defect in the germline DNA, which provides the first hit in the multistep pathway to malignant transformation. This explains why familial cancers tend to occur at an earlier age than sporadic cancers. The best understood example of this is in familial retinoblastoma, in which there is a germline defect in the *Rb* gene on chromosome 13. A mutation to the remaining normal *Rb* gene occurring during the period of rapid fetal eye-cell proliferation is sufficient to allow development of a malignant retinal tumor.

The most important gene in human malignancies appears to be the tumor suppressor gene *p53*, which has been called "guardian of the genome." *p53* is thought to prevent division in stressed or damaged cells until they have had time to complete their repair processes. Absence or inactivation of *p53* allows damaged or defective cells to proliferate without control. *p53* alteration or inactivation has been noted in cancer of the colon, lung, esophagus, breast, liver, brain, reticuloendothelial tissues, hematopoietic tissues, and sarcomas; this gene is abnormal in Li-Fraumeni cancer family syndrome. Other oncogenes prominent in human malignancies include *ras,* found in 33 to 95% of all adenocarcinomas, and c-*myc,* detected in lymphomas and many types of carcinoma, including lung cancer, breast cancer, and neuroblastoma.

Some Oncogenes Associated with Human Cancer

MALIGNANCY	ONCOGENE (CHROMOSOME)	COMMENT
Breast cancer	c-*erbB-2* or *neu* (17q), *p53* (17p13), *Rb* (13q14), c-*myc*	Mechanism of neoplastic change not yet well defined
Burkitt's lymphoma	c-*myc* (8q24), Ig heavy chain (14q32), κ chain (2p11), λ chain (22p11)	Translocation places c-*myc* next to promotors for Ig heavy or light chain genes, causing increased transcription of c-*myc* mRNA
CML	c-*abl* (9q), *bcr* (22q)	Translocation causes fusion product of the two genes, with ↑ tyrosine kinase activity of chimeric protein
Colon cancer	APC or MCC (5q), *ras* (12p and others), DCC (18q), *p53* (17p13)	Multistep progression from adenomatous polyp to malignancy
Follicular lymphoma	*bcl-2* (18q21), Ig heavy chain (14q32)	(14;18) translocation found in 85% of follicular and 20% of diffuse B-cell lymphomas
Pancreatic adenocarcinoma	*ras, p53*	*ras* implicated in 90% of cases
Promyelocytic leukemia	Retinoic acid receptor (17), c-*myl* (15)	(15;17) translocation causes activation of retinoic acid receptor by fusion to c-*myl*
Small-cell lung cancer	*p53, Rb,* c-, N-, and L-*myc,* unknown gene on 3p21	Mechanism of transformation not well defined

Abbreviations: APC = adenomatous polyposis coli, *bcr* = breakpoint cluster region, DCC = deleted in colorectal carcinoma, MCC = mutated in colorectal cancers.

References: Nowell PC: Cancer, chromosomes, and genes. Lab Invest 66:407–417, 1992.
Wynford-Thomas D: Oncogenes and anti-oncogenes: The molecular basis of tumor behavior. J Pathol 165:187–201, 1991.
Lane DP: *p53,* guardian of the genome. Nature 358:15–16, 1992.

OSTEOARTHRITIS

OA is a noninflammatory articular condition distinguished by deterioration of cartilage in association with new bone formation. It is the most common type of human arthritis. The prevalence of OA increases with age. By age 40, 90% of subjects in an autopsy study had pathologic changes in a weight-bearing joint. Studies of plain x-rays of the hands and feet show an OA prevalence of 85% among subjects 75 to 79 years old.

Mechanical factors clearly play a role in the development of OA. Trauma is perhaps the most commonly identified. It can be in the form of joint laxity (such as hypermobility syndromes), injury, or destruction caused by another joint disease (gout or RA). Obesity clearly is an associated epidemiologic factor in OA of the knee. Metabolic disorders such as ochronosis, hemochromatosis, and Wilson's disease are uncommon but well-known predisposing factors to the development of OA. Hyperparathyroidism and DM are more common predisposing conditions.

The influence of genetic factors has been known for many years. The familial tendency toward Heberden's nodes is well established. More recently, genetic defects in cartilage structure have helped to add new insights into pathogenesis.

Early pathologic changes in articular cartilage include proliferation of chondrocytes and a flaking of cartilage. As the process continues, there is eventual wearing to the underlying bone. New bone formation is a hallmark of OA. Bone also proliferates in subchondral tissue where cartilage has completely been denuded. Cysts commonly are seen beneath this ebernated bone.

Clinically, patients generally become symptomatic after age 40. Pain exacerbated by motion of the joint and relieved with rest is characteristic. Morning stiffness is present but rarely lasts more than 30 minutes. Sites of involvement are commonly those of previous trauma or surgery. Distal interphalangeal and carpal metacarpal joint involvement are also common areas. Hips, knees, and both lumbar and cervical spine likewise are often involved. Physical examination generally reveals reduced range of motion, crepitus, and tenderness with motion. Joint effusion can be present as well. Deformity may occur with collapse of joint surfaces. It occurs with cartilage loss and new bone formation resulting in malalignment.

Classical radiographic findings include joint space narrowing and subchondral sclerosis. Osteophytes are seen at the margins and sites of ligamentous attachments. Subchondral cysts and altered shape of bone are noted. Laboratory data remain nonspecific. Data including ESR in general are normal. Synovial fluid has low levels of inflammation and generally less than 2,000 WBCs.

Treatment includes management of any predisposing factors that exacerbate the condition. Weight reduction can significantly reduce pain of OA in hips, knees, and back. In addition, obesity is considered an important factor upon failure of total joint replacements. Thus, weight reduction is an important modality itself and in helping to ensure the success of other important therapies. Physical and occupational therapy can provide temporary relief and can also furnish information helpful in preventing injury or managing the pain and disability already present. Strengthening of supporting musculature also helps maintain range of motion.

Most commonly, physicians rely on medication including NSAIDs and mild narcotics. Systemic steroids are of little use and generally are avoided. Intra-articular injections are known to be efficacious, although the frequency must be fewer than three injections per year because of the effect on articular cartilage metabolism.

A number of surgical procedures have evolved for treatment of OA. Conservative arthroscopic debridement of cartilage has been noted to reduce pain and joint locking. In unicompartment disease of the knees, an osteotomy (removal of a wedge of bone from the tibia, femur, or both) can be successful in returning alignment to normal.

Although the foregoing modalities are helpful, they do not restore the articular cartilage, and, ultimately, many patients may need total joint replacement. Arthroplasty is reserved for patients with intractable pain and without relief of disability. Depending on the location, total joint replacements have variable success rates. Pain relief and functionality have been generally acceptable in the shoulders, hips, and knees. Elbows and ankle replacement have been less successful.

Reference: Pellettier JP: Osteoarthritis: Update on diagnosis and treatment. J Rheum 18(Suppl 27):1–149, 1991.

OSTEOMALACIA

Osteomalacia is one of the histologic categories of osteopenia, a condition defined clinically and radiologically as a generalized decrease in bone density. Unlike osteoporosis, in which there are proportional reductions in both bone matrix and mineralization, osteomalacia is characterized by defective mineralization of a normal amount of matrix. In childhood, this condition is referred to as **rickets** and involves the growth plate. Symptoms include diffuse bone pain and muscular weakness, and patients often present with fractures of the wrist, hip, or vertebrae following minor trauma. Laboratory evaluation should include measurement of serum Ca^+ and PO_4^-, serum creatinine, serum alkaline phosphatase (usually elevated, unlike in cases of osteoporosis), serum 25(OH)–vitamin D, and 24-hr urinary Ca^+ excretion. X-ray findings include bowing of the long bones, indistinct bone cortices, pseudofractures (Looser's transformation zones) in the femoral neck, ribs, or clavicles, and subperiosteal resorption in the phalanges or tips of the clavicles.

Conditions Associated with Osteomalacia

A. Disorders in the vitamin D endocrine system
  1. Decreased bioavailability
    Insufficient sunlight exposure
    Nutritional deficiency
    Nephrotic syndrome (urinary loss)
    Malabsorption (fecal loss)
  2. Abnormal metabolism
    Liver or renal disease
    Vitamin D–dependent rickets type I
    Tumoral hypophosphatemic osteomalacia
    Hypoparathyroidism (?)
    Chronic acidosis (?)
    Anticonvulsants
B. Disorders of phosphate homeostasis
  1. Decreased intestinal absorption due to malnutrition, malabsorption, or antacids containing aluminum hydroxide
  2. Increased renal loss
    X-linked hypophosphatemic rickets
    Tumoral hypophosphatemic osteomalacia
    Paraproteinemias
    Wilson's disease
    Glycogen storage diseases
    Neurofibromatosis

Table continued on next page.

Conditions Associated with Osteomalacia (Cont.)

C. Calcium deficiency
   1. Dietary insufficiency
   2. Excessive renal loss (?)
   3. Malabsorption (?)
D. Primary disorders of bone matrix
E. Inhibitors of mineralization
   1. Aluminum
   2. Etidronate
   3. Phenytoin (?)
   4. Fluoride (?)

? = The association of the disease to osteomalacia or the mechanism by which it produces osteomalacia is not established.

From Bikle DD: Osteomalacia and rickets. In Wyngaarden JB, et al (eds): Cecil Textbook of Medicine, 18th ed. Philadelphia, W.B. Saunders, 1988, p 1480 with permission.

Nutritional deficiency of vitamin D may be corrected with vitamin D_2 2,000 to 4,000 IU/day for several months until bone healing is documented by radiologic and biochemical measurements, followed by maintenance dosage with 200 to 400 IU daily. Associated Ca^+ deficiency may be corrected with 24 to 32 oz of milk daily and 1 to 2 gm of oral elemental Ca^+ daily or (if severe and symptomatic) IV Ca^+ (20 mg elemental Ca^+/kg/day). If low 25(OH) vitamin D levels cannot be corrected after 4 weeks of dietary supplementation and increased sunlight exposure, malabsorption should be suspected and treated with vitamin D_2 at a dose of 50,000 to 100,000 IU orally each day along with periodic measurement of serum 25(OH) vitamin D levels and 24-hr urinary Ca^+ and serum Ca^+ values to detect early vitamin D toxicity. An increase in urinary Ca^+ excretion is a marker for bone healing and will usually occur before hypercalcemia. IM vitamin D supplementation may be necessary at times. Renal osteodystrophy is best managed with either calcitriol 0.5 to 1.0 µg PO daily or dihydrotachysterol 0.25 to 0.5 mg daily.

OSTEOMYELITIS

Osteomyelitis is infection that can develop in any bone of the body. The three major types are differentiated in the following table.

The diagnosis of osteomyelitis remains challenging. In cases of hematogenous spread, changes on x-ray may not appear for at least 10 days. In such cases, three-phase technetium bone scanning may provide earlier clues. Precise identification of the infecting organism is crucial in management, as the patient is being committed to prolonged antibiotic therapy. Bone biopsy must be strongly considered, especially in cases of chronic osteomyelitis in which sinus tract cultures are frequently misleading. Mycobacterial and fungal infections must be considered in appropriate cases.

Optimal treatment schedules have not been clearly defined. For acute osteomyelitis, parenteral antibiotics are given in high doses for 4 weeks per traditional treatment schedules. However, some newer studies suggest that sequential parenteral/oral therapy may be effective. For chronic osteomyelitis, prolonged oral antibiotic regimens have shown promise. Complications of untreated disease may include secondary amyloidosis and epidermoid carcinoma in a draining sinus.

Major Types of Osteomyelitis

FEATURE	HEMATOGENOUS	SECONDARY TO CONTIGUOUS FOCUS OF INFECTION	DUE TO VASCULAR INSUFFICIENCY
Age distribution (yr)	Peaks at 1–20 and ≥50	≥50	≥50
Bones involved	Long bones Vertebrae	Femur, tibia, skull, mandible	Feet
Precipitating factors	Trauma (?) Bacteremia	Surgery Soft-tissue infections	DM Peripheral vascular disease
Bacteriology	Usually only one organism *S. aureus* Gram-negative organisms	Often mixed infection *S. aureus* Gram-negative organisms Anaerobic organisms	Usually mixed infections *S. aureus* or *epidermidis* Streptococci Gram-negative organisms Anaerobic organisms
Major clinical findings			
Initial episode	Fever Local tenderness Local swelling Limitation of motion	Fever Erythema Swelling Heat	Pain Swelling Erythema Drainage Ulceration
Recurrent episode	Drainage	Drainage Sinus	(Same)

From Norden CW: Osteomyelitis. In Mandel GL, et al (eds): Principles and Practice of Infectious Diseases, 3rd ed., New York, Churchill Livingstone, 1990, p 923, Table 1, with permission.

OSTEONECROSIS

Osteonecrosis is the death of bone because of inadequate nutrient blood flow. Once infarction of cancellous bone occurs, the repair process is usually unable to replace it completely. With continued stress, nonviable bone will fracture and eventually collapse. Interruption of flow can occur secondary to mechanical disruption of vessels, inflammation, deposited materials, radiation injury, or embolic phenomenon. In sickle-cell anemia, for example, clumps of RBCs embolize, blocking flow. Similarly, nitrogen bubbles are felt to embolize, leading to the osteonecrosis seen in deep-sea divers (caisson disease, the bends). Finally, some have hypothesized that increased venous pressure can lead to reduced arterial flow. Particularly obscure is the mechanism by which use of glucocorticoids leads to osteonecrosis.

A number of conditions are associated with osteonecrosis (see following table). Pancreatitis and gout are sometimes included in this list, although alcoholism has been hypothesized as the true association in many such patients. Finally, there remains a cadre of patients who have no obvious risk factors and for whom the label of idiopathic osteonecrosis is most appropriate.

Conditions Associated with Avascular Necrosis

Traumatic
Fracture of the femoral neck
Traumatic dislocation of the hip
Trauma to the hip without fracture or dislocation
Reconstructive hip surgery (including cap arthroplasty, surface replacement arthroplasty, cuneiform osteotomy of the femoral neck, and synovectomy)
Hip manipulation (including treatment of congenital dysplasia of the hip and use of traction in the correction of slipped epiphysis)

Nontraumatic
Juvenile
  Slipped capital femoral epiphysis
  Legg-Calvé-Perthes disease
  Idiopathic juvenile avascular necrosis
Adult
  Systemic steroid administration
  Excessive alcohol intake
  Chronic liver disease
  Renal transplantation
  SLE and other collagen vascular disorders
  Caisson disease or decompression sickness
  Exposure to high altitude
  Sickle-cell disease and sickle-cell variants
  Miscellaneous hemoglobinopathies and coagulopathies
  Ileitis and colitis
  Pancreatitis
  Metabolic bone disease
  Hyperlipidemias
  Burns
  Pregnancy
  Gout
  Gaucher's disease
  Sarcoidosis
  Tumors
  Chemotherapy and other toxic agents
  Fabry's disease
  Arteriosclerosis and other vascular occlusive disorders
  Radiation
  Smoking

From Steinberg ME, et al: Osteonecrosis. In Kelly WN, et al (eds): Textbook of Rheumatology, 4th ed. Philadelphia, W.B. Saunders, 1993, p 1630, with permission.

Sites of involvement vary considerably, often depending on any underlying predisposing factor. The distribution can vary, although the most commonly recognized sites include the femoral head, humeral head, and tibial plateau. About 50% of patients with osteonecrosis of the hip may develop bilateral lesions. Other sites (e.g., humeral head, knees) are involved in 15% of patients with osteonecrosis of the femoral head. Lesions may affect any part of a bone.

Late in the presentation, plain x-ray can be diagnostic. Crescent-shaped radiolucent areas and osseus collapse are quite characteristic. CT can define the extent of disease and allow earlier detection than plain x-ray. Reduced blood flow initially manifests itself as a cold spot on nuclear scintigraphy. With time, as the repair process occurs, an increase in uptake is noted, producing a hot spot. As marrow fat is replaced with fibrous tissue, MRI can note the change and reveal abnormalities even before bone scanning.

Treatment regimens are controversial. Rarely patients have a mild enough course to do well with NSAIDs or mild pain killers. Generally, operative intervention is required. Some procedures designed to decompress the bone, with either core removal or osteotome, are not universally acclaimed as successful. Recently a revascularization procedure has shown early promising results. The most successful pain control has been with total joint replacement.

References: Mankin HJ: Nontraumatic necrosis of bone (osteonecrosis). N Engl J Med 326:1473–1479, 1992.

Resnick D, et al: Osteonecrosis: Diagnostic techniques, specific situations and complications. In Resnick D, et al (eds): Diagnosis of Bone and Joint Disorders. Philadelphia, W.B. Saunders, 1988, p 3190.

OSTEOPOROSIS

Osteoporosis is a major problem in postmenopausal white females. Other risk factors include leanness, cigarette use, gastric resection, premature menopause, heavy ethanol use, steroid use, and hyperthyroidism. African-American females apparently have heavier peak bone density and less of a problem with osteoporosis. Estrogen-mediated bone loss affects mostly trabecular bone in the first 20 years after menopause and is additive to age (senile)-related bone loss (which affects both trabecular and cortical bone).

The major impact of osteoporosis in older women is hip fracture. One-third of women who reach the age of 90 will have had a hip fracture. Vertebral crush fracture is common but usually less debilitating. By the time x-rays show osteoporosis, at least 30 to 40% of bone mass is already lost. Calcium intake decreases markedly with age (80% of patients over the age of 75 take in less calcium than recommended). Calcium supplementation of 1.0 to 1.5 gm/day is needed in women. Vitamin D deficiency is not rare, especially in the elderly who are housebound or institutionalized and therefore have limited exposure to sunlight. Weight-bearing exercise prevents bone mass loss. But bone mass may decrease rapidly when an exercise program is stopped.

Treatment of Vertebral Crush Fractures

- Pain relief in acute episode
- Avoidance of immobility
- Avoidance of unnecessary lifting
- Minimal use of corsets and braces
- Preventive measures (removal of rugs, obstacles)
- Calcitonin is a very useful drug in decreasing the pain

Other Problems Associated with Osteoporosis

Multiple myeloma	Hyperparathyroidism
Male hypogonadism	Vitamin D deficiency
Phenytoin use	Malabsorption

Reference: Mitlak BH, et al: Diagnosis and treatment of osteoporosis. Annu Rev Med 44:265–277, 1993.

OTITIS MEDIA

Otitis media, as the name implies, is inflammation of the middle ear. The incidence of otitis media peaks within the first 4 years of life and diminishes rapidly thereafter, but it does remain a potential illness throughout life. The diagnosis is made by acute symptoms (fever, local pain or drainage, hearing impairment) associated with the presence of middle ear fluid.

Bacteriology of Acute Otitis Media in Adults

ORGANISM	NO OF PATIENTS*	%
Haemophilus influenzae	9	26
Streptococcus pneumoniae	7	21
Moraxella catarrhalis	1	3
Streptococcus pyogenes	1	3
Staphylococcus aureus	1	3
Others†	9	26
No growth	9	26

* Cultures of middle ear aspirates from three patients grew more than one organism (*H. influenzae* and *S. aureus; S. pneumoniae* and *S. epidermidis; S. aureus* and *S. epidermidis*).

† Other bacteria that were isolated in pure or mixed culture from the middle ear aspirates and not from the middle ear canal included *Propionibacterium acnes, Enterobacter agglomerans, Staphylococcus epidermidis,* and group G streptococcus.

From Celin SE, et al: Bacteriology of acute otitis media in adults. JAMA 266:2249–2252, 1991, p 2250, with permission.

Empirical therapy depends on the prevalence of beta-lactamase-producing organisms in the local area. In most locales, amoxicillin, or trimethoprim-sulfamethoxazole in the penicillin-allergic patient, is adequate. If there are other concerns of frequency of administration or higher prevalence of beta-lactamase, other therapeutic options include the combination of amoxicillin and clavulanic acid, cefixime, or cefuroxime axetil.

OVARIAN CANCER

Ovarian cancer is the most common cause of death from gynecologic malignancies in women in the United States, with an estimated death toll in 1992 of 13,000. Serous cancers account for 35 to 50% of the tumors, and mucinous for 6 to 10%. Peculiar to the malignancy is the so-called borderline tumor or noninvasive type of tumor, which constitutes one-fourth to one-third of the serous and 40 to 50% of the mucinous tumors. Survival is significantly better even in late stages for these borderline tumors.

The risk factors include low parity, but not necessarily infertility. There appears to be a preventive effect from oral contraceptives, especially among women not already protected by pregnancy. The risk of this cancer increases with the total time between menarche and menopause, excluding the time of pregnancy, lactation, or oral contraceptive administration. Estrogen replacement therapy does not affect the incidence. Some risk factors mentioned in older literature but hard to confirm include asymptomatic mumps and talc containing asbestos in dusting powders applied to the perineal area or sanitary napkins. A familial ovarian cancer syndrome has also been described.

The International Federation of Gynecology and Obstetrics (FIGO) has formulated a staging system. In outline, they are (I) ovarian, (II) pelvic, (III) peritoneal, and (IV) metastatic disease. At the present time, the overall 5-year survival is approximately 37% and is markedly dependent on the FIGO stage.

STAGE	SURVIVAL
I (favorable pathology)	>90%
II	60–80%
III	15–20%
IV	<5%

(The actual percentage of patients in stage II is decreasing and patients often are upgraded to III after staging.)

The advent of widespread use of CT scans of the pelvis and abdomen has considerably changed the picture of this disease in recent years, although the paucity of early symptoms and the lack of reliable screening tests cause many cases not to be recognized until the later stages. However, abdominal ultrasound has been an effective tool in examining the ovaries during the search for ovarian cancer. Increasing sophistication in the use of laparoscopy, with its attendant ability to biopsy the ovaries with a minimum of surgical complications, has also added greatly to diagnostic acumen in this disease. The tumor markers used in this disease, CA-125 and DF3, are not consistently reliable as screening tests but are mainly used in following the course of the disease and response to therapy.

Treatment is complicated because it depends on stage, histology, age, and the patient's desire for further childbearing. Because often patients are young and still wish to have children, a unilateral oophorectomy may be considered. Serous tumors are associated with the highest incidence of bilateral disease, and bilateral salpingo-oophorectomy and hysterectomy are recommended unless the tumor is of early-stage borderline pathology. This group of patients requires careful and frequent follow-up and should have excision of residual adnexa and uterus after completion of childbearing. An independent primary endometrial carcinoma may occur concurrently with ovarian cancer in up to 20% of cases, so endometrial curettage is always indicated. Serous papillary carcinoma of the endometrium as well as other primary endometrial pathologies occasionally metastasizes to the ovary and mimics ovarian primaries. Size of residual disease is a critical factor in subsequent therapy and prognosis. Peritoneal lesions of greater than 1.5 cm portend poor survival.

Chemotherapy is useful in treatment of ovarian cancer, and the new drug taxol has shown promise in early studies, yielding a 30% response rate. Standard agents of cisplatin, doxorubicin, and cyclophosphamide show response rates of more than 50% and median survivals of 24 months. Patients in stage III or IV with complete response to chemotherapy confirmed by second-look laparotomy had a 4-year survival at upwards of 85% in one study. Unfortunately, other studies have failed to confirm those results. One study showed only a 30% 5-year survival in patients who had a negative second-look laparotomy. Adjuvant therapy in early stages has been tried and appears promising, with 5-year disease-free survivals of 80%. Time to progression after initial resection remains an important variable. For periods of less than 14 months, median survival time is 6.5 months, whereas for more than 14 months, the median survival is 12 months.

P

PACEMAKER SYNDROME

Pacemaker syndrome refers to the symptom complex of palpitations, dizziness, lightheadedness, and nausea that results from ventricular-pacing-induced hypotension. Pacemaker syndrome is a complication of single-chamber ventricular pacemakers that is most likely to occur in patients who have underlying CHF (or moderate to severe LV systolic dysfunction), who are over 65 years old, or who have LVH. These patients commonly have impaired LV diastolic function. As a result, they are likely to have a greater atrial contribution to ventricular filling. In normal adults, active atrial contraction contributes 10 to 20% of the total ventricular filling. In patients over the age of 65 or with LVH or CHF, the atrial contribution to ventricular filling may be as high as 40%. Thus, in these patients, loss of AV synchrony, as during ventricular pacing, may acutely and significantly reduce ventricular filling, resulting in both a drop in cardiac output and hypotension.

Pacemaker syndrome can be prevented by dual-chamber pacing, which can preserve AV synchrony, or by adding a new feature to a ventricular single-chamber (such as VVI—ventricular-inhibited) pacemaker called **hysteresis.** Hysteresis is characterized by an escape interval that is greater than the pacing interval of the pacemaker. This feature allows the patient to remain in a spontaneous, nonpaced sinus rhythm as long as possible and reduces the need for ventricular pacing, thus reducing the recurrence of pacemaker syndrome. If hysteresis is not effective in controlling pacemaker syndrome, replacement of a VVI with a dual-chamber (and thus atrial-sensed and atrial-triggered) pacemaker may be necessary.

PAGET'S DISEASE

Osteitis deformans (Paget's disease) is a skeletal disease of unknown etiology. The disease occurs in approximately 3% of people over the age of 40, with a slight male predominance. The prevalence can reach 10% in populations over age 80. Although Paget himself felt the disease was caused by chronic inflammation, the accumulating data suggest that a slow virus may be involved. Bone remodeling is abnormal, leading to an irregular and disorganized pattern recognizable by x-ray.

Patients are often asymptomatic, and pagetic bone is commonly encountered on an incidentally obtained x-ray. When symptoms are present, patients may notice pain or deformity. Pain may be unrelated to exercise and commonly occurs at night. Increasing bone size may lead to symptoms. Bowing of the long bones and enlargement of the skull are frequently noted. The sacrum and spine (particularly the lumbar spine) are the most common areas involved. Other less frequently involved sites include the femur (right more often than left), cranium, sternum, and pelvis.

The intense enlargement and sclerosis of bone can lead to several well-known complications. Compressive neuropathies including hearing loss and spinal cord compression can occur. Articular complications including both asymptomatic hyperuricemia and classic gout, pseudogout, and degenerative arthritis are seen. Fractures of involved bone most often occur in the femur, tibia, and humerus. Increased bone vascularity and turnover may rarely lead to high-output cardiac failure with classical symptoms of dropsy. The development of sarcoma and giant cell tumors in pagetic bone is well described.

The disease affects all aspects of bone metabolism. It begins with increased osteoclastic activity leading to resorption of bone. Radiographically, osteolytic lesions such as osteoporosis circumscripta are seen on skull films. Subsequently, new bone is added, albeit in a disorganized (woven bone) form. There are no haversian systems within pagetic bone. Eventually, osteoblastic activity quiets, and radiographically sclerotic lesions are present.

Laboratory data often show elevated alkaline phosphatase, with the bony isoenzyme fractions elevated. Elevated 24-hr urine hydroxyproline excretion reflects bony destruction. Immobilization is the primary risk factor for significantly elevated serum calcium and phosphorus. Occasionally, an associated hyperparathyroidism can also lead to hypercalcemia. Without these predisposing factors, calcium and phosphorus are generally normal.

When x-ray lesions are noted, metastatic cancer should also be considered. Disseminated prostate and breast cancer are the most likely to radiographically resemble Paget's disease. Occasionally, a hemangioma of bone may be sclerotic and be mistaken for pagetic bone.

If Paget's is coincidentally discovered and the patient is asymptomatic, no treatment is necessary. In symptomatic patients, calcitonin, by decreasing osteoclast activity, is perhaps the most useful medication but must be taken parenterally. Antibodies can develop to the salmon hormone, a problem overcome by substituting human calcitonin. Nausea, flushing, and dizziness may accompany each injection. Alternative medications include the bisphosphonates. Although many are currently undergoing trials, etidronate (Didronel) is the only one currently available in the United States. Like calcitonin, it impairs osteoclast activity. In addition, however, it reduces osteoblastic function. It must be given cyclically, usually administered in 3- to 6-month time intervals. This medication is well tolerated but poorly absorbed and must be taken on an absolutely empty stomach. Although most patients obtain good relief, about 15% may have a paradoxical increase in pain. Occasionally, surgical intervention has to be undertaken, particularly if pathologic fractures are present or if the physician is concerned about the presence of sarcoma. In general, prognosis is good and medical treatment useful.

Reference: Hosking DJ: Advances in the treatment of Paget's disease. Drugs 40:829, 1990.

PAIN, CHRONIC

Chronic pain is defined as a nociceptive sensation lasting for more than 6 months. Persistent pain causes disability and loss of function, frequently accompanied by depression, insomnia, anxiety, social withdrawal, and financial distress. Narcotic dependency may develop from attempts at pain control.

Pain is a perception unique to each patient, as painful stimuli are modulated through an individual's affective and cognitive processes. Before treatment of a patient with chronic pain, it is essential to fully understand the significance of the pain to the patient's life. Important questions to address include the location, intensity, and character of the pain; exacerbating or alleviating factors; associated emotional components (suffering); change in behavior, mood, or social interaction since the pain began; and results of therapy, including medications used currently and in the past.

The character of pain and its distribution in relation to the physical exam are helpful to know in an evaluation of the nature of a chronic pain syndrome. In patients with prominent psychiatric factors or drug-seeking behavior, the pain description may not correspond to logical anatomic patterns, or the pain may last beyond the expected healing time for a prior injury or surgery. However, it is important to remember, too, that pain with atypical patterns may be referred from visceral sites, and pain can persist for years after surgical sectioning of nerves if nerve endings do not grow back properly.

It is useful to divide chronic pain into chronic benign pain and chronic pain caused by malignancy, as the therapeutic approach differs between the two.

Chronic benign pain may originate from diverse conditions including low back or spinal cord injury, reflex sympathetic dystrophy, peripheral neuropathy, degenerative joint disease, postherpetic neuralgia, phantom limb pain, and adhesive arachnoiditis. Sometimes there is no definable physical etiology.

Treatment of chronic benign pain syndromes consists of a multidisciplinary approach involving some or all of the following modalities:

- Physical therapy and rehabilitation
- Psychologic counseling
- Behavior modification
- Biofeedback, stress management
- Detoxification from narcotics
- Medications: antidepressants, NSAIDs
- Orthotic devices (back braces, etc.)
- Transcutaneous stimulators (TENS unit), spinal cord stimulation
- Trigger-point injections

Tricyclic antidepressants such as doxepin and amitriptyline have a primary analgesic effect in certain types of pain, especially neuropathic or deafferentation pain. They are also valuable in treating associated depression, anxiety, and insomnia, all of which may intensify the patient's perception of the pain. NSAIDs provide analgesia and reduce local tissue irritation. As the response to NSAIDs is highly individual, several drugs of this class may need to be tried before finding the one that works for a particular patient. It is important to give an adequate therapeutic trial (2–3 weeks) before determining that a medication does not work. Anticonvulsants can be helpful for lancinating neuropathic pain.

Opiates are generally not recommended in the treatment of chronic benign pain. If psychiatric factors are important in the pain syndrome, then the use of narcotics may worsen the situation by introducing the problem of drug addiction. However, in certain painful conditions (e.g., spinal cord injury), the use of oral, parenteral (PCA pump), or epidural narcotics may be required for optimal pain control.

Chronic pain caused by malignancy (cancer pain) is a special situation. Several types of pain occur in cancer patients: pain from cancer, pain from the treatment of cancer (i.e., surgery or radiotherapy), and pain from preexisting or newly developed benign conditions (e.g., constipation, decubitus ulcers). It is important to recognize the source of pain in order to treat it appropriately.

The first line of therapy in cancer pain is to address the malignancy. Palliative radiotherapy can be very effective in pain relief. Chemotherapy can sometimes reduce painful tumor expansion. The mainstay of pain treatment, however, is medication, often involving the narcotic analgesics. The ladder approach is recommended, depending on the severity of the pain:

- Mild pain: nonnarcotic (e.g., acetaminophen or NSAID)
- Moderate pain: weak narcotic (e.g., codeine) ± NSAID or
  acetaminophen
- Severe pain: strong narcotic (e.g., morphine) ± NSAID or
  acetaminophen

Combining a narcotic with a nonnarcotic has a synergistic effect and allows pain relief while minimizing the side effects from opiates. The NSAIDs are recommended for pain caused by bony metastases, as prostaglandins may mediate the osteolytic and osteoclastic effects of bone metastases. Pain originating from nerve destruction responds better to tricyclic antidepressants or anticonvulsants such as amitriptyline (Elavil), phenytoin (Dilantin), and carbamazepine (Tegretol). Pain originating from epidural spinal cord compression may respond dramatically to steroid treatment.

Since most cancer pain recurs as soon as the analgesic wears off, it is best to give regular doses of a long-acting narcotic to keep the pain continuously suppressed. The patient should also be supplied with a short-acting narcotic to use in case of breakthrough pain. The oral route is preferable in most patients. For individuals with GI tract obstruction, fistula, or intractable nausea and vomiting, analgesics may be administered by rectal suppository, transdermal patch, sublingually, or by PCA pump. The epidural route may be necessary in patients with severe pain who experience intolerable systemic side effects from oral narcotics. (Also see Analgesics, Narcotic.)

Following are guidelines for the use of analgesics in management of cancer pain.

- Choose a specific drug for a specific type of pain.
- Know the clinical pharmacology of the drug prescribed—duration of effect and
  equianalgesic dose for route prescribed.
- Administer the analgesic on a regular basis after initial titration of the dose.
- Use drug combinations to provide additive analgesia and reduce
  side effects.
- Avoid combinations that increase sedation without enhancing
  analgesia (e.g., diazepam + chlorpromazine).
- Anticipate and treat side effects—constipation, nausea and
  vomiting, sedation.
- Respect individual differences: adjust dose in children, the
  elderly, and patients with organ dysfunction.
- Manage the tolerant patient: use combinations of drug therapy
  and anesthetic/neurosurgical procedures, or switch to an alternative narcotic
  analgesic with one-half the equianalgesic dose.
- Prevent and treat acute withdrawal by tapering drugs.

Reference: Foley KM, et al: Analgesic drug therapy in cancer pain: Principles and practice. Med Clin North Am 71:207–232, 1987.

PANCREATITIS

Acute Pancreatitis

Acute pancreatitis is defined as an inflammatory process in the pancreas that is theoretically reversible, in contrast to chronic pancreatitis, which implies a chronic inflammatory disease that is irreversible. Pathologically, acute pancreatitis is characterized by areas of fat necrosis and edema, which may be mild or severe. Complications of acute pancreatitis include pancreatic abscess, phlegmon, pseudocyst formation, and fistula. Additionally, recurrent attacks may lead to chronic scarring and progression to chronic pancreatitis.

Clinically, patients typically present with abdominal pain, nausea, and vomiting. The pain tends to be rapid in onset and escalates over several hours to maximum intensity. The pain is often located in the epigastrium or the left upper quadrant and may radiate into the back or chest. The pain is typically made worse by eating. Physical findings depend in part on the severity of the attack. Severe disease may be manifested by cardiovascular collapse, whereas in more moderate to mild disease, the bulk of findings are located within the abdomen. Typically there is mild abdominal distention combined with tenderness in the upper abdomen with or without signs of peritoneal irritation. Bowel sounds are generally diminished or absent. In cases of hemorrhagic pancreatitis, ecchymoses of the flank (Grey Turner's sign) or periumbilical ecchymoses (Cullen's sign) may be present.

The diagnosis is suggested clinically and supported by laboratory tests, including elevation of serum amylase and lipase, as well as pancreatic edema with surrounding inflammation on ultrasound or CT scan.

Causes of Acute Pancreatitis

Common bile duct stones	Alcohol
Tumor	Infection (mumps virus, coxsackievirus,
Drugs	parasites, *Mycoplasma pneumoniae*)
Hypertriglyceridemia	Post ERCP
Trauma	Scorpion bites
Autoimmune disease	Pancreas divisum
Hypercalcemia	Penetrating duodenal ulcer
Hereditary pancreatitis	Idiopathic (15%)

Drugs Associated with Acute Pancreatitis

Azathioprine	Calcium	Tetracycline
Pentamidine	Furosemide	Thiazide diuretics
Ethacrynic acid	Sulfonamides	Procainamide
Estrogens	Chlorthalidone	Valproic acid
Methyldopa	Nitrofurantoin	6-Mercaptopurine
L-asparaginase		

Ranson's Criteria

Ranson and coworkers initially described a variety of clinical features, identified within the first 24 to 48 hrs after admission to the hospital, that can be used to predict the severity of an attack of pancreatitis as manifested by the duration of hospitalization, the likelihood of complications, and mortality. The criteria are listed in the table below. Although they do not predict the outcome in any individual patient, they can be used at bedside to identify patients at high risk for mortality or poor outcome.

Ranson's Criteria in Acute Pancreatitis

I. Admission criteria	II. During initial 48 hrs
Age >55 yrs	Hematocrit decrease >10%
WBC count >16,000/mm^3	BUN rise >5 mg/dl
Blood glucose >200 mg/dl	Serum calcium <8 mg/dl
LDH >350 IU/L	PO$_2$ <60 mm Hg
SGOT >250 IU/dl	Base deficit >4 mEq/L
	Fluid sequestration >6 L

Reference: Ranson JHC, et al: Prognostic signs and non-operative peritoneal lavage in acute pancreatitis. Surg Gynecol Obstet 143:209, 1976.

Chronic Pancreatitis

Chronic pancreatitis is defined as an inflammatory disease of the pancreas characterized by persistent and often progressive lesions resulting in chronic scarring of the gland and the ducts. Chronic pancreatitis theoretically may be a result of any of the causes associated with acute pancreatitis. In general, however, alcohol accounts for between 70 and 80% of all cases of chronic pancreatitis. Additional causes include tropical (nutritional) pancreatitis, hereditary pancreatitis, hyperparathyroidism, ductal obstruction related to tumors and pseudocysts, abdominal trauma, pancreas divisum, and idiopathic forms of pancreatitis.

Diagnostic Tests

Nearly all patients with acute pancreatitis have elevation of the serum amylase. Typically, amylase rises rapidly after the onset of the acute attack and declines toward normal over the next 3 to 5 days. Elevation of serum lipase generally accompanies hyperamylasemia, but it remains elevated for a longer period of time than serum amylase and may be used in cases when amylase is normal due to delay in obtaining laboratory studies. Lipase is also useful in confirming that amylase elevation is due to pancreatic disease. Renal clearance of amylase has been used in the past as an indicator of pancreatitis; however, there are significant incidences of falsely normal ratios in patients with acute pancreatitis and of false positives in the absence of acute pancreatitis.

Plain films of the abdomen may be used to detect nonpancreatic diseases that may simulate acute pancreatitis, including pneumonia, bowel obstruction, and perforated viscus. In cases of chronic pancreatitis, calcification may be seen in the pancreatic bed. In acute pancreatitis, nonspecific findings of diffuse ileus may be seen. Ultrasonography may reveal pancreatic edema, pseudocysts, bile duct stones, or ductal dilatation, but often adequate examination is precluded due to gaseous distention of bowel loops. CT scan may be particularly useful in the evaluation of a patient with pancreatitis, since interpretation is not affected by bowel gas. CT scan can be used to help define the severity and extent of the inflammatory process, as well as to detect complications associated with acute pancreatitis (pseudocysts, phlegmon, abscess).

Tests for Chronic Pancreatitis

I. *Measurement of pancreatic exocrine secretion*
   Secretin or cholecystokinin stimulation or the Lundh test meal: used to stimulate pancreatic secretion and collect pancreatic juice for enzyme and bicarbonate determination (levels reduced in pancreatic insufficiency)
   Indirect measurement of pancreatic secretion:
     Bentiromide test
     Dual Schilling test
     Fecal chymotrypsin concentration
II. *Imaging techniques of the pancreas*
   Plain film of the abdomen (calcification)
   Ultrasound (dilated pancreatic duct, calcification)
   CT of the abdomen (dilated duct, calcification, cystic lesions)
   ERCP (most sensitive and specific test, gold standard, ductal irregularities, stones, etc.)

PARANEOPLASTIC SYNDROMES

Paraneoplastic syndromes are remote effects caused by a primary tumor or its metastases. There are three known ways in which a tumor can cause a paraneoplastic syndrome:

1. A tumor may secrete a biologically active substance not normally produced by the cell of origin (ectopic or inappropriate hormone production).
2. A tumor may secrete increased amounts of a substance normally produced by its cell of origin.
3. Healthy cells may secrete mediators such as antibodies or cytokines in response to the tumor.

Known Paraneoplastic Syndromes

SIGN OR SYMPTOM	MEDIATOR	MALIGNANCIES
Ectopic hormones		
Cancer cachexia	IL-1, TNFα, IL-6	Diverse
Cushing's syndrome	ACTH	Lung cancer, esp. SCLC; carcinoid tumor
Erythrocytosis	Erythropoietin	Hepatoma, cerebellar hemangioblastoma
Fever	IL-1, IL-6, TNFα	Hodgkin's disease, hypernephroma
Gynecomastia	β-HCG	Germ cell tumors, lung cancer
Hypercalcemia	PTHrP	SCC of lung, esophagus, and head and neck; renal cell carcinoma; others
Hypercalcemia	IL-1, TNFα and β	Multiple myeloma, leukemia, lymphoma
Hypercalcemia	1,25 $(OH)_2$ vitamin D	Adult T-cell leukemia (HTLV I)
Hypoglycemia	Somatomedins (prob.)	Mesenchymal tumors, hepatoma
Leukemoid reaction	Colony-stimulating factors[1]	Cancer of lung, stomach, pancreas; Hodgkin's disease
SIADH	ADH	Lung cancer, especially SCLC
	ANP	SCLC

Table continued on next page.

Known Paraneoplastic Syndromes (Cont.)

SIGN OR SYMPTOM	MEDIATOR	MALIGNANCIES
Excess normal cellular products		
Amyloidosis	Ig or calcitonin fragments	Multiple myeloma, medullary thyroid carcinoma
Dysproteinemia	Igs	Multiple myeloma, lymphoma
Erythrocytosis	Erythropoietin	Hypernephroma
Hypoglycemia	Insulin	Insulinoma
Watery diarrhea	VIP	Islet-cell tumor of pancreas
Zollinger-Ellison syndrome	Gastrin	Gastrinoma
Reaction to tumor		
Dementia	Angiogenic peptides[2] (prob.)	Lung cancer
Dermatomyositis	C5b-9 on microvasculature	Lung, stomach, ovary
Eaton-Lambert syndrome	Ab to calcium channel	SCLC, stomach, ovary
Encephalomyelitis	Anti-Hu antibody	Lung
Myasthenia gravis	Ab to AChR	Thymoma, lymphoma, breast
Opsoclonus/myoclonus	Anti-Ri antibody	Neuroblastoma, SCLC, breast
Retinopathy	Ab to rods and cones	SCLC, melanoma
Sensory neuropathy	Anti-Hu antibody	SCLC
Subacute cerebellar degeneration	Anti-Hu antibody	SCLC
	Anti-Yo antibody	Ovary, breast, uterus
Thrombophlebitis	Activation of coagulation	GI adenocarcinoma, lung, breast
Etiology unknown		
Acanthosis nigricans	–	Gastric, other abdominal adenocarcinoma
Autonomic and GI neuropathy	–	SCLC
Bazek's syndrome	–	Head and neck, lung, esophagus
Clubbing	–	Lung, kidney, many others
Erythema gyratum repens	–	Lung, esophagus, breast
Hypertrophic pulmonary osteoarthropathy	–	Lung cancer (except SCLC), intrathoracic metastasis
Leser-Trélat sign	–	Lymphoma, GI adenocarcinoma
Limbic encephalitis	–	Lung cancer, Hodgkin's disease
Oncogenic osteomalacia	–	Mesenchymal tumors
Sensorimotor neuropathy	–	Lung, GI, breast cancer
Subacute motor neuropathy	–	Lymphoma
Subacute necrotic myelopathy	–	Lung, kidney cancer

[1]G-CSF, GM-CSF, M-CSF, IL-1, IL-3.
[2]Acidic and basic fibroblast growth factors, TNF, TGF α and β, IL-1β.

Abbreviations: Ab, antibody; AChR, acetylcholine receptor; ANP, atrial natriuretic peptide; PTHrP, parathyroid hormone–related protein; SCC, squamous-cell carcinoma; SCLC, small-cell lung cancer; TGF, transforming growth factor.

In the first two categories listed in the table, treatment or removal of the cancer may improve the paraneoplastic syndrome. Thus, both SIADH in small-cell lung cancer and Zollinger-Ellison syndrome in gastrinoma are often reversible. In many of the CNS paraneoplastic syndromes, however, symptoms may be independent of the course of the malignancy. For example, in paraneoplastic cerebellar degeneration, antibodies against tumor antigens cross-react with antigens on cerebellar Purkinje's cells. The ensuing destruction of Purkinje's cells is irreversible because the cerebellar cells are incapable of regenerating.

Reference: Bunn PA, et al: Paraneoplastic syndromes. In DeVita V et al (eds): Cancer. Principles and Practice of Oncology, 3rd ed. Philadelphia, J.B. Lippincott, 1989, pp 1896–1933.

PARATHYROID GLANDS: HYPERPARATHYROIDISM

Hyperparathyroidism is more common in women than men (2:1 ratio), and its incidence in persons over 65 is 1%. Most patients are asymptomatic, having had an increased serum calcium discovered on incidental screening. Symptoms of mild hyperparathyroidism consist of fatigue, weakness, dementia, depression, anorexia, and constipation. On serum assay, PTH may be elevated, but it is important to know what portion of the PTH molecule is being assayed, since increased levels of inactive portions are common but of uncertain importance. It is also important to measure ionized Ca^{++} in patients whose serum Ca^{++} is at the upper limits of normal or minimally elevated. The urgency of treatment is great only in those with significantly increased serum Ca^{++} or with other severe symptoms (specifically, skeletal, renal, GI, or neuromuscular problems). The long-term effects of asymptomatic increases in PTH are unknown.

This is a surgical disease, and parathyroid surgery is well tolerated by all age groups. Surgery is recommended for patients with a markedly elevated serum Ca^{++} (even if asymptomatic); prior life-threatening episodes of hypercalcemia; kidney stones; reduced renal function; markedly elevated urinary calcium excretion; or reduced bone mass. A number of minimally symptomatic patients report feeling markedly better after parathyroid surgery.

Patients who are not surgical candidates should be treated with estrogens and hydration. It is important to ensure preservation of renal function and to avoid thiazide diuretics in these persons.

Reference: Deftos LJ, et al: Management of hyperparathyroidism. Annu Rev Med 44:19–26, 1993.

PARKINSON'S DISEASE

Parkinson's disease is a degenerative condition that impairs motor control. It affects approximately 1% of all people over the age of 60, making it one of the commonest neurologic conditions in the elderly. The characteristic clinical features are:

1. Tremor
2. Rigidity
3. Bradykinesia
4. Postural instability

The tremor of Parkinson's disease is most prominent at rest and is a very coarse, large-amplitude, fairly slow (3–5 Hz) tremor. It seldom changes significantly with movement, but it tends to worsen with stress and diminish with relaxation.

Rigidity is manifested as an increase in the tone of the muscles, causing a stiffness throughout the range of movement. There is a characteristic cogwheeling to the tone. The bradykinesia is a slowness of movement, but there is also a paucity of movements: patients appear frozen and statuelike. They have masked facies, with little expression. The gait is characteristically stooped and shuffling, and patients turn en bloc rather than pivoting or turning quickly. Parkinson's patients have a tendency to fall forward or backward (retropulsion), and they have poor postural reflexes.

Parkinson's disease is caused by a gradual loss of dopamine-containing cells in the substantia nigra of the basal ganglia, at the top of the brain stem. This involvement of the basal ganglia, or extrapyramidal system, leads to the motor difficulties so characteristic of this disease. The cause of this sporadic condition is unknown, but oxidative breakdown may play a role. The fortuitous observation of Parkinson's disease induced in drug addicts by MPTP, a byproduct of meperidine (Demerol) synthesis, led to an animal model of parkinsonism caused by oxidation of MPTP, with subsequent damage to dopamine-containing cells in the substantia nigra. Prevention of oxidation by monoamine oxidase inhibitors such as selegiline (Deprenyl, Eldepryl) may slow the progression of the disease.

Therapy for Parkinson's disease requires the replacement of dopamine, usually in the form of Sinemet, a compound containing L-dopa (which the body converts into dopamine) and carbidopa (which prevents metabolism of the L-dopa and allows it to reach the CNS without undue side effects). A sustained-release formula of 50 mg of carbidopa combined with 200 mg of L-dopa constitutes standard therapy, given two or more times per day.

Other therapies include:

1. *Sinemet,* whose regular format, without the sustained-release properties, can be given as 10/100- or 25/250-mg pills up to six times per day, or as often as needed.
2. *Dopamine agonists,* such as bromocriptine (Parlodel) or pergolide.
3. *Anticholinergic agents,* such as benztropine (Cogentin) or trihexyphenidyl (Artane). These are especially useful for the tremor of Parkinson's disease.

A distressing feature of the therapy of Parkinson's disease is the development of toxicity from the medications. Sensitivity often develops to Sinemet and other dopamine agonists, leading to dopamine hyperactivity with resultant dyskinesias and dystonias, causing the patient to move too much, rather than too little. There may similarly be a sudden wearing-off of the response to these agents, causing the patient to freeze abruptly. Treatment may therefore result in the on-off phenomcnona exhibited by fluctuations between hyperactivity and freezing. Lower doses of dopamine, often spread out more evenly, may be needed to minimize these complications.

The diagnosis of Parkinson's disease is clinical, based upon the characteristic features. MRI, spinal fluid tests, and laboratory tests are usually normal.

References: Agid Y: Parkinson's disease: Pathophysiology. Lancet 337:1321, 1991.
Clough CG: Parkinson's disease: Management. Lancet 337:1324, 1991.

PARVOVIRUS B19 INFECTION

Parvovirus was first discovered in 1975 and since then has been linked to several childhood and adult syndromes. It was found to be the causative agent of a common childhood disease, erythema infectiosum (fifth disease). Children with erythema infectiosum typically have fever and a slapped-cheek rash on the face. In adults, initial infection is marked by fever, adenopathy, and arthropathy and is typically followed by fatigue, depression, and joint pains. The joint pains may persist for years. Parvovirus infections occur in the late winter and early spring.

Parvovirus is also responsible for aplastic crises in patients with hemoglobinopathies including sickle-cell disease, hereditary spherocytosis, pyruvate kinase deficiency, thalassemia, and autoimmune hemolytic anemia. Parvovirus infection typically causes a brief, 1- to 2-week bone marrow suppression that is insignificant in patients with normal RBC survival but can be devastating in patients with decreased RBC survival. Parvovirus infection in pregnant women can cause hydrops fetalis, fetal malformations, and spontaneous abortions.

There is no specific therapy for parvovirus infection other than RBC transfusion for those with aplastic crisis. It can be diagnosed through acute (IgM) antibody detection. Infection with parvovirus results in lifelong immunity to future infection.

Reference: Rotbart HA: Human parvovirus infection. Annu Rev Med 41:25–34, 1990.

PEPTIC ULCER DISEASE

A peptic ulcer is a circumscribed defect of the mucus membrane penetrating through the muscularis mucosa and occurring in areas exposed to acid and pepsin. PUD occurs in stomachs that hypersecrete acid, in patients taking harmful drugs (NSAIDs), or in patients secreting a relatively normal amount of acid but with a stomach infected with *Helicobacter pylori*. In younger patients and those secreting a high level of acid, PUD tends to occur in the duodenal bulb; in older patients and those secreting less acid or taking NSAIDs, it occurs in the stomach.

Patients with PUD can typically present with burning epigastric pain made better by food and made worse by an empty stomach. However, symptoms vary, and almost any upper-GI-related symptom can be caused by PUD. Patients presenting with suggestive symptoms should be placed on an H_2 blocker, sucralfate or antacids.

If the patient is under 40 years of age and a 6-week course of therapy cures the disease, nothing more needs to be done. If the patient has recurrent disease, is unresponsive to treatment, or is over 40, an upper GI endoscopy should be done to check for cancer and to diagnose *H. pylori* infection. Patients with an ulcer who are *H. pylori* positive should finish a course of therapy for the ulcer and then be placed on metronidazole 250 mg QID, bismuth subsalicylate (Pepto Bismol) two tablets QID, and tetracycline 250 mg QID for 2 weeks to eradicate the *H. pylori*. Patients with PUD and *H. pylori* have a 90% 1-year relapse rate; in patients in whom *H. pylori* is eradicated there is less than a 12% recurrence. If *H. pylori* is not present, then the patient should be questioned about NSAID use. If there is no NSAID use, a serum gastrin should be ordered to look for Zollinger-Ellison syndrome. A gastric ulcer should be followed to healing, with gastroscopies every 2 months in order to exclude gastric cancer.

The **indicators for surgery** in PUD are perforation, obstruction, suspicion of cancer, bleeding, disabling recurrences, and inability to heal with medical therapy. A gastric ulcer that has not healed despite 6 months of therapy and eradication of *H. pylori* has about an 8% chance of being cancerous and should be resected. In ulcers that are continually symptomatic after 6 months of treatment and *H. pylori* eradication, one should suspect a hypergastrin syndrome, surreptitious use of ulcer-causing drugs, or cancer. After these conditions are excluded, patients should be considered for ulcer surgeries, which include superselective vagotomy or Billroth's procedures.

Reasons for Recurrence of PUD After Surgery

CAUSE	TREATMENT
Incomplete vagotomy	H_2 blockers
Retained antrum	H_2 blockers or surgery
Zollinger-Ellison syndrome	Omeprazole or surgery
Helicobacter pylori infection	Eradication with antibiotics
NSAID use	Misoprostol or stop NSAID
Silk surgical sutures	Sucralfate
Antral G-cell hyperplasia	H_2 blockers or antrectomy
Hypercalcemia	Treat underlying cause
Cushing's syndrome, adrenal tumor	Treat underlying cause

Recurrent ulcers present with pain or bleeding, and diagnosis is best made by endoscopy.

PERICARDITIS

Acute Pericarditis

Acute pericarditis is a clinical syndrome characterized by three features:

1. Chest pain
2. Pericardial friction rub
3. ECG abnormalities

Chest pain due to acute pericarditis can be differentiated from chest pain due to myocardial ischemia by its quality, duration, precipitating factors, and relation to changes in posture or to physical activity as illustrated in the table that follows. Unlike chest pain due to myocardial ischemia, chest pain due to acute pericarditis is sharp and pleuritic, lasts several hours, increases with recumbency, and is relieved by sitting up and leaning forward.

Pericardial versus Ischemic Pain

	ISCHEMIA	PERICARDITIS
Location	Retrosternal; left shoulder, arm	Precordium; left trapezius ridge
Quality	Pressure, burning, buildup	Sharp, pleuritic; or dull, oppressive
Thoracic motion	No effect	Increased by breathing, rotating thorax
Duration	Angina; 1–15 min Unstable angina: $^1/_2$ hr to hrs	Hours or days
Effort	Stable angina: usually Unstable angina or infarction: usually not	No relation
Posture	No effect; may sit, belch, use Valsalva or knee-chest position for relief	Leaning forward for relief; aggravated by recumbency

From Fowler NO: Acute pericarditis. In Fowler NO (ed): The Pericardium in Health and Disease. Mt. Kisco, NY, Futura Publishing Co., 1985, p 158, with permission.

The classic physical finding in acute pericarditis is a pericardial friction rub. This is a scratching, grating, high-pitched sound, which Victor Collin first described as "the squeak of leather of a new saddle under the rider." The pericardial friction rub may have up to three components: presystolic, ventricular systolic, and early diastolic. Although a pericardial friction rub may be heard in the majority of patients with acute pericarditis, it is commonly an evanescent sound and often changes in quality or severity from one physical examination to another.

The classic ECG findings in acute pericarditis are ST-segment elevation, T-wave inversion, and PR-segment depression. The earliest ECG changes are the ST-segment elevation and PR-segment depression followed by T-wave inversion. Unlike acute MI, acute pericarditis is characterized by diffuse ST-segment elevation rather than ST-segment elevation localized to specific ECG leads. The classic ECG characteristics of acute pericarditis are illustrated in the following figure.

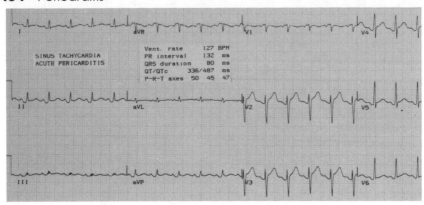

ECG changes in a patient with acute pericarditis.

Acute pericarditis can result from a number of diverse etiologies:

1. Idiopathic
2. Viral infection: coxsackievirus A and B, adenovirus, echovirus, mumps, varicella, hepatitis B and HIV/AIDS
3. Mycobacterial infection such as tuberculosis
4. Bacterial infection such as *Staphylococcus, Streptococcus,* gram-negative bacteremia, *Neisseria,* and *Legionella*
5. Fungal infection such as histoplasmosis, *Candida,* and blastomycosis
6. Acute MI
7. Uremia with or without hemodialysis
8. Radiation
9. Neoplastic disease such as lung and breast cancer, lymphoma, and leukemia
10. Autoimmune diseases such as acute rheumatic fever, SLE, RA, scleroderma, and polyarteritis nodosa
11. Drugs such as hydralazine, procainamide, dilantin, isoniazid, and penicillin
12. Trauma such as chest trauma, pacemaker insertion, thoracic surgery, esophageal rupture, and pancreatic-pericardial fistula
13. Post–MI (Dressler's) and postpericardiotomy syndromes
14. Dissecting aortic aneurysm
15. Myxedema
16. Chylopericardium

Constrictive Pericarditis

Constrictive pericarditis is a chronic disease characterized by fibrosis and/or calcification of the pericardium resulting in restriction of filling of the heart. The symmetrical constricting effect of the fibrotic and calcified pericardium results in elevation of all diastolic pressures, namely the LV, RV, and pulmonary arterial pressures. Due to the elevated venous pressure, early ventricular filling occurs in an abnormally rapid manner. However, the stiff, noncompliant pericardium abruptly halts ventricular filling. As a result, the classical auscultatory and hemodynamic hallmarks of constrictive pericarditis result from the unimpeded, early rapid-filling phase and the subsequent sudden cessation of ventricular filling. This pattern of filling is reflected in the characteristic dip-and-plateau configuration of both LV and RV pressure tracings, the prominent and steep y descent, and the diminished x descent. This is in contrast to cardiac tamponade, which is characterized by absent or blunted y descent and a preserved x descent, because ventricular filling is restricted throughout diastole. In other words, the impedance to ventricular filling in cardiac tamponade is pandiastolic, whereas restriction to filling of the ventricles in constrictive pericarditis is early diastolic.

Constrictive pericarditis can also be differentiated from cardiac tamponade in the hemodynamic changes during respiration. In patients with cardiac tamponade, inspiration causes an exaggerated filling of the RV, thereby shifting the interventricular septum to the left. As a result, LV volume is decreased and stroke volume is reduced, resulting in a significant fall in systolic BP by >10 mmHg. In constrictive pericarditis, the inspiratory fall in intrathoracic pressure is not transmitted to the heart because the pericardial space is obliterated. As a result, there is minimal if any increase in venous return to the RV and little if any shift of the interventricular septum to the left. Thus, during inspiration in patients with constrictive pericarditis, there is no significant fall in systolic BP. Thus, pulsus paradoxus—the inspiratory drop in systolic BP by >10 mmHg—is present in patients with cardiac tamponade but not in patients with constrictive pericarditis. Kussmaul's sign—a paradoxical inspiratory increase in venous pressure—is present in patients with constrictive pericarditis but not in patients with cardiac tamponade.

PERIPHERAL NEUROPATHY

Peripheral neuropathy is the commonest neurological problem found on a general medical ward. Its high incidence may reflect the fact that neuropathies often complicate systemic diseases, such as DM and uremia.

Clinically, a peripheral neuropathy may be recognized by characteristic signs and symptoms as follows.

1. *Weakness:* The weakness is distal, involving the hands and feet primarily. Many neuropathies are asymmetric (e.g., carpal tunnel syndrome, peroneal nerve palsy), whereas others cause symmetric, stocking-and-glove symptoms.
2. *Sensory changes:* Numbness is common with most neuropathies. Pain, paresthesias, and burning dysesthesias may also occur.
3. *Atrophy and fasciculation*
4. *Decreased reflexes:* The tone may also be slightly diminished.
5. *Trophic changes:* Many neuropathies affect the autonomic nerves, causing changes in temperature, sweating, loss of hair and nails, shining skin, etc.

The differential diagnosis of neuropathy is very extensive. A useful mnemonic is DANG THE RAPIST:

D = diabetes
A = alcohol
N = nutrition
G = Guillain-Barré

T = trauma
H = hereditary
E = environmental

R = remote effects of cancer
A = amyloid
P = porphyria
I = infectious and inflammatory
S = systemic
T = tumor

Together, DM and alcohol account for over 50% of all peripheral neuropathies in America. Nutritional problems include vitamin B_{12} and thiamine deficiency. Guillain-Barré syndrome is technically a radiculopathy, but it usually presents clinically as a peripheral neuropathy. Trauma is one of the commonest causes of neuropathy, especially entrapment or compression of a nerve. Hereditary neuropathies are extremely common and their diagnosis often requires formal nerve conduction velocity (NCV) studies on family members, because the symptoms may be mild and a family history may therefore be negative. Environmental factors include toxins such as rapeseed oil, tryptophan (eosinophilia-myalgia syndrome), and drugs such as phenytoin. The remote effects of cancer include a pure sensory neuropathy. Amyloid often affects the peripheral nerves, especially the autonomic nervous system. Porphyria causes a motor neuropathy primarily. Infectious causes include HIV neuropathy and syphilis. Inflammatory neuropathies are also common, including polyarteritis nodosa and SLE. Systemic causes, related to general medical illnesses, include uremia and hypothyroidism. Tumors can cause neuropathy directly (not only as paraneoplastic syndromes), especially by infiltration of the nerves.

The workup for peripheral neuropathy includes electrophysiologic testing:

1. **NCV:** Nerves normally conduct impulses at a speed of 55 m/sec and if that conduction is slowed, it suggests that the nerves are impaired. Significant slowing especially suggests damage to the myelin around the nerve (demyelinating neuropathy).

2. **EMG:** When a needle electrode is placed within the muscle, it can record muscle contractions. If the muscle is denervated, fibrillations and fasciculation are seen, and abnormal, high voltage, polyphasic muscle potentials may appear. Evidence of denervation without much nerve conduction slowing suggests that the axon of the nerve itself has been damaged (axonal neuropathy).

Treatment of peripheral neuropathies generally involves therapy of the underlying cause.

Reference: Schaumberg HH, et al: Disorders of Peripheral Nerves. Philadelphia, F.A. Davis, 1983.

PERIPHERAL VASCULAR DISEASE

Peripheral vascular disease usually presents with intermittent claudication in the calves, thighs, or buttocks or with Leriche's syndrome. In the elderly it may present as necrosis of peripheral tissues. The risk factors are those of atherosclerosis anywhere in the body and include cigarette smoking, DM, HTN, and hyperlipidemia. In patients with established claudication, 80% will have a relatively stable course, 10% will have other manifestations of atherosclerotic cardiovascular disease, and 10% will progress to ulcers, gangrene, vascular surgery, or amputation.

The absence of hair on the legs is associated with chronic ischemia. The physical exam should include auscultation for femoral or abdominal arterial bruits. The diagnosis can be made by comparing ankle BP to brachial BP (through measurement of systolic BP by palpation or Doppler). In normal patients, ankle BP should equal brachial BP. An ankle-to-brachial systolic BP ratio of less than 0.5 is consistent with PVD. However, moderate intermittent claudication can occur with a ratio of 0.8 to 0.5. Falsely normal ankle systolic BP may occur in patients with heavily calcified arteries that are not easily compressed by the sphygmomanometer cuff.

Medications do not appear to be helpful in decreasing pain. The first component of treatment is to stop smoking. Regular walking programs increase the time to pain by improving muscle function. Over a 3- to 6-month period, walking distance increases twofold to fivefold. Angioplasty has a 2-year 75% limb salvage even in oldest patients. Arteriograms should be reserved for those patients being considered for surgery or angioplasty.

Reference: Woods BO: Clinical evaluation of the peripheral vasculature. Cardiol Clin 9:413–427, 1991.

PERITONITIS, SPONTANEOUS BACTERIAL

Ascites, especially cirrhotic ascites, occasionally becomes infected without an apparent source; this is called spontaneous bacterial peritonitis (SBP). The pathogenesis of SBP is related to a low concentration of opsonins in the ascitic fluid, which allows infection with native gut flora. Clinical presentation can be subtle, because the fluid masks signs of peritonitis. Therefore, any patient with ascites who has fever, increased weakness, change in mental status, or any change in condition that requires a hospital visit should be tested for SBP. The test consists of diagnostic paracentesis, the obtaining of a cell count to determine the percentage of PMNs, and the inoculation of blood culture bottles with 10 cc of ascitic fluid. Patients with >500 PMNs per ml almost always have SBP. Those with >250 have about a 60% chance of having SBP and should be treated. No other chemical tests are needed for diagnosis. However, SBP of ascitic fluid caused by abscess or perforation is suggested by a glucose <50 mg/dl or an ascitic fluid LDH level greater than the serum LDH upper limit of normal. Once patients are diagnosed with SBP, they should be treated empirically with ticarcillin clavulanate, ampicillin/sulbactam, or a third-generation cephalosporin for 7 to 10 days. Antibiotics can be changed once culture results are known. The most common organisms are *Streptococcus pneumoniae,* group A streptococcus, and Enterobacteriaceae.

PHARYNGITIS

Pharyngitis can be caused be numerous agents, including bacteria such as *Streptococcus pyogenes, Haemophilus influenzae,* and *Neisseria gonorrhoeae;* viruses such as EBV, HSV, and coxsackievirus; and other organisms such as *Mycoplasma pneumoniae, Chlamydia,* and *Candida albicans. Mycobacterium tuberculosis* rarely causes pharyngitis but should be considered in the differential diagnosis, as should primary or secondary syphilis. Fortunately, diphtheria is declining but can occur in patients with inadequate immunity.

When evaluating the patient who complains of a sore throat, one should quickly identify those with streptococcal infection, who require therapy to prevent acute rheumatic fever. Untreated streptococcal infection can also lead to peritonsillar abscess. Streptococcal infection can be suspected from the clinical history and examination. Four signs and symptoms are associated with a high probability of streptococcal infection: swollen, tender anterior cervical nodes; fever; tonsillar exudates; and lack of cough. Patients with all four symptoms should be treated presumptively for streptococcal pharyngitis and do not require additional testing. Patients seen in the ED should be treated presumptively if they have at least three of the symptoms. Office or clinic patients with three or fewer of the symptoms should undergo diagnostic testing with rapid antigen tests in the office. Patients with a positive rapid antigen test should be treated. Patients with a negative rapid antigen test should have a throat culture done and be treated if the culture is positive.

Penicillin is the antibiotic of choice and can be given as penicillin V 250–500 mg QID for 10 days. IM benzathine penicillin (1.2 million units) is also effective and may be more useful in the patient unlikely to complete a full course of oral antibiotic therapy. Erythromycin can be used in penicillin-allergic patients. (See also Sore Throat.)

Reference: Centor RM, et al: Throat cultures and rapid tests for diagnosis of group A streptococcal pharyngitis in adults. In Sox HC Jr (ed): Common Diagnostic Tests: Use and Interpretation. Philadelphia, American College of Physicians, 1990.

PHEOCHROMOCYTOMA

Pheochromocytomas represent one of the most important categories of secondary HTN: surgically curable if recognized, frequently fatal if not. These tumors originate from chromaffin cells in the adrenal medullae in 90% of cases. The remaining 10% are found in sympathetic nerves in extra-adrenal sites, usually in the abdomen, chest, or neck. Extra-adrenal pheochromocytomas are malignant in 30 to 40% of cases, far more commonly than adrenal tumors. Usually pheochromocytomas secrete both norepinephrine and epinephrine, although some secrete only one of those catecholamines or, rarely, dopamine. These tumors are most commonly associated with paroxysmal HTN, although they are identified as the cause of sustained diastolic HTN in approximately 0.05% of cases.

Pheochromocytoma Pearls

6 H's:	Hypertension	Heart consciousness
	Headache	Hypermetabolism
	Hyperhidrosis	Hyperglycemia

Table continued on next page.

Pheochromocytoma Pearls (Cont.)

95% will have:	Headache or hyperhidrosis or palpitation
Rough rule of 10:	10% familial 10% bilateral (adrenal) 10% malignant 10% multiple (other than bilateral adrenal) 10% extra-adrenal 10% occur in children
MEN, type-2 triad:	Medullary thyroid carcinoma Bilateral—familial pheochromocytoma (frequent) Hyperparathyroidism (50%)
MEN, type-3 sextet:	Medullary thyroid carcinoma Bilateral—familial pheochromocytoma (frequent) Mucosal neuromas Thickened corneal nerves Marfanoid habitus Alimentary-tract ganglioneuromatosis (very rarely hyperparathyroidism)
4 C's:	Cholelithiasis Cushing's syndrome (very rare) Cutaneous lesions Cerebellar hemangioblastoma (very rare)

From Manger WM, et al: Pheochromocytoma. In Laragh JH, et al (eds): Hypertension: Pathophysiology, Diagnosis and Management. New York, Raven Press, 1990, p 1650, with permission.

The most reliable screening test is a measurement of 24-hr urinary total metanephrines (metanephrine plus normetanephrine). CT scans accurately detect 95% of these tumors.

Prior to surgery, patients with a documented pheochromocytoma should undergo screening for medullary thyroid carcinoma and hyperparathyroidism. Phentolamine is the drug of choice for managing associated hypertensive crises during surgery (3–5 mg IV bolus followed by an infusion of sodium nitroprusside or phentolamine). Surgery for this condition is best handled by a team with expertise in this difficult field.

PITUITARY GLAND: HYPOPITUITARISM

Pituitary hormone deficiency may involve one or several of the pituitary hormones.

Classification of Hypopituitarism

I. Isolated (single pituitary hormone deficiency):
1. Congenital deficiency of GNRH (absence of puberty, deficient gonadal function, and low plasma LH and FSH; associated with anosmia)
2. Isolated acquired TSH deficiency, evidence of hypothyroidism, poor TSH response to TRH (may be seen in pituitary apoplexy)

    3. Isolated ACTH deficiency, causing selective glucocorticoid deficiency, absence of hyperpigmentation, or volume contraction. Its main features are failure to thrive, tendency to water intoxication, hyponatremia, generalized weakness, inability to respond normally to stress, and hypoglycemia. Plasma cortisol level is low and does not rise after insulin-induced hypoglycemia.

    4. Isolated growth hormone deficiency (cause of short stature). Pituitary apoplexy may cause one, two, or more deficiencies.

II. Panhypopituitarism (more common than isolated pituitary deficiency):

    1. Destruction of the pituitary by a pituitary tumor, craniopharyngioma, or metastatic tumor to the hypothalamic-pituitary region.

    2. Sheehan's syndrome (or postpartum pituitary infarction) is characterized by lack of lactation, low prolactin level, nonresponsiveness to TRH stimulation, and other deficiencies.

    3. Empty sella turcica may be associated with variable degrees of hypopituitarism.

    4. Other causes: granulomatous diseases (e.g., sarcoidosis), infections, radiotherapy.

Clinical Features

The clinical features of panhypopituitarism are due to deficiencies of thyroid hormone, glucocorticoid, and sex hormone. Growth hormone and gonadotropins are often the first hormones to become deficient. Involvement of the hypothalamus causes vasopressin deficiency (diabetes insipidus), characterized by polyuria, nocturia, and increased thirst. Clinical manifestations of hypopituitarism include constipation, fatigue and drowsiness, weakness, weight loss, hypoglycemic symptoms, nausea and vomiting, decreased libido, menstrual abnormalities, infertility, impotence, atrophy of the breasts, atrophic vagina and labia, dyspareunia, small prostate, and soft testes. Failure to lactate in the postpartum period may be indicative of Sheehan's syndrome. There are often postural hypotension, hypothermia, and slow pulse. The skin features are often characteristic and include pallor; waxy, soft skin with fine wrinkles; absence of tanning; decreased axillary and pubic hair; decreased facial hair in the male; and pale nipples and areolae. There may be decreased sweating and decreased sebum.

Evaluation of Pituitary Function

    1. Insulin tolerance test to assess cortisol and growth hormone responses to insulin-induced hypoglycemia (0.15 units/kg weight is administered IV and growth hormone and cortisol levels measured every 15 min).

    2. TFTs (free thyroxine index, free T_4, TSH, and TRH stimulation test to assess TSH responsiveness to TRH).

    3. Measurement of prolactin, FSH and LH, and testosterone; semen analysis in males.

    4. Pituitary adrenal function may be alternatively assessed by an 8 a.m. cortisol and 11-deoxycortisol measurement in response to metyrapone.

Management includes replacement of the major deficient hormones: L-thyroxine therapy for hypothyroidism, dose 0.1 to 0.2 mg once daily, and hydrocortisone 20 to 30 mg daily; testosterone cypionate or enanthate 200 to 300 mg IM every 2–3 weeks in men; conjugated estrogens 0.625 to 1.25 mg per day on days 1–24 and medroxyprogesterone acetate 5 to 10 mg per day on days 10–24 for women.

PITUITARY TUMORS

The size of a pituitary tumor varies from a few millimeters to a few centimeters. Lesions of <1 cm are considered to be *microadenomas* (very common in unselected populations); larger tumors are *macroadenomas*. Circumstances in which a pituitary tumor may be discovered include:

1. An imaging procedure obtained in a fairly asymptomatic individual for an unrelated reason (e.g., skull x-ray, CT scan, or MRI of the head showing either enlargement of the sella turcica or evidence of a pituitary abnormality).
2. Visual disturbances, headaches, or other neurologic abnormalities (mostly with macroadenomas exceeding 1 cm in diameter).
3. Features of hormone excess, particularly hyperprolactinemia (e.g., galactorrhea, amenorrhea), features of cortisol excess (e.g., Cushing's disease), or features of growth hormone excess (acromegaly).
4. Presenting features of hypopituitarism due to a destruction in the hypothalamic-pituitary region.
5. In the setting of a pituitary apoplexy (severe headaches, visual disturbances, acute or subacute neurological manifestations).

Types of Pituitary Tumors

---

1. Prolactinoma may be a microadenoma or a macroadenoma.
2. Growth-hormone-secreting tumors are usually macroadenomas.
3. Cushing's disease (the pituitary tumor is often very small and may not be identified by MRI or CT scan).
4. TSH-secreting tumors cause TSH-induced hyperthyroidism. They are often macroadenomas and are characterized by hyperthyroidism and either a detectable or an elevated baseline TSH level. The measurement of alpha TSH subunit and the response of TSH and alpha TSH subunit to TRH stimulation allows establishment of the diagnosis.
5. FSH- and LH-secreting tumors are often associated with hypogonadism, visual impairment, and headaches.
6. Chromophobe adenoma is the traditional name for a large number of tumors that do not produce functional hormones. Nearly 70% of macroadenomas secrete hormone fragments, especially the alpha or beta chain of glycoprotein hormones (FSH, LH, or TSH). The fragments may be identified by immunostaining of the tumor tissue and may be measured in the blood. Nearly 30% of macroadenomas do not produce excess hormone and are called nul tumors.

Clinical features of prolactinoma include inappropriate lactation especially when accompanied by amenorrhea, anovulation, and infertility. Hyperprolactinemia may contribute to bone mineral loss.

Differential Diagnosis of Hyperprolactinemia

Pituitary disease	Vascular causes
Prolactinomas	Neurogenic causes
Acromegaly	Chest wall lesions

Table continued on next page.

Differential Diagnosis of Hyperprolactinemia (Cont.)

Empty sella turcica syndrome	Spinal cord lesions
Hypothalamic diseases	Breast stimulation
Craniopharyngiomas	Pregnancy
Meningiomas	Hypothyroidism
Dysgerminomas	Chronic renal failure
Other tumors	Cirrhosis
Sarcoidosis	Idiopathic hyperprolactinemia
Medications, (e.g., phenothiazines, tricyclic antidepressants, reserpine)	Eosinophilic granuloma

Levels of prolactin higher than 250 ng/ml are suggestive of a prolactinoma. Modest elevations of prolactin should suggest other causes such as drugs.

The manifestations of acromegaly are enlarged sella, headache, visual impairment, rhinorrhea, papilledema, and pituitary apoplexy. Manifestations due to growth hormone excess are acral growth, soft tissue growth, hypermetabolism, hyperhidrosis, hypertrichosis, prognathism, arthritic manifestations, osteoporosis, visceromegaly, hyperpigmentation, weight gain, goiter, impaired glucose tolerance, and diabetes.

Management of Pituitary Tumors

1. Transsphenoidal or transfrontal surgery depending on size of the tumor
2. Drug therapy:
   a. Prolactinomas: dopamine agonists, bromocriptine
   b. Acromegaly: bromocriptine and somatostatin analogues

PLEURAL EFFUSIONS

Pleural effusions are often asymptomatic. If the effusion accumulates rapidly or is large, the most common symptoms are dyspnea, cough, and pleuritic chest pain. Small effusions (less than 500 cc) frequently have minimal findings on exam and the CXR may reveal blunting of the costophrenic angle. Larger effusions (1,500 cc), with concomitant atelectasis, may demonstrate bronchial breath sounds, egophony, inspiratory lag, diminished breath sounds, fremitus, and dullness to percussion. The CXR may reveal opacification and the upper margin may form a meniscus along the lateral wall. Larger effusions may cause complete opacification, and shift the mediastinum toward the unaffected lung.

Classification of pleural effusions: The key to diagnosing and differentiating the cause of a pleural effusion lies in determining whether the effusion is transudative or exudative. The mechanism of formation of transudative pleural fluid (low protein, normal pleura) is generally caused by imbalances in the Starling forces that control the formation and resorption of normal pleural fluid. Exudates (high protein) are the result of a diseased pleura, generally as the result of inflammation or malignancy. Therefore, a diagnostic thoracentesis is required to evaluate the fluid.

Tests that may be indicated and may help differentiate the cause of the effusion include those in the following table.

Characteristics of Transudates and Exudates

	TRANSUDATES	EXUDATES
Typical appearance	Clear	Clear, cloudy, or bloody
Protein (absolute value) (g/dl)	<3.0	>3.0
Protein (fluid/serum ratio)	<0.5	>0.5
LDH (absolute value) (IU/L)	<200	>200
LDH (fluid/serum ratio)	<0.6	>0.6
Glucose (mg/dl)	>60	Variable, often <60
WBC count (total) (/ml)	<1,000	>1,000
PMNs	<50%	Usually >50%
RBC count (/ml)	<5,000	Variable

Differential Diagnosis of Pleural Effusions

I. Transudative pleual effusions
A. CHF
B. Cirrhosis
C. Nephrotic syndrome
D. Superior vena caval obstruction
E. Fontan procedure
F. Urinothorax
G. Peritoneal dialysis
H. Glomerulonephritis
I. Myxedema
J. Pulmonary emboli
K. Sarcoidosis

II. Exudative pleural effusions
A. Neoplastic disease
  1. Metastatic disease
  2. Mesothelioma
B. Infectious diseases
  1. Bacterial infections
  2. TB
  3. Fungal infections
  4. Parasitic infections
  5. Viral infections
C. Pulmonary embolization
D. Gastrointestinal disease
  1. Pancreatic disease
  2. Subphrenic abscess
  3. Intrahepatic abscess
  4. Intrasplenic abscess
  5. Esophageal perforation
  6. Abdominal surgical procedures
  7. Diaphragmatic hernia
  8. Endoscopic variceal sclerotherapy
E. Collagen vascular diseases
  1. Rheumatoid pleuritis
  2. SLE
  3. Drug-induced lupus
  4. Immunoblastic lymphadenopathy
  5. Sjögren's syndrome
  6. Familial Mediterranean fever
  7. Churg-Strauss syndrome
  8. Wegener's granulomatosis

F. Drug-induced pleural disease
  1. Nitrofurantoin
  2. Dantrolene
  3. Methysergide
  4. Bromocriptine
  5. Amiodarone
  6. Procarbazine
  7. Methotrexate
  8. Practolol
G. Miscellaneous diseases and conditions
  1. Asbestos exposure
  2. Postpericardiectomy or post-MI syndrome
  3. Meigs' syndrome
  4. Yellow nail syndrome
  5. Sarcoidosis
  6. Pericardial disease
  7. Fetal pleural effusion
  8. Uremia
  9. Trapped lung
  10. Radiation therapy
  11. Ovarian hyperstimulation syndrome
  12. Postpartum pleural effusion
  13. Amyloidosis
  14. Electrical burns
  15. Iatrogenic injury
H. Hemothorax
I. Chylothorax

From Light RW: Pleural Diseases. Philadelphia, Lea & Febiger, 1990, p 76, with permission.

Causes of Malignant Pleural Effusions in Two Different Series

TUMOR	SPRIGGS AND BODDINGTON*		ANDERSON*	
	N	%	N	%
Lung carcinoma	275	43	32	24
Breast carcinoma	157	25	35	26
Lymphoma and leukemia	52	8	34	26
Ovarian carcinoma	27	4	9	7
Sarcoma (including melanoma)	13	2	5	4
Uterine and cervical carcinoma	6	1	3	2
Stomach carcinoma	18	3	1	1
Colon carcinoma	9	1	0	0
Pancreatic carcinoma	7	1	0	0
Bladder carcinoma	7	1	0	0
Other carcinoma	23	4	6	4
Primary unknown	40	6	8	6
	634		133	

*Data from Spriggs AI, Boddington MM: The Cytology of Effusions, 2nd ed. New York, Grune & Stratton, 1968; and Anderson CB, Philpott GW, Ferguson TB: The treatment of malignant pleural effusions. Cancer 33:916–922, 1974.

From Light RW: Pleural Diseases. Philadelphia, Lea & Febiger, 1990, p 98, with permission.

Malignancies can cause pleural effusions by a variety of mechanisms, including direct and indirect effects of the cancer.

Mechanisms by Which Malignant Disease Leads to Pleural Effusions

Direct result
 1. Pleural metastases with increased permeability
 2. Pleural metastases with obstruction of pleural lymphatic vessels
 3. Mediastinal lymph node involvement with decreased pleural lymphatic drainage
 4. Thoracic duct interruption (chylothorax)
 5. Bronchial obstruction (decreased pleural pressures)
 6. Pericardial involvement
Indirect result
 1. Hypoproteinemia
 2. Postobstructive pneumonitis
 3. Pulmonary embolism
 4. Postradition therapy

From Light RW: Pleural Diseases. Philadelphia, Lea & Febiger, 1990, p 99, with permission.

*Characteristics of Pleural Effusions in Different Disorders**

CONDITION	TYPICAL FINDINGS
CHF	Transudate; protein may increase with diuresis or chronicity; right side more frequent but often bilateral; may localize in fissure (pseudotumor)
Pneumonia	Exudate; bacterial infections: in $1/3$ of patients (more with pneumococcus and gram negatives), cells mainly polymorphonuclears. Viral infections: less common, usually small, cells mainly mononuclear. May be eosinophilic (>10%) in either; designated an empyema when organisms or gross purulence present
Malignancy	Exudate: lymphocytic, often hemorrhagic, with malignant cells in fluid or on pleural biopsy; often large and symptomatic; frequency: lung > breast > lymphoma > others
Pulmonary embolism	Exudate (75%) or transudate (25%); may be hemorrhagic; occurs in $1/3$ to $1/2$ of patients
TB	Exudate: lymphocyte predominant, high protein; eosinophilia (>10%) rare; unilateral; small to moderate in majority; usually no associated parenchymal abnormality on CXR; tubercle bacilli demonstrable in 10% on smear, 25% on culture, 50–75% on pleual biopsy; presentation either acute (<1 wk, fever, chest pain) or subacute; can be asymptomatic
Cirrhosis	Transudate; usually right-sided; can be massive and symptomatic, even without marked ascites
RA	Exudate; leukocyte count variable; glucose often very low (<15 mg/dL); LDH may be very high; may contain high cholesterol level and/or crystals; effusion occurs in 5% of patients, more commonly in men; may persist for months and require repeated drainage
SLE	Exudate; leukocyte count variable; glucose near serum level; fluid complement levels (C3, C4 components) typically low; LE cells may be present; effusion occurs in $1/3$ to $1/2$ of patients; often bilateral, usually small and of short duration
Drug-induced effusion	Exudate; in drug-induced lupus, characteristics are similar to those in naturally occurring lupus; uncommon otherwise; often eosinophilic
Dressler's syndrome	Exudate; in setting of pleuropericarditis following myocardial infarction, trauma, or surgery involving pericardium
Benign asbestos-related effusion	Exudate; cells variable, often serosanguineous; may be eosinophilic (>10%); sometimes bilateral; can recur; usually small to moderate in size; asymptomatic in $2/3$; related to amount of exposure; shorter lag time than with other asbestos-related conditions
Pancreatitis	Exudate with high amylase (of pancreatic origin); usually small-to-moderate size; typically left-sided but may be bilateral
Intraabdominal abscess	Exudate; leukocyte count (polymorphonuclears) often very high; glucose >60 mg/dL; sterile
Esophageal perforation	Rapidly increasing exudate, often with air-fluid level; epithelial cells, sometimes with food particles; high amylase (of salivary origin); may be on either side or bilateral; usually acute presentation with severe pain, toxicity, prostration

*In roughly descending order of frequency in clinical practice.

From Pierson D: Disorders of the pleura, mediastinum and diaphragm. In Wilson JD, et al (eds): Harrison's Principles of Internal Medicine, 12th ed., New York, McGraw-Hill, 1991, p 1112, with permission.

PLEURISY

Pleurisy is an older term for the inflammation of the pleura caused by TB. However, pleuritis, a more appropriate term for inflammation of the pleura, may be caused by pneumonia, TB, pulmonary infarction, viruses, or neoplasm. The symptom of pain on inspiration or movement of the chest wall is classic for pleuritis. The diagnosis is aided by the presence of other symptoms such as cough, fever, chills, hemoptysis, history of TB or exposure to TB, or weight loss. The CXR is also helpful in the diagnosis. Pleural disease in the absence of physical and CXR findings may be of viral origin, such as epidemic pleurodynia (Bornholm disease). Parenchymal disease on CXR suggests an infectious process such as acute bacterial pneumonia. Pleural effusion on the CXR, in the absence of parenchymal disease, suggests postprimary TB, subdiaphragmatic abscess, mesothelioma, or primary bacterial infection of the pleural space. Disease outside the chest may also cause pleuritic pain. Occasionally, rheumatoid arthritis may cause exudative pleural effusions, which are rarely painful. A subphrenic abscess may cause pleuritic chest pain as well as fever and an exudative pleural effusion. Pancreatitis can cause a left-sided pleural effusion with a high amylase concentration in up to 15% of patients with acute pancreatitis or pancreatic pseudocysts.

Treatment is directly dependent on the underlying disease, so a diagnosis must be made. Sputum for cytology, bacterial, and fungal cultures should be obtained. However, aspiration of pleural effusions and/or pleural biopsy may be necessary. It is important to remember that a clinical diagnosis of empyema requires chest tube drainage, without which thick pleural adhesions are very common and later require decortication to allow normal respiratory function. Separation of pleural effusions into transudates and exudates is useful for diagnosis and treatment (see Pleural Effusions, p 472).

Laboratory Studies of Pleural Fluid

TEST RESULT	CONDITIONS SUGGESTED
WBC count >10,000//L	Empyema, parapneumonic effusion, pancreatitis, malignancies, TB
Lymphocytosis	TB, malignancy
Eosinophilia	Traumatic hemothorax, asbestosis, paragonimiasis
pH <7.0	Complicated parapneumonic effusion
RF 1:320	RA
Elevated amylase	Pancreatitis, ruptured esophagus
Glucose <60 mg/dl	Parapneumonic effusion, TB, malignancy, rheumatoid effusion, hemothorax
TG >110 mg/dl	Chylothorax

Reference: Light RW: Pleural Diseases. Philadelphia, Lea & Febiger, 1990.

PNEUMOCOCCAL PNEUMONIA

Streptococcus pneumoniae is the most common cause of community-acquired pneumonias requiring hospitalization. Approximately 5–7% of adults are colonized by *S. pneumoniae* in the upper respiratory tract. Disease is thought to be acquired by aspiration of these organisms and is more frequent in winter and early spring.

Patient characteristics that predispose to pneumonia:

1. Alcoholism
2. Pulmonary disease
3. Heart disease (esp. CHF)
4. Lymphoma and myeloma
5. Asplenia/splenic dysfunction
6. Autoimmune diseases
7. Malignancy
8. Liver disease (cirrhosis)
9. Renal disease
10. Seizure disorder
11. HIV infection
12. Immunosuppression
13. Hypogammaglobulinemia

Clinical Findings and Diagnosis

A. The classically described presentation of a sudden onset of pleuritic chest pain with one shaking chill and production of rust-colored sputum is unusual.
B. CXRs demonstrate a bronchopneumonia pattern in 60% and lobar consolidation in 40%.
   1. Up to one-third of patients have detectable pleural effusions.
   2. Total CXR resolution may take up to 6 weeks to occur.
C. Up to one-third of patients have positive blood cultures. Patients with splenic dysfunction and HIV infection are even more likely to be bacteremic.
D. Gram stain of sputum demonstrates lancet-shaped, gram-positive diplococci.

Factors that Increase Mortality in Pneumococcal Pneumonia

- Very young age or age >50 years old
- Multilobar disease
- Bacteremia
- Significant underlying illness

CHF	Hodgkin's disease
COPD	Alcoholism
Splenic dysfunction	Sickle-cell anemia
Cirrhosis	Renal failure
Multiple myeloma	

- Delay in onset of therapy

PNEUMOCONIOSIS

Occupational and Environment-Related Disease

The key to diagnosing and preventing occupational and environmentally related lung disease is obtaining a pertinent and complete history.

Key Elements of an Occupational and Environmental History

Present illness (for each element of problem list)
Symptoms related to work
Other employees similarly affected
Current exposure to dusts, fumes, chemicals, biologic hazards
Prior first report of work injury
Work history
Describe all prior jobs, typical workday, change in work process
Work site
Ventilation, medical and industrial hygiene surveillance, employment examinations,
protective measures
Union health and safety; moonlighting; days missed work last year, why; prior worker
compensation claims
Past history
Exposure to noise, vibration, radiation, chemicals, asbestos
Environmental history
Present and prior home and work locations
Jobs of significant others
Hazardous wastes/spills exposure
Air pollution
Hobbies: painting, sculpture, welding, woodworking
Home insulation/heating
Home and work cleaning agents
Pesticide exposure
Do you wear seat belts?
Do you have firearms at home or work?
Review of systems
Specific emphasis
Shift changes, boredom, reproductive history

From Becker CE: Key elements of the occupational history for the general physician. West J Med 137:581–582, 1982, with permission.

Hypersensitivity pneumonitis: Although this is an infrequently encountered clinical syndrome, there are over 50 known causes of hypersensitivity pneumonitis. The immune hypersensitivity reaction results from repeated inhalation of particulate antigens derived from fungal, bacterial, animal protein, or chemical sources. There are two distinct clinical syndromes: acute and subacute/chronic. In the acute syndrome, symptoms develop 4 to 10 hrs after exposure and resolve during the next 24 hrs. In the chronic syndrome, symptoms develop insidiously and progressively.

Clinical Syndromes of Hypersensitivity Pneumonitis

Bacteria	Fungi
Farmer's lung: *Micropolyspora*	Malt worker's lung: *Aspergillus* sp.
Bagassosis: *Thermoactinomyces*	Cheese washer's lung: *Penicillium* sp.
Animal proteins	Reactive chemicals
Bird breeder's lung: avian proteins	TDI hypersensivity: TDI

Pneumoconiosis: This group of interstitial lung diseases results from the inhalation of inorganic dusts. Some of the more common entities are:

Asbestosis	Silicosis
Berylliosis	Coal workers' pneumoconiosis
Siderosis	Talc pneumoconiosis
Stannosis	Hard-metal pneumoconiosis

PNEUMOCYSTIS CARINII PNEUMONIA

Diagnosis and X-ray Pattern

Suspicion is the key to the diagnosis of PCP. One must suspect or know of a profound immunosuppressive state and recognize the sometimes subtle complaints. In a patient already known to be infected with HIV, this may not be difficult to do. In the patient with no prior clinical evaluation who comes off the street, it can be next to impossible without the heightened suspicion.

The most common presenting complaints are fever, dyspnea, chest tightness, and a persistent dry cough. These symptoms may persist for extended periods of time. On physical exam the only remarkable findings may be fever, tachypnea, and few dry rales. More severe cases may present with cyanosis.

A table to help differentiate clinical conditions based upon CXR findings follows. Note that it is unusual for PCP to cause hilar adenopathy or pleural effusion.

CXR Findings in AIDS Patients with Respiratory Disease

CXR PATTERN	ILLNESS
Normal	No disease
	Pneumocystis carinii pneumonia
	Disseminated fungal infection
Focal infiltrate	Pyogenic pneumonia
	Tuberculosis
	Cryptococcal pneumonia
	Pneumocystis carinii pneumonia
Pleural effusion	Kaposi's sarcoma
	Pyogenic pneumonia
	Tuberculosis
Mediastinal adenopathy	Tuberculosis/*Mycobacterium avium* complex
	Lymphoma
Interstitial infiltrate	*Pneumocystis carinii* pneumonia
	Tuberculosis
	Lymphocytic interstitial pneumonia
	Nonspecific pneumonitis
	Pyogenic pneumonia

From Chaisson RE, et al: Clinical manifestations of HIV infection. In Mandell GL, et al (eds): Principles and Practice of Infectious Diseases, 3rd ed. New York, Churchill Livingstone, 1990, p 1073, with permission.

Treatment and Prophylaxis

Without treatment, PCP is progressive and fatal. Early diagnosis and treatment can halt that progression and provide a cure with minimal morbidity. There are two mainstays of both the treatment and prophylactic regimens: trimethoprim-sulfamethoxazole (TMP/SMX) and pentamidine. A third agent, atovaquone, has recently received FDA approval as an alternative therapy. The two tables that follow give dosing, administration, and cost information.

Acute treatment: In the patient not known to be sulfa sensitive and without limiting hematologic or hepatic abnormalities, TMP/SMX is the agent of choice. Initial therapy can be administered orally unless nausea and vomiting would make successful administration unlikely. Toxicity is common, but usually not severe. GI upset and mild rash, frequently accompanied by fever, are often noted. The rash can be self-limited and does not automatically necessitate a change of therapy. Leukopenia, anemia, and hepatitis are more bothersome, and patients should be monitored for these complications.

In patients unable to tolerate TMP/SMX, pentamidine has been the next choice in therapy. Due to the possibility of hypotension in response to a too rapid infusion, an infusion pump should be used. Impaired renal function and alterations in glucose control are the primary toxicities. Renal toxicity, if discovered early, is usually reversible with withdrawal of the drug. Hypoglycemia may appear at any time in the course of therapy and results from hyperinsulinemia secondary to pancreatic beta-islet cell toxicity. In a patient on pentamidine, the appearance of

Drugs to Treat PCP*

DRUG	TOTAL DAILY ADULT DOSE	ROUTE	HOURS BETWEEN DOSES	DAYS OF THERAPY	COST FOR 21 DAYS ($)†
Specific agents					
Trimethoprim/	15–20 mg/kg	IV or	6–8	21	798 (IV),
sulfamethoxazole	75–100 mg/kg	PO			13 (PO)
Pentamidine isethionate	4 mg/kg	IV	24	21	2,079
Trimethoprim and	15–20 mg/kg	PO	8	21	50
dapsone	100 mg	PO	24	21	
Trimetrexate	45 mg/m^2	IV	24	21	2,624
Clindamycin and	1.8 g	PO	8	21	223
primaquine	15 mg	PO	24	21	
Atovaquone	2250 mg	PO	8	21	504
Ajunctive agents					
Prednisone	40 mg	PO	12	5	
	40 mg	PO	24	5	
	40 mg	PO	24	11	3

*Drugs grouped as pairs in the left-hand column are given in combination. TMP/SMX is the preferred regimen for patients with PCP who can tolerate it.

†As estimated from the Red Book (1994); prices are lowest prices for generic drugs.

Adapted from Masur H: Drug therapy: Prevention and treatment of *Pneumocystis* pneumonia. N Engl J Med 327:1853–1860, 1992.

mental status changes should immediately raise the issue of hypoglycemia and mandate a finger stick glucose level. Hyperglycemia and diabetes appear later and can be permanent.

Atovaquone (Mepron, 566C80) was recently approved by the FDA for use in AIDS-associated PCP in those patients intolerant of TMP/SMX. It provides an alternative oral regimen, making hospitalization or outpatient IV therapy with pentamidine less neccssary. It has been given this alternative designation as opposed to an outright approval due to concern about secondary bacterial infections in the study groups receiving atovaquone when compared to the TMP/SMX groups. Adverse events have been reported to be mainly rash, nausea, and diarrhea. Tolerance for this agent was much better than that for either TMP/SMX or pentamidine with equivalent efficacy. Absorption is dependent upon fat content and it is recommended that the medication be taken with a high-fat meal.

Steroid therapy has been shown to decrease mortality, respiratory failure rates, and clinical deterioration in AIDS-PCP. This therapy should be given to all patients with <70 mm Hg or a $P_aO_2/P_{(A-a)}O_2$ >35 mm Hg. Therapy with oral prednisone is recommended, but IV methylprednisolone can be used if oral administration is not possible.

Prophylaxis: All patients with a prior episode of PCP need prophylaxis to prevent recurrent pneumonia (secondary prophylaxis). This is true whether or not the patient is taking zidovudine. In addition, all patients with a CD4+ count ≤200 or a CD4+ lymphocyte percentage <17% need prophylaxis to prevent an initial episode of PCP (primary prophylaxis). Of all AIDS cases reported to CDC in 1990, PCP was the AIDS- defining illness in 49%. Estimated lifetime frequency of PCP in AIDS patients has been 75 to 85%. Thus, this somewhat basic intervention has probably

Drug Regimens Used in Antipneumocystis Prophylaxis

AGENT	ADULT DOSE (MG)	ROUTE	DOSE INTERVAL	MONTHLY COST ($)*
TMP/SMX	160/800†	Oral	Daily	5
	160/800	Oral	BID, 2 or 3 days/wk	3
	80/400	Oral	Daily	2
Pentamidine isethionate	4‡	Iv	Monthly	99
	300	Aerosol (Respirgard)	Monthly	99
	60	Aerosol (Fisoneb)	Every other week	40
Pyrimethamine-sulfadoxine	50/1000	Oral	Every other week	8
Dapsone	100	Oral	Daily in 1 or 2+ divided doses	6
Pyrimethamine-dapsone	75/200	Oral	Weekly	6

*As estimated from the Red Book (1994); prices are lowest prices for generic drugs.

†Preferred regimen for patients who can tolerate it. This dose is equivalent to one double-strength tablet.

‡Per kilogram of body weight.

Adapted from Masur H: Drug therapy: Prevention and treatment of *Pneumocystis* pneumonia. N Engl J Med 327:1853–1860, 1992.

had the greatest impact on the decreased morbidity and increased survival of HIV-infected patients.

The drug of choice for PCP prophylaxis is TMP/SMX. When taken in a compliant fashion, its efficacy approaches 100%. In the recent past, fairly toxic doses of this medication were used and a large proportion of patients were intolerant of the drug. The currently used doses minimize that problem. Reasons to prefer this drug for prophylaxis include its efficacy, ease of administration, and low cost. Additionally, it may provide adequate prophylaxis against toxoplasmosis, although it is not appropriate treatment for active toxoplasmosis. Dosage is currently in a state of flux, but a dose of one double-strength tablet (160/800 mg) each day is effective. Many clinics have now cut this back to one tablet every other day with complete protection. Even with the decreased dose, 10 to 15% of patients experience adverse effects severe enough to need alternative therapy.

Aerosolized pentamidine is the most common alternative therapy; indeed in many clinics it was the first-line drug. However, with greater experience, limits of this therapy are becoming clear. The efficacy is probably 80 to 85% per year, resulting in a fair number of episodes of PCP. Techniques to improve drug distribution within the lungs can improve the efficacy somewhat. In addition, extrapulmonary pneumocystis disease has been well described, and aerosolized therapy is not effective in preventing it because there is little or no systemic activity following inhalation.

Any patient starting aerosolized therapy needs to have a recently documented PPD, a new CXR, and a sputum submitted for AFB smear and mycobacterial culture. Therapy should be initiated only after a negative smear is documented.

These deficiencies of aerosolized pentamidine have led some clinicians to again explore the possibilities of IM injections of pentamidine. This route of administration had been abandoned earlier due to concern about both sterile abscesses at the injection site and systemic toxicity. Trials of atovaquone for prophylaxis are also under way.

PNEUMONIA

Aspiration Pneumonia

Aspiration of oral or gastric contents into the tracheobronchial tree produces variable syndromes depending on the type and volume of material aspirated. Aspiration of oral contents with large numbers of infectious organisms causes necrotizing pneumonia, which may progress to lung abscess with or without empyema. Aspiration of gastric contents with a pH <3 produces a chemical burn pneumonitis. Aspiration of large particulate matter can obstruct the trachea or large airways.

Aspiration of Oral Contents

A condition predisposing to aspiration is almost always present. These can be broadly categorized as (1) altered mental status (either acutely, as with seizure, or chronically) and (2) disruption of the normal mechanical function of the pharynx and larynx.

In patients who aspirate outside the hospital, the clinical course may span several weeks, with symptoms consisting of low-grade fever, cough, production of foul-smelling sputum, and weight loss. Because the right bronchus is straighter than the left, aspiration pneumonia occurs more commonly on the right, and because the anatomic localization is determined by gravity, the posterior segments are involved in patients who aspirate in the recumbent position and the basal segments of the lower lobes are involved in patients who aspirate in the erect position. The normal mouth flora consists mostly of anaerobes (most of which are sensitive to penicillin), and hence in normals these anaerobes account for most of the lung infections associated with aspiration.

In chronically ill patients, especially those in hospitals and nursing homes, the mouth becomes colonized with resistant anaerobes and gram-negative aerobic enteric rods. Penicillin G (12–20 million units per day IV in a normal-sized person with normal renal function) is the treatment of choice for aspiration pneumonia acquired outside the hospital. A combination beta-lactam antibiotic plus beta-lactamase inhibitor (e.g., ampicillin-sulbactam) is often recommended for hospital-acquired aspiration pneumonia. Long-term antibiotic treatment is required, and resolution of fever and weight gain are clinical indicators of successful therapy. If a lung abscess fails to drain, bronchoscopy should be performed to look for an obstructing carcinoma. Percutaneous drainage procedures are usually not required.

Aspiration of Gastric Contents (Mendelson's Syndrome)

Aspiration of solutions with a pH <3 results in an instantaneous chemical burn of the airways and lung parenchyma. Serumlike fluid passes from the intravascular space through the damaged alveolocapillary membrane into the alveoli, eventually neutralizing the pH of the aspirated fluid. Clinical manifestations depend on the pH and the volume aspirated. Usually there is bilateral involvement of lower lobes. Tachypnea, cough, wheezing, rales, fever, and hypoxia are present. Treatment consists of tracheal suctioning and supplemental oxygen. Some patients require mechanical ventilation. If large particulate matter was present in the aspirate, bronchoscopic removal is necessary to relieve obstruction. Although much has been written for and against the use of steroids, most experts do not recommend their use. Bacteria play no role in the lung injury, and antibiotics should not be given until there is evidence of lung infection.

References: Finegold SM: Aspiration pneumonia. Rev Infect Dis 13(Suppl 9):S737–S742, 1991.

DePaso WJ: Aspiration pneumonia. Clin Chest Med 12:269–284, 1991.

Chronic Pneumonia

Differential Diagnosis of Chronic Pneumonia*

PATHOGEN	PREDISPOSING FACTORS	RADIOLOGIC APPEARANCE
Mycobacterium tuberculosis	Age Immunosuppressive therapy, AIDS Hemodialysis Repeated exposure to infected person	Primary disease: Hilar adenopathy, pleural effusion, upper lobe infiltrate Postprimary disease: Fibrocavitary infiltrate in apical or posterior segments of upper lobe
Cryptococcus neoformans	Lymphoreticular and hematologic malignancies Renal transplant Corticosteroid therapy Diabetes mellitus AIDS	Multiple, rounded densities without discrete borders Cavitary lesions with air/fluid levels Alveolar or interstitial infiltrates
Aspergillus fumigatus, A. flavus, Mucor, Rhizopus	Myelosuppression Immunosuppression	Variable: Patchy infiltrates Bronchopneumonia Multiple nodules Cavitation
Pseudomonas pseudomallei	Skin abrasions Residing in endemic area, e.g., Southeast Asia	Involving upper lobes Consolidation followed by cavitation Pleural effusions uncommon Chronic disease resembles TB
Pneumocystis carinii	AIDS Malignancy Congenital immunodeficiency Therapeutic immunosuppression	Diffuse bilateral infiltrates Infiltrates coalesce with time, air bronchograms develop Cavitation rare Hilar adenopathy and pleural effusion absent
Nocardia asteroides	Corticosteroid therapy Pulmonary alveolar proteinosis Malignancy Immunosuppression, AIDS	Confluent bronchopneumonia Progression to consolidation Cavitation and pleural effusion frequent
Histoplasma capsulatum	Residing in endemic area, e.g., Ohio and Mississippi River valleys Immunosuppression, AIDS	Acute: ≥1 patches of pneumonitis with hilar and mediastinal lymph node enlargement; calcification of healed lesions Chronic: Apical fibrocavitary lesions; miliary infiltrates occur with dissemination
Coccidioides immitis	Diabetes mellitus Pregnancy Immunosuppression, AIDS Certain ethnic groups (blacks) Residing in endemic area, e.g., southwestern U.S.	Nonspecific alveolar infiltrate Bilateral hilar adenopathy Abscess formation with thin-walled peripheral cavity

*This table continues horizontally on opposite page.

Differential Diagnosis of Chronic Pneumonia (Cont.)

ASSOCIATED SIGNS AND SYMPTOMS	KEY LABORATORY METHODS AND DATA
Vary from asymptomatic with a conversion of PPD skin test to critically ill, e.g., productive cough, hemoptysis, diaphoresis, fever, weight loss; extrapulmonary involvement frequent, i.e., kidney, bone, joints, peritoneum, CNS	Positive PPD Positive sputum smear for AFB Positive culture for tubercle bacillus
Constitutional symptoms dominate, i.e., fever, malaise, chest pain, weight loss; headache may suggest CNS lesion; scant sputum production; physical findings in lung minimal	Serologic testing for cryptococcal capsular antigen useful India ink preparation helpful Histologic evidence desirable Positive sputum culture
Fever, dyspnea, nonproductive cough frequent; pleuritic chest pain with hemoptysis occurs; wheezing, rales, and pleural friction rub less common	High index of suspicion required Demonstration of fungus histologically and by tissue culture No clinically useful serology available
Clinical disease may be acute, subacute, or chronic; cough may be productive with hemoptysis; fever with rigors and chest pain common; rales in area of pneumonitis	Microscopic exam of sputum reveals organism with methylene blue Organism grows readily on routine lab media Serology useful in diagnosis
May be self-limited and mild in healthy children < age 4; fatal diffuse pneumonia in premature or malnourished infants; immunocompromised patient has severe pneumonia with fever, nonproductive cough with progressive dyspnea and cyanosis	Definitive diagnosis requires demonstration of organism in infected lung material Cyst wall stained by methenamine silver nitrate or toluidine blue 0 stains Progressive hypoxemia Serology not diagnostically useful
More frequent in men; fever, weight loss, productive cough with hemoptysis; may disseminate, particularly to brain with abscess formation	Gram-positive rods that do not form spores Partially acid-fast using modified Ziehl-Neelsen stain Lab should hold cultures 2–4 wks Serology, skin testing not useful for diagnosis
Acute asymptomatic pulmonary infection in children with hilar lymphadenopathy, transient dissemination, and subsequent calcification; chronic cavitary form in patients with COPD; progressive dissemination in infants and immunosuppressed adults	Fourfold rise in titers of histoplasmin complement fixation Sputum culture has low yield Skin test not useful for diagnosis and may cause seroconversion Tissue culture and staining useful
Most primary infections are asymptomatic or resemble another atypical pneumonia; nonproductive cough, fever, chills, malaise, anorexia; erythema nodosum and erythema multiforme occur; chronic progressive disease with hemoptysis and dissemination occurs in immunocompromised patient	Positive sputum culture diagnostic Elevated complement-fixing antibody titer is a hallmark of disease Skin testing has only limited clinical value but does not affect serology

Table continued on next page.

Differential Diagnosis of Chronic Pneumonia (Cont.)*

PATHOGEN	PREDISPOSING FACTORS	RADIOLOGIC APPEARANCE
M. avium-intracellulare complex, *M. kansasii, M. fortuitum, M. chelonei*	Middle-aged men with COPD Exposure to dust AIDS Ankylosing spondylitis	Often indistinguishable from TB Thin-walled cavities with dense surrounding infiltrate Pleural thickening over involved lung
Candida albicans	Immunosuppressive agents Broad-spectrum antibiotics Hyperalimentation Invasive monitoring devices	Finely nodular diffuse infiltrates Microabscess formation not evident Homogeneous infiltrate rare

*This table continues horizontally on opposite page.

Community-Acquired Pneumonia

Community-acquired pneumonia is most often caused by *Streptococcus pneumoniae,* but many other agents may also cause disease. The diagnosis is suspected from the patient's history and confirmed by physical examination, CXR, and sputum Gram stain and culture. Therapy is directed at the causative agent. Pneumococcal polysaccharide vaccine is effective in preventing pneumonia caused by most serotypes of *S. pneumoniae.*

Diagnosis
History
Fever
Abdominal pain
Cough productive of yellow-green
  or bloody sputum

Dyspnea
Malaise
Pleuritic pain

Physical examination
Vital signs: elevated temperature, tachycardia, tachypnea
General: cyanosis (if severe pneumonia)
Lungs: crackles, egophony, pectoriloquy, dullness to percussion (if pleural
  effusion present)

Laboratory tests
Sputum Gram stain and culture
Elevated WBC count

CXR showing consolidation
  and/or pleural effusion

Causative Agents
Bacteria
  Streptococcus pneumoniae
  Haemophilus influenzae
  Klebsiella pneumoniae
  Staphylococcus aureus

Viruses
  Influenza
  Adenovirus
  Varicella zoster
Other
  Mycobacterium tuberculosis
  Aspiration

Fungi
  Histoplasma
  Coccidioides
Nonbacterial
  Mycoplasma pneumoniae
  Legionella pneumophila
  Chlamydia
  Coxiella burnetii

Differential Diagnosis of Chronic Pneumonia (Cont.)

ASSOCIATED SIGNS AND SYMPTOMS	KEY LABORATORY METHODS AND DATA
Cough, chills, weight loss, fever, minimal findings on chest exam; infections tend to be indolent; extrapulmonary lesions rare	Repeatable positive sputum culture with compatible clinical picture Requires >100 colonies/culture to be significant Skin testing of no value
Fever, cough with hemoptysis; extrapulmonary foci in conjunction with underlying disease dominate clinical picture; arterial oxygen normal	Definitive diagnosis requires tissue biopsy with positive histology *Candida* in sputum may be normal flora Blood cultures occasionally positive Current serology not reliable

Modified from Infectious Diseases, Pneumonia, Part II: Differential diagnosis of chronic pneumonia. In Roche Handbook of Differential Diagnosis. Hoffman-LaRoche, 1983, pp 14–17, with permission.

PNEUMOTHORAX

Differential Diagnosis of Pneumothorax

1. Spontaneous
   a. Primary: occurs in healthy individuals
   b. Secondary: complication of underlying lung disease
2. Traumatic
   a. Iatrogenic
   b. Noniatrogenic
3. Catamenial (associated with menses)

Causes of Secondary Spontaneous Pneumothorax

1. COPD	6. Interstitial lung disease
2. Asthma	Sarcoidosis
3. Cystic fibrosis	Eosinophilic granuloma
4. Infection (pneumatocele, abscess)	7. Marfan syndrome
5. Tuberculosis	8. Malignancy
	9. Endometriosis

Treatment of Spontaneous Pneumothorax

The goals of treatment for pneumothorax are to remove air from the pleural space and to prevent recurrence. The recurrence rates for both primary and secondary spontaneous pneumothorax are similar. The recurrence rate for a second spontaneous pneumothorax ranges from 10 to 50%, and approximately 60% of those patients will have a third recurrence. After three episodes, the recurrence rate exceeds 85%. Therefore, repeated spontaneous pneumothorax should be treated by pleurodesis or surgical intervention, including parietal pleurectomy. In patients with primary spontaneous pneumothorax, a small pneumothorax is usually well tolerated and may occasionally be treated conservatively. However, in patients with underlying lung disease (secondary), a pneumothorax may be poorly tolerated and life threatening.

Therapeutic options for spontaneous pneumothorax include:
   1. Observation may be considered in a small, primary pneumothorax but may have a higher rate of recurrence than other treatments.

2. Supplemental O_2 accelerates the rate of resorption and may be considered in a small, primary pneumothorax being managed by observation.
3. Aspiration is considered by many the initial therapy of choice in a small, primary pneumothorax.
4. Tube thoracostomy.
5. Tube thoracostomy with instillation of sclerosing agent is recommended both as initial therapy in secondary pneumothorax and for treatment of a second primary pneumothorax.
6. Open thoracotomy is reserved for persistent air leaks and a recurrent pneumothorax despite previous sclerosis.

Reference: O'Rourke JP, Yee ES: Civilian pneumothorax: Treatment options and long-term results. Chest 96: 1302–1306, 1989.

POISONING

Common Poisoning Syndromes

SYNDROME OR AGENTS	SYMPTOMS AND SIGNS
Anticholinergic syndromes Antihistamines, antiparkinson medication, atropine, scopolamine, amantadine, antipsychotics, antidepressants, antispasmodics, mydriatics, skeletal-muscle relaxants, many plants (notably jimson weed and *Amanita muscaria*)	Delirium with mumbling speech, tachycardia, dry flushed skin, dilated pupils, myoclonus, slightly ↑ temperature, urinary retention, and ↓ bowel sounds; seizures and dysrhythmias may occur in severe cases
Sympathomimetic syndromes Cocaine, amphetamine, methamphetamine (and its derivatives 3,4-methylene-dioxy-methamphetamine, and 2,5-dimethoxy-4-bromoamphetamine) and OTC decongestants (phenylpropanolamine, ephedrine, and pseudoephedrine)	Delusions, paranoia, tachycardia (or bradycardia if the drug is a pure alpha-adrenergic agonist), hypertension, hyperpyrexia, diaphoresis, piloerection, mydriasis, and hyperreflexia; seizures, hypotension, and dysrhythmias may occur in severe cases
Opiate, sedative, or ethanol intoxication Narcotics, barbiturates, benzodiazepines, ethchlorvynol, glutethimide, methaqualone, meprobamate, ethanol, clonidine, guanabenz	Coma, respiratory depression, miosis, hypotension, bradycardia, hypothermia, pulmonary edema, ↓ bowel sounds, hyporeflexia, and needle marks; seizures may occur after overdoses of some narcotics, notably propoxyphene
Cholinergic syndromes Organophosphate and carbamate insecticides, physostigmine, edrophonium, some mushrooms	Confusion, CNS depression, weakness, salivation, lacrimation, urinary and fecal incontinence, GI cramping, emesis, diaphoresis, muscle fasciculations, pulmonary edema, miosis, bradycardia or tachycardia, seizures
Salicylates Aspirin, methyl salicylate (wintergreen oil), various OTC medications	Tinnitus, decreased hearing, vertigo, nausea, vomiting, hyperventilation, confusion, tachycardia, hyperpyrexia, lethargy, seizures, coma, shock, pulmonary edema

Table continued on next page.

Common Poisoning Syndromes (Cont.)

SYNDROME OR AGENTS	SYMPTOMS AND SIGNS
Acetaminophen	<24 hrs: anorexia, nausea, vomiting, diaphoresis 24 48 hrs: hepatic tenderness 2–5 days: jaundice, coagulopathy, encephalopathy
Isopropyl alcohol	Headache, dizziness, poor coordination, confusion, abdominal pain, nausea, vomiting, miosis, respiratory depression, hypotension, loss of DTR, coma
Methanol	Headache, nausea, vomiting, dizziness, respiratory depression, lethargy, dilated pupils, impaired vision, and hyperemia of optic disc
Ethylene glycol	Headache, nausea, vomiting, ataxia, stupor, coma, convulsions, cardiac failure, pulmonary edema, oliguria, and hypothermia
Petroleum distillates Kerosene, charcoal lighter, gasoline, turpentine	Local irritation of mucus membranes of mouth and pharynx, vomiting, diarrhea, respiratory impairment, pulmonary edema, lethargy, and seizures
Lithium	Tremor, fasiculations, dizziness, fatigue, abdominal pain, dysarthria, ataxia, lethargy, flaccid paralysis, dysdiadochokinesia, nystagmus, and coma
Marijuana	Disorientation, confusion, panic, auditory and visual hallucinations
Phencyclidine (PCP)	Bizarre or violent behavior, lethargy, agitation, confusion, blank stares, nystagmus, hypertension, tachycardia, bizarre posturing, writhing or grimacing, hyperthermia, bronchospasms, ↑ secretions, seizures
Iron	0–6 hours: vomiting, diarrhea, hypotension, tachypnea, tachycardia, GI hemorrhage, seizures, lethargy, shock, or coma 12–48 hrs: coma, coagulopathy, or shock 2–5 days: jaundice and hypoglycemia 2–6 weeks: pyloric scarring; gastric outlet or small bowel obstruction

Modified from Kulig K: Initial management of ingestions of toxic substances. N Engl J Med 326:1678, 1992.

POLYARTERITIS NODOSA

After the 1866 publication by Kusmaul and Maier, most vasculopathies were described as periarteritis nodosa, which ultimately changed to polyarteritis nodosa

(PAN). Differences in clinical presentation have gradually allowed more discrete diagnoses. PAN today is characterized as a multisystem inflammatory disease of medium-sized vessels. It occurs with an incidence of 0.2 to 2/100,000, affecting men twice as commonly as women. Onset is usually in the 50s or 60s.

The vessels involved range from those branching off the aorta to the arterioles, although small and medium-sized vessels are most commonly involved. Reasons for the commonly observed predilection for involvement at bifurcation points remain unknown. Pathologically, the injury is panmural, with inflammation followed by fibroblastic proliferation. Thrombus and aneurysm formation may occur. Ultimately, with luminal occlusion, organ ischemia and infarction occur.

In the kidneys, inflammation of arcuate and interlobar arteries is the most common. Glomerular involvement is less frequent. GI tract vessel involvement can lead to bowel ischemia and hepatitis. Occasionally PAN can manifest itself initially as acalculous cholecystitis. Involvement of the vaso vasorum can lead to ischemic lesions of the peripheral nerves. Testicular involvement is relatively uncommon.

Clinical manifestations include constitutional symptoms (fever, malaise, and weight loss). Arthralgias occur in 50 to 75% of patients. Frank arthritis can occur and in general is asymmetric and nondeforming. Skin lesions are seen in 25 to 50% of patients and include palpable purpura, infarctive lesions, and nonhealing ulcerations. Peripheral neuropathy occurs almost as often as arthralgia and may be the initial manifestation. Progress is generally asymmetric, and multiple mononeuropathies are common. CNS involvement may lead to seizure or infarction. HTN or active urinary sediment suggests renal involvement. As noted, abdominal pain most often accompanies gut ischemia. Diffuse pain, abdominal distention, and evidence of obstruction suggest mesenteric vascular collapse. Coronary artery involvement can lead to MI.

Laboratory data are generally both nonspecific, and nondiagnostic. ESR and other measures of acute phase reactants are usually elevated. Normochromic anemia is also common. Serum albumin is frequently reduced. Antineutrophil cytoplasmic antibodies occur in patients with PAN. Both the perinuclear and cytoplasmic staining patterns are described. Up to half of patients are HBsAg positive. Those in the latter group are generally not clinically different from those without detectable HBsAg.

The diagnosis is made by identifying the clinical syndrome associated with confirmation of the presence of active vasculopathy by either angiography or biopsy of the involved organ: skin, sural nerve, kidney, or muscle. Angiography can reveal either arterial saccular or fusiform aneurysms or simply narrowing or tapering of the arteries. This procedure is most appropriate if there is abdominal involvement clinically but may be positive even if the patient is asymptomatic.

Treatment should be aggressive. Occasionally the clinical manifestations may be mild and glucocorticoids alone can be sufficient. Prednisone in doses of 40 to 60 mg daily are usually effective. Clinical follow-up is important and any progression of disease or initially widespread or active disease will require cytotoxic medication. When added, cyclophosphamide at a dose of 1 to 2 mg/kg PO is effective. Data show daily oral medication is somewhat more efficacious than monthly IV infusion. Some advocate the addition of an antiplatelet medication as well.

Reference: Conn DL: Polyarteritis. Rheum Dis Clin North Am 16:341–362, 1990.

POLYMYALGIA RHEUMATICA AND TEMPORAL ARTERITIS

PMR is a systemic rheumatic condition of uncertain etiology that is diagnosed on the basis of its clinical presentation. Patients develop at least 4 to 6 weeks of aching, particularly in the neck, shoulder, and hip regions. Onset is usually insidious, but occasionally it can be dramatic. Gelling is common and morning stiffness, reminiscent of RA in intensity, is seen. Other clinical manifestations of the disease include constitutional symptoms, such as low grade fever, weight loss, and fatigue. There may be proximal muscle aches but strength is preserved and there is no histologic evidence of active inflammatory myopathy. Patients also have localized tenderness of the joints, and data suggest a low-level synovial inflammation may be present.

Laboratory data are generally normal with the exception of an elevated ESR. Levels can be 50 to more than 100 mm per hr. Patients can often have a normochromic normocytic anemia. Serologically, there is no increased incidence in RF or ANA over age-matched controls. There is no histological evidence of muscular inflammation, and thus creatinine kinase, aldolase, and serum transaminases are not elevated. No x-ray features are diagnostic.

There is some controversy about the relationship between PMR and temporal arteritis. The percentage of patients with PMR who have temporal arteritis is reported to vary between 15 and 40%. Conversely, symptoms of PMR are common in patients with temporal arteritis. In fact, up to 50% of patients with classical temporal arteritis may have symptoms of PMR, which may be the presenting features of the illness.

Clinically, patients with temporal arteritis are similar to those with PMR. Fever, malaise, anorexia, weight loss, and night sweats can all occur. Presentation as fever of unknown origin is not uncommon, particularly in the very elderly. Headache is the most common complaint overall. Achiness of the jaw with chewing or long telephone conversations (jaw claudication) is characteristic and may occur secondary to facial and maxillary artery occlusion. Numbness of the tongue can occur, making speaking difficult. Sore throat pain, retroauricular pain, and, if vestibular involvement occurs, vertigo, tinnitus, and nystagmus can be present. Ophthalmological involvement is the most serious aspect of temporal arteritis. Blindness, due to involvement of the short posterior ciliary artery resulting in ischemic optic neuritis, occurs in 17% of patients. Once visual acuity is diminished, recovery is uncommon. Other uncommon ophthalmologic events include iritis with central retinal vein occlusion, episcleritis, scintillating scotomata, and ptosis. Intracranial arteritis rarely occurs. About 10 to 15% of patients with temporal arteritis can have giant-cell inflammation of other large and medium-size arteries in the neck.

Histologically, patients with temporal arteritis have a granulomatous inflammation of the vessel. Because the disease does not occur uniformly, the presence of skip lesions can make diagnosis on the basis of biopsy difficult. Thus, a negative biopsy does not necessarily mean the entity is absent.

In patients with the clinical syndrome of PMR, particularly in association with fever or jaw claudication, temporal artery biopsy should be considered. Large segments should be obtained because of skip regions. Some investigators have advocated bilateral biopsies, but this increases the risk of blindness on the basis of the biopsy itself. Arteriography has not generally been helpful. Treatment of patients with PMR usually consists of modest doses of oral glucocorticoids. Specific recommendations vary, but 15–20 mg of daily prednisone usually will quiet symptoms and return the ESR to normal. Temporal arteritis is also treated with daily glucocorticoids in patients with severe systemic complaints; or, with patients with active eye disease, some advocate doses up to 100 mg daily. More commonly, doses of 30–40 mg daily can provide relief. Although the ESR usually returns to normal, clinical symptoms are the most reliable way to follow patients. Most patients do well with about 2 years of treatment. Care must be taken to prophylax against osteoporosis.

Reference: Chuang TY, et al: Polymyalgia rheumatica: A 10 year epidemiologic and clinical study. Ann Intern Med 97:672–680, 1982.

POLYMYOSITIS

Polymyositis and dermatomyositis are destructive diseases affecting striated muscle fibers. These diseases are of unknown etiology and usually present with symmetrical weakness of proximal limb and trunk muscles. Dermatomyositis is associated with a scaly, erythematous rash over the hand, elbow, and knee joints and/or the classic heliotrope rash of the upper eyelids. Female-to-male ratio is 2:1. Polymyositis is at least three times more common than dermatomyositis. The two conditions may occur as idiopathic primary illnesses or in association with other conditions as in the following classification scheme.

Classification of Polymyositis and Dermatomyositis

GROUP	DESCRIPTION
1	Primary idiopathic polymyositis
2	Primary idiopathic dermatomyositis
3	Dermatomyositis or polymyositis associated with neoplasia (especially in patients greater than age 50 yr)
4	Childhood dermatomyositis or polymyositis associated with vasculitis
5	Polymyositis or dermatomyositis associated with connective tissue disorder (overlap group)

Diagnosis is based on classic clinical findings associated with an elevated serum creatine phosphokinase level, abnormal EMG tracings, and muscle biopsy demonstrating degenerating muscle fibers. Surprisingly, the ESR often shows poor correlation with disease activity. Treatment includes prednisone, usually at a starting dose of 60 mg a day, and physical therapy. Occasionally immunosuppressant therapy with azathioprine or methotrexate is needed to control activity of these diseases. Long-term therapy is usually necessary, but a high survival rate is expected in the absence of malignancy.

POSTHERPETIC NEURALGIA

Postherpetic neuralgia is defined as neuropathic pain that is a sequela of herpes zoster (shingles) episodes. It presents as pain that is present in the affected dermatome more than 2 months after the initial episode. It is more common following more severe and painful episodes of zoster. It occurs in less than 10% of healthy persons younger than 50 but is three to five times more common in older persons. Symptoms usually resolve within the first year.

Treatment: Capsaicin cream (0.025–0.075%) topically for 14–28 days decreases pain by stopping reaccumulation of substance P. However, 30% of capsaicin users cannot tolerate the drug. Avoid narcotic analgesics if possible. Amitriptyline is often effective, especially when started early in the episode. The usual dose is lower than the typical antidepressant dose and is given at bedtime. The initial dose should be low and then increased every 3 to 5 days until either side effects occur or pain control is achieved. It may be combined with transcutaneous electrical nerve stimulation. Desipramine may also work, as may other antidepressants.

Postherpetic neuralgia can sometimes be very difficult to treat and debilitating for the patient despite the aforementioned therapies. In those patients, rather than trying numerous antiseizure medications, we refer them to chronic pain clinics for definitive management.

Reference: Rowbotham ML: Treatment of postherpetic neuralgia. Semin Derm 11:218–222, 1992.

PREGNANCY

Medical Complications

Hypertension

HTN during pregnancy can be classified as follows: (1) chronic HTN, (2) preeclampsia/eclampsia, (3) preeclampsia and chronic HTN, and (4) transient HTN. In any form, HTN during pregnancy is abnormal and should be addressed aggressively. It is defined as a rise in systolic BP >30 mmHg or in diastolic BP >15 mmHg over prepregnancy levels.

Preeclampsia presents the greatest danger to the fetus. It is unique to pregnancy, generally occurring after 20 weeks of gestation, and is associated with proteinuria, edema, hemoconcentration, hypoalbuminuria, hepatic dysfunction, and coagulation abnormalities. There is a marked increase in peripheral vascular resistance secondary to an exaggerated response to circulating angiotensin II and catecholamines. Preeclampsia is more common in nulliparous women, gestations with multiple fetuses, multiparous women with previous episodes of preeclampsia, and women with underlying HTN. Poor prognostic factors include systolic BP >160, diastolic BP >110, proteinuria >2 gm/day, increased serum creatinine or serum transaminases, and decreased platelet count. Eclampsia is defined as preeclampsia complicated by seizures. The risk of maternal cerebral hemorrhage and death with eclampsia is substantial. Preeclampsia with chronic HTN has a poorer prognosis than either condition alone. Transient HTN is defined as an elevated level of BP during pregnancy without subsequent development of signs or symptoms of preeclampsia.

Treatment reduces both maternal and fetal risks. Because reduced intravascular volume has been documented, the use of diuretics is relatively contraindicated. Hydralazine and alpha methyldopa remain the cornerstones of treatment. ACE inhibitors are contraindicated as well, because they can cause fetal renal dysfunction. Delivery remains the treatment of choice for eclampsia.

Peripartum Cardiomyopathy

The development of CHF during pregnancy is, fortunately, a rare event. Peripartum cardiomyopathy (PPCM), which occurs usually in the third trimester or early postpartum period, can be dramatic, with all the classic signs and symptoms of dropsy. Evaluation shows LV dilatation with elevated pulmonary and arterial and wedge pressures. Endomyocardial biopsy often shows some inflammation, although the exact etiology remains unknown. The prognosis is generally good, with 50% of patients returning to normal cardiac function. Recurrence with subsequent pregnancies is well documented. Treatment is supportive, with inotropes, vasodilators, and diuretics. Digitalis is used, although intoxication is more common in PPCM patients than other patients with dilated cardiomyopathy. There is little experience with nitrates in pregnancy, and ACE inhibitors have been shown to cause a reduction in fetal renal function. Hydralazine is widely and safely used when vasodilatation is required. Because there is an increased risk of thromboembolic disease, anticoagulation with heparin is recommended.

Diabetes

In the case of either new-onset DM during pregnancy (gestational DM) or the impact of pregnancy on existing DM (progestational DM), management can have a profound impact on fetal outcome and maternal health. Specifically, DM is associated with macrosomia, increased risks of other congenital malformations, and neonatal metabolic abnormalities (principally hypoglycemia and hypocalcemia). There appears to be an increase in maternal mortality, HTN, and the rate of C-sections in women with DM. Additionally, there are data to suggest that the complications of diabetes (such as retinopathy and nephropathy) progress during pregnancy. Ketosis during pregnancy is associated with a high rate of fetal wastage and CNS congenital abnormalities.

The diagnosis is best accomplished with an oral glucose tolerance test. Control of sugars should be reasonably stringent because tight control of sugars before and during pregnancy reduces complications. Dietary recommendations should conform with those for normal-pregnancy weight gain requirements. Glycemic targets are noted in the table the follows. Insulin, when required, is probably best used in multidose regimens with both short- and long-acting preparations. Control should not be relaxed at delivery. Diabetic ketoacidosis at delivery is associated with a high risk of fetal respiratory distress syndrome. Some authorities advocate slow IV infusion (1 or 2 units regular insulin/hr), with hourly glucose checks.

Target Blood Glucose Levels in Pregnancy

Fasting	60–90 mg/dl
Preprandial	60–105 mg/dl
1 hr postprandial	70–140 mg/dl
2 hrs postprandial	60–120 mg/dl
2 to 4 AM	>60 mg/dl

From O'Sullivan MJ, et al: Diabetes and pregnancy. In Gleicher N, et al (eds): Principles and Practice of Medical Therapy in Pregnancy, 2nd ed., Norwalk, CT, Appleton & Lange, 1992, p 367, with permission.

Thyroid Disease

Graves' disease is the most common cause of hyperthyroidism during pregnancy. Diagnosis can be difficult because the signs of pregnancy can sometimes overlap the signs of thyroid disease. Nonoverlapping signs and symptoms such as resting tachycardia, weight loss, and eye signs take on greater importance. The course of Graves' disease can fluctuate during pregnancy as well. Patients with severe morning sickness or trophoblastic disease constitute a unique subset of hyperthyroid patients. Although many of these patients present with clear biochemical evidence of hyperthyroidism (see later), clinical hyperthyroidism is less common. Congenital hyperthyroidism can occur in fetuses born to mothers with Graves' disease. The mechanism for this uncommon phenomenon is thought to be placental transfer of maternal thyroid-stimulating immunoglobulin.

The prevalence of hypothyroidism in pregnant women in the United States is about 0.6%. Most commonly, either Hashimoto's thyroiditis or previous ablative treatment for hyperthyroidism is the traceable etiology. When hypothyroid patients do become pregnant (somewhat rare because there is decreased fertility in this condition), the condition can have serious consequences. Low-birth-weight infants, stillbirths, pre-eclampsia, and abruptio placentae have been associated. As with hyperthyroidism, many of the symptoms of disease occur with pregnancy. Fatigue, constipation, muscle cramps, fluid retention, and carpal tunnel syndrome can occur during pregnancy or hypothyroidism. Thus, bradycardia, thick brittle hair, cold intolerance, delayed reflexes, and hoarse voice take on added importance. Treatment with thyroid hormone ought to be aggressive in patients with a low risk of occult heart disease.

In the postpartum period, subacute lymphocytic thyroiditis can be seen. It is an autoimmune process of unknown cause. Early on, release of T_4 and T_3 secondary to damage to the gland produces a condition clinically indistinguishable from Graves' disease, except for a markedly reduced thyroid uptake (usually >20% in Graves'). This study should be done only in nonnursing mothers because ^{125}I is found in breast milk.

Just as the clinical signs and symptoms of thyroid disease can be misleading, laboratory data can likewise be difficult to interpret. Serum T_3 and T_4 are elevated in pregnancy because of the significant elevation in thyroid-binding globulin (TBG) caused by elevated levels of estrogen during pregnancy. Perhaps the most useful diagnostic laboratory test is the TSH level. Even slight elevations of this supersensitive assay can suggest hypothyroidism. Because HCG can stimulate the thyroid, T_4 levels rise in patients with severe morning sickness or gestational trophoblastic disease. These patients have falsely low TSH and the biochemical picture of hyperthyroidism.

Propylthiouracil is the drug of choice for treating hyperthyroidism during pregnancy. High doses block thyroid hormone synthesis. It crosses the placenta and can cause inhibition of the fetal thyroid. Iodine can be effective very early but is rarely used, since it is taken up by fetal thyroid and can cause fetal goiter. Beta-blockers can relieve symptoms and will decrease extrathyroidal conversion of T_4 to T_3. However, some fetal effects have been reported with beta-blockers. Radioactive iodine has no role during pregnancy as it crosses the placenta.

Thromboembolism

This is a common occurrence in pregnancy (estimated to be 0.5%). Superficial thrombophlebitis is most common and is seen more frequently in patients with venous varicosities. DVT also occurs more frequently during pregnancy. PE occurs in 12 to 15% of pregnant patients with established DVT. Ovarian, pelvic vein thrombosis, or cerebral infarctions are also more frequent during pregnancy. Increased levels of circulating clotting factors, as well as decreased venous return (stasis) from the lower limbs, contribute to hypercoagulability in pregnant women.

The diagnosis of thrombosis during pregnancy is difficult. Clinical signs are notoriously inaccurate. DVT must be considered in all patients who present with an acutely swollen and tender calf, yet up to 50% of such patients may ultimately be found to have normal flow. Pelvic thrombophlebitis most often occurs postpartum and is related to uterine infection. Ovarian vein thrombophlebitis can occasionally provide more clinical clues, with fever, abdominal pain, nausea, and vomiting. Right-sided thrombosis is considerably more common than left. Doppler studies and impedance plethysmography are the procedures of first choice for diagnosis. ^{125}I scanning is contraindicated during pregnancy and the postpartum period because it crosses the placenta and is concentrated in breast milk. Treatment can be instituted on the basis of these tests if the diagnosis is unequivocally positive. Some experts note that with proper shielding, radiation to the fetus is quite low and therefore x-ray venography to confirm DVT is less risky than empiric treatment if earlier tests are equivocal. Ventilation perfusion scanning can be safely done during pregnancy when pulmonary embolism is suspected. Pulmonary arteriography exposes the fetus to considerable radiation but should be considered if there is a contraindication to anticoagulation in the presence of a high-probability lung scan. Additional reasons to pursue arteriography include suspected PE in a patient with another pulmonary disease resulting in an abnormal CXR or massive PE requiring suction embolectomy.

Warfarin crosses the placenta, is associated with congenital malformations, and has no role in pregnancy. Heparin is used but requires careful monitoring. Maintaining the APTT at 1.5 to 2 times normal is generally satisfactory. Subsequently, SC administration (often 5,000–10,000 units) twice daily also provides adequate anticoagulation. Complications are the same as in nonpregnant patients receiving heparin. At delivery, IV infusion can be continued although careful monitoring is required. An APTT of 1.5 times the control generally does not lead to bleeding complications. Just prior to delivery, if the APPT is greater than 1.5 times the control, protamine sulfate can be administered until hemostasis is achieved after delivery. Heparin should be continued postpartum because of the high risk for subsequent thrombosis. Patients receiving SC heparin should continue this treatment through delivery. Epidural anesthesia is contraindicated because of the risk of hematoma formation.

Other factors: Alcohol and smoking can have profound impact on the health of the fetus and should be addressed during pregnancy by a consulting internist.

PRESIDENTS' ILLNESSES

George Washington (1732–1799)

1751	Smallpox while in the Barbados.
1752	Tuberculosis.
1761	Malaria or typhoid.
1786	Quinine treatment for malaria.
1799	Died of a throat infection complicated by treatment with blood letting, calomel, and antimony tartrate.

John Adams (1735–1826)

	Enjoyed good physical health.
	Experienced episodes of depression.
	Cardiac failure late in life.
1826	Died, at age 91, of cardiac disease.

Thomas Jefferson (1743–1826)

1774	Severe dysentery.
1783	Beginning of recurrent severe headaches.
1794–1826	Rheumatism, back pains. Question of diabetes late in life.
1826	Died in a coma.

James Madison (1751–1836)

1772	Strange episodes of seizures.
1788	Malaria.
1813	Malaria during his presidency.
	Late in life severe arthritis of hands and arms.

1834	Deaf in one ear, failing eyesight.
1836	Died, unknown cause.

James Monroe (1758–1831)

1776	Seriously wounded at Battle of Trenton.
1823	Transitory seizure disorder.
1831	Died of a chronic pulmonary infection.

John Quincy Adams (1767 1848)

1814	Brief episode of depression.
1846	Sustained a stroke.
1848	Had a second stroke at his desk in U.S. House of Representatives, became comatose, and died two days later.

Andrew Jackson (1767–1845)

1780	Smallpox while a prisoner of the British in Revolutionary War.
1806	Sustained a near-fatal chest wound in a pistol duel. The wound never healed and he was left with periodic draining of a lung abscess through the bronchus and recurrent pulmonary hemorrhage the rest of his life.
1813	Left arm shattered by gunshot wound in tavern brawl in Nashville, leading to chronic osteomyelitis.
1813	Dysentery while commanding army in War of 1812.
1845	Died of right ventricular failure, presumably due to chronic pulmonary disease.

Martin Van Buren (1782–1862)

	Suffered from gout, otherwise good health.
1862	Died of pulmonary disease, unknown type.

William Henry Harrison (1773–1841)

	May have had peptic ulcer disease.
1841	Died of pneumonia and the complications of treatment by purging one month after his inauguration.

John Tyler (1790–1862)

	Suffered from repeated attacks of diarrhea.
1862	Died of a stroke.

James Knox Polk (1795–1849)

1812	Had operative removal of bladder stone by perineal approach. Contracted malaria while president.
1849	Died of cholera during an epidemic in Nashville.

Zachary Taylor (1784–1850)

1809	Contracted yellow fever as an army officer stationed in New Orleans.
1810	Malaria.
1850	While president, he died of a diarrheal illness.

Millard Fillmore (1800–1874)

	Enjoyed good health except for obesity.
1874	Died of a cerebral vascular accident.

Franklin Pierce (1804–1869)

	Long-standing excessive use of alcohol.
1848	Sustained a fracture of pelvis and dislocated left knee when thrown from horse while serving in the Mexican War.
1848	Malaria, dysentery.
1860s	Probable cirrhosis with ascites.
1869	Died in a coma (hepatic coma?).

James Buchanan (1791–1868)

	Congenital divergent strabismus.
	Had severe attacks of gout.
1868	Developed heart failure, died of terminal pneumonia.

Abraham Lincoln (1809–1865)

	Color blind, possible Marfan syndrome.
1835	Malaria, episode of depression.
1841	Depression.
1863	Mild case of smallpox.
1865	Assassinated by bullet to head.

Andrew Johnson (1808–1875)

	Episodes of kidney stones.
1865	Intoxicated at his inauguration as vice president.
1865	Malaria.
1873	Cholera, during epidemic in Tennessee.
1875	Died of a cerebral vascular accident.

Ulysses S. Grant (1822–1885)

1843	Probable tuberculosis after graduation from West Point.
	Excessive use of alcohol for many years.
1858	Malaria.
1884	Cancer of the throat, leading to his death in 1885.

Rutherford B. Hayes (1822–1893)

1849	Peritonsillar abscess.
1862	Bullet wound of left elbow while serving as lieutenant colonel in Union Army.
1893	Probable cause of death was acute myocardial infarction.

James A. Garfield (1831–1881)

1881	Shot in the back by an assassin, resulting in internal hemorrhage and later wound infection, sepsis, and parotid gland abscess. He died 80 days after the assassin's attack.

Chester A. Arthur (1830–1886)

	Obesity.
1883	Malaria.
1883	Probable gallbladder disease.
1885	Glomerulonephritis, cardiac failure.
1886	Died of a cerebral vascular accident.

Grover Cleveland (1837–1908)

	Typhoid fever, marked obesity, gout.
1893	While president, cancer involving the left hard palate area and left antrum was surgically removed on board a ship near Manhattan. He later used a prosthetic left upper jaw.
1908	Cardiac failure, probably died of coronary occlusion.

Benjamin Harrison 1833–1901

	Enjoyed good health.
1901	Died of pneumonia following influenza.

William McKinley (1843–1901)

	Obesity.
1901	Bullet wound to upper abdomen from gun of assassin causing two holes in the stomach (repaired by surgery) and necrosis of the pancreas from which he died 9 days after the assault.

Theodore Roosevelt (1858–1919)

	Severe asthma as a child, very myopic, obesity.
	Boxing injury while president led to retinal hemorrhage, detachment, and marked loss of vision.
1912	Chest wound from bullet shot by assailant during the presidential campaign.
	Chronic rheumatoid arthritis.
1913	Critically ill with multiple severe wound infections from injuries sustained on exploration trip of Amazon River and complicated later by osteomyelitis of femur.
1918	Mastoiditis, leading to unilateral deafness.
1919	Sudden death, probably due to coronary occlusion.

William Howard Taft (1857–1930)

	Massive obesity, weight 330 pounds.
1901	Dengue fever while in the Philippine Islands.
1901	Perirectal abscess.
1903	Amebic dysentery.
	Hypertension, benign prostatic hypertrophy.
1922	Cystoscopy for bladder stones.
1923	Angina pectoris.
1929	Cerebral arteriosclerosis with memory loss.
1930	Died in a coma.

Woodrow Wilson (1856–1924)

	Chronic gastritis, heartburn, chronic headaches.
	Left ophthalmic artery thrombosis, nearly blind.
1906	Bronchial asthma in later life.
1919	Cerebrovascular accident while President.
1924	Died of massive cerebral infarction.

Warren G. Harding (1865–1923)

1923	Left ventricular failure.
1923	Died of coronary artery occlusion and bronchopneumonia.

Calvin Coolidge (1872–1933)

	Bronchial asthma.
1933	Died probably of coronary artery disease.

Herbert Hoover (1874–1964)

1964	Cause of death uncertain.

Franklin D. Roosevelt (1882–1945)

1918	Influenza pneumonia.
1921	Poliomyelitis, leaving him with severe weakness of both legs.
1937	Hypertension while president.
1944	Bronchopneumonia.
1945	Died of massive cerebral hemorrhage.

Harry S. Truman (1884–1972)

1894	Diphtheria with temporary paralysis.
	Periodic headaches in adult life.
1954	Cholecystectomy and appendectomy.
1963	Herniorrhaphy.
1972	Died of multiorgan failure at age 88 years.

Dwight D. Eisenhower (1890–1969)

1955	Heart attack.
1956	Ileitis requiring surgery.
1957	Mild stroke affecting speech briefly.
1966	Cholecystectomy.
1969	Died following seventh myocardial infarction.

John F. Kennedy (1917–1963)

	Back injury from playing football.
1943	War injury to his back.
1947	Addison's disease found.
1954	Spinal fusion operation for prior injuries to back.
1955	Second back operation.
1963	Died of bullet wound of brain.

Lyndon B. Johnson (1908–1973)

1955	Severe myocardial infarction.
1973	Died of a heart attack.

Richard M. Nixon (1913–1994)

1973	Phlebitis
1994	Died of a stroke.

Gerald R. Ford (1913–   )

James E. Carter (1924–)
Ronald Reagan (1911–)
1981	Bullet wound to chest.
1985	Malignant polyp of colon removed.
1987	Prostatic surgery.

George H. Bush (1924–)
1991	Hyperthyroidism, atrial fibrillation.

William J. Clinton (1946–)

References: Marx R: The Health of the Presidents. New York, G.P. Putnam's Sons, 1960.
Lundberg GA: Closing the case in JAMA on the John F. Kennedy autopsy. JAMA 268:1736–1738, 1992.

PRESSURE ULCERS

Pressure ulcers are seen in 1 to 3% of hospitalized patients. About 50% of pressure ulcers occur in patients over age 70 and two-thirds of them develop in the hospital. Their presence is associated with a sixfold increase in the probability of death.

Pathophysiology: Pressure is key. Lying on a regular mattress, with pressure over the sacrum and greater trochanter, can result in 100 to 150 mm Hg of skin pressure, which is adequate to produce tissue hypoxia. Shear forces (sliding), friction, and moisture alter the skin's integrity and contribute to ulcer formation.

Staging:
- I. Nonblanching erythema, skin intact
- II. Partial thickness skin loss
- III. Full thickness, may involve subcutaneous tissue
- IV. Deep, full thickness extending into muscle or bone

(Grade III and IV ulcers allow for easy access of bacteria into the blood stream and are often primary sites for sepsis.)

Prevention:
- Change patient's position every 2 hrs but **avoid all pressure on preexisting pressure ulcers.** With pressure ulcer, an ounce of prevention truly is worth a ton of cure.
- Avoid shear: Minimize the time the patient spends in a head-up position (sitting up in bed at an angle of 30° or greater).
- Use at least 4 inches of foam to spread pressure.
- Keep skin clean and dry.
- Maintain nutritional status.
- Do not use donut-type cushion. (It decreases blood flow to the center area.)
- High-tech air-loss, air-fluidized, or water beds are not necessary for prevention but are good for treatment, especially of patients with large ulcers.

Risk factors for development of pressure ulcer:

Immobility or restraints	↓ Skin sensitivity
↓ Albumin (marker of poor nutrition)	Previous pressure ulcer
Fractures	Fecal/urinary incontinence
Impaired cognition	

Treatment: For stages I and II, avoid all pressure, and keep the ulcer clean. For stages III and IV, initial ulcer debridement followed by avoiding all pressure, wet-to-dry dressing with chlorpactin two to four times a day until all necrotic tissue is removed. Then maintain a moist environment with an oxygen-permeable closure.

If cellulitis is present, treat systemically with antibiotics. If visible bone is present, consider osteomyelitis, remembering that a swab of the ulcer may not yield the pathogen causing the osteomyelitis or cellulitis. Instead, injection followed by aspiration under the ulcer margin of sterile saline has been shown to be better in isolating specific wound pathogens. Optimize the patient's nutrition (may use tube feeding at times to accomplish this). Normalize hemoglobin and BP control, and treat spasm of limbs.

The role of surgery in terms of myocutaneous flaps or primary wound closure is uncertain.

Goode PS, et al: The prevention and management of pressure ulcers. Med Clin North Am 73:1511–1524, 1989.

PROSTATE

Benign Prostatic Hypertrophy

BPH is defined as hyperplasia of both the stromal and glandular components of the prostate. It is due to long-standing stimulation by a combination of androgenic and nonandrogenic growth factors. It is seen in 90% of men over age 80 in all races and environments, except for eunuchs and men with congenital absence of 5α-reductase activity (no dihydrotestosterone).

Symptoms are relatively nonspecific and consist of **obstructive** symptoms (hesitancy, need to strain, decreased force of stream, decreased caliber of stream, dribbling, urinary retention, feeling that one needs to void shortly after voiding, and increased postvoid residual volume) and **irritative** symptoms (increased frequency, urgency, nocturia, and dysuria). However, in patients with obstructive symptoms, fully 25% do not have obstruction on urodynamic studies but have bladder (detrusor muscle) pathology. The presence of irritative symptoms reveals even less about the prostate and usually reflects detrusor instability.

Digital exam does not reliably size the median lobe of the prostrate, so one cannot rule out urethral obstruction merely by assessing the lateral prostatic lobes on exam. On digital rectal exam of a patient with BPH, the prostate should have the same firmness as the thenar eminence or the tip of the nose, for normal prostate or BPH. If it feels firmer (like a knuckle), think about cancer. Urodynamics can help measure the degree of obstruction. An average urine flow rate of less than 10 cc/sec is definitely abnormal and is consistent with obstruction. Transrectal ultrasonography can be used to measure prostatic size, the presence of prostatic carcinoma (hypoechoic areas), and bladder size

Surgery is indicated for decreased renal function, hydronephrosis, recurrent UTIs, urinary retention, or the need for chronic catheterization. Balloon dilation of the prostate has a high recurrence rate and bleeding is common so that procedure is not recommended except in special circumstances. Transurethral resection of the prostate is well tolerated and useful for prostates 25 to 100 gm in size. Retrograde ejaculation after surgery is common, but urinary incontinence is not. However, in patients without specific indication for TURP, watchful waiting in patients with BPH may be the best therapy choice. Symptom improvement in response to TURP is less than 80% in those over age 80.

Medications that should be used cautiously in patients with BPH include alpha-adrenergic agonists (↑ bladder sphincter tone), OTC cold preparations, and alpha-adrenergic nasal sprays; anticholinergic agents decrease detrusor function.

Medical therapy includes prazosin (2–4 mg/day) or terazosin. These selective alpha-blockers can relieve symptoms by reducing the tonic component of obstruction. Finasteride is a 5α-reductase inhibitor that blocks conversion of testosterone to dihydrotestosterone. With prolonged use, approximately 50% of patients experience an improvement in obstructive symptoms and a decrease in prostate mass as measured by ultrasound.

To determine whether a hypertrophied prostate is causing obstruction, a postvoid residual volume is obtained by catheterizing the patient immediately after voiding. In patients with joint prosthesis, intravascular graft, valvular heart disease, or prosthetic valves, antibiotic prophylaxis should precede catheterization. A postvoid residual volume >50 to 200 cc is abnormal and warrants an ultrasound evaluation for hydronephrosis and urologic consultation.

Reference: DuBerc CE, et al: Diagnosis and management of benign prostatic hypertrophy. Adv Intern Med 37:55–83, 1991.

PROSTATIC CANCER

Prostatic cancer is the second most common cancer in males in the United States and the third most common cause of male cancer deaths. Its incidence has increased in recent years, particularly in blacks, although there has been a decrease in mortality. The disease is uncommon in the young, but incidence increases sharply to more than 1,000 per 100,000 man-years for the U.S. male population aged 85 years and over. The average age at diagnosis is 73 years. Age-related changes in testosterone levels, increased incidence of BPH, and increased incidence of prostatic cancer have all been examined for interrelation, but to date data remain inconclusive on the specific causes of prostate cancer. Early diagnosis is made by rectal examination of the prostate and the finding of a nodule, although the tumor marker PSA has been shown to discover early disease undetectable by physical exam. However, because the pathological incidence of prostate cancer far exceeds its clinical incidence, use of PSA leads to detection of disease that needs no treatment. Tumors are staged microscopically by the Gleason grading system, which considers the degree of glandular differentiation of the tumor and its relationship to the prostate stroma under low-power magnification. Anatomic staging is according to a four-stage system, A–D, although a TMN system has been designed. Staging utilizes a CT scan of pelvis, bone scan, CXR, PSA, and surgical lymph node sampling (in all but A1 and D2 disease). Treatment and survival depend on the stage of the disease.

Although chemotherapy has been used in late-stage disease, it has generally been ineffective. However, hormonal therapy has been expanded in the past 10 years, and several agents are now used very effectively in treatment of systemic disease. Classical agents such as estrogens inhibit the release of LHRH from the hypothalamus, thereby decreasing FSH and LH and diminishing testosterone output. LHRH analogues inhibit testosterone production by feedback inhibition of FSH and LH. Ketoconazole inhibits steroid synthetic pathways in the testes and adrenal glands.

Therapy and Prognosis for Prostate Cancer

STAGE	TREATMENT	SURVIVAL
A1	Transurethral resection followed by a close observation; many advocate radical surgery	Equivalent to that of the general population in patients older than 70 yrs
A2 (surgically staged)	Radiation therapy or radical prostatectomy	5-yr and 10-yr survival rates lower than those of the general population
B (surgically and non-surgically staged)	Radical prostatectomy Radiation therapy	5 yr: 77%; 10 yr: 61%; 15 yr: 40% 5 yr: 75%; 10 yr: 57%; 15 yr: 28%
C (surgically and non-surgically staged)	Radiation therapy	5 yr: 64%; 10 yr: 35%; 15 yr: 20%
D0	Treatment of local symptoms, if necessary	Related to the development of systemic relapse
D1	For urinary obstruction: transurethral prostatectomy or radiation therapy Systemic treatment (controversial): close observation alone or early endocrine therapy	Related to the development of distant metastases, which occur within 5 yrs in 80% of patients who do not receive any systemic treatment
	Radical prostatectomy, lymph node dissection, and orchiectomy	Preliminary survival data are encouraging in selected patients
D2	Close observation for asymptomatic disease Hormonal therapy for symptomatic disease: orchiectomy, DES, LHRH analogues, antiandrogens, or combined hormonal treatment Chemotherapy for hormone-refractory disease Palliative radiation therapy for symptomatic areas	Median survival, 2.5 yrs

From Garnick MS: Urologic cancer. In Rubenstein E, et al: Scientific American Medicine. New York, Scientific American, 1989, p 12.IX.4, with permission.

Antiandrogens block the binding of dihydrotestosterone (DHT) to its cytoplasmic receptor and thus prevent the conversion of DHT to testosterone. Androgen deprivation produces subjective improvement in about 80% of patients and objective evidence of tumor regression in nearly 50%.

Radiation therapy is used both for treatment of metastatic and symptomatic bony disease and for prevention of the gynecomastia that occurs with many of the hormonal therapies.

Diagnostic Use of PSA levels

PSA is a serine protease found only in the prostate.[1] Its normal function involves liquefaction of the seminal gel. The serum PSA level is an extremely sensitive test for prostate disease. The level is elevated in BPH, prostatitis, prostate cancer, and other inflammatory conditions of the prostate.

PSA can be used as a screening test for prostate cancer, although the false-positive rate is high because it is such a sensitive test. Diagnostic accuracy is increased when coupled with a digital rectal exam and transrectal ultrasound. In men older than 50 years of age:

1. If serum PSA is <4 ng/ml, the likelihood of prostate cancer is low, especially when coupled with a negative rectal exam.
2. If serum PSA is between 4 and 10 ng/ml, there is a 25% chance of having prostate cancer.
3. If serum PSA is >10 ng/ml, the chance is almost 60% of having prostate cancer.
4. Rectal exam or prostate massage increases the serum PSA 1.5 to 2 fold. For maximum accuracy, levels should not be drawn immediately after prostate manipulation.

In general, the serum PSA level corresponds with tumor burden. Advanced disease is uncommon if PSA is less than 4 ng/ml, and bone or lymph node metastases are unusual if PSA is less than 20. A very high PSA level at the time of diagnosis predicts a poor prognosis.

PSA levels are sensitive indicators of the clinical course after therapy for localized prostate cancer. With a serum half-life of 2.2 to 3 days, PSA levels should return to normal by 3 weeks after curative surgery or radiotherapy. Rising levels accurately predict relapse and may precede other evidence of disease progression by 12 to 18 months.

PSA is a much more sensitive and specific test than acid phosphatase or prostatic acid phosphatase. The latter two tests are no longer generally recommended in the standard evaluation of prostate disease.

---

[1]Recently, small amounts of PSA have been detected in salivary glands.
Reference: Andriole GL: Serum prostate-specific antigen: The most useful tumor marker. J Clin Oncol 10:1205–1207, 1992.

PROSTATITIS

Acute prostatitis is uncommon in the elderly, but common in young men. It presents acutely with chills, fever, and low back or residual pain. Patients complain of irritative or obstructive symptoms of voiding, and exam reveals a tender, warm, and swollen prostate. It is important to treat acute bacterial prostatitis completely, as chronic prostatitis is difficult to treat once established. Nonbacterial prostatitis common in middle age is often due to *Chlamydia*. Treated with tetracycline or erythromycin, relapses are common.

Chronic bacterial prostatitis is more common in old men and is a cause of recurrent UTIs. It presents as mild low back pain, urinary urgency and frequency, nocturia, and perineal discomfort. The prostate is usually minimally tender on exam but may be normal, and often concretions are found.

Pathophysiology: Any change in ejaculatory frequency leads to an inflamed prostate, which may produce congestion or retention of infected prostatic fluid.

Intraprostatic urinary reflux may allow seeding of prostate by bladder or urethral organisms. Common pathogens in acute and chronic bacterial prostatitis are *Escherichia coli* or other coliforms, *Pseudomonas, Enterococcus,* and *Staphylococcus aureus.*

Diagnosis: Prostate massage yields expressate with more than 15 WBC/HPF in prostatitis. Macrophages may be laden with fat droplets. Culture of urine often yields the responsible pathogen. This can be followed by a specimen taken after prostate massage.

Treatment: Requires 6 to 12 weeks of TMP/SMX, 1 double-strength tablet PO BID of carbenicillin, or an oral quinolone (ciprofloxacin 500 BID $\times$ 30 days or norfloxacin 400 mg BID $\times$ 30 days) depending on the culture results. Treatment is successful in approximately 50 to 60% of cases. The presence of prostatic calculi (concretions) increases the likelihood of antibiotic failure. Infected prostatic calculi requires a surgical procedure.

Prostatodynia is a condition presenting with the symptoms of prostatitis, but without infection. It is either due to hyperactivity or spasm of prostatic smooth muscle or due to chemical prostatitis from urine reflux. It can be treated with prazosin (1–2 mg once or twice a day), but treatment may need to be continued indefinitely.

Reference: Meares EM: Prostatitis. Med Clin North Am 75:405–424, 1991.

PROTEINURIA

Differential Diagnosis and Evaluation

Normal urine contains not more than 150 mg of protein per day, and only a small fraction of this is of serum origin. The major component is Tamm-Horsfall protein, a component of glycocalyx secreted by the renal tubule. Normally, a small amount of albumin and other plasma proteins are filtered by the glomerulus but are reabsorbed and catabolized in the proximal tubules. Proteinuria refers to an abnormal amount or type of protein in the urine. Glomerular basement membrane acts as a size barrier, preventing the filtration of proteins with an MW >70,000, and as a charge barrier because its negative charge repels the filtration of negatively charged albumin and other plasma proteins.

Proteinuria >3.5 gm/24 hrs is referred to as nephrotic syndrome, although the term is often used to denote the presence of hyperlipidemia and hypoalbuminemia. Tubular proteinuria refers to the urinary presence of protein that is filtered in normal amounts by the normal glomeruli but not reabsorbed due to malfunction of the proximal tubule. In its full-blown form, in addition to proteinuria, all other components of Fanconi's syndrome are also seen. This form of proteinuria is seen in multiple myeloma, amyloidosis, acute tubular necrosis, transplant rejection, and allergic interstitial nephritis. Overflow proteinuria results from an increase in the filtered load of certain proteins. Examples include Bence Jones protein, hemoglobin, myoglobin, and β-2 microglobulin. The following table lists common causes of nonnephrotic-range proteinuria.

Differential Diagnosis of Nonnephrotic Proteinuria

Renal parenchymal origin
Obstructive/reflux nephropathy
Interstitial nephritis
Glomerulonephritis
Primary: minimal lesion disease, membranous GN, focal sclerosis, acute poststrepto-
coccal GN, mesangiocapillary nephritis
Secondary: DM, SLE, Henoch-Schönlein purpura, amyloidosis, Goodpasture's syn-
drome, AIDS
Renal transplantation
Drug toxicity
Sickle-cell disease
Acute pyelonephritis
Alport's syndrome
Partial lipodystrophy
Orthostatic proteinuria
Other causes
Essential HTN, CHF, acute febrile illness, serum sickness, pregnancy, severe obesity,
neoplasia
Overflow proteinuria
Multiple myeloma, hemoglobinuria, myoglobinuria, trauma, sepsis, monocytic and myelo-
monocytic leukemia

Evaluation of the patient with proteinuria: Routine screening for proteinuria is done by dipstick technique, which detects albumin only when the albuminuria is at least 30 mg/dl. The method is therefore somewhat insensitive, and more sensitive radioimmunoassay techniques may be necessary if accurate assessment is needed. It is important to note that proteins other than albumin are not detected by the dipstick method. For example, the Ig fragments excreted in the urine of patients with myeloma are not detected by calorimetric method but are detected by a sulfosalicylic acid test, which forms a precipitate with Bence Jones proteins. Dipstick detection of proteinuria in a concentrated urine (specific gravity >1.025) has uncertain diagnostic significance. The importance of early detection of proteinuria lies in the fact that in certain forms of progressive renal diseases, especially DM nephropathy, prompt treatment of HTN and maintenance of euglycemia slow the progression of renal failure in patients who have microalbuminuria.

The next step in evaluation of patients with proteinuria is a 24-hr urine collection for quantification. At least two such measurements should be made in order to ensure accuracy of measurements. This procedure is also utilized to measure endogenous creatinine clearance as well as the compliance of the patient. If the collection is complete, the average amount of creatinine would be 15 mg/kg in a female and 20 mg/kg in a male.

Orthostatic proteinuria refers to the presence of protein in the urine in the daytime, when the patient is active and upright, whereas protein is normal in the nighttime, when the patient is recumbent. The condition is easily diagnosed by splitting the 24-hr urine collection into two parts and documenting the proteinuria only in the daytime collection. The condition is benign and does not require any further workup.

Serum and urine electrophoresis are ordered mainly to document the presence or absence of a monoclonal protein spike characteristic of myeloma or amyloidosis and also to document the presence of light chains in the urine. If albumin is the predominant protein present in the urine, it is referred to as selective proteinuria. Selective proteinuria is associated with minimal change disease; nonselective proteinuria is seen in more severe forms of glomerular injury. A renal ultrasound is necessary to document the size of the kidneys and to exclude obstruction and reflux nephropathy.

Renal biopsy remains the final important step in the establishment of diagnosis in patients with proteinuria, especially if the diagnosis is not obvious from the other tests. In lupus nephritis, biopsy is performed to learn the nature and extent of renal involvement and also to guide the prognosis and therapy. If the kidney is small and/or scarred, it is unlikely that biopsy will be of any benefit, especially if renal function is severely impaired.

PRURITUS

Pruritus is a frequent problem in general medicine and often has simple etiologies and solutions. However, since it can also be associated with significant systemic disease, it should not be dismissed lightly. No specific characteristics of the itching are helpful in diagnosis, so a precise Hx & PE and lab exam are necessary to verify a diagnosis. Patients with obvious skin lesions are the easiest to diagnose, because they usually have primary dermatologic disease. Occasionally, skin biopsies are necessary to categorize the diagnosis. The presence of pruritus without an obvious skin lesion may be associated with many other conditions.

Conditions in which Generalized Pruritus without Diagnostic Skin Lesions May Occur

Metabolic and endocrine conditions	Renal disease
Hyperthyroidism	Chronic renal failure
Diabetes mellitus	Hematologic disease
Carcinoid	Polycythemia vera
Malignant neoplasms	Paraproteinemia
Lymphoma and leukemia	Iron deficiency
Abdominal cancer	Hepatic disease
CNS tumors	Obstructive biliary disease
Multiple myeloma	Pregnancy (intrahepatic cholestasis)
Mycosis fungoides	Psychogenic states
Drug ingestion	Transitory:
Opium derivatives	Periods of emotional stress
Subclinical drug sensitivities	Persistent:
Infestations	Delusions of parasitosis
Pediculosis corporis	Psychogenic pruritus
Scabies*	Neurotic excoriation
Hookworm (ancylostomiasis)	Miscellaneous conditions
Onchocerciasis	Dry skin (xerosis)
Ascariasis	"Senile" pruritus†
Trichinosis	Mastocytosis
Certain zoonoses	Pregnancy-related disorders

*Diagnostic lesions may be present.

†Unexplained intense pruritus in patients over 65 years without obvious "dry skin" and with no apparent emotional stress.

From Fitzpatrick TB, et al (eds): Dermatology in General Medicine, 3rd ed. New York, McGraw-Hill, 1987, p 81, with permission.

Evaluation of the patient should include a detailed Hx & PE laboratory tests (including CBC, ESR, urinalysis, and fasting glucose, as well as liver, thyroid, and renal function tests), CXR, Pap smear, stool for ova and parasites, and stool guaiac. Psychogenic pruritus occurs as a reaction to stress but is a diagnosis of exclusion. Psychological tests are often helpful. Geriatric patients often have dry skin usually noted mostly at night and often beginning on the back. Drug reactions should never be excluded. Frequent offenders are aspirin, opiates and their derivatives, chlorpromazine (via cholestasis), and quinidine. Scabies causes intense itching and affects the web spaces of the hands and feet most often. The insect can be found in the clothing, particularly along the seams. Generalized pruritus may be the first sign of biliary cirrhosis, lymphoma, and, infrequently, carcinoma. It is also associated with advanced uremia.

Treatment of pruritus must be directed at the etiology in order for it to be successful. However, a few diseases permit palliative therapy. UV-B light is useful in uremia, and cholestyramine has been found to be helpful in cholestasis. Topical menthol/phenol combinations in an emollient constitute a temporary treatment. Topical anesthetics containing benzocaine should not be used because they may cause dangerous sensitization to the agent.

PSEUDOINFARCTION

Differential Diagnosis of Pseudoinfarction Q Waves

The classic ECG hallmark of MI is the presence of pathologic Q waves, defined as negative initial deflections wider than 40 msec in duration and greater than a third of the R wave (positive deflection) in the same lead. Although pathologic Q waves are generally indicative of an old or healed MI, several clinical syndromes can result in the appearance of Q waves on a 12-lead ECG in the absence of an MI. Such Q waves are referred to as pseudoinfarction Q waves, should generally be suspected in patients with no known history of CAD or MI, and may thus be confused with pathologic Q waves due to clinically unrecognized MI. The differential diagnosis of pseudoinfarction Q waves includes the following.

1. **Hypertrophic cardiomyopathy:** Q waves in patients with hypertrophic cardiomyopathy usually result from septal hypertrophy (and thus typically appear in leads I, AVL, V5, or V6) or represent delta waves due to associated preexcitation syndrome (in which case they may appear in any lead). Hypertrophic cardiomyopathy should be suspected in the presence of severe LVH or biventricular hypertrophy, age under 30 years, and a family history of sudden death at a young age or of a known family history of hypertrophic cardiomyopathy.

2. **Preexcitation syndrome** (such as Wolff-Parkinson-White): Q waves may appear in any lead in patients with preexcitation syndromes, and since these Q waves represent negative delta waves, their location is particularly helpful to identify the location of the accessory pathway causing the preexcitation syndrome. Preexcitation syndrome should be suspected in a young patient with a pathologic Q wave, a short P-R interval, and a wide QRS complex on a 12-lead ECG.

3. **Hyperkalemia:** Q waves may appear in patients with severe hyperkalemia (serum K^+ >7 mEq/L) and are often associated with other ECG findings of hyperkalemia such as tall tented T wave, prolonged P-R interval, decreased amplitude or absent P waves (due to sinoatrial block), or wide QRS complex. The

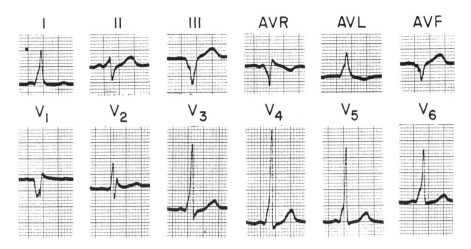

Type B WPW syndrome in a 26-year-old woman with no other evidence of organic heart disease. The delta wave and major portion of the QRS complex in lead V1 are downward. A pseudoinfarction pattern is present in leads III and AVF. (From Chou T-E: Electrocardiography in Clinical Practice, 2nd ed. Orlando, Grune & Stratton, 1986, p 509, with permission.)

pathologic Q waves of hyperkalemia, like other ECG manifestations of hyperkalemia, disappear completely after resolution of the hyperkalemia.

4. **LV hypertrophy:** Q waves appear in the precordial leads V1, V2, and, rarely, V3 as well as in patients with severe LVH. These Q waves are often accompanied by tall R waves in the lateral precordial ECG leads V5 and V6 and left axis deviation.

5. **Left bundle branch block:** Q waves in the precordial leads V1 and V2 are commonly present in patients with a complete LBBB, in the absence of MI. The diagnosis of old or acute MI is often not possible on a 12-lead ECG.

6. **Cardiac sarcoid or amyloid:** Rarely, pathologic Q waves may not be explained by any of the foregoing, common causes of pseudoinfarction Q waves, and cardiac infiltration with sarcoid or amyloid may be the underlying etiology. These are distinctly rare causes of Q waves on a 12-lead ECG.

PSEUDOMEMBRANOUS COLITIS

Diarrhea occurring during or shortly after a course of antibiotics is very common, with a frequency approaching 10%. A small percentage of such diarrhea is pseudomembranous colitis. Pseudomembranous colitis is due to overgrowth of the anaerobe *Clostridium difficile,* with elaboration of a number of toxins, resulting in watery diarrhea. *C. difficile* is part of colon flora in approximately 5% of healthy humans, and this prevalence may double in hospitalized patients. Less than 5% of pseudomembranous colitis cases are seen in the absence of previous antibiotic therapy. All antibiotics can cause pseudomembranous colitis.

The condition usually presents with five or more loose, mucous-laden stools per day. One-third of patients have fecal leukocytes. Patients may alternate by a few days with diarrhea and a few days without. Practically, the diagnosis is made by detection of *C. difficile* toxin in stool, but the gold standard is biopsy at colonoscopy.

Treatment: Both metronidazole (250–500 mg PO TID or QID) or vancomycin (125–250 mg PO QID) can be used. Avoid antiperistaltic drugs because *C. difficile* toxins are antiperistaltic on their own. Cholestyramine may bind the toxin, minimally decreasing symptoms. Isolation of patients is important in order to stop patient-to-patient spread.

Reference: Silva J: Update on pseudomembranous colitis. West J Med 151:644–648, 1989.

PSORIATIC ARTHRITIS

Psoriasis is a common disease, affecting about 2% of the U.S. population. It is currently recognized that about 5% of patients who have psoriasis will develop an associated inflammatory arthropathy. Onset of the arthritis usually occurs in the fifth decade, and both men and women are equally affected. The skin disease usually precedes the arthropathy, and nail involvement may predict arthropathy. Approximately 30% of psoriasis patients without arthritis have extensive nail pitting, and about 80% of patients with arthritis associated with psoriasis have nail disease.

The etiology of psoriasis is unknown. Genetic factors clearly play a role. Up to 70% of monozygotic twins are concordant for the skin disease as well as the arthropathy. Dizygotic twins have a concordance rate of half that of monozygotic twins. HLA Cw6 is noted to have a high incidence in patients with skin disease, although its absence significantly increases the risk for arthropathy. In a study by Winchester and colleagues, 20% of HIV patients had psoriasiform lesions. Three percent of that population had definite psoriatic arthritis. Other studies show rates of about 5 to 10% of skin disease and 1 to 2% for the development of arthropathy, implying an increased risk for both skin disease and arthropathy compared to the general population.

In psoriasis patients, the distinct subtypes of arthritis are recognized by the pattern of joints involved. Oligoarticular involvement occurs most commonly and is characterized by the asymmetric involvement of relatively few joints. Dactylitis (sausaging) of digits occurs commonly. Classic psoriatic arthritis involves the distal interphalangeal joints. Psoriatic nail changes are most strongly associated with this pattern of arthritis. A symmetric polyarthropathy that mimics RA is well documented and occurs in about 15% of psoriasis patients who develop arthritis. Occasionally, the peripheral arthropathy can be intense and destructive, resulting in osteolysis of the phalanges and metacarpals. Often termed arthritis mutalans, this pattern of articular involvement occurs in about 5% of psoriasis patients with arthritis. Finally, a sacroiliitis and spondylitis can occur, clinically indistinguishable from ankylosing spondylitis.

Classically, x-rays show the so-called pencil-in-cup deformity. Distal phalanges are destroyed in association with a cupping of the proximal phalanges. Acroosteolysis (erosion of the terminal tufts) can be seen. Classic bamboo spine is relatively rare.

Laboratory data in general are nonspecific. The ESR and other acute-phase reactants are often elevated. Patients with psoriasis and arthritis who have circulating RF are felt to have the coincident RA and psoriasis rather than the arthritis of psoriasis. About 40% of patients with the spondylitic features are found to be HLA B27 positive. There is no association of HLA B27 with peripheral arthritis patterns and psoriasis. Hyperuricemia occurs in about 20% of patients with psoriasis and is thought to be related to the cell turnover that occurs with active skin disease. The diagnosis can sometimes be difficult. Not every episode of joint pain in patients with psoriasis is psoriatic arthritis.

Progression of disease is generally slow and indolent. One study showed less deformity and disability in patients with arthritis associated with psoriasis than in patients with RA. Nonetheless, about 5% of patients develop arthritis mutalans. Treatment of mild disease can be accomplished with NSAIDs. More severe disease is best treated with methotrexate. Glucocorticoids are best avoided because there is commonly an intensification of disease with withdrawal. Recent studies have shown benefit from cyclosporine A.

References: Arnett FC, et al: Psoriasis and psoriatic arthritis associated with human immunodeficiency virus infection. Rheum Dis Clin North Am 17:59–78, 1991.

Winchester R, et al: Implications from the occurrence of Reiter's syndrome and related disorders. Scand J Rheumatol 74(suppl):89–93, 1988.

PULMONARY EMBOLISM

PE is a potentially life-threatening complication of venous thrombosis. Over 90% of PEs arise from venous thrombosis of the lower extremities at sites above the calf veins. Over 500,000 cases of PE occur per year, with approximately 50,000 fatalities. Because the diagnosis cannot be made clinically, once a PE is suspected, the appropriate diagnostic tests should be performed. A recent review of PE mortality from the PIOPED (Prospective Investigation of Pulmonary Embolism Diagnosis) study found a mortality rate of 2.5%, with most deaths occurring during the first week. These results underscore the importance of early diagnosis and treatment.

Signs and Symptoms

1. Dyspnea	8. Low-grade fever
2. Feeling of "impending doom"	9. With large embolism
3. Palpitations	Fixed split S_2
4. Hemoptysis	S_3 or S_4 gallop
5. Pleuritic chest pain	Dilated neck veins
6. Tachypnea	Cyanosis
7. Tachycardia	Hypotension

Laboratory Test Results in Patients with PE

1. CXR: most often reported as "normal"
   Atelectasis/volume loss
   Localized edema
   Vascular cutoff sign
   Consolidation (pulmonary infarct)
2. ECG: sinus tachycardia most common abnormality
   S_1Q_3 pattern
   Right axis deviation
   Right-sided strain pattern
3. ABG: P_aCO_2 usually decreased
   P_aO_2 usually decreased but may be above 80 mm Hg
   Increased A-a oxygen gradient ($P_{(A-a)}O_2$)

Diagnosis of PE

1. VQ scan: The VQ scan can establish the diagnosis with a high degree of certainty in those patients with high probability or a normal scan. However, only a minority of patients have these results, and further testing (noninvasive testing of the lower extremities or angiography) may be indicated.
    a. A normal scan excludes patients with clinically significant PE.
    b. A high probability scan indicates at least an 85% probability of PE.
    c. Either a low clinical suspicion combined with a low-probability scan or a high-probability scan combined with a high clinical suspicion improves diagnostic accuracy.
2. Pulmonary angiography: This test is the gold standard to which all other tests are compared.

Treatment of PE

1. Anticoagulation
2. Inferior vena caval interruption (filters)
3. Thrombolytic agents
4. Embolectomy

References: Carson JL, et al: The clinical course of pulmonary embolism. N Engl J Med 326:1240–1245, 1992.

Moser KM: Venous thromboembolism. Am Rev Respir Dis 141:235–249, 1990.

The PIOPED Investigators: Value of the ventilation/perfusion scan in acute pulmonary embolism. Results of the prospective investigation of pulmonary diagnosis (PIOPED). JAMA 263:2753–2759, 1990.

PULMONARY FIBROSIS

Interstitial Lung Disease

Interstitial lung disease (ILD) refers to a heterogeneous group of disorders with similar clinical and radiologic features. The CXR is the usual starting point for diagnostic evaluation. Fibrotic changes are usually widespread, involving both of the lungs, although not necessarily affecting every part of the lungs or all parts uniformly. Most ILD is associated with widespread fibrotic changes, small lung fields, and restrictive defects on PFTs. However, as will be noted later, some radiographic features may be more specific for several types of ILD.

Approximately 85 to 90% of patients present with symptoms of varying degrees (usually dyspnea and/or dry cough) and an abnormal CXR. Much less commonly, patients present with symptoms and a normal CXR or are referred for an abnormal CXR but are asymptomatic.

Physical findings may be unimpressive. Common findings include bibasilar rales, clubbing (notably in idiopathic pulmonary fibrosis or familial fibrosis), and findings of pulmonary HTN in advanced disease. Specific diagnoses may be associated with physical findings that will aid in diagnosis (e.g., telangiectasia in scleroderma, lymphadenopathy and parotid enlargement in sarcoid, arthritis in connective tissue diseases).

There are over 100 causes of ILD and they are often classified according to **known** etiology (e.g., drug induced, pneumoconioses) versus **unknown** etiology (e.g., sarcoidosis, idiopathic pulmonary fibrosis). The following classification lists some of the more common and interesting causes of ILD.

Classification of ILD by Etiology

I. Idiopathic fibrotic diseases
   Idiopathic pulmonary fibrosis
   Lymphocytic interstitial pneumonitis
   Acute interstitial pneumonitis
   Bronchiolitis obliterans organizing pneumonia

II. Connective tissue diseases

SLE	Rheumatoid arthritis
Scleroderma	Ankylosing spondylitis
Sjögren's syndrome	Others less commonly

III. Primary diseases

Sarcoidosis	ARDS
Lymphangitic carcinoma	Eosinophilic granulomatosis
Systemic vasculitides	Alveolar microlithiasis
Lymphangioleiomyomatosis	Neurofibromatosis
Eosinophilic pneumonia	Other rare diseases

IV. Drug related

Oxygen	Radiation
Chemotherapy	Antiarrhythmic agents (amiodarone, others)
Antibiotics (nitrofurantoin, others)	Anti-inflammatory agents (aspirin, gold, others)
Narcotics (morphine, cocaine, others)	

V. Occupational

Pneumoconiosis	Hypersensitivity pneumonitis

ILD and Associated Findings by Etiology

I. ILD associated with spontaneous pneumothorax

1. Eosinophilic granuloma	3. Neurofibromatosis
2. Lymphangioleiomyomatosis	4. Tuberous sclerosis

II. ILD associated with increased lung volumes

1. Eosinophilic granuloma	4. Neurofibromatosis
2. Tuberous sclerosis	5. Chronic hypersensitivity pneumonitis
3. Sarcoidosis	

III. ILD associated with upper lobe predominance

1. Ankylosing spondylitis	4. Berylliosis
2. Eosinophilic granuloma	5. Neurofibromatosis
3. Silicosis	6. Chronic sarcoidosis

IV. ILD associated with lymphadenopathy

1. Sarcoidosis	3. Berylliosis
2. Lymphoma	4. Lymphangitic carcinoma

References: Crystal RG, et al: Interstitial lung disease of unknown etiology: Disorders characterized by chronic inflammation of the lower respiratory tract. N Engl J Med 310: 154–166, 1984.

Stokes LT, et al: Lungs and connective tissue disorders. In Murray JF, et al (eds): Textbook of Respiratory Medicine. Philadelphia, W.B. Saunders, 1988, pp 1462–1485.

PULMONARY FUNCTION TESTS

Indications:

1. Screening to separate subjects with normal lungs from those with cardiopulmonary disease.
2. Early detection of lung disease.
3. Evaluation of patients with dyspnea.

4. Evaluation of patients prior to surgical procedures so as to assess risk for postoperative morbidity.
Thoracic operations
Upper abdominal operations
Heavy smokers
Obese patients
Preexisting lung disease
Elderly patients
5. Assessment of disability
6. Objective evaluation of patients undergoing specific therapy to assess pulmonary response to the treatment.
7. Periodic evaluation of workers in occupations associated with known pulmonary hazards
8. Monitoring the progression of lung disease

Spirometry: Useful information can be obtained from spirometry (*spirare* = to breathe, *metron* = measurement). The most valuable information obtained from spirometry is as follows:

1. *FVC:* Forced vital capacity is the largest volume measured during a maximum expiration made as rapidly as possible (forced) following a maximum inspiration.
2. *FEV$_1$:* Forced expiratory volume in 1 sec is the volume that is exhaled during the first 1 sec of the FVC maneuver.
3. *FEV$_1$/FVC:* This ratio describes the percentage of total exhalation that occurs during the first second of forced expiration. The ratio is normally >75%, meaning that, in the absence of airway obstruction, 75% or more of the FVC should be exhaled in the first second.
4. *FEF$_{25-75\%}$:* The mean forced expiratory flow measures the flow in the middle portion of the FVC curve (from 25 to 75% of FVC). It is relatively independent of effort and represents flow in the small airways.
5. *MVV:* The maximal voluntary ventilation measures the volume expired during a series of rapid deep respirations over 12 to 15 sec. The MVV measures both inspiratory and expiratory capacity and would be reduced with obstruction or weakness.

Glossary for Static Lung Volumes and Capacities

	SYMBOL	DEFINITION
Volumes		
Residual volume	RV	The volume of air remaining in the lungs after maximum expiration
Expiratory volume	ERV	The maximum volume of air expired from the resting end-expiratory level
Tidal volume	TV*	The volume of air inspired or expired with each breath during quiet breathing
Inspiratory reserve volume	IRV	The maximum volume of air inspired from the resting end-inspiratory level
Capacities		
Inspiratory capacity	IC	The maximum volume of air inspired from the end-expiratory level (the sum of IRV and TV)
Vital capacity	VC	The maximum volume of air expired from the maximum inspiratory level

Table continued on next page.

Glossary for Static Lung Volumes and Capacities (Cont.)

	SYMBOL	DEFINITION
Inspiratory vital capacity	IVC	The maximum volume of air inspired from the maximum expiratory level
Functional residual capacity	FRC	The volume of air remaining in the lungs at the end-expiratory level (the sum of RV and ERV)
Total lung capacity	TLC	The volume of air in the lungs after maximum inspiration (the sum of all volume compartments)

*The symbol TV is traditionally used for tidal volume to indicate a subdivision of static lung volumes. However, the symbol V_T is used for tidal volume in formulas for gas exchange.

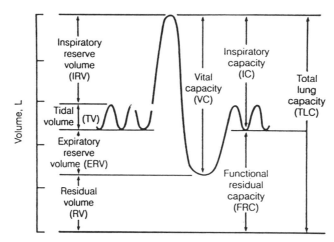

The subdivisions of lung volume as recorded by a spirometer. The record is generated on paper calibrated for volume in the vertical direction and time in the horizontal. The term *capacity* is applied to a subdivision composed of two or more volumes. (From Grippi MA, et al: Pulmonary function. In Fishman AP: Pulmonary Diseases and Disorders. New York, McGraw-Hill, 1988, p 2471, with permission.)

DL_{CO}: The carbon monoxide diffusion capacity is a function of the lung volume, the quantity of hemoglobin binding sites in the pulmonary capillaries, any alteration of the pulmonary interstitium, and the inequality of gas and perfusion within the lungs. This test may be helpful in patients with pulmonary fibrosis, pulmonary vascular disease, emphysema, pulmonary hemorrhage, or unexplained symptoms of dyspnea and in those at risk for developing diffusion problems because of occupation, medication, or other risk factors.

Characteristics of Obstructive and Restrictive Disease

Obstructive Ventilatory Defect

CHARACTERISTICS	SUPPLEMENTAL DATA
→ or ↓ VC	↑ RV
↓ maximum expiratory airflow	↑ airway resistance
	Abnormal distribution of inspired gas
↓ MVV	Significant response to bronchodilator
	↓ DL_{CO}
	↓ lung elastic recoil

Common Causes of Obstructive Ventilatory Defect

Upper airway	Central and peripheral airway
Pharyngeal and laryngeal tumors,	Bronchitis
edema, infections	Bronchiectasis
Foreign bodies	Bronchiolitis
Tumors, collapse and stenosis of	Bronchial asthma
the trachea	Parenchymal disease
	Emphysema

Restrictive Ventilatory Defect

CHARACTERISTICS	SUPPLEMENTAL DATA
↓ VC	↓ TLC
Relatively → expiratory flow rates	↓ lung compliance
	Chronic alveolar hyperventilation
Relatively → MVV	↑ $P_{(A-a)}O_2$ (A–a O_2 gradient)
	Abnormal distribution of inspired gas
	↓ DL_{CO}

Common Causes of Restrictive Ventilatory Defect

Interstitial lung diseases	Chest wall diseases
Interstitial pneumonitis	Injury
Fibrosis	Kyphoscoliosis
Pneumoconiosis	Spondylitis
Granulomatosis	Neuromuscular disease
Edema	Space-occupying lesions
Pleural diseases	Tumors
Pneumothorax	Cysts
Hemothorax	Extrathoracic conditions
Pleural effusion, empyema	Obesity
Fibrothorax	Peritonitis
	Ascites
	Pregnancy

Symbols used: ↑ = increased, ↓ = decreased, → = normal

From Welch MH: Ventilatory function of the lungs. In Guenter CA, et al (eds): Pulmonary Medicine. Philadelphia, J.B. Lippincott, 1977, pp 72–123, with permission.

Gold WM, et al: Pulmonary function testing. In Murray JF, et al (eds): Textbook of Respiratory Medicine. Philadelphia, W.B. Saunders, 1988, pp 611–682.

PULMONARY HYPERTENSION

Primary Pulmonary Hypertension

Normal pulmonary arterial systolic BP is 25 mm Hg, diastolic is 10 mm Hg, and mean pressure is 15 mm Hg. By definition, pulmonary HTN exists if the mean pulmonary arterial pressure exceeds 25 mm Hg. Disorders with pulmonary HTN are classified based on the underlying pathophysiologic mechanism of the elevated pulmonary arterial pressure:

1. Elevated left atrial pressure
   LV failure:
       Systolic dysfunction: LV ischemic heart disease, congestive cardiomyopathies
       Diastolic dysfunction: restrictive cardiomyopathies
   Mitral valvular disease:
       Rheumatic mitral stenosis and/or regurgitation
       Occlusion of mitral orifice by:
           Left atrial myxoma
           Thrombus
2. Pulmonary venous disease
   Pulmonary veno-occlusive disease
3. Pulmonary vascular disease
   Primary pulmonary HTN (plexiform arterial lesions)
   Multiple pulmonary emboli
   Pulmonary hypertension with portal venous HTN
   Familial pulmonary HTN
   Immunologic disorders:

SLE	Scleroderma
Raynaud's phenomenon	Polyarteritis nodosa
Wegener's granulomatosis	Rheumatoid arthritis
Arteritis, associated with HIV	Dermatomyositis

   Drugs and toxins:
       Aminorex, an anorectic agent
       Talc, in IV drug abusers
       Bush tea, from the seeds of *Crotalaria fulva*
   Pulmonary arterial occlusions:

Schistosomiasis	Sickle-cell anemia (rare)
Filariasis	Metastatic malignancies (rare)

4. Respiratory disorders
   Interstitial lung disease:

Pulmonary fibrosis	Sarcoidosis
Asbestosis	

   COPD
   Alveolar hypoventilation:
       Marked obesity (pickwickian syndrome)
       Kyphoscoliosis
       Respiratory muscle dysfunction
   ARDS
5. High-altitude disease
6. Congenital heart disease
   Left-to-right shunting of blood:

Patent ductus arteriosus	Atrial septal defect
Eisenmenger's syndrome	Truncus arteriosus
Aortic-pulmonary septal defect	
Peripheral pulmonary arterial stenosis	Aneurysm of sinus of Valsalva, communicating with the right side of the heart

In patients with pulmonary HTN due to elevated left atrial pressure or pulmonary venous disease, the pulmonary capillary wedge pressure is elevated, whereas it is normal in pulmonary HTN due to other causes.

When pulmonary HTN is due to a respiratory disorder, severe arterial hypoxemia is usually present with the P_aO_2 less than 55 mm Hg. Significant sustained pulmonary HTN results in physical findings such as:

1. Accentuated second heart sound (S_2) at the base of the heart.
2. Murmur of pulmonic regurgitation (i.e., early decrescendo diastolic murmur along the left sternal border).
3. Right ventricular heave.
4. Murmur of tricuspid regurgitation (i.e. pansystolic murmur, increased with inspiration, located in the fourth intercostal space at the left sternal border).
5. Third heart sound (S_3) over the right ventricle.
6. Jugular venous distension.

Reference: Rich S: Primary pulmonary hypertension. Prog Cardiovasc Dis 31:205–238, 1988.

Treatment with Calcium Antagonists

Primary pulmonary HTN is an uncommon disease of unknown etiology that is relentlessly progressive and incurable. The treatment has consisted of oral anticoagulants and vasodilators and has been based on the assumption that the disease may be due to pulmonary vasoconstriction or recurrent pulmonary embolization. Although there are several published reports on the effectiveness of vasodilators in patients with primary pulmonary HTN, the evidence that vasodilators have long-term efficacy in reducing pulmonary artery pressure (PAW) and pulmonary vascular resistance (PVR) is scarce.

The first report of the promising role of high doses of calcium antagonists in these patients was published in July 1992. A total of 64 patients who were treated with high doses of calcium channel blockers and who responded with a reduction of PAW and PVR by >20% were followed up for up to 5 years. The calcium antagonist used in those patients was nifedipine (average daily dose of 172 mg) or diltiazem (average daily dose of 720 mg). After 5 years, 94% of 17 patients who responded were alive compared to 55% who did not respond. The survival of the patients who responded was significantly greater than that of a historical control group, the NIH registry. This is illustrated in the figure that follows. It was the first study that suggests that high doses of calcium channel blockers in patients with primary pulmonary HTN who respond with reductions in PAW and PVR may improve survival over a 5-year period.

Based on the results of this study and others that showed an improvement in survival in patients with primary pulmonary HTN who were treated with oral anticoagulation, it is now recommended that a patient who responds to calcium channel blockers with a 20% or greater reduction in PAW and PVR with high doses of calcium channel blockers should be continued on the agent. Nonresponders should be treated with oral anticoagulation.

Reference: Rich S, et al: The effect of high doses of calcium-channel blockers on survival in primary pulmonary hypertension. N Engl J Med 327:76–81, 1992.

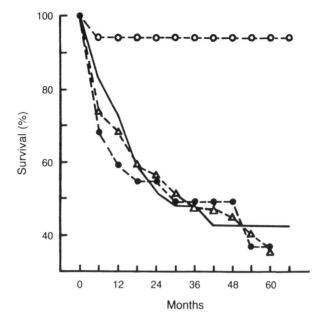

Kaplan-Meier estimates of survival among patients who responded to treatment (open circles), those who did not respond (solid line), and patients enrolled in the NIH registry (solid circles and triangles). The percentages were calculated every 6 months for 5.5 years. The rate of survival was significantly better in the patients who responded ($p = 0.003$) than in the other groups. (From Rich S, et al: The effect of high doses of calcium-channel blockers on survival in primary pulmonary hypertension. N Engl J Med 327:76–81, 1992, p 79, with permission.)

Secondary Pulmonary Hypertension

Pulmonary HTN results from increased blood flow at one of several sites within the circulation. A marked increase in pulmonary blood flow, even in the absence of an increase in resistance to blood flow, can result in pulmonary HTN. The causes can thus be classified as follows:
1. Increased resistance to pulmonary venous drainage
    a. Elevated LV diastolic pressure
    b. Mitral valve disease
    c. Pulmonary venous obstruction due to congenital pulmonary vein stenosis, anomalous pulmonary venous drainage with obstruction, mediastinal stenosis, or veno-occlusive disease.
2. Increased resistance through the pulmonary vascular bed
    a. Parenchymal pulmonary disease
    b. Eisenmenger's syndrome
3. Increased resistance through the large pulmonary arteries
    a. Pulmonary thromboembolism
    b. Peripheral pulmonic stenosis
4. Hypoventilation
5. Miscellaneous causes such as high altitude and IV drug abuse

In some patients with pulmonary HTN, no cause is discernible, in which case pulmonary HTN is called idiopathic or primary. The diagnosis of primary pulmonary HTN should be made after extensive evaluation of the cardiovascular and pulmonary systems for any secondary causes of pulmonary HTN. The most common causes of secondary pulmonary HTN are parenchymal pulmonary disease (obstructive or restrictive) and intracardiac shunts such as atrial or ventricular septal defects complicated by Eisenmenger's syndrome.

PULMONARY INFILTRATES

Drug and Noninfectious Causes

Drug and Noninfectious Causes of Pulmonary Infiltrates

Rheumatic disorders
1. Rheumatoid arthritis
2. Polymyositis/dermatomyositis
3. SLE
4. Sjögren's syndrome
5. Progressive systemic sclerosis
6. Ankylosing spondylitis

Immunologic diseases
1. Goodpasture's syndrome

Occupational pulmonary diseases
1. Coal workers' pneumoconiosis
2. Silicosis
3. Heavy metal exposure: cadmium, beryllium tungsten, cobalt, aluminum
4. Asbestosis
5. Irritant gases: ammonia, sulfur dioxide, HCl, chlorine gas, phosgene, NO

Eosinophilic pneumonias
1. Parasitic infections: *Ascaris lumbricoides, Necator americanus, Ancylostoma duodenale, Trichinella spiralis, Fasciola hepatica, Strongyloides stercoralis, Dirofilaria immitis, Wucheria malayi, Toxocara canis*
2. Chemical induced
3. Associated with asthmatic syndrome: asthma, mucoid impaction of bronchi, bronchopulmonary aspergillosis
4. Associated with hypersensitivity disorders and systemic angiitis: polyarteritis nodosa, allergic angiitis and granulomatosis (Churg-Strauss disease)
5. Drug induced: penicillamine, colchicine, methysergide, ergonovine, terbutaline, ritodrine

Malignancy
1. Leukemia
2. Multiple myeloma and Waldenström's macroglobulinemia
3. Lymphoma
4. Lymphangitic spread: lung, stomach, breast, colorectal, pancreas

Metabolic disorders
1. Amyloidosis
2. Inborn errors of metabolism: Niemann-Pick disease, Gaucher's disease, Fabry's disease, mucopolysaccharidoses, glycogen storage disorders, GM_1 gangliosidosis, metachromatic dystrophy

Miscellaneous
1. Gastric acid aspiration
2. Oxygen toxicity
3. Pulmonary edema
4. Pulmonary hemorrhage
5. Pulmonary infarction
6. Pulmonary leukoagglutination
7. Sarcoidosis
8. Histiocytosis X
9. Idiopathic pulmonary fibrosis
10. Vasculitis (Wegener's granulomatosis)
11. Diffuse interstitial pneumonitis
12. Lymphangioleiomyomatosis
13. Tuberous sclerosis
14. Radiation
15. Pulmonary alveolar proteinosis
16. Bronchiolitis obliterans

PYELONEPHRITIS

Pyelonephritis denotes infection of the renal parenchyma. The kidney becomes infected either by bacteria infecting the lower urinary tract that ascend to the kidney or by hematogenous spread from a distant source. Enterobacteriaceae (*Escherichia coli*) are the most common infecting organisms. Pyelonephritis is more common in sexually active women but can also occur in older men with prostatitis.

Although pyelonephritis is usually associated with so-called toxic symptoms such as flank pain, high fever, chills, dysuria, nausea, and vomiting, it is difficult to distinguish between pyelonephritis and bladder infection with clinical and culture findings. Urine cultures are positive in both bladder and renal parenchymal infections.

When suspected, pyelonephritis has usually been managed with IV antibiotics requiring hospitalization. Recent data suggest that outpatient, oral antibiotic therapy is effective in patients who do not have an underlying condition such as pregnancy, immunocompromise, DM, or other chronic, debilitating illness. Patients who are severely ill with hypotension, dehydration, and mental status changes or who have comorbid conditions should be hospitalized.

For outpatients, norfloxacin, trimethoprim-sulfamethoxazole, and amoxicillin-clavulanate are reasonable choices for 14 days of therapy. The exact efficacy of these regimens requires further study. Antibiotic therapy should be changed appropriately based on culture results. Patients followed as outpatients require close follow-up through either office visits or phone contact.

Patients requiring hospitalization should receive ampicillin or cefazolin plus an aminoglycoside. Patients generally defervesce within 72 hours but can remain acutely ill for 3 to 4 days. Complications of pyelonephritis include perinephric abscess.

Reference: Pinson AG, et al: Oral antibiotic therapy for acute pyelonephritis: A methodologic review of the literature. J Gen Intern Med 7:544, 1992.

PYODERMA GANGRENOSUM

This is an ugly skin ailment that has been associated with diverse conditions including ulcerative colitis, regional enteritis, hepatitis, RA, and hematological disorders such as myeloproliferative disease and multiple myeloma. The classic lesion of pyoderma gangrenosum begins as an erythematous, tender nodule that rapidly ulcerates. The margins are bluish, edematous, overhanging, and surrounded by erythema. They may enlarge to 10 cm or larger, and they heal with cribriform scaring. The lesions may arise acutely, often occur on the lower extremities, and may develop in areas of trauma. The chronic ulcer must be differentiated from vasculitis, fungal infections, lesions associated with iodide and bromide ingestion, factitious skin lesions, and ulcerated necrobiosis lipoidica diabeticorum. The skin biopsy is not diagnostic, and therefore pyoderma gangrenosum remains a clinical syndrome.

In hematologic disorders, pyoderma gangrenosum sometimes assumes a bullous form and has been described as atypical pyoderma gangrenosum in patients with leukemia or myeloproliferative disease. In those cases, there may be an overlap with neutrophilic dermatosis or Sweet's syndrome. In Sweet's syndrome, the typical presentation is that of an acute febrile disorder with painful, cutaneous plaques located usually on the upper extremities, head, and neck. Cutaneous leukemia can be differentiated by the presence of blasts and other young cells rather than mature neutrophils in the biopsy. The treatment of the underlying disorder may result in improvement in pyoderma, but good response can also be obtained with administration of corticosteroids.

QT INTERVAL

Prolongation, Recognition, and Differential Diagnosis

The QT interval duration varies according to heart rate. To correct for variations in the QT interval due to changes in heart rate, a corrected QT interval (QT_c) can be calculated as the ratio of the measured QT interval divided by the square root of the R-R interval. A normal QT_c interval ranges between 360 and 440 milliseconds.

The QT interval is prolonged in the following clinical situations:

1. Electrolyte disturbances
   a. Hypokalemia
   b. Hypomagnesemia
   c. Hypocalcemia
2. Drugs
   a. Antiarrhythmic drugs: Type I (A or C)
   b. Tricyclic antidepressants

The importance of the recognition of a prolonged QT interval lies in the predisposition of patients with a prolonged QT interval to potentially life-threatening ventricular cardiac arrhythmias such as V tach and V fib. A unique type of V tach associated with a prolonged QT interval is torsades de pointes, a polymorphic V tach. Prolongation of the QT interval to greater than 50% over the baseline QT interval should be avoided in patients receiving type IA antiarrhythmic drugs such as quinidine, procainamide, or disopyramide. It is also recommended to initiate antiarrhythmic drug therapy in the hospital and to observe the patient for any evidence of a proarrhythmic effect. Proarrhythmia is defined as a significant increase in the number of ventricular arrhythmias ($\geq$4-fold) and/or the new appearance of V tach during initiation of an antiarrhythmic drug.

R

RADIATION THERAPY

Radiation therapy consists of the use of ionizing radiation to cause lethal damage to the DNA of cancer cells. The cells are not killed directly, but they die when they attempt to reproduce. There are two ways of administering radiotherapy:

1. Teletherapy, in which external units beam ionizing radiation on a target volume that includes the tumor
2. Brachytherapy, in which a radioactive material is implanted into a tumor (interstitial therapy) or placed in a body cavity next to the tumor (intracavitary therapy)

Much of radiotherapy is done with electromagnetic radiation in the form of photon beams. Particulate radiation with electrons, neutrons, and protons is also commonly used. Agents employed for brachytherapy include radioactive isotopes of gold, iridium, or iodine.

In external beam radiotherapy, the depth of the radiation dose depends on the energy of the beam. Clinically used energies range from 85 kV, for therapy of tumors on the body surface, to 35 million volts, for treatment of tumors within the body.

Characteristics of Radiotherapy Modalities

SOURCE	ENERGY	HALF-VALUE LAYER*	USED IN TREATING
Superficial x-rays	85–140 kV	0.5–3 cm	Skin cancers
Orthovoltage x-rays	180–400 kV	3–6 cm	Skin and surface cancers
Megavoltage x-rays			
^{60}Co	1.25 MeV	11 cm	Deep cancers
Linear accelerator	4–25 MeV	11–20 cm	Deep cancers
Electrons	6–35 MeV	1–8 cm	Skin cancers
Neutrons	16–50 MeV	13–15 cm	Deep cancers

*Thickness of a specific material that reduces the intensity of the radiation beam by 50%; a measure of depth of penetration.

From Parker RG, et al: Principles of radiotherapy and chemotherapy. In Casciato A, et al (eds): Manual of Clinical Oncology, 2nd ed. Boston, Little, Brown, 1988, p 14, with permission.

Cancers vary widely in their sensitivity to radiation. The hematopoietic malignancies are very sensitive, and they respond to low doses of radiation. In contrast, the sarcomas are relatively insensitive, requiring much higher doses for cell killing. The absorbed radiation dose is measured in rads or centigrays (cGy): 1 rad = 1 centigray, and 1 gray = 100 rad. The dose of radiation that can safely be administered to a particular tumor depends on the radiation tolerance of the surrounding healthy tissue. Tissues with dose-limiting sensitivity to radiation damage include the eye, bone marrow, liver, kidney, lung, heart, brain, and spinal cord. To spare normal tissues, the shrinking field or boost technique is commonly employed. The largest area of potential tumor involvement is treated with a limited dose of radiation. The radiation field is then coned down so as to provide a maximal dose to the known sites of tumor involvement.

Radiotherapy is more effective in tissues that are well oxygenated, because of the formation of reactive oxygen intermediates that cause lethal damage to the DNA. It is recommended that patients receiving radiotherapy maintain an Hct of 30% or above in order to ensure adequate oxygenation of cells. For the same reason, radiation therapy is more effective in small tumors, because more of the cancer cells have an adequate blood supply. For large tumors, it is best to reduce tumor bulk with chemotherapy or surgery before beginning therapy. The effects of radiotherapy can be enhanced by the concomitant use of radiosensitizers. Commonly used radiosensitizers include 5-fluorouracil, cisplatin, hydroxyurea, and bleomycin. Radiosensitizing drugs such as dactinomycin and doxorubicin should be used with caution because of their potential for increased toxicity.

The acute side effects of conventional-dose radiotherapy include mild fatigue, anorexia, nausea, and bone marrow suppression. Often there is erythema and desquamation of the overlying skin. If there is rapidly proliferating normal tissue in the radiation field, local toxicities will occur (e.g., mucositis in head and neck irradiation, esophagitis after irradiating the mediastinum). Radiation pneumonitis presents as cough, pulmonary infiltrates, dyspnea, and fever. The diagnosis is made by observing the shape of the CXR infiltrate, which conforms to the shape of the radiation field. Treatment involves the use of prednisone 40 to 60 mg/day tapered over a 4- to 6-week period. Delayed effects of radiation therapy such as constrictive pericarditis, pulmonary fibrosis, and encephalomalacia can occur months to years after treatment.

RED EYE

Differential Diagnosis

The differential diagnosis of a nontraumatic red eye includes acute conjunctivitis, acute keratitis (inflammation of the cornea), acute uveitis (the uvea consists of the iris, ciliary body, and choroid considered together), acute glaucoma, spontaneous subconjunctival hemorrhage, and hordeolum (stye). The following table presents the symptoms and signs of each of these.

Differential Diagnosis of the Red Eye

	ACUTE CONJUNCTIVITIS	ACUTE KERATITIS	ACUTE UVEITIS	ACUTE GLAUCOMA
Pain	0 to +	++ to ++++	++	++++
Photophobia	0	+++	+++	+
Blurred vision	0	++	+ to +++	++++
Discharge	++ to ++++	0 to +++	0	0
Conjunctival injection	Diffuse	Diffuse	Circumcorneal	Diffuse
Cornea	Clear	Variable	Usually clear	Steamy
Pupillary light response	Normal	Normal	Poor	Absent

Adapted from Riordan EP, et al: The eye. In Schroeder SA, et al: Current Medical Diagnosis and Treatment, 30th ed. East Norwalk, CT, Appleton & Lange, 1991, p 103.

Conjunctivitis, by far the most common cause of red eye, can be caused by bacterial (*Streptococcus pneumoniae, Staphylococcus aureus, Haemophilus aegyptius, Moraxella lacunata, Neisseria gonorrhoeae*), chlamydial, and viral (especially adenovirus) infections, as well as by hay fever and keratoconjunctivitis sicca (dry eye)—a common disorder in elderly women. Nongonococcal bacterial conjunctivitis has a self-limited course of 10 to 14 days, which can be shortened to 2 to 3 if a sulfonamide ophthalmic solution is applied. Gonococcal conjunctivitis can be diagnosed by examination of a smear of the exudate: it is an ophthalmological emergency because it can quickly progress to corneal ulceration if left untreated. IV antibiotics (penicillin or cefotaxime) are required. Spontaneous subconjunctival hemorrhage, while its appearance may be dramatic, is of no clinical significance. It often occurs with coughing and disappears within 7 to 10 days. A stye is treated with warm compresses and topical antibiotics. Incision or attempts at manual drainage of the stye are not recommended.

Acute keratitis can be caused by bacteria (*Pseudomonas aeruginosa, Streptococcus pneumococcus, Moraxella* sp., staphylococci), herpes simplex, fungi, and *Acanthamoeba*. Prolonged wearing of soft contact lenses is often the precipitating factor in bacterial and *Acanthamoeba* keratitis. Without prompt and effective treatment, acute keratitis can have devastating consequences. Immediate referral to an ophthalmologist is necessary.

The intraocular inflammation seen with acute uveitis is classified as anterior uveitis, posterior uveitis, or panuveitis. The eye tends to be redder when anterior uveitis is present than with posterior uveitis. Uveitis is a local manifestation of a systemic disease. Disorders in which uveitis can occur include (among others) ankylosing spondylitis, Behçet's syndrome, ulcerative colitis, Crohn's disease, sarcoidosis, tuberculosis, and syphilis. Prompt referral to an ophthalmologist is necessary. Collaboration between the internist and the ophthalmologist is necessary for the evaluation and long-term management of the disease.

Acute glaucoma (angle closure glaucoma) is an ophthalmological emergency that can lead to permanent visual loss within 2 days. Pain is often extreme and patients see halos around lights. Patients can appear systemically ill and have nausea, vomiting, and abdominal pain.

Reference: Wilhelmus KR: The red eye. Infect Dis Clin North Am 2:99–116, 1988.

REITER'S SYNDROME (REACTIVE ARTHRITIS)

Reactive arthropathy is one of the HLA B27–associated spondyloarthropathies. It was from Hans Reiter's 1916 description of a young German calvary officer that the syndrome gets its name. Reiter's is diagnosed on the basis of the clinical picture. The classical triad for Reiter's syndrome is an active inflammatory arthropathy in association with conjunctival inflammation after a bout of diarrhea or urethritis. The urethritis may be persistent and has been shown to occur without sexual exposure. Reiter's syndrome is seen, with increased frequency and severity, in patients infected with HIV.

Recently, electron microscopic studies have shown particles of *Chlamydia,* long believed to be one of the etiologic agents in Reiter's, in inflamed synovium. An intact organism has neither been identified nor grown in culture. *Yersinia* antigens in synovial fluid from patients with reactive arthritis suggest that these findings have meaning. The clinical features usually include onset of articular inflammation 2 to 4 weeks after a diarrheal illness or sexual exposure. Urethritis is usually a transient and mucopurulent discharge with mild dysuria. It is generally more common in men. The conjunctivitis is usually bilateral and occurs coincidentally with the urethritis. Occasionally, a more severe ocular involvement including acute anterior uveitis is present. Intense ocular pain, photophobia, and redness are also present. The arthritis is usually the last feature of the triad to appear and most commonly affects the lower limbs. Sausaging of the digits (dactylitis) is common. Evaluation of the synovial fluid reveals inflammation. The articular involvement is generally asymmetric and oligoarticular. An enthesopathy is present as with all spondyloarthropathies. Inflammation at the tendinous insertions leads to heel pain. Plain x-rays may reveal erosions at the calcaneus. The sacroiliac joints can be involved as well, leading to low back pain.

Extra-articular manifestations include keratoderma blennorrhagicum, a papulosquamous skin eruption most common on the palms and soles. Circinate balanitis can also be present. There are shallow, painless ulcerations on the glans or shaft of the penis. They can appear as dry, scaling plaques in circumcised males. Onycholysis is also present and is difficult to distinguish from fungal infection of the nails.

Reiter's is often a chronic disease leading to disability. Treatment includes NSAIDs. As with most spondyloarthropathies, the acidic medications such as indomethacin may have some advantage. More aggressive cases of Reiter's have been successfully calmed with azathioprine.

References: Granfors K, et al: *Yersinia* antigens in synovial-fluid cells from patients with reactive arthritis. N Engl J Med 320:216–222, 1989.

Schumacher HR, et al: Light and electron microscopic studies on the synovial membrane in Reiter's syndrome. Arthritis Rheum 31:937–946, 1988.

RENAL FAILURE

Acute Renal Failure

About 5% of hospitalized patients develop ARF, which is defined as a rapid decline in renal function leading to retention of nitrogenous metabolites, salt, and water in the body. The serum creatinine and urea nitrogen usually rise by 0.5 mg and 10 mg/dl/day, respectively, in most cases of significant ARF. The syndrome often leads to oliguria—urine output <400 ml/day—but at least a third of cases may exceed that limit (nonoliguric ARF). Complete cessation of urine output, or anuria, is rather uncommon and is seen with total urinary obstruction. ARF can result from prerenal or postrenal causes, as well as factors that affect the kidneys themselves.

The diagnosis of ARF is one of exclusion. Prerenal factors should be carefully looked for and treated, since they account for up to half of all cases of ARF in some studies. A careful history should be obtained to exclude exposure to nephrotoxins (particularly NSAIDs, aminoglycosides, radiocontrast media, and ACE inhibitors). UA, especially urinary indices, is very helpful in the evaluation of the cause of ARF.

A renal ultrasound is obtained in all relevant cases to exclude urinary tract obstruction and to delineate the kidneys' size and shape.

Causes of Acute Renal Failure

PRERENAL	POSTRENAL
Hypovolemia	Urethral obstruction
Hemorrhage	Bladder neck obstruction
GI losses	Prostatic hypertrophy
Third space	Bladder carcinoma
Burns	Bladder infection
Peritonitis	Functional: neuropathy or ganglionic blocking
Traumatized tissue	agents
Diuretic abuse	Obstruction of ureters, bilateral
Impaired cardiac function	Intraureteral
CHF	Sulfonamide and uric acid crystals, blood
Myocardial infarction	clots, pyogenic debris, stones, edema
Pericardial tamponade	Necrotizing papillitis
Acute pulmonary embolism	Extraureteral
Peripheral vasodilation	Tumor: cervix, prostate
Bacteremia	Endometriosis
Antihypertensive drugs	Periureteral fibrosis
Increased renal vascular resistance	Accidental ureteral ligation during pelvic
Anesthesia	operation
Surgical operation	Pelvic abscess or hematoma
Hepatorenal syndrome	Ascites, pregnancy
Renal vascular obstruction (bilateral)	

Selected Causes of Intrarenal Acute Renal Failure

Glomerular diseases
  Rapidly progressive glomerulonephritis
  Postinfectious glomerulonephritis
  Focal glomerulosclerosis associated with AIDS
Tubulointerstitial nephritis
  Hypersensitivity reactions: penicillins, sulfonamides, fluoroquinolones, etc.
  Associated with systemic infections (*Legionella,* systemic exposure to organic solvents,
    Toxoplasma, etc.)
Acute tubular necrosis
  Ischemia, hypotension, septicemia, postoperative patients
  Direct drug toxicity: aminoglycoside, cisplatin, amphotericin, contrast agents, cyclosporine
  Myoglobin or hemoglobin
  Renal cortical necrosis
  Acute tubular necrosis in pregnancy
  Hypercalcemia
Vascular diseases
  Renal artery occlusion
  Acute vasculitis
  Malignant hypertension
  Atheroembolic disease, multiple cholesterol emboli syndrome

Urinary Indices in Acute Renal Failure

INDEX	PRERENAL	ACUTE TUBULAR INJURY
Urinary osmolality, mOsm/kg H_2O	>500	<350
Urinary sodium, mEq/L	<20	>40
Urine/plasma creatinine ratio	>40	<20
Fractional sodium excretion	<1	>1

Management: All reversible factors such as volume depletion, urinary obstruction, and infection should be carefully sought and treated. After ensuring euvolemia, a trial of diuretics (furosemide 80–200 mg IV or mannitol 12.5–25 gm IV) is justified to convert oliguric to nonoliguric renal failure because the latter has a better prognosis. Once ARF is established, restrict fluids to match the output plus insensible losses. Frequent monitoring of BUN and serum electrolytes is necessary. Adequate attention must be paid to nutritional status, especially in catabolic patients. Nephrotoxic agents and magnesium-containing compounds should be avoided. Indications for dialysis include severe and resistant hyperkalemia, fluid overload, metabolic acidosis (<7.2), uremic encephalopathy, and pericarditis.

Despite adequate management of ARF, its mortality remains high (20–50% in medical settings and 60–70% in surgical settings). During the recovering phase of ATN, close monitoring of fluid and electrolyte status is necessary because 25% of all deaths in ARF occur in the diuretic phase.

Reference: Hakim RM, et al: Hemodialysis in acute renal failure. In Brenner BM, et al (eds): Acute renal failure, 2nd ed. New York, Churchill Livingstone, pp 768–808, 1988.

Diagnosis and Bedside Estimation of Creatinine Clearance

Once the presence of renal dysfunction is confirmed, attention should be directed to establishing the etiology. The diagnostic process starts with a complete Hx & PE, UA with examination of the urine sediment by the physician, serum BUN and creatinine, serum electrolytes, and urine Na^+ and creatinine. The factors that can result in renal dysfunction are classified as prerenal, renal, and postrenal (see tables on p 529).

Prerenal causes are those resulting from a decrease in effective renal perfusion. Most commonly this is secondary to intravascular volume depletion. Volume losses can be external, as with protracted vomiting, diarrhea, or hemorrhage, or they can be internal, as with retroperitoneal bleeds or peritoneal fluid accumulation secondary to peritonitis. However, ineffective renal perfusion and consequent prerenal azotemia is also caused by conditions such as CHF and cirrhosis, in which effective perfusion is low even in the face of a normal or even expanded intravascular volume. Prerenal causes are obvious from the Hx & PE. Confirmatory lab values include

- BUN/serum creatinine ratio approaching 20:1 (normal is 10:1)
- Urine Na^+ of <10 mEq/L
- Fractional excretion of Na+ (FE_{Na+}) of <1
  $$FE_{Na+} = [(U_{Na+}/S_{Na+}) - (U_{Cr}/S_{Cr}) \times 100]$$

Renal causes are those that lead to decreased function by producing intrinsic renal disease. The renal dysfunction results from damage to any of the parenchymal structures, including the glomeruli, tubules, vascular structures, or interstitium. The most common causes of renal parenchymal injury in hospitalized patients are severe reduction in renal plasma flow (from hypotension) and nephrotoxic agents such as radiographic contrast agents and aminogyloside antibiotics. Due to loss of concentrating ability, the urine shows a high specific gravity; urine Na^+ and FE_{Na+} are high because of loss of the ability to conserve Na^+. The BUN/creatinine ratio approximates 10.

Postrenal causes are those in which renal dysfunction is due to obstruction of the flow of urine from the renal pelvis. Unless the patient has a solitary kidney, obstruction does not produce a significant rise in BUN unless both kidneys are obstructed. Therefore, at the level of the renal pelvis or ureter, bilateral obstruction is required. However, bladder neck or urethral obstruction leads to postrenal azotemia. Marked reduction (not necessarily absolute) in urine flow suggests the possibility of urinary obstruction. Urinary findings are not specific, but bladder catheterization may be diagnostic if the obstruction is urethral or at the bladder neck.

Estimation of the GFR is the most commonly used method of assessing the severity of renal dysfunction. In clinical practice, the creatinine clearance (C_{Cr}) is used to reflect the GFR:

$$C_{Cr} \text{ (or GFR)} = (U_{Cr} \times 24\text{-hr urine volume}) - P_{Cr}$$

Valid estimates of renal function depend on the presence of a steady-state situation. If the patient suffers an acute loss of renal function, the plasma creatinine (P_{Cr}) will not have had time to reach its maximum value, and calculations based on that low creatinine will overestimate the GFR. Also, serum creatinine can be misleading in older patients: Age-related renal changes reduce GFR, but aging is also associated with reduction in muscle mass and production of creatine. Thus, in older patients, serum creatinine can remain in the reference range even with a significant decline in the GFR. A commonly used formula for bedside estimation of GFR takes age into account:

$$\text{GFR (ml/min)} = [(140 - \text{age}) \times \text{weight in kg}] - (72 \times P_{Cr})$$

Reference: Conger JD, et al: Acute renal failure: Pathogenesis, diagnosis, and management. In Schrier RW (ed): Renal and Electrolyte Disorders, 4th ed. Boston, Little, Brown, 1992, pp 495–537.

Chronic Renal Failure

CRF is defined as progressive and irreversible decline in renal function (GFR). Elevation of serum creatinine is usually not obvious until the GFR falls to <50% of normal. Clinical symptoms usually manifest when the GFR falls below 20 ml/min. When the GFR is <5 ml/min, the term *end-stage renal disease (ESRD)* is used. The common causes of ESRD in the United States are as follows.

Major Causes of Chronic Renal Failure

Diabetes mellitus	31%
Hypertension	27%
Glomerulonephritis	14%
Cystic renal disease	3.6%
Obstructive uropathy	5.7%
Others	5.7%
Unknown	13%

1990 Annual Data Report of U.S. Renal Data Systems, National Institutes of Health, National Institute of Diabetes, Digestive and Kidney Diseases. Bethesda, NIH, 1990.

Clinical Features: CRF results in functional derangements of various organ systems in the body collectively referred to as the uremic syndrome. *Azotemia* refers to retention of nitrogenous wastes; *uremia* refers to the clinical manifestations resulting from azotemia.

The Uremic Syndrome

1. Electrolyte disorders
   a. Potassium: hyperkalemia, total body depletion
   b. Sodium: salt-losing nephrophathy, sodium retention
   c. Acidosis: metabolic acidosis with high "anion gap," type IV renal tubular acidosis (hyporeninemic hypoaldosteronism)
   d. Calcium: tendency toward hypocalcemia—phosphate retention and secondary hyperparathyroidism, with vitamin D deficiency
   e. Phosphate: hyperphosphatemia contributes to disorders of calcium metabolism
   f. Magnesium: accumulation due to excessive intake
   g. Aluminum: accumulation due to excessive intake
2. Cardiovascular abnormalities
   a. Accelerated atherosclerosis
   b. Hypertension
   c. Pericarditis
   d. Myocardial dysfunction
3. Hematologic abnormalities
   a. Anemia: erythropoietin deficiency, iron deficiency
   b. Leukocyte dysfunction: infection
   c. Hemorrhagic diathesis: defective platelet function
4. Gastorintestinal disorders
   a. Anorexia, nausea, vomiting, gastroparesis
   b. Gastrointestinal bleeding
   c. Disorders of taste
5. Renal osteodystrophy
   a. Osteomalacia
   b. Osteitis fibrosa (secondary hyperparathyroidism)
   c. Osteosclerosis
   d. Osteoporosis
6. Neurologic abnormalities
   a. Central nervous system: insomnia, fatigue, psychological symptoms, asterixis
   b. Peripheral neuropathy: stocking-glove sensory neuropathy
7. Myopathy: especially of proximal muscles
8. Impaired carbohydrate tolerance: peripheral resistance to insulin, hypoglycemia
9. Endocrine and metabolic disorders
   a. Glucose intolerance: insulin resistance, insulin degradation, hypoglycemia
   b. Other endocrine disorders: fertility, sterility
   c. Hypothermia
10. Hyperuricemia: clinical gout is rare; pseudogout occurs
11. Pruritus, soft tissue calcification, uremic frost

From Warnock DG: Chronic renal failure. In Wyngaarden JB, et al (eds): Cecil Textbook of Medicine, 19th ed. Philadelphia, W. B. Saunders, 1992, p 533, with permission.

Evaluation of the patient with CRF: Careful assessment by Hx & PE should be made to delineate the factors responsible for the etiology of renal failure. In addition, reversible factors aggravating CRF should be actively sought and treated. These are listed as follows:

Aggravating Factors for Progression of Renal Disease

1. Vascular volume depletion
   a. Absolute: aggressive use of diuretics, GI fluid losses, dehydration
   b. Effective: low cardiac output, renal hypoperfusion with atheroembolic disease, ascites with liver disease, nephrotic syndrome
2. Drugs: aminoglycosides, prostaglandin synthesis inhibitors in setting of renal hypoperfusion, diuretics in dosage to cause volume depletion
3. Obstruction
   a. Tubular: uric acid, Bence Jones protein
   b. Posttubular: prostatic hypertrophy, necrotic papillae, ureteral stones
4. Infections: sepsis with hypotension, UTI
5. Toxins: radiographic contrast material
6. Hypertensive crises
7. Metabolic: hypercalcemia, hyperphosphatemia

Some renal parenchymal diseases are amenable to treatment and they include acute hypertensive nephropathy, analgesic nephropathy, hemolytic-uremic syndrome, hypercalcemic nephropathy, interstitial nephritis, lupus nephritis, multiple myeloma, oxalate nephropathy, pyelonephritis, rapidly progressing glomerulonephritis with crescents, renal vein thrombosis, and Wegener's granulomatosis.

Management: After the reversible factors have been identified and treated, management of CRF includes careful monitoring and treatment of fluid and electrolyte status. In general, fluid intake should be restricted to match urine output plus insensible losses. Diuretics should be used if the patient is edematous. Loop diuretics are preferred, for, unlike the thiazides, they remain effective in patients with GFR <25 ml/min. Higher doses of loop diuretics may be needed in CRF, as they compete with organic anions for tubular secretion. HTN should be adequately controlled, and ACE inhibitors and calcium channel blockers seem to be very effective in that aspect. Dietary Na^+ should be restricted (2–6 gm/day) in patients with edema, CHF, and uncontrolled HTN. Dietary K^+ is restricted in patients with GFR <5 ml/min. Dietary protein restriction (0.6 gm/kg/day) may be protective against further loss of renal function.

Treatment of anemia by means of iron and folic acid supplements and, more recently, recombinant human erythropoietin is warranted. Hypocalcemia is treated with calcium and vitamin D_3 (0.25–0.5 µg/day) supplements. Hyperphosphatemia should be controlled with dietary phosphate restriction and phosphate binders such as calcium carbonate, calcium acetate, and aluminum hydroxide preparations. If the symptoms of uremia are not controlled by these conservative measures and especially when the quality of life deteriorates with advancing azotemia, renal replacement therapy with dialysis or transplantation should be considered.

Reference: Kalhr S, et al: The progression of renal disease. N Engl J Med 318:1657, 1988.

Continuous Ambulatory Peritoneal Dialysis

During the past two decades, several advances in the development of peritoneal access and better understanding of the peritoneal membrane as a dialysis membrane have facilitated the evolution of peritoneal dialysis as a viable option in chronic dialytic therapy. The principle consists of infusing the dialysate (usually about 2 liters) into the peritoneal cavity through a surgically inserted catheter by gravity and allowing the fluid to equilibrate for a certain amount of dwell time. The retained metabolites in the patient's body then undergo equilibration with the dialysate, which is subsequently drained out. In CAPD, the patient manually performs these exchanges for four or five cycles a day, whereas in continuous cyclic PD, three or four exchanges are performed by an automated cycler in the nighttime and in a single all-day ambulatory exchange. The dialysate usually consists of hypertonic dialysate with 1.5, 2.5, or 4.25% dextrose solutions.

Indications and Contraindications for Chronic PD

I. Indications
- Cardiovascular instability (hypotension, arrhythmias)
- Inadequate/unreliable vascular access
- Contraindication to systemic heparinization
- Patient preference
- Logistics (poor access to hemodialysis)

II. Major contraindications
- Peritoneal fibrosis, resection, or adhesions
- Pleuroperitoneal communication (hydrothorax)
- Recent abdominal surgery
- Severe catabolic states
- Recent aortic prosthesis (infection)
- Colostomy or nephrostomy (infection)
- Respiratory compromise

III. Minor contraindications
- Peripheral vascular disease
- Hernias or diverticular disease
- Hyperlipidemia
- Obesity

IV. Contraindications for self-care
- Physical or mental handicaps (including blindness)

Chronic PD has several advantages and disadvantages with respect to hemodialysis as follows:

Advantages of PD
- Minimal risk of disequilibrium syndrome
- Less hemodynamic stress per treatment
- Improved clearance of middle molecules
- No systemic anticoagulation
- Transfusion requirements minimized
- Technically more simple
- Patient independence (chronic therapy)

Disadvantages of PD
- Less effective treatment of hypercatabolic ARF
- Less efficient solute/fluid removal
- Increased risk of infection
- Catheter malfunction
- High protein/amino acid loss in dialysate
- Worsening hypertriglyceridemia

The main complication of chronic PD is the occurrence of peritonitis. About 60% of patients undergoing CAPD develop peritonitis in the first year of therapy. The incidence of peritonitis is approximately 1.5 to 2 episodes per patient per year. The peritonitis usually manifests as abdominal pain and tenderness, fever, and cloudy peritoneal dialysate that contains >100 WBC/mm^3 with >50% neutrophils. The PD fluid should be Gram stained and cultured. About 70% of cases are due to gram-positive cocci, and 20% are due to enteric gram-negative organisms. The presence of two or more organisms should make one suspect perforation of a hollow viscus.

Treatment consists of intraperitoneal or IV loading with appropriate antibiotic and maintenance doses added to the peritoneal dialysate bags. Recurrent bacterial, fungal, or TB peritonitis, with or without attendant loss of PD function, necessitates removal of the peritoneal catheter and initiation of chronic hemodialysis. Other complications associated with CAPD include hernias, hyperglycemia, hyperlipidemia, hypoalbuminemia (mean daily protein loss in PD is 10–20 gm), and abdominal viscus perforations. Other problems associated with CAPD include catheter obstruction, tunnel infections, and exit-site leaks.

The advent of automated cyclers has made continuous cyclic PD quite popular because cyclers allow total freedom during the daytime. Overall, chronic PD offers an excellent alternative to hemodialysis as a form of renal replacement therapy.

Hemodialysis

Hemodialysis is the currently predominant mode of therapy of ESRD. It is estimated that there are over 90,000 patients on chronic hemodialysis in the United States. Home hemodialysis requires the presence of a motivated partner and a congenial home situation. Although the in-home modality is cheaper than in-center hemodialysis, the number of patients on home hemodialysis has remained rather constant in the past few years.

The principle of hemodialysis involves circulation of the patient's blood in an artificial dialyzer at a rate of 200 to 300 ml/min while a dialysate flows (usually in the opposite direction) at a rate of 500 ml/min, clearing the blood of various solutes. The dialyzers are usually made of cuprophane or polysulfone compounds. Vascular access is usually provided through an AV fistula or a synthetic or bovine graft that has been surgically implanted. The dialysate usually contains acetate or HCO_3^- as a base, in order to correct metabolic acidosis. HCO_3^- is preferred over acetate in patients with liver disease who cannot convert acetate to HCO_3^- and in patients who are hemodynamically unstable. To attain optimal therapy, 3- to 4-hour sessions are

Complications of Chronic Hemodialysis

ACUTE COMPLICATIONS	CHRONIC COMPLICATIONS
Hypotension	Anemia
Dialyzer reactions	Transfusion-related diseases (e.g., hepatitis,
Bleeding	HIV)
Hypoxemia	Renal bone disease
Disequilibrium syndrome	Acquired cystic disease
Arrhythmias	Dialysis pericarditis
Leukopenia	Accelerated atherosclerosis
Electrolyte disturbances	Amyloidosis, dialysis dementia

needed three times a week. Once the patient has been initiated to chronic hemodialysis, therapy is continued on an outpatient basis.

Common complications associated with AV access include thrombosis, infection, ischemia of the limb, and high-output CHF. As in patients with prosthetic heart valves, antibiotic prophylaxis should precede any procedure that causes bacteremia.

Overall, long-term survival in patients on chronic hemodialysis has improved significantly since more effective and safer techniques of hemodialysis have evolved. The major improvements include development of faster techniques of dialysis (high-efficiency and high-flux dialyzers), development of human recombinant erythropoietin for the treatment of anemia of dialysis, and use of vitamin D_3 preparations and new phosphate binders in the treatment of renal bone disease.

Prerenal Azotemia

Prerenal azotemia is a common and usually avoidable occurrence in the hospitalized elderly. There are five major reasons the elderly are more prone to prerenal azotemia than younger adults. All except one result from normal, age-related changes in the body.

1. Elders have **10 to 15% less total body water** than younger adults. There are somewhat smaller decreases in plasma volume and ECF volume. Total body water decreases because as people age, lean body mass decreases, with a proportionate increase in body fat. Fat has less water than muscle. Besides predisposing the elderly to prerenal azotemia, these changes in body composition shrink the volume of distribution of drugs that distribute mainly into lean body mass and may predispose the elderly to drug toxicity.

2. Age-related changes in the kidney mean that elders have **decreased urine-concentrating ability** during states of water deprivation. During water deprivation, elders cannot achieve as high a urine osmolality as younger adults can. This is thought to be related to medullary washout and the relative insensitivity of the collecting ducts to antidiuretic hormone in the aged kidney.

3. There are age-related changes in the kidney, and the elderly have **impaired Na^+ conservation** by the kidney. Elders placed on a very low Na^+ diet excrete more Na^+ in their urine than do younger adults. An inability to conserve salt normally may be very important in states in which intravascular volume is threatened, because "where salt goes, so goes the water." Some believe age-related decreases in autonomic nervous system activity may play a role in elders' impairment of Na^+ conservation.

4. Elders have a **decrease in thirst, with resultant hypodipsia.** This has been found in circumstances of water deprivation. Decreased drive to ingest fluids in the face of age-related losses in the kidney's ability to conserve salt and water exacerbate prerenal azotemia.

5. The elderly are often receiving **drugs** that predispose to prerenal azotemia. The most common class of these is the diuretics. Because of their efficacy in the elderly, their acceptable side effect profile, and their low cost, diuretics continue to be a mainstay in the treatment of HTN, a very common condition in the elderly. They induce a chronic state of mild volume depletion, which is well tolerated until

the patient is placed in clinical circumstances that further threaten intravascular volume.

Fever, delirium, inability to get to oral fluids because of the bedfast state (e.g., as with hip fracture), use of bladder catheters that predispose to pyelonephritis, the propensity of elderly men to have subclinical degrees of bladder neck obstruction from prostatic hypertrophy, and use of nephrotoxic agents all work to increase the likelihood of prerenal azotemia in the hospitalized elderly.

Reference: Porush JG, et al: Renal Disease in the Aged. Boston, Little, Brown, 1991.

RHABDOMYOLYSIS

The syndrome of rhabdomyolysis is due to the acute necrosis of muscles. It presents with symptoms of weakness, pain, and swelling of muscles. Myoglobin is released into the circulation, leading to myoglobinuria.

In patients with rhabdomyolysis, elevated serum levels of certain enzymes that are present in muscles are detected, such as creatine kinase (CK), aldolase, LDH, and SGOT. Potassium, phosphate, uric acid, and lactic acid enter the circulation from the necrotic muscles, leading to hyperkalemia, hyperphosphatemia, hyperuricemia, and metabolic acidosis with an excessive anion gap. As calcium is deposited in necrotic muscle, hypocalcemia may be detected. With severe rhabdomyolysis, acute renal failure is common, with multiple causative factors including myoglobinuria, volume depletion, hypotension, and acidosis. Rhabdomyolysis varies in severity from a mild condition to a critical illness.

Causes of Rhabdomyolysis

Trauma to muscles	Infectious disorders
Crush injuries to limbs	Clostridial myonecrosis
Vascular occlusive disease	Streptococcal myonecrosis
Ischemic muscle necrosis	Septic shock
Anterior tibial syndrome	Trichinosis
Myopathies	Postinfectious
Polymyositis	Infectious mononucleosis
Muscular dystrophy	Coxsackie virus infection
Dermatomyositis	Influenza
Haff disease (Baltic Sea area)	Toxic conditions
Muscle enzyme deficiencies	Alcoholic myopathy
Myophosphorylase	Malignant hyperthermia
Phosphofructokinase	Neuroleptic malignant syndrome
Phosphoglycerate mutase	Withdrawal of anti-parkinsonian drugs
Phosphoglycerate kinase	Overdosage of drugs
Lactic dehydrogenase	Barbiturates
Carnitine palmityltransferase	Amphetamines
Metabolic derangements	Narcotics
Hypernatremia	Phencyclidine (PCP, angel dust)
Hypokalemia	Repeated epileptic seizures
Water intoxication	Severe electrical injury
Hypophosphatemia	

RHEUMATIC DISEASE

Use of the Laboratory in Diagnoses

The manifestations of rheumatic disease are often enigmatic, and diagnosis requires the clinical acumen of a savvy internist. There is rarely a test or procedure that will objectively establish a diagnosis analogous to the way coronary catheterization can confirm the diagnosis of CAD. Nonetheless, our ability to document the immune response, by detecting autoantibodies or measuring complement levels, can provide information suggesting diagnosis (antinative DNA or anti-Sm in lupus), pathogenesis, and etiology of disease (antiacetylcholine receptor in myasthenia gravis).

Acute-phase reactants: The concentration of some plasma proteins (called acute-phase proteins) is substantially increased (up to 25%) with inflammation. The major acute-phase proteins in humans are C-reactive protein (CRP) and serum amyloid A protein (SAA), but ferritin, fibrinogen, complement components, and haptoglobin also fit the definition. The most common measures of these reactants are the ESR and direct measurement of CRP. Although a general estimation of tissue injury or inflammation is sometimes obvious after careful examination, the ESR can often be useful in initially directing attention toward inflammatory disease.

Rheumatoid factor (RF): RF is an autoantibody directed against antigenic determinants of the Fc fragment of Ig. Although usually IgM, RFs of all isotypes have been documented, and they are found in many diseases. Cryoglobulins commonly have RF activity. In addition to their presence in many nonrheumatic diseases, it is well-known that these factors can be absent in RA (so-called seronegative RA). Higher titers of RF are associated with more severe and active joint disease, the presence of nodules, and more frequent extra-articular disease manifestations. Although RF may decline or disappear with successful therapy, sequential clinical examination is a more useful monitor of disease activity.

Antinuclear antibodies (ANA): In 1948, Hargraves described the lupus erythematosus cell; although the test is still available, its current importance is primarily historical. In 1957 Friou first demonstrated ANAs by immunofluorescent staining. Originally described as a single entity, ANAs were soon found to represent a group of antibodies directed against different nuclear constituents, which can be subdivided into those antibodies directed against DNA (double-stranded [native] or single-stranded DNA), against histones, and against other nonhistone nuclear antigens.

Anti-double-stranded (native) DNA antibodies recognize the deoxyribose phosphate backbone of DNA. When present, these antibodies are highly specific for SLE, and they may be accurate markers for disease activity. Often the titers become elevated in SLE patients with nephritis. Conversely, single-stranded DNA antibodies recognize purines and pyrimidines and do not react with native DNA. They are not useful diagnostic markers because they occur in other disease states.

Because antihistone antibodies occur in >96% of patients with drug-induced lupus, these antibodies were initially thought to be a specific marker for this condition. They are also noted to occur in idiopathic lupus (up to 80%), thus limiting their diagnostic usefulness. Antibodies to nonhistone nuclear proteins can also be important. Sometimes grouped together as antiextractable nuclear antigen (ENA), these proteins were originally found in the nucleus of cells (extractable in the laboratory with saline buffer). Nowadays many antigens fit that description, however, and the term has little specificity.

Anti-Sm(ith)[1] antibody is found almost exclusively in SLE and is an excellent disease marker. There is some evidence that patients with anti-Sm have CNS disease with higher frequency. Another so-called ENA—anti-U1 RNP—may be a marker for a specific overlap syndrome (SLE and systemic sclerosis) called mixed connective tissue disease. With time, many patients with anti-U1 RNP eventually develop SLE, polymyositis, or systemic sclerosis.

Anti-Ro (Sjögren's syndrome A[SSA]) and anti-La (Sjögren's syndrome B[SSB]) are antibodies to intracellular protein/RNA complexes that regulate RNA polymerase III. Anti-Ro often occurs with anti-La, but anti-La always occurs in the presence of anti-Ro. Anti-Ro antibodies are found in approximately 40% of SLE patients, 70% of Sjögren's patients, and 20% of RA patients. Anti-La is less frequently found: in 15% of SLE patients and in 40% of Sjögren's patients. Anti-Ro is associated with neonatal lupus (both dermatitis and cardiac disease). Because of transplacental transfer of antibody, these antibodies are believed to deposit in fetal atrial and conducting tissue, leading to congenital heart block. In Sjögren's syndrome patients, the presence of these antibodies can predict leukopenia, anemia, vasculitis, and cryoglobulinemia.

Nearly all patients (96%) with systemic sclerosis have ANA. About 70 to 80% of patients with the CREST variant of systemic sclerosis have anticentromere antibodies (ACA). Anticentromere can have prognostic significance as well. Patients who present with idiopathic Raynaud's phenomenon and a positive ACA are predictive of a greater chance of progression to CREST than those who do not have this circulating antibody.

Anti–Scl 70 occurs commonly in systemic sclerosis. This antigen is DNA topoisomerase I, an enzyme that supercoils DNA. Two-thirds of patients with anti–Scl 70 had scleroderma, and 70% of patients with scleroderma tested positively for anti–Scl 70.

Antineutrophilic cytoplasmic antibodies (ANCA): ANCA are found in patients with systemic arteritis and glomerulonephritis (including Wegener's granulomatosis and polyarteritis nodosa). Two patterns of staining are noted. The cytoplasmic (C-ANCA) pattern stains proteinase 3, a product of azurophilic granules. It is frequently associated with a systemic vasculopathy (Wegener's granulomatosis or polyarteritis nodosa). The perinuclear (P-ANCA) staining pattern is believed at least in part to be artifactual. Nonetheless, an associated antibody to myeloperoxidase (another azurophilic granule constituent) is noted. Its presence may be more specific for renal-limited vasculitis. There are also data to suggest that elevations in C-ANCA are associated with disease activity and can be predictive of relapses of disease. A recent prospective study has shown fewer relapses and lower total doses of immunosuppressive drugs in patients with Wegener's when treatment was instituted following a rise in ANCA titer. In addition to being an accepted serologic marker for disease, ANCA has recently been hypothesized as having a more direct pathogenic role in promoting necrotizing vascular lesions by generating neutrophil activation.

Complement: The complement system comprises a group of plasma proteins that interact to increase vascular permeability, attract leukocytes, enhance phagocytosis, immobilize cells at the site of inflammation, and attack membranes, all of which facilitate cell lysis and death. Hereditary deficiencies (C1, C2, C4) are associated with SLE, whereas absent C3 is linked with life-threatening infections. Assuming that no hereditary complement deficiency exists, measurement of C3, C4 and CH_{50} provides a sensitive test for complement consumption. Measurement may be a useful guide to development of acute illness and efficacy of therapy. Recently it has been suggested that the monitoring of complement split products (C3a and iC3b) may be helpful in predicting flares of lupus. These measurements are currently experimental and not uniformly available but may become commonly ordered laboratory tests.

HLA B27: HLA B27 is an allele of the class I histocompatibility genes and, for reasons that are unknown, is strikingly associated with the seronegative spondyloarthropathies (ankylosing spondylitis, Reiter's syndrome, spondyloarthropathy of inflammatory bowel disease). Hypotheses for that association include:

1. B27 acts as a receptor site for an infective agent.
2. B27 is a marker for the immune-response gene that determines susceptibility to an environmental trigger.
3. B27 may induce tolerance to a foreign antigen with which it cross-reacts.

The usefulness of this marker in diagnosis is limited. If a patient with clinically obvious disease was found to be B27 negative, it would be unlikely to cause a change in diagnosis or therapy; in that clinical situation, a positive test would not add useful information. In a patient with an atypical presentation, a positive HLA B27 might alert suspicion but would certainly not allow a specific diagnosis to be made.

------

[1]These antibodies were originally identified by the first two letters of the last name of the patient in whom they were found.

Reference: Hardin JA: The molecular biology of antibodies. In Schumacher HR Jr (ed): Primer of Rheumatic Diseases, 9th ed. Atlanta, The Arthritis Foundation, pp 32–35, 1988.

RHEUMATIC FEVER

Rheumatic fever is a disease caused by an unusual interaction between an antecedent group A streptococcal infection and the human immune system. The rate of disease has dropped steadily during the past quarter century; sociologic factors, changes in virulence of the streptococcus, and antimicrobial use have contributed to the decline. In association with recent outbreaks, nearly half to two-thirds of patients had no prior history of pharyngitis.

Although streptococcal pharyngeal infections are associated with the development of rheumatic fever, streptococcal infections elsewhere in the body have only rarely been documented to produce rheumatic fever. In addition to severity of infection, duration of throat carriage of the bacterium may also play a role. There is usually about one month's time between onset of the infection and rheumatic fever. Molecular mimicry has been hypothesized as the pathogenic mechanism of rheumatic fever. Specific M-types 5, 6, 18, and 24 are associated with rheumatic fever. Interestingly, type 5 cross-reacts with antigens on heart sarcolemma and myosin.

Clinical Manifestations: The illness most commonly strikes children and teenagers. The streptococcal infection may be inapparent in up to one-third of patients. Males and females are affected with equal frequency. Arthritis and carditis are symptoms common in children and teenagers. A migratory polyarthropathy is the most common presenting manifestation of the disease, usually with abrupt onset of pain in a given joint, maximizing 12 to 24 hours after onset. Joint pain is usually accompanied by fever and appears more severe than examination would indicate. As the pain diminishes, another joint will be affected, and the initial joint may be completely asymptomatic.

Occasionally, articular involvement may linger, making distinction from other chronic inflammatory arthropathies difficult. Knees and ankles are the joints most frequently affected, although all joints have been reported. Occasionally, an intense arthralgia without articular swelling can be seen.

Up to three-quarters of children and teenagers with rheumatic fever may develop cardiac disease, although only 15% of adults are so affected. Cardiac failure (myocarditis), changing murmurs, and pericarditis are the most commonly seen manifestations, but heart block can also occur. Valvular involvement is serious, and the extent of long-term damage appears related to severity of the acute valve disease.

The rash of rheumatic fever occurs rarely in adults and in less than a third of children. The classical erythema marginatum almost never occurs unless associated with polyarthritis. Appearing as salmon-colored, nonpurpuric macules over the trunk and extremities, it is evanescent but usually presents with fever. Nodules are not seen in adults and present only quite rarely even in children. Sydenham's chorea (St. Vitus' dance) has occurred in up to half of afflicted children in the past but occurs in less than 5% today. When present, it is usually bilateral and characterized by abrupt, purposeless movements, which disappear with sleep.

Diagnosis: Lab data usually show evidence of previous streptococcal infection. Cultures can be positive and are important in establishing the diagnosis. ESR and C-reactive protein are usually elevated. Synovial fluid evaluation can commonly show significant numbers of inflammatory cells. Although complements are also reduced in the fluid, this is a nonspecific finding and probably ought not to be measured. Occasionally, mild abnormalities in hepatic function are seen. Diagnosis can sometimes be difficult because of the lack of absolutely distinguishing features.

Although originally designed for administrative purposes during World War II, the 1944 Jones criteria for the diagnosis of rheumatic fever have been revised. Like many diagnostic criteria, they remain most useful for diagnosis when applied to populations of patients rather than to individual patients.

The differential diagnosis should include Reiter's syndrome or reactive arthropathy. Lyme disease—a vasculopathy—and Kawasaki's disease can also be confused. In children, juvenile arthritis can mimic this, and even in adults, Still's disease can be quite difficult to distinguish.

Treatment: In general, the disease is self-limited. Chorea may develop as long as two months after the acute pharyngitis. Recurrences are most likely to occur in patients who had carditis during the initial episode, and they usually occur in the first two years. Treatment is best instituted with antimicrobials during the acute streptococcal pharyngeal disease. Once rheumatic fever is initiated, aspirin remains a reliable anti-inflammatory. Clear prospective studies with other NSAIDs are not available. Although glucocorticoids can usually be avoided, they can sometimes add significant benefit if carditis is present. Subsequently, antimicrobial prophylaxis remains important. This is best achieved with monthly administration of benzathine penicillin, although a more recent study suggests that perhaps an injection every three weeks may be most effective. Duration for prophylaxis remains unclear. Recent suggestions include continuation for five years after the last attack. Should rheumatic heart disease develop, then patients should receive indefinite prophylaxis.

Reference: Dajani AS, et al: The special writing group of the Committee on Rheumatic Fever, Endocarditis, and Kawasaki Disease of the Council on Cardiovascular Disease in the Young of the American Heart Association. Guidelines for the diagnosis of rheumatic fever; Jones criteria 1992 update. JAMA 68:2069–2073, 1992.

RHEUMATOID ARTHRITIS

Etiology and Clinical Manifestations

RA is a chronic systemic inflammatory disease characterized by nonsuppurative inflammation of diarthrodial joints. Although often accompanied by extra-articular manifestations, arthritis represents the major expression of the disorder. The name is attributed to Sir Alfred Garrod and was coined in an effort to distinguish the disease from gout. Recently revised diagnostic criteria are shown in the table that follows. Although helpful when applied to populations for study, they are less useful when applied to the diagnosis of individual patients.

1988 Revised ARA Criteria for Classification of Rheumatoid Arthritis*

CRITERIA	DEFINITION
Morning stiffness	Morning stiffness in and around the joints lasting at least 1 hr before maximal improvement
Arthritis of three or more joint areas	At least three joint areas have simultaneously had soft tissue swelling or fluid (not bony overgrowth alone) observed by a physician. The 14 possible joint areas are (right or left) PIP, MCP, wrist, elbow, knee, ankle, and MTP joints
Arthritis of hand joints	At least one joint area swollen as above in wrist, MCP, or PIP joint
Symmetric arthritis	Simultaneous involvement of the same joint areas (as in 2) on both sides of the body (bilateral involvement of PIP, MCP, or MTP joints is acceptable without absolute symmetry)
Rheumatoid nodules	Subcutaneous nodules, over bony prominences, or extensor surfaces, or in juxta-articular regions, observed by a physician
Serum rheumatoid factor	Demonstration of abnormal amounts of serum rheumatoid factor by any method that has been positive in less than 5% of normal control subjects

Table continued on next page.

1988 Revised ARA Criteria for Classification of Rheumatoid Arthritis* (Cont.)

CRITERIA	DEFINITION
Radiographic changes	Radiographic changes typical of RA on posteroanterior hand and wrist radiographs, which must include erosions or unequivocal bony decalcification localized to or most marked adjacent to the involved joints (osteoarthritis changes alone do not qualify)

*For classification purposes, a patient is said to have RA if he or she has satisfied at least four of the above seven criteria. Criteria 1 through 4 must be present for at least 6 weeks. Patients with two clinical diagnosis are not excluded. Designation as classic, definite, or probable rheumatoid arthritis is *not* to be made. PIP = proximal interphalangeal; MCP = metacarpophalangeal; MTP = metatarsophalangeal.

From Harris ED: Clinical features of rheumatoid arthritis. In Kelly WN, et al (eds): Textbook of Rheumatology, 4th ed. Philadelphia, W. B. Saunders, 1993, p 874, with permission.

RA has a worldwide distribution, with a prevalence rate of about 1%. Age of onset is commonly between 40 and 60, with a peak in the range of 45 to 54. Although both sexes are affected, RA is estimated to occur up to three times more commonly in women. Genetic factors play a role in the development of RA. This is clear based on familial clustering of disease, including increased incidence in monozygotic twins (concordance rate of about 30–50%). Most patients with RA carry HLA DR1 or DR4.

Lack of complete concordance even in monozygotic twins also suggests a role for environmental factors. The search for that exposure risk has been one of the most persistent hunts in all of rheumatic disease research. Epstein-Barr virus (EBV) has been suggested as a possible agent that might stimulate RA. Some homology has been demonstrated between a viral protein and a shared epitope on the third hypervariable region of $DR\beta_1$ of the DR4 and DR1 proteins. This raises the possibility that molecular mimicry may play a role in RA. The role of noninfectious environmental factors, including hormonal influences, has been explored.

Articular Involvement

The synovial membrane is the primary site of inflammation. Initially, the synovium becomes swollen and edematous, with proliferation of the synovial membrane. A mononuclear cell infiltrate, mostly of T lymphocytes, occurs. As the disease progresses, the synovial membrane grows into the joint (pannus) and is associated with destruction of articular cartilage and subchondral bone. The predominant cell in the synovial fluid is the PMN. Immune complexes and RF are detectable in synovial fluid. Synovial fluid glucose and complement are both known to be reduced.

The onset of disease is usually slow and insidious. Patients experience symmetric tenderness and swelling. Pain that is lessened with rest but stiffness after rest (gelling) remain cardinal features of the disease. Disease can begin in a single inflamed joint or be polyarticular. Onset in the winter or around the time of a stressful life event is common. Fatigue and weakness often precede classical articular swelling. Most commonly, patients experience exacerbations of joint pain and swelling followed by periods of relative calm. At the other end of the spectrum, patients can have persistent and unrelenting disease activity despite aggressive treatment, leading inexorably to joint destruction.

Joint involvement in the hands usually occurs in symmetric fashion. Distal interphalangeal joint (DIP) involvement occurs in up to a third of patients, casting doubt on the notion that this manifestation can help distinguish psoriatic arthritis from RA. Proximal interphalangeal (PIP) joint and metacarpophalangeal (MCP) joint involvement occurs in nearly all cases. Deformities of the hand occur because active inflammation leads to destruction and altered tendon mechanics. The swan neck deformity describes flexion at the MCP and DIP joints with extension at the PIP joints. This results from inflammation and subsequent contraction of muscles and tendons. Flexion contracture at the PIP with extension of the DIP is referred to as the boutonniere deformity. The pathogenesis of this deformity is thought to relate to an injury of the extensor tendon.

Wrist and carpal bones are often involved at presentation, and their destruction can lead to subluxation at the wrist. Ulnar styloid erosions are characteristic. Inflammation at the wrist can lead to median nerve compression with resultant carpal tunnel syndrome. Involvement of the forefoot is also common. Early in the disease, the metatarsal arch may collapse, leaving the second to fourth metatarsal heads to bear weight (rather than the first and fifth). Rheumatoid nodules may appear on the Achilles tendon and can rarely contribute to rupture. Ankle involvement is less common than foot involvement. The knees are ultimately affected in over 50% of RA patients. Erosion and mechanical instability may follow, also leading to gait instability. Baker's (popliteal) cyst formation commonly complicates long-standing RA of the knee.

When the axial skeleton is involved, it is generally confined to the cervical segments. When the odontoid becomes eroded, there can be subluxation at the atlantoaxial joint, leading to spinal cord compression.

Reference: Harris ED Jr: Rheumatoid arthritis: Pathophysiology and implications for therapy. N Engl J Med 322(18):1277–1289, 1990.

Extra-articular Manifestations

Although the primary expression of RA is arthritis, a number of nonarticular features of the illness can occur. Perhaps the most common extra-articular feature encountered is circulating RF. About 80% of patients with classical RA have these antibodies against the Fc portion of the Ig molecule (most commonly IgM, but all isotypes have been documented), but the exact role these factors play in the pathogenesis of RA is unclear. One study found that although volunteers receiving transfusions from patients with high-titer RF would seroconvert, no disease of any kind developed, and the RF cleared without sequelae. Although some have suggested that patients with high-titer RF have more aggressive disease, lack of circulating RF does not guarantee a mild course. In addition, it should be remembered that RF can be found in the circulation of patients with other conditions and is not diagnostic of RA.

Another extra-articular feature of RA consists of nodules, which are found in 30 to 40% of RA patients. Nodules are not unique to RA patients; similar lesions are found in patients with granuloma annulare and SLE. Gouty tophi can also be mistaken for rheumatoid nodules. The nodules are not found in patients without circulating RF. They appear nearly anywhere on the body, most often at sites of pressure (commonly on the elbows or, in bedridden patients, the occiput or the sacrum). They have been described in the eye, on heart valves, and in the lung. The nodules in the lung can often be mistaken for having an isolated carcinoma.

Histologically there is a central area of necrosis surrounded by palisading histiocytes, which in turn is surrounded by chronic inflammatory cells.

Vasculitis can complicate RA, most commonly presenting in patients with long-standing disease and high-titer RF. Early onset of vasculitis suggests aggressive disease and poor prognosis. Weight loss and fever can herald the onset of vasculitis, although the articular disease can be quiescent. The most common manifestations are cutaneous lesions such as digital infarctions and lower limb ulcerations. Active involvement of the heart and lungs is well described in association with the vasculopathy of RA. Renal and GI involvement are rare. The lesions may be indistinguishable from those of polyarteritis nodosa.

Pericardial involvement is the most common cardiac manifestation of RA. Up to 50% of seropositive nodular RA patients may have some evidence of pericardial inflammation when sensitive echocardiographic techniques are used, but this is rarely symptomatic, and progression to tamponade or constriction is uncommon. Other cardiac manifestations of RA include valvulitis, myocarditis, and coronary arteritis. Occasional rhythm disturbances have been reported, with heart block being the most common.

Pulmonary disease most commonly presents as pleuritis, developing in 20% of RA patients. Evaluation of pleural fluid shows changes similar to those in pericardial fluid, specifically, the presence of RF, high numbers of inflammatory cells, low glucose, and low levels of complement. Pulmonary rheumatoid nodules have been described. In coal miners unlucky enough to develop seropositive RA, pulmonary rheumatoid nodules, and interstitial pulmonary lung disease, the eponym Caplan's syndrome is applied. Fibrosing alveolitis with progression to pulmonary HTN has been documented. When compared to RA patients without interstitial disease, the mortality of patients with pulmonary disease is increased, with a 5-year survival of 50%. The rarest pulmonary complication of RA is bronchiolitis obliterans that presents abruptly—with short-windedness—and progresses rapidly to a fatal conclusion.

Ocular involvement usually occurs as scleritis or episcleritis. Scleral involvement in RA is rare. Nodules can be present, and scleral thinning and bluish scars can be seen. Perforation is a rare but serious complication.

Felty's syndrome—a complication of seropositive RA with splenomegaly and granulocytopenia—occurs in 1 to 3% of RA patients. The etiology is unknown, but patients with Felty's syndrome are thought to have more severe articular disease and suffer more frequent extra-articular complications. Recurrent infections develop as the neutropenia becomes severe. Felty's syndrome in a patient without splenomegaly or without active synovial inflammation has been reported. Splenectomy has been successful in the acute setting, but long-term evaluation of this treatment has been disappointing.

References: Ziff M: The rheumatoid nodule. Arthritis Rheum 33(6):761–767, 1990.

Bacon PA: Extra-articular rheumatoid arthritis. In McCarty DJ (ed): Arthritis and Allied Conditions, 11th ed. Philadelphia, Lea & Febiger, pp 1967–1998, 1989.

General Treatment with Disease-Modifying Antirheumatic Drugs

There have been significant advances in recent years in the treatment of RA. The introduction of disease-modifying antirheumatic drugs (DMARDs) and improvement in surgical technique together contribute to improving the quality of life.

Perhaps the most important change, however, is in the approach to treatment rather than in the details of medication use. Traditionally applied DMARDs seem to have little impact on outcome. In fact, 50% of patients with 10 years of active disease are disabled. Although contrary to traditionally held views, RA does influence mortality. Thus, early institution of an aggressive approach to the treatment of RA has been advocated. It is hoped that early institution of DMARDs will allow less progression of disease, prevent disability, and lessen the disease's impact on mortality.

Glucocorticoids: In 1950 Dr. Philip Hench shared the Nobel prize for the "cure" of RA with glucocorticoids. The positive effects were profound and easily demonstrated, but the toxicities were nearly as dramatic. The development of Cushing's syndrome, loss of bone mass because of accelerated osteoporosis, and associated osteonecrosis were among the most devastating toxicities. Despite these problems, when used judiciously in low doses orally, intra-articularly, or occasionally parenterally, the positive effects often outweigh the negative. Deflazacort, an analogue of prednisone not yet available in the United States, was demonstrated to be equal to prednisone in efficacy but with fewer adverse effects on both glucose and bone metabolism.

Gold: Earlier this century, RA was assumed to be due to chronic infection. Thus, when experimental information suggested that gold might be useful in treating TB, it was a natural theoretical extension to investigate its usefulness in chronic arthritis. Currently, both injectable and oral preparations are available and have efficacy in treating RA. Recently, some have questioned the usefulness of chrysotherapy-based efficacy, toxicity, cost, and the monitoring necessary.

IM chrysotherapy is initiated with a test dose of 10 mg. If tolerated, a repeat dose of 25 mg is given in 1 week. Most regimens then recommend subsequent weekly 50-mg doses. Response often occurs once a cumulative dose of 500 mg has been reached. Subsequently, the interval between injections is increased, and a maintenance schedule of 50 mg monthly is most commonly used, although one published study found equal efficacy using 25-mg doses. Oral gold has been touted as less toxic.

Toxicity can be serious, and careful monitoring is required. Mucocutaneous toxicities including aphthous stomatitis and rash are most common. An unusual reaction consisting of flushing, vertigo, and shortness of breath called the nitritoid reaction is associated with injectable gold sodium thiomalate and requires a change to another formulation. Proteinuria can occur in up to 10% of patients receiving IM gold, and thus UA should be performed prior to each injection. Bone marrow depression with thrombocytopenia, granulocytopenia, and rarely aplastic anemia are the most serious toxicities. CBC monitoring before each injection is critical. Diarrhea may occur at the institution of oral gold treatment but responds to an increase in dietary bulk together with dose reduction.

Antimalarials: These drugs have been shown to interfere with antigen-antibody complexes, with nucleic acid biosynthesis, and with the function of lymphocytes and monocytes. The exact mechanism of action for these drugs is unknown. Currently, chloroquine, quinacrine, and hydroxychloroquine are available. Hydroxychloroquine in doses of 200 mg BID is most commonly used in the United States.

Ocular toxicities include retinal staining, corneal deposits, and ciliary body dysfunction. Long-standing retinal lesions are rare but may not be reversible, and they require regular ophthalmologic reviews. Nonocular toxicities include myopathy and some mild skin pigmentary changes.

D-penicillamine: D-penicillamine was first used in patients with RA after it was shown to cause dissociation of certain macroglobulins, including RF. Reduction in RF titers was observed, and clinical studies have confirmed its efficacy. As with gold and the antimalarials, the exact mechanism of effectiveness remains unknown. Side effects are remarkably similar to those of gold, including rash and mucous membrane involvement. Bone marrow suppression (most commonly thrombocytopenia) is reported. Proteinuria is present in up to 20% of patients. Discontinuation of the drug is required with onset of toxicity.

Methotrexate (MTX): MTX's antifolate action is hypothesized to be the source of its effectiveness. MTX leads to a reduction in circulating RF titers but not to significant changes in total number or percentage of mononuclear cells or their subsets. Without evidence of dramatic impact on either the humoral or cellular arms of the immune system, some have hypothesized that MTX functions as an effective anti-inflammatory drug rather than as an immunomodulator.

Whatever the mechanism of action, however, it is one of the most efficacious DMARDs available. It begins to reduce the number of painful and swollen joints within 4 to 6 weeks. Doses vary from about 7.5 to 15 mg administered once weekly. Although the oral preparation is usually well tolerated, occasionally patients benefit from parenteral administration. Toxicity includes stomatitis, alopecia, bone marrow suppression, and idiopathic pulmonary toxicity. Finally, inflammation and scaring of the liver may occur with MTX. Data strongly suggest that alcohol consumption increases the likelihood of this complication.

Azathioprine (AZA): Some have suggested that AZA's inhibition of monocyte function may be responsible for its effect on the immune system and thus its efficacy in RA. The primary toxicity is bone marrow suppression. Less commonly, hepatopathy or drug fever can occur.

Cyclophosphamide: Cyclophosphamide is one of the few medications that have truly been shown to be disease modifying or remittive, but it is also one of the most toxic. Short-term toxicities include bone marrow suppression, nausea, vomiting, and hemorrhagic cystitis (whose incidence can be reduced with aggressive hydration and concomitant use of mesna). Long-term risks include the development of bladder carcinoma, lymphoma, or leukemia.

Cyclosporine A (CSA): CSA is a noncytotoxic immunomodulatory drug that inhibits activation of the T-helper/inducer lymphocyte. Although not currently approved by the U.S. Food and Drug Administration for RA, several trials have shown significant clinical improvement. Patients with the greatest immune deficit seemed most responsive to this medication. Investigators noted redevelopment of the original defective lymphocyte function when CSA treatment was withdrawn. Renal insufficiency (maybe due to concomitant NSAID use), HTN, and hirsuitism often lead to its discontinuation.

Fish Oils: Arachidonic acid is the precursor of prostaglandins (E_2) and leukotrienes (B_4), which have potent proinflammatory effects. Substituted dietary omega-3 fatty acids (the principal component of fish oil) competitively inhibits arachidonic acid utilization and becomes a substrate for production of alternative products (prostacyclin I_3, leukotriene B_5, and thromboxane A_3), which are less effective mediators of inflammation. One study of patients with active RA compared dietary supplementation with two different dosages of fish oil and olive oil (placebo). The number of tender joints and number of swollen joints decreased in high and low groups compared to placebo. No changes in hemoglobin, ESR, or RF were noted. Little toxicity was noted, although a change in body odor is recognized.

Immunomodulators: Because RA patients have large numbers of activated T lymphocytes infiltrating the synovium and because previous treatment regimens aimed at reduction in T-cell populations (thoracic duct drainage, leukapheresis, total lymphoid irradiation, and CSA use) have led to clinical improvement, the use of monoclonal antibodies to modify T-cell populations in the treatment of patients with RA has been undertaken. Several investigators have administered anti-CD4 monoclonal antibody to patients with intractable RA, and clinical improvement was evident by day 7 and lasted up to 6 months. Adverse effects included chills and fever (lymphokine-release syndrome) and rash or urticaria.

$DAB_{486}IL-2$ is a protein product of a fusion gene. The resulting protein contains diphtheria toxin fused to IL-2. Because activated cells have increased IL-2 receptors, these fusion proteins selectively bind to these cells and reduce this population. In one small study, mean grip strength improved compared to placebo.

New and advanced treatments for RA are constantly being found and studied. Ultimately, however, joint replacement remains an effective way of maintaining function or reducing pain. Judiciously applied rest, heat, and cold modalities can provide significant relief of symptoms, although they do not change the long-term outcome of disease.

Reference: Skeith KJ, et al: New horizons in the medical treatment of rheumatoid arthritis. Curr Opin Rheum 4:365–371, 1992.

RHINITIS, ALLERGIC

Allergic rhinitis may occur seasonally—when a susceptible patient is exposed to pollens and grasses—or perennially—when allergens exist constantly in the environment (such as dust mites or molds). Symptoms include nasal congestion; sneezing; nasal discharge; itchiness of the eyes, nose, and palate; and sore throat. Symptoms usually begin in childhood but can occur at any age. Patients with allergic rhinitis are susceptible to recurrent upper respiratory infections and sinusitis.

On physical exam, the nasal mucosa is usually pale and boggy and the eyes may appear inflamed. There are usually no signs of infection unless the patient has a coexisting viral infection or sinusitis. Skin testing can be used to detect the specific allergen.

Symptoms of allergic rhinitis are best relieved by avoidance of the allergen. Sometimes this requires meticulous attention to the home environment, particularly if the patient is allergic to dusts and molds. Medications such as antihistamines (terfenadine and chlorpheniramine) and decongestants (ephedrine, pseudoephedrine, and phenylpropanolamine) are helpful. If nasal spray decongestants are used, patients should limit their use to 3 to 4 days to avoid an increase in symptoms due to rhinitis medicatosum. Intranasal corticosteroid sprays are particularly helpful for these patients. Patients who are unable to avoid allergen exposure and have persistent symptoms may need immunotherapy.

Reference: Approach to the patient with chronic nasal congestion and discharge. In Goroll AH, et al (eds): Primary Care Medicine: Office Evaluation and Management of the Adult Patient. Philadelphia, J.B. Lippincott, 1987.

RING-ENHANCING LESIONS ON CT AND MRI SCANS

The most common causes of ring enhancement are metastatic neoplasm or infectious brain abscess (bacterial, fungal, parasitic, or TB). Ring enhancement with contrast on brain CT or MRI scans usually implies disruption of the blood-brain barrier. However, lesions that initially enhance homogeneously may develop central necrosis as they enlarge, changing their enhancement pattern to peripheral or ringlike. All of the following can cause ring-enhancing lesions:

Causes of Ring-Enhancing Lesions

Infections
  Bacteria: aerobes (*Staphylococcus, Streptococcus*), anaerobes (*Bacteroides, Streptococcus*), Lyme disease, syphilis
  Mycobacteria and higher bacteria: TB, *Actinomyces, Nocardia*
  Fungi: *Aspergillus, Blastomyces, Candida, Coccidioides, Cryptococcus, Mucor, Paracoccidioides, Sporothrix*
  Parasites: *Amoeba, Echinococcus, Schistosoma, Taenia solium* (cysticercosis), *Toxoplasma*
Neoplasms
  Primary: astrocytoma, chordoma, choroid plexus tumor, craniopharyngioma, ependymoma, ganglioneuroma, glioblastoma multiforme, hamartoma, hemangioblastoma, lymphoma, neuroblastoma, teratoma
  Metastatic: breast, choriocarcinoma, colon, hepatoma, lung, lymphoma, melanoma, prostate, renal-cell carcinoma
Miscellaneous
  Vascular lesions: giant aneurysm, hematoma, infarct
  Other: lymphomatoid granulomatosis, multiple sclerosis (rarely), radiation necrosis, sarcoidosis, Wegener's granulomatosis

The characteristics of the MRI or CT image can help to narrow the list of possibilities. Benign CNS tumors typically lack surrounding edema and tend to have homogeneous or heterogeneous contrast enhancement. In addition, many of the CNS tumors are found in characteristic locations (e.g., ependymoma, craniopharyngioma). Very few primary CNS tumors present as multiple lesions (these include hamartomas, glioblastoma multiforme, and lymphoma). Malignant melanoma has a characteristic appearance on MRI (hyperintense on short TR/TE images and isointense on long TR/TE images).

CT or MRI can also provide clues that help to distinguish brain abscess from malignant neoplasm. Ring enhancement of a brain abscess is usually smooth and thin walled and may be thinner along the medial margin of the lesion. Enhancement around brain metastases tends to be thick and/or nodular. A mature brain abscess develops a collagen capsule that appears on MRI as a low-intensity ring on the unenhanced T2 weighted image. This is not seen in malignant lesions.

References: Salzman C: Value of the ring-enhancing sign in differentiating intracerebral hematomas and brain abscesses. Arch Intern Med 147:951–952, 1987.

Quisling RG: Neoplasms, cysts and other focal intracranial masses, and intracranial inflammations and infestation. In Correlative Neuroradiology, 2nd ed. New York, John Wiley & Sons, 1985, pp 339–409.

S

SARCOIDOSIS

Sarcoidosis is a systemic illness that affects multiple body organs and is pathologically associated with noncaseating granulomas. These granulomata are not diagnostic, and they can be seen in other illnesses including fungal disease, brucellosis, and Hodgkin's disease. The incidence is slightly higher in women than men, and onset is usually before age 40. In the United States it has been recognized with a higher frequency in African-Americans than in whites, but this association does not hold on a worldwide basis, with about 79% of cases being diagnosed in whites.

Although the etiology is unknown, a number of points can be made about the mechanism of disease production. Evaluation of T-cell population in bronchoalveolar lavage has shown an increased number of helper T cells (CD4+). This is in sharp contrast to their reduced levels in peripheral circulation. Current hypothesis holds that macrophages are stimulated by an unknown antigen and that they secrete interleukin I (IL-1), leading to activation and recruitment of T cells. Activated T cells secrete IL-2, leading to continued T-cell activation and recruitment of monocytes, in turn leading to the formation of granuloma.

Sarcoidosis most commonly affects the lungs and is recognized by hilar adenopathy and pulmonary parenchymal involvement. A staging system based on the CXR has been established. In stage I disease, bilateral hilar adenopathy alone is present. Stage II patients have both hilar adenopathy and pulmonary parenchymal involvement. Stage III patients have parenchymal involvement only. The staging is both descriptive and prognostic. Only 25% of patients with stage I disease will have continued activity (or progression) after 2 years. Patients with stage I disease also have a much lower incidence of extrapulmonary involvement. Patients presenting with stage II disease are more likely to be symptomatic, and only half will have remission after 2 years of disease activity. Presentation with stage III disease is uncommon. Two-thirds of stage III patients will still have active disease after 2 years.

Many patients are asymptomatic (especially with stage I disease), and diagnosis can be established only after a workup that is initiated because of an abnormality found on an incidentally obtained CXR. The most common clinical manifestations include fatigue and generalized malaise. Pulmonary symptoms include shortness of breath and cough. Lofgren's syndrome defines a subset of patients presenting acutely with fever, erythema nodosum, hilar adenopathy, and intense arthralgia. Musculoskeletal manifestations are relatively uncommon, but asymptomatic granulomas can be found in muscle. Occasionally, tender or palpable nodules are noted. A proximal myopathy has also been described. When hypercalcemia also complicates sarcoidosis, involved muscles can show some calcification. Patients with sarcoidosis and myopathy do have elevated creatine phosphokinase levels, and muscle biopsy can be diagnostic.

Sarcoid nodules in the muscles can be visualized with MRI, although MRI is not diagnostic in itself. Bone or osseous lesions, mainly in the small bones of the hands and feet, occur in less than 15% of patients. Phalangeal cysts may be helpful in diagnosis, but they are not unique. Lytic lesions and large cysts of the vertebral bodies are seen. The cortex of bone is usually intact, but occasionally granulomas (which are felt to be the source of the cysts) do erode into the joints. When these destructive bony lesions are associated with nodular cutaneous masses, a clinical picture of dactylitis sometimes called lupus pernio may be present. Articular involvement occurs in about 5% of patients and can rarely be the initial manifestation. Ankle and knees are the most common joints involved. The joints can be swollen, and the synovial fluid often has an inflammatory appearance. Cultures are negative and no crystals are noted. Subcutaneous nodules can be found in the synovium. Heel pain is another characteristic rheumatic finding in sarcoidosis. Vasculitis, affecting large and small blood vessels, can occur in sarcoid. Occasionally, sarcoidosis can affect exocrine glands, mimicking Sjögren's syndrome. The diagnosis is made on biopsy of a salivary gland and transbronchial lung biopsy.

The diagnosis is based on both recognition of the clinical features and demonstration of noncaseating granulomas in tissue (most often the lung). Other causes of tissue granuloma and hilar adenopathy should be excluded. These can include TB or fungal infections such as histoplasmosis. Lymphoma or metastatic cancer can occasionally mimic sarcoidosis in presentation. Angiotensin-converting enzymes (ACEs) are often elevated in patients with active pulmonary disease, including sarcoidosis, making ACEs more helpful as a disease activity marker than as a diagnostic marker.

Glucocorticoids are generally used in patients with active symptomatic disease. Modest doses can usually control symptoms, and treatment can usually be withdrawn in about 1 year. Occasionally, higher doses are required to treat complications such as hypercalcemia.

Reference: Thomas PD, et al: Current concepts of pathogenesis of sarcoidosis. Am Rev Respir Dis 135:747, 1987.

SCHILLING TEST

The standard Schilling test measures vitamin B_{12} absorption and is used to detect intrinsic-factor deficiency in patients with pernicious anemia. The test results are often abnormal in patients with genetic defects in vitamin B_{12} absorption; with bacterial overgrowth of the small bowel; following extensive destruction, resection, or bypass of the terminal ileum; and with pancreatic insufficiency.

Stage one of the standard Schilling test consists of an oral dose of radiolabeled vitamin B_{12} given simultaneously with an IM injection of 1 mg nonradiolabeled B_{12}. The urine is collected for 24 hrs and the amount of radioactivity is measured. Patients with normal absorption of B_{12} and normal renal function will excrete greater than 7% of the radioactively labeled B_{12} in 24 hrs.

In **stage two,** the test is repeated after oral administration of 60 mg intrinsic factor. Patients with pernicious anemia normalize the level of urinary radiolabeled B_{12}.

Small intestinal bacterial overgrowth may cause B_{12} malabsorption and an abnormal result in stage one of the Schilling test due to bacterial utilization of the vitamin. This is not corrected with intrinsic factor in stage two. After 1 week of treatment with a broad-spectrum antibiotic (**stage three**) to eliminate the intestinal bacteria, stage one of the Schilling test should normalize. Normal B_{12} absorption also requires normal pancreatic exocrine function. Pancreatic proteases are required for the cleavage of vitamin B_{12} from R-protein. If pancreatic insufficiency exists, B_{12} malabsorption may occur. Normalization of B_{12} absorption after administration of pancreatic enzyme therapy (**stage four**) suggests a pancreatic origin of B_{12} malabsorption.

SEIZURES

Seizures can be classified into four major types:

1. Generalized
   A. Absence
   B. Tonic-clonic
2. Partial
   A. Simple
   B. Complex

Generalized absence seizures, also called **petit mal,** occur almost exclusively in childhood and are very rare in adults. They usually consist of brief lapses of consciousness, or staring spells, that occur without warning, that last several seconds, and that result in an abrupt return to reality, lacking any postictal confusion or other deficit. Although brief, these spells may occur hundreds of times per day, considerably disrupting daily function. The EEG shows a very characteristic pattern of spikes and slow waves occurring at a rate of 3/sec diffusely over the brain. Treatment is usually successful, using either ethosuximide (Zarontin) or valproic acid (Depakote).

Generalized tonic-clonic seizures, also called **grand mal** seizures, are what most laypersons conceive a seizure to be, namely, the sudden onset of stiffening (tonic) contraction of the muscles of the arms and legs, with accompanying loss of consciousness. There may be a cry (as air is forced out of the lungs) and evacuation of the bladder. Muscle activity gradually gives way to clonic jerking followed by cessation of the seizure, usually within 90 to 120 sec. There is seldom a preceding aura. Consciousness is generally not regained immediately but may take several minutes, or even hours. Postictally, there are general confusion and lethargy. Primary generalized seizures are most common in childhood and may respond particularly to valproic acid. In adults, seizures with these clinical features often arise from a particular focus of epileptic activity, such as that caused by a stroke or a brain tumor, and they may therefore be referred to as secondarily generalized seizures. Other causes include drugs (especially alcohol and cocaine), trauma, and metabolic derangements. Treatment may be most effective with phenytoin (Dilantin), carbamazepine (Tegretol), or phenobarbital.

Partial simple seizures are also known as **focal seizures** because they involve only one isolated region of the cortex. For instance, damage in the motor strip may trigger neuronal firing and seizures affecting the opposite face, arm, or leg. The seizure activity does not spread, but rather remains localized, so that only a focal area is affected and consciousness is thus never lost. Usually, such seizures arise in the context of a focal brain lesion, such as a stroke, tumor, or scar from head trauma. Phenytoin, carbamazepine, primidone (Mysoline), and phenobarbital may all provide excellent control.

Partial complex seizures are also known as **psychomotor seizures** or temporal lobe seizures, for they often arise from the temporal lobe. Although the seizure discharge remains localized, consciousness is impaired if not lost completely. However, motor manifestations may be minimal, without tonic-clonic jerking, but rather with automatisms consisting of lip smacking, staring, pulling at clothes, or other automatic semipurposeful actions. The seizure may begin as an aura, often consisting of an unusual odor or a mental disturbance, such as déjà vu. Within a few seconds, consciousness is lost and the patient shows automatic movements. The symptoms may persist for several minutes, after which there is a postictal period of confusion, bewilderment, and fatigue. Partial complex seizures are the commonest seizure in adulthood and usually are caused by focal damage in the temporal or frontal lobes, such as from a stroke, tumor, or head injury. Often, they can be traced back to perinatal hypoxia or birth difficulties. Therapy is with carbamazepine,

Major Properties of Anticonvulsants

DRUG	HALF-LIFE (hr)	STEADY STATE (days)	DOSE (mg)	THERAPEUTIC RANGE (mg/dl)	SIDE EFFECTS
Carbamazepine (Tegretol)	10–30	10	400–1,800	4—12	Diplopia, dizziness $\downarrow$Sodium = SIADH Myelosuppression Hepatic Rash Psychotropic
Phenytoin (Dilantin)	9–40	7–21	150–600	10–20	Nystagmus, ataxia Uglification:$\uparrow$gums, facies, hair Myelosuppression Hepatic Rash Lymphoma Neuropathy Lupus syndrome Teratogenic
Phenobarbital	50–160	30	30-240	15–45	Sedation Hepatic Rash
Primidone (Mysoline)	4–12	30 for øbarb	250–1,500	5–15	Sedation
Valproic acid (Depakote)	8–20	4	600–3,000	50– No ceiling	Nausea Weight gain Tremor Alopecia Hepatic, $\uparrow$ammonia Pancreatitis $\downarrow$Platelets Teratogenic
Ethosuximide (Zarontin)	20–70	7–14	500–1,500 (10–25 mg/kg/day)	40–100	Nausea Sedation

phenytoin, primidone, or phenobarbital, but these are the most difficult seizures to control completely. Occasionally, refractory patients may need temporal lobectomy.

The major medications for adult seizures are phenytoin, carbamazepine, primidone, and phenobarbital. These medications differ in their pharmacokinetics, toxicity, convenience, and expense, but all are approximately equal in their ability to suppress seizures. Decisions regarding proper drug management are thus based less on efficacy than on other properties.

References: Scheuer ML, et al: The evaluation and treatment of seizures. N Engl J Med 323:1468, 1990.

Gram L: Epileptic seizures and syndromes. Lancet 336:161, 1990.

SENSITIVITY, SPECIFICITY, AND PREDICTIVE VALUE OF DIAGNOSTIC TESTS

The terms *sensitivity, specificity,* and *positive* or *negative predictive values* are frequently used in the assessment of a test and its ability to rule in or rule out a given condition (also called the accuracy of the test). To be able to use these values, it is necessary to understand how they are derived. Because a test can be positive or negative (if we disregard inconclusive results) and a patient either has or does not have a condition, there are four possible outcomes in any test situation. These are reflected as follows:

	Disease Present	Disease Absent	
Test +	a	b	a = true positive b = false positive
Result −	c	d	c = false negative d = true negative

The above terms are derived from the table. Their definitions and derivations are as follows:

$$\text{Sensitivity} = \frac{a}{a + c} = \text{the percentage of patients with the disease in whom the test is positive (``\% positive in disease'')}$$

$$\text{Specificity} = \frac{d}{b + d} = \text{the percentage of persons without the disease in whom the test is negative (``\% negative in health'')}$$

$$\text{Positive Predictive Value} = \frac{a}{a + b} = \text{the percentage of patients with a positive test result who actually do have the disease}$$

$$\text{Negative Predictive Value} = \frac{d}{c + d} = \text{the percentage of patients with a negative test result who really do not have the disease}$$

SEPSIS

Sepsis results from overwhelming tissue or bloodstream invasion by certain microorganisms and their toxic products. As septic shock has a 50 to 75% mortality rate, prompt recognition and treatment of the syndrome are essential.

According to a recent consensus, **sepsis** is defined as a response to infection manifested by two or more of the following conditions:

- Temperature >38°C or <36°C
- Heart rate >90 bpm
- Respiratory rate >20 breaths/min or P_aCO_2 <32 mm Hg
- WBC count >12,000 cells/mm^3, <4,000 cells/mm^3, or >10% immature (band) forms

Severe sepsis is characterized as sepsis associated with organ dysfunction, hypoperfusion, or hypotension. Lack of perfusion of vital organs in sepsis leads to lactic acidosis, oliguria, and acute altered mental status, among other findings.

Septic shock is defined as severe sepsis with hypotension (systolic BP of <90 mm Hg or a reduction of >40 mm Hg from baseline without other causes for hypotension).

I. **Organisms causing septic shock**
   A. Gram-negative bacteria: *Escherichia coli, Klebsiella, Enterobacter, Proteus, Pseudomonas, Serratia, Neisseria*
   B. Gram-positive bacteria: *Staphylococcus, Streptococcus pneumoniae*
   C. Uncommon: opportunistic fungi, mycobacteria, *Falciparum malaria,* dengue, herpesviruses
II. **Pathophysiology**
   A. Microbial factors
      1. Gram-negative organisms: endotoxin (lipopolysaccharide)
      2. Gram-positive organisms: peptidoglycans, exotoxins (staphylococcal toxic shock protein)
   B. Host factors
      1. Cytokines (TNF,[1] IL-1, IL-6, and IL-8)
      2. Coagulation cascade
      3. Kinin system, vasoactive peptides (histamine)
      4. Complement cascade
      5. Release of enzymes and oxidants from PMNs
      6. Acute-phase proteins synthesized by the liver
      7. Leukocyte and endothelial cell adhesion molecule expression
      8. Catecholamines
      9. Arachidonic acid metabolites

---

[1]Tumor necrosis factor is believed to be the principal mediator of septic shock.

III. **Signs and symptoms of sepsis**

Acrocyanosis	Ileus	Organ dysfunction
Capillary leakage	Lactic acidosis	Skin lesions
Chills	Leukocytosis	Somnolence
↓↓Systemic vascular	Mental status changes	Tachycardia
resistance	Myalgias	Tachypnea
Fever or hypothermia	Myocardial depression	Vasodilation
Hypotension	Nausea, vomiting, diarrhea	

IV. **Organ dysfunction, often multiple**
 A. Brain: mental status changes
 B. Cardiovascular: functional hypovolemia (low SVR, ↑ cardiac output), refractory hypotension
 C. Lungs: ARDS, respiratory failure
 D. Kidneys: oliguria, azotemia, acute tubular necrosis
 E. GI: hemorrhagic necrosis of the intestine
 F. Liver: hepatic necrosis
 G. Hematopoietic: thrombocytopenia, DIC
V. **Diagnosis**
 A. Blood cultures positive in 50–60%; other site of infection may be documented
 B. Gram stain of buffy coat
VI. **Treatment**[2]
 A. IV antibiotics
 B. Hemodynamic support: fluid resuscitation, pressors, Swan-Ganz catheter to assess volume status
 C. Respiratory support: oxygen, RBC transfusion to maintain oxygen-carrying capacity, intubation for respiratory failure, PEEP
 D. Acidosis: sodium bicarbonate for pH <7.20
 E. DIC: replacement of clotting factors and platelets for major episodes of bleeding
 F. Renal support: diuretics, low-dose dopamine, dialysis for renal failure
 G. Experimental modalities: anti-endotoxin antibodies, ibuprofen, anti-TNFα antibodies

---

[2]Note that the use of glucocorticoids has not been shown to improve survival.
Reference: American College of Chest Physicians/Society of Critical Care Medicine Consensus Conference: Definitions for sepsis and organ failure and guidelines for the use of innovative therapies in sepsis. Crit Care Med 20:864–874, 1992.

SEXUALLY TRANSMITTED DISEASES

There are many infectious diseases that are transmitted through sexual contact, including gonorrhea, syphilis, chancroid, granuloma inguinale, nongonococcal urethritis (NGU), pelvic inflammatory disease (PID), lymphogranuloma venereum (LGV), herpes simplex virus infection, hepatitis B, hepatitis C, human immunodeficiency virus (HIV) infection, chlamydial infection, and trichomonas infection. Common STDs seen in the ambulatory setting are listed in the table that follows. All patients with an STD should be screened for HIV infection and syphilis.

Sexually Transmitted Diseases

INFECTION	SIGNS AND SYMPTOMS	DIAGNOSIS	TREATMENT
Neisseria gonorrhoeae			
Urethra	Dysuria, urinary urgency, pyuria, hematuria, lower abdominal discomfort, purulent urethral exudate	Gram-neg. diplo-cocci in PMNs on Gram stain;[1] culture	Ceftriaxone 250 mg IM[2] plus treatment for *Chlamydia*
Cervix	Vaginal discharge, lower pelvic pain, abnormal uterine bleeding	Culture	Same as above
Pharynx	Sore throat, exudate	Culture	Same as above
Anorectal	Anal discharge, tenesmus, pain	Culture	Same as above

Table continued on next page.

Sexually Transmitted Diseases (Cont.)

INFECTION	SIGNS AND SYMPTOMS	DIAGNOSIS	TREATMENT
Systemic	Joint pain, fever, tenosynovitis, hemorrhagic papules	Culture	Ceftriaxone 1.0 gm IV daily for 7–10 days[3]
Chlamydia trachomatis			
Urethra or cervix	Lower abdominal pain, dysuria, mucopurulent discharge, fever	Fluorescent antibody stain or enzyme immunoassay	Doxycycline 100 mg BID for 10 days[4]
Herpes simplex			
Penis, vagina, cervix	Prodrome: fever, malaise, lymphadenopathy, burning, paresthesia. Lesions: painful, shallow ulcerations on penis or vagina	Culture or cytological smear	Acyclovir 200 mg 5 times a day for 7 days (initial attack) or 5 days (recurrence), analgesia; moist compresses
Trichomonas vaginalis			
Urethra	Dysuria, urethral discharge, dysuria, urinary frequency and urgency	Saline wet prep	Metronidazole 2 gm once
Vagina	Vaginal burning, pruritus, frothy discharge, dysuria, urinary frequency and urgency	Saline wet prep	Same
Condyloma acuminata			
Penis or anorectal	1- to 2-cm flat or coalesced warts	Physical exam	20% tincture of podophyllum applied to involved area
Cervix or vagina	Vaginal discharge, 1-to 2-cm flat or coalesced warts	Physical exam	Same
Treponema pallidum			
Primary	Painless ulcer with raised edges at site of sexual contact (chancre)	Dark field exam, serology	Penicillin G benzathine 2.4 million U IM[5]
Secondary	Maculopapular rash usually on palms and soles, lymphadenopathy, fever, condyloma latum	Dark field exam, serology	Same
Tertiary	Multiple symptoms depending on organ system involved	Serology; CSF exam	Penicillin G 2–4 million U IV q 4 hrs × 10–14 days[5]

[1]Useful only for diagnosis of infection in men. Cultures should be obtained in women.

[2]Alternatives: spectinomycin 2 gm IM or ciprofloxacin 500 mg orally once.

[3]May use IV for 2–3 days, then complete 7- to 10-day course with cefuroxime axetil 500 mg orally BID.

[4]Alternative: erythromycin 500 mg orally QID × 7 days.

[5]Alternative therapies may be less effective. Patients with concurrent HIV infection may need additional therapy.

SHINGLES

Shingles represent the reactivation of latent herpes zoster infection. By age 15, 90% of the U.S. population will have had the primary infection (chickenpox) and harbor the virus. Shingles begins with a prodrome of pain or hyperaesthesia along the affected dermatome. There are usually low-grade fever and malaise for 3 to 5 days followed by the eruption of pruritic vesicles that crust over and heal in the next 2 to 3 weeks. About 50% of the time it is in the thoracic area. With increased age comes an increase in frequency of trigeminal nerve involvement. The virus can spread hematogenously, not only to the skin but also to visceral organs. The onset in otherwise apparently healthy, younger (<50 years) patients should lead to HIV testing, but involved cancer evaluations are not warranted.

Treatment: In cases of disseminated disease or in posttransplant or profoundly immunocompromised persons, the best treatment is acyclovir. In a normal, younger person with localized lesions, treatment with acyclovir is probably unnecessary. Acyclovir (400–800 mg IV or PO five times a day) should be started in the first 2 days (within 48 hrs of the appearance of the skin lesions); it will result in a decrease in the formation of new lesions, in the duration of pain, and in the incidence of postherpetic neuralgia. The role of a vaccine to prevent reactivation by boosting the immune system is unknown. Hypertonic soaks can be used to treat vesicles and erosions until crusting occurs (10- to 15-min soaks 4 or 5 times a day). If the lesions become purulent, then either topical or systemic antibiotics should be started. Prednisone (40 mg/day for 10–14 days) decreases both the pain and the risk of postherpetic neuralgia, but the risk/benefit ratio must be considered. If the dermatome involved is in the distribution of the ophthalmic nerve, steroids plus IV acyclovir should be started. This constitutes a relative emergency because blindness is frequently the end result. Postherpetic neuralgia is a major problem (see Postherpetic Neuralgia).

Reference: Straus SE: Shingles: Sorrows, salves, and solutions. JAMA 269:1836–1839, 1993.

SHORTNESS OF BREATH

Shortness of breath, or dyspnea, is a frightening and discomforting symptom for patients. Its causes are multiple, and the differential diagnosis can be aided by classifying the symptoms into several categories. Patients should be questioned about trauma, and the details about length of symptoms and precipitating factors should be obtained. Useful laboratory studies may include CXR, ABGs, and ECG. If indicated, PFTs and cardiac testing may yield significant information.

Management begins early, and immediate ventilatory assistance may be necessary in the presence of either apnea, reduced vital capacity less than twice the tidal volume in patients with neuromuscular diseases, somnolence in patients with COPD, or ARDS.

Physical exam should note the presence or absence of stridor or inspiratory wheezing, suggesting upper airway obstruction. Trauma to, or foreign body obstruction of, the upper airway causing respiratory compromise often requires early tracheostomy. Glottic edema can occur with a hypersensitivity reaction to drugs such as penicillin, food such as shellfish, or insect bites, or in the syndrome of hereditary angioedema. The most common cause of inspiratory stridor in children is infectious tracheobronchitis. In adults, acute epiglottitis with *Haemophilus influenzae* type B is preceded by a febrile upper airway infection. Chronic upper airway obstruction may be caused by cancer of the larynx or subglottis, fibrotic stenosis from previous trauma, vocal cord paralysis, or sarcoid or rheumatoid arthritis involving the larynx.

Expiratory stridor results when distal airways become narrowed. Tears in the trachea from trauma can narrow the lumen, and subcutaneous or mediastinal emphysema may be found on physical exam. Bronchoscopy is the best diagnostic tool. Acute allergic reactions in asthmatics can cause abrupt shortness of breath. Foreign bodies in the trachea, CHF, and PE may also cause expiratory wheezing.

Chronic wheezing is most often the result of COPD and occurs in most people after 20 or more pack-years of smoking. It is accompanied by chronic mucoid sputum production, and the CXR may show emphysema. Patients with bronchiectasis usually produce large amounts of purulent sputum. Increasing shortness of breath in a patient who already has COPD may indicate the development of an intrathoracic malignancy.

If physical exam reveals rales rather than wheezes and there is no history of trauma, acute CHF may account for shortness of breath. If fever is an accompanying symptom, pneumonia should be strongly considered. Both CXR and sputum examination are also useful. Both bacterial and tuberculous pneumonia can present in this way, and in immunocompromised patients, other unusual organisms such as *Pneumocystis* should be considered.

Diminished or absent breath sounds suggests increased intrapleural fluid or air, as in chylothorax, empyema, or pneumothorax. Hypotension in this setting should lead to the possibility of a tension pneumothorax. Gradual onset of severe shortness of breath in an asthmatic with diminished breath sounds on exam signifies acute respiratory decompensation, and such patients often need immediate intubation.

Shortness of breath with normal breath sounds may occur in the setting of trauma with fractured ribs or with fat embolism. Acute pulmonary embolism should also be considered, as should hyperventilation syndrome. Lung scans, if time permits, are helpful.

Shortness of breath on exertion is seen with COPD, primary pulmonary HTN, or pulmonary HTN secondary to multiple PEs. It can be seen with interstitial pulmonary diseases, such as sarcoidosis, eosinophilic granuloma, and idiopathic pulmonary fibrosis. It is also seen with failure of the respiratory muscles as occurs in myasthenia gravis and muscular dystrophy. (See also Dyspnea.)

SICKLE-CELL DISEASE

Hemoglobin S is caused by a single mutation that results in the replacement of glutamate by valine in the sixth amino acid of the beta chain of the protein. When hemoglobin S is deoxygenated, a gel or tactoid is formed, which results in distortion of the RBC into a sickle shape. In individuals homozygous for Hb S, repetitive deoxygenation causes irreversibly sickled erythrocytes. These are a hallmark of the sickle hemoglobinopathies and were first reported by Herrick in the peripheral blood of a black dental student from the West Indies.

The sickle hemoglobinopathies include homozygous SS, SC, S β-thalassemia, and other, less common conditions such as SD–Los Angeles. At birth, children are protected by high concentrations of fetal hemoglobin (Hb F), but within 6 months the manifestations of the disease may appear. Many states now have in place sickle screening programs that identify affected children and notify parents to seek appropriate medical attention.

The diagnosis may be suspected in patients with hemolytic anemia and characteristic sickle cells on the peripheral blood film. Hemoglobin electrophoresis confirms the diagnosis and is an important aid in the identification of double heterozygotes for Hb S and C or β-thalassemia.

Complications

Sickle-cell disease is marked by periodic vasoocclusive disease or crises (see later discussion). Organ dysfunction also occurs. The first loss is the spleen, which is usually infarcted to a nubbin within the first 6 years of life. During that time, children may experience sudden sequestration events that may be life threatening. The absence of the spleen also renders these children more susceptible to infection with encapsulated organisms, primarily pneumococci. Such children should receive penicillin prophylaxis, and all patients should receive a polyvalent pneumococcal vaccine. When patients present with fever, a high index of suspicion for pneumococcal sepsis should be maintained, particularly when hypotension is present. Prompt institution of antibiotics is necessary. Splenic sequestration, splenic infarction, and hyposplenism may be observed in adults with SC, SB_+, and SB_0 thalassemias.

Sickle-cell disease is also a hemolytic disorder marked by significant anemia, which is usually well tolerated. Chronic hemolysis is attended by the formation of pigment gallstones, indirect hyperbilirubinemia, and increased requirements for folate. Thus folate supplementation is the rule, and many patients experience symptomatic cholelithiasis and require cholecystectomy. Patients with chronic hemolysis do not tolerate infections with parvovirus B19, a virus with a relative predilection for erythroid progenitor cells. Infections with parvovirus result in a transient pure red cell aplasia, which is tolerated in hematologically normal individuals. Arrest of erythropoiesis in a hemolytic disorder such as sickle-cell disease is called an **aplastic crisis.** Such patients present with profound anemia with the nearly total absence of reticulocytes from the peripheral blood. Transfusions are lifesaving under these circumstances. As patients age, there is deterioration of certain organ systems. Renal failure is an increasingly important problem and a recent review suggests that HTN is an early sign. Hematuria and renal papillary necrosis are also seen. Aseptic necrosis of the femoral heads leads to significant disability, although hip replacement is often successful. Retinopathy is also a problem and necessitates periodic evaluation by an ophthalmologist.

Pregnancy is attended by a greater risk to mother and fetus, but many women with sickle-cell disease are able to have children. However, the pregnancy is best managed by those familiar with such high-risk individuals. Routine transfusion therapy during pregnancy, once the rule, has now become more selectively applied to women who are experiencing difficulty.

Sickle ankle ulcers are not as commonly seen now, but when they occur, they require a diligent effort on the part of the patient to change wet to dry dressings or manage an Unna's paste boot. Occasionally, systemic antibiotics are required if there are signs of either lymphangitis or fever. Some patients may improve with skin grafts, and if they do not, a trial of transfusion therapy in extremely recalcitrant ulcers may be undertaken.

Reference: Sergeant GR: Sickle Cell Disease. New York, Oxford University Press, 1985.

Crises

The most frequent complication of sickle-cell disease requiring hospitalization in the adult patient is the pain crisis. It seems logical to suppose that vasoocclusion is due to clogging of the microvasculature by rigid, irreversibly sickled cells, but the frequency of sickle pain does not correlate with the number of sickled cells and it is hard to understand why crises begin and end without specific treatment when irreversibly sickled cells are always present. The initiation and termination of sickle vasoocclusive crises are likely to be intimately linked to changes in the endothelium or in regulation of blood flow in the microvasculature.

Patients vary widely in the number, severity, and duration of these episodes, which may affect the back, abdomen, chest, or extremities. The pain is often quite severe and described as gnawing or boring. Crises may begin as pain localized to an area, then may subside only to appear elsewhere. Bone pain is also frequently part of a pain crisis. Occasional patients present with painful shin lesions that produce local swelling, tenderness, and warmth. This picture mimics superficial thrombophlebitis, although the exquisite tenderness is a distinguishing feature.

There is a group of well sickle-cell patients who are seldom seen in the ED, whereas another group with frequent crises accounts for one-third of hospital visits. In the group of older patients (over 20 years), mortality was increased in those with more frequent crises. Why some patients do badly while others do well and yet all of whom have the same homozygous disease is a puzzle. The influence of other genes (α-thalassemia, for example) or factors related to the microvasculature may be determinants of the severity of sickle-cell disease.

Once a crisis has begun, the duration is quite variable. Patients may treat themselves at home with acetaminophen or codeine. If the pain does not subside, treatment in the ED is sought. If there is no response to IM or IV narcotics after 2 to 6 hrs of treatment, then admission for continued administration of narcotics in sufficient doses to control pain is required. The duration of hospitalization may be short or prolonged—up to 3 weeks in some instances. If hospitalization is required, the typical stay is 1 week. Patients will return for additional treatment if discharged prematurely.

These patients face not only pain but also the anxiety that the physician in the emergency room will not treat the pain aggressively. ED personnel all too often label sickle-cell patients as ED abusers and drug seekers. The absence of objective clinical signs and the need to rely on the patient's history alone make it difficult for an inexperienced physician to feel comfortable with the need for frequent administration of morphine or meperidine. Control of precipitating factors offers limited benefit to most patients, although in some individuals, crises occur in the setting of infection, pregnancy, temperature changes, stress, acidosis, or dehydration. Hydration during the summer months is particularly important because most of these patients cannot concentrate urine well. When admitted for treatment of pain crises, patients need a brief administration of isotonic fluids, although most can tolerate oral liquids if the nursing staff is able to encourage them. Transfusion in the treatment of an ordinary pain crisis is unnecessary and may sensitize the recipient so that future transfusion therapy, when critically needed, will be hampered by difficulty in cross-matching blood.

Certain vasoocclusive phenomena require special care in evaluation and treatment and often require admission. Chest syndrome should be suspected when patients present with dyspnea in association with chest pain or chest wall tenderness. ABGs and a CXR are prudent steps. Vasoocclusion of the lung vasculature and pneumonia have similar appearance, so treatment with antibiotics is often rendered. If hypoxemia is present and cannot be corrected by administration of oxygen, then transfusions or an exchange transfusion is of benefit.

Priapism is a condition to be endured by men with sickle-cell anemia, and treatment of this condition is unsatisfactory. Some patients have an antecedent period of multiple brief episodes of painful tumescence (stuttering priapism). During the acute attack, very aggressive treatment of pain along with fluids may help. If the painful erection is sustained, consultation with a urologist and consideration of an exchange transfusion may improve matters. Unfortunately, impotence is a common outcome after one or more episodes of priapism.

Right upper quadrant abdominal pain is also a challenge for the physician and may be due to a sickle hepatic vasoocclusive process, hepatitis, or gallstones and cholelithiasis. Abdominal ultrasound examination represents an important diagnostic study.

CNS sickle-cell disease includes stroke, TIAs, aneurysm, and seizures and represents a true emergency in these patients. Both a careful evaluation by a neurologist and the early institution of exchange transfusion and continued transfusion therapy to maintain the sickle hemoglobin below 30 to 50% are essential in the management of sickle CNS disease.

The benefits of modern molecular biology have been slow to accrue to the treatment of sickle-cell disease. Some children have undergone successful allogeneic bone marrow transplantation, and positive results have been encouraging. However, many sickle-cell patients do relatively well for many years without this treatment, and so patient selection is difficult.

Certain drugs, such as hydroxyurea, can turn back the developmental switch that shifts hemoglobin F production in the fetus to adult hemoglobin S. This increase in hemoglobin F levels can reduce the sickling process.

References: Ballas SK: Treatment of pain in adults with sickle cell disease. Am J Hematol 34:49–54, 1990.

Rodgers GP, et al: Augmentation by erythropoietin of the fetal hemoglobin response to hydroxyurea in sickle cell disease. N Engl J Med 328:73–80, 1993.

SINUSITIS

Predisposing Factors for Sinusitis

Environmental	Systemic
Cigarette use	Cystic fibrosis
Altitude change (e.g., air travel)	Kartagener's syndrome
Environmental pollution	Nasotracheal intubation
Anatomic	Viral infection
Nasal polyps	Allergic rhinitis
Nasal septal deviation	Miscellaneous
Adenoid hypertrophy	Nasal decongestant abuse
Intranasal foreign bodies or tumors	Trauma

Diagnosis of Sinusitis

History
- Fever
- Purulent nasal drainage
- Facial pain over lower forehead (frontal sinuses) or upper cheek (maxillary sinuses) that increases when bending over

Physical examination
- Vital signs: elevated temperature, tachycardia
- General: appearance generally ill
- HEENT: Tenderness to palpation over lower forehead or upper cheek, opacity of involved sinuses with transillumination, purulent nasal drainage in nares

Laboratory tests
- Sinus x-rays showing mucosal thickening, sinus opacification, or air-fluid level
- CT scan of sinuses

Usual pathogens: *Haemophilus influenzae, Branhamella catarrhalis,* viruses (rare), *Streptococcus pneumoniae,* other streptococci, fungi (rare)

Treatment: oral or nasal decongestants (e.g., pseudoephedrine), analgesia, and antibiotics (for toxic patients): amoxicillin, trimethoprim-sulfamethoxazole, cephalosporin, amoxicillin-clavulanic acid, and erythromycin

SKIN CANCER

The generalist physician should examine the entire skin surface of all patients regularly for any suspicious lesions, particularly in the areas such as the back, posterior shoulder, and buttocks that are not easily examined by patients. Patients frequently ask about specific lesions. All patients should also receive counseling about sun exposure plus specific recommendations to wear a hat and long sleeves and to use sunscreen (at least 15 SPF) if exposed to the sun for a long period.

The various types of skin cancers include basal cell carcinoma (BCC), squamous cell carcinoma (SCC), and melanoma. Actinic keratoses, although benign, do have the potential to develop into malignancies. Malignant melanomas may also develop in preexisting nevi or moles.

Treatment of skin cancers centers on early detection while the lesion remains localized and amenable to resection. BCCs are the most common form of skin cancer and appear as slow-growing, pearly growths with telangiectasias covering the surface. They are caused by sunlight exposure and are therefore most common in sun-exposed areas, such as the face, neck, and forearms. BCCs rarely metastasize.

SCCs also occur in sun-exposed areas and frequently arise from actinic keratoses. Also, SCCs can be found in areas that had previous injury, such as leg ulcers, burns, and radiation-treated areas. Unlike BCCs, these cancers usually have scale and slight pigmentation. They bleed easily when scratched.

Melanomas are the most deadly type of skin cancer, but they may easily be confused with benign nevi. Any nevus that is darkly pigmented with an irregular outline or has bled should be carefully evaluated. Also, any nevus that has changed in appearance should be biopsied. Melanomas tend to be very dark and have irregular outlines with outward spreading. Patients with melanoma may also develop symptoms of itching, ulceration, and bleeding. Malignant melanomas can metastasize but there is a 60 to 80% 5-year survival rate in those with early detection.

Actinic keratoses look like red, scaling, crusty lesions on the face, neck, hands, and forearms. When found, they should be removed by freezing with liquid nitrogen or topical therapy with 5-fluorouracil. These patients also need to be followed carefully for development of any other skin cancers.

Reference: Lamberg SI: Common problems of the skin. In Barker LR, et al (eds): Principles of Ambulatory Medicine, 3rd ed. Baltimore, Williams & Wilkins, 1991.

SLEEP APNEA

Apnea refers to a pause in respiration lasting longer than 10 sec. The upper limit of normal is five episodes of apnea per hour. The severity of apnea is determined by a combination of the number of apneic episodes per hour (apnea index), the number of apneic episodes and hypopneic episodes (decreased respiration associated with arterial desaturation of 4%), the severity of arterial desaturation, the length of apnea, cardiac events during apnea, and, very important, the patient's symptoms and concurrent medical condition.

Apnea is divided into three categories: obstructive apnea, central apnea, and mixed apnea (which has elements of both obstructive and central apnea). Central and obstructive sleep apnea are differentiated by a lack of respiratory effort in central apnea versus *ineffective* respiratory effort due to upper airway obstruction in obstructive sleep apnea. The figure and table that follow demonstrate the different airflow and respiratory patterns and the clinical characteristics of the two conditions.

Apnea Type

The relationship between airflow and respiratory effort in both central and obstructive apnea is demonstrated. During a central apnea there is cessation of airflow for at least 10 seconds with no associated ventilatory effort. An obstructive apnea is defined as a similar cessation of airflow, but with continued respiratory effort. From White DP: Central sleep apnea. Med Clin North Am 69:1206–1208, 1985, with permission.

Clinical Characteristics of Patients with Sleep Apnea

CENTRAL	OBSTRUCTIVE	
Normal body habitus	Commonly obese	Intellectual deterioration
Insomnia: hypersomnia rare	Daytime hypersomnia	Sexual dysfunction
Awaken during sleep	Rarely awaken during	Morning headache
Snoring mild and intermittent	sleep	Nocturnal enuresis
Depression	Loud snoring	
Minimal sexual dysfunction		

From White DP: Central sleep apnea. Med Clin North Am 69:1208, 1985, with permission.

Consequences of Obstructive Sleep Apnea

Restless sleep	Associated with HTN
Excessive daytime sleepiness	Pulmonary HTN
Intellectual deterioration	Cor pulmonale
Personality changes	Nocturnal arrhythmias
Behavioral disorders	Unexplained nocturnal death
Chronic hypoventilation	

Treatment Options for Obstructive Sleep Apnea

1. Weight loss
2. Avoidance of alcohol and sedatives
3. Avoidance of the supine sleeping position
4. Tricyclic antidepressants
5. Nasal CPAP or BiPAP (bilevel positive airway pressure)
6. Surgical options
   Uvulopalatopharyngoplasty
   Septoplasty
   Correction of malformations
   Tracheostomy
7. Oral/dental devices

References: Association of Sleep Disorders Centers and the Association for the Psychophysiological Study of Sleep: Diagnostic classification of sleep and arousal disorders. Sleep 2:1–137, 1979.

Bradley TD, et al: Pathogenesis and pathophysiology of obstructive sleep apnea syndrome. Med Clin North Am 69:1170, 1985.

SODIUM

Calculation of Sodium Deficits

Na^+ determines the ECF volume in the body. The kidneys regulate the amount of Na^+ in the body and therefore regulate the extracellular volume.

The best way to grasp the concepts underlying Na^+ excess and Na^+ depletion is to realize that these terms mean volume disorders: Na^+ excess means extracellular **volume excess.** Na^+ depletion means extracellular **volume depletion.**

Na^+ excess is manifested by edema; thus CHF, cirrhosis, and nephrotic syndrome are all states associated with Na^+ (volume) excess. Na^+ depletion is manifested by orthostatic hypotension and tachycardia, poor skin turgor, and, in severe cases, shock.

Although some laboratory tests may *support* the diagnosis of a Na^+ (volume) disorder, no lab test reliably indicates the Na^+ (volume) status in the body. Besides the physical examination, the only way to assess Na^+ (volume) balance is by means of a measurement of CVP or PCWP.

Na^+ (volume) deficits occur in patients with fluid losses through the skin or GI tract. These fluids vary in terms of Na^+ content, with sweat having 65 mEq/L, gastric juice having 20 to 100 mEq/L, bile having 150 mEq/L, and pancreatic juice, ileal fluid, and colonic fluid having 120 to 140 mEq/L. Na^+ can also be lost via the kidneys. Under normal circumstances, the kidneys vary their excretion of Na^+ to match dietary intake, but excess Na^+ losses (volume losses) can be caused by diuretics. Rare causes of renal Na^+ losses are salt-losing nephritis and adrenal insufficiency.

The lab tests that support diagnosis of a Na^+ (volume) deficit include an elevated hematocrit and plasma protein concentration. The most helpful test is the urine Na^+. If renal function is normal and diuretics have not been ingested, a urine Na^+ <15 mEq/L supports the diagnosis of a Na^+ (volume) deficit. The serum Na^+ concentration is of no help in the diagnosis of Na^+ (volume) deficit, because it is normal in pure volume (Na^+) depletion. Serum Na^+ tells only about the water balance, never about Na^+ balance. In a patient with a Na^+ (volume) deficit, an abnormal serum Na^+ concentration means that a concomitant disorder of *water* balance exists.

The treatment of Na^+ (volume) deficit consists of infusion of isotonic saline. There are no easy formulas to calculate the Na^+ (volume) deficit. One to 2 liters of isotonic saline should be infused over the first hour if hypotension or signs of shock are present.

Reference: Burnell JM, et al: The problem of sodium and water needs of patients. J Chron Dis 11:189–198, 1960.

SORE MOUTH

Sore mouth is a common symptom, often not brought to the attention of physicians and often treated with self-medications. For the most part, simple remedies are effective. Thus it is important to do a thorough exam when a patient's mouth is sore enough to cause the person to seek medical care.

A careful description of the discomfort together with a complete physical exam often leads to the correct diagnosis. A complaint of burning tongue when no lesions are apparent may be due to smoking, early glossitis, or heavy metal poisoning. Trauma must always be considered. Bimanual palpation of the tongue and the floor of the mouth may reveal masses that are not able to be visualized.

Pain deep in the tongue may be due to stones in the salivary ducts, foreign bodies, or neoplasms. Neoplasms can also be seen in the floor of the mouth, and it is important that the patient remove dentures for examination of areas under them for possible lesions causing the pain. Foreign bodies such as fish bones should be looked for carefully.

If superficial lesions are seen, they may appear to be bruises from biting of the tongue during seizures or during encounters of violence. Ulcers occur frequently in the mouth. The National Institute of Dental Research has classified aphthous ulcers into minor, major, and herpetiform types. Unfortunately, the categorization has not helped in treatment, and therapy for these often very painful lesions is symptomatic and supportive.

Carcinoma, tuberculous granulomas, herpes simplex, Vincent's stomatitis, leukoplakia, thrush, and irritation from dentures are all fairly apparent on exam. Since many of these lesions appear much the same on first exam, biopsy should be considered in any lesions that do not improve in 7 to 10 days.

Generalized disorders can cause pain in the mouth. These include pellagra, riboflavin deficiency, scurvy, atrophic glossitis, leukemia, lichen planus, scarlet fever, heavy metal poisoning, syphilis, diphenylhydantoin toxicity, uremia, pernicious anemia, sensitivity to some antibiotics, and Behçet's syndrome.

After treatment of underlying causes, symptomatic treatment includes viscous lidocaine, tetracycline, and peroxide and chlorhexidine gluconate (Peridex) oral rinses.

SORE THROAT

Sore throat may be acute or chronic. Acute pharyngitis presents with the full range of symptoms, from mild discomfort to inability to swallow saliva. Exam of the throat may reveal redness or exudates. The tonsils and posterior pharyngeal wall can also be involved. It is important to confirm the diagnosis by noting features peculiar to specific diseases, such as the white patches associated with *Candida,* the pseudomembrane of diphtheria, or the ulcers and anaerobic odor of fusobacterial infections. A complication of acute pharyngitis is peritonsillar abscess, also known as quinsy. This is an infection with *Streptococcus pyogenes* (or *Staphylococcus aureus),* and it presents with severe enlargement of the tonsils and peritonsillar edema that may occlude the airway. Fever and chills are usually present. Treatment requires incision and drainage of the abscess.

Sore throat is frequently caused by viruses, generally the same ones that cause the common cold: influenza virus, rhinovirus, some adenoviruses, respiratory syncytial viruses, Epstein-Barr virus, echovirus, and poliovirus.

Chronic sore throat may be caused by neoplasms in the throat area. Carcinoma of the tonsil and nasopharyngeal carcinoma are the most common cancers found. Risk factors include smoking and alcohol, so patients with this history and complaints of sore throat should be examined carefully.

Benign causes of sore throat are mouth breathing, exposure to such irritants as tobacco smoke, subacute thyroiditis, inflamed thyroglossal duct cyst, postsurgical trauma, and glossopharyngeal neuralgia.

Nonreflux esophagitis as is seen with monilial and herpes esophagitis can present with sore throat as the initial complaint. This may also occur with ulcers of the esophagus such as can be seen in Barrett's esophagus.

Treatment of sore throat depends on the source. If symptoms of viral illness predominate, symptomatic therapy may be all that is indicated. If illness is prolonged beyond several days or if pus is seen, antibiotics should be added. If an abscess is located, incision and drainage should be carried out. Other causes must be treated according to their etiologies. (See also Pharyngitis.)

Etiology of Pharyngitis

I. Infectious

  A. Treatable

    Group A *Streptococcus pyogenes*   *Francisella tularensis*
    Haemophilus influenzae   *Candida*
    H. parainfluenzae   *Cryptococcus*
    Neisseria gonorrhoeae   *Histoplasma*
    N. meningitidis   *Mycoplasma pneumoniae*
    Corynebacterium diphtheriae   *Streptococcus pneumoniae*
    Spirochaeta pallida   *Staphylococcus aureus*
    Fusobacterium   Gram-negative bacilli

  B. Untreatable

    1. Primary

        Influenza virus   Echovirus
        Rhinovirus   Herpes simplex
        Coxsackievirus A   Reovirus
        Epstein-Barr virus

    2. Manifestation of systemic disease

        Poliovirus   Viral hepatitis
        Measles   Rubella
        Chicken pox   Pertussis

II. Noninfectious

  A. Trauma by heat, sharp objects, etc.
  B. Inhalation of irritants
  C. Dehydration: mouth breathing
  D. Glossopharyngeal neuralgia
  E. Subacute thyroiditis
  F. Psychogenic causes
  G. Monomyelocytic leukemia
  H. Immunosuppressed state

Modified from Weinstein L: Diseases of the upper respiratory tract. In Wilson JD, et al (eds): Harrison's Principles of Internal Medicine, 11th ed. New York, McGraw Hill, 1987, p 1112.

SPINAL STENOSIS

Narrowing of the spinal canal that produces pain and occasionally neurologic sequelae is termed spinal stenosis. The source of such narrowing can vary. Congenital conditions, such as diffuse intervertebral skeletal hyperostosis (DISH) or other, less exuberant forms of degenerative arthritis can lead to a narrower canal. Up to 30% of patients with spinal stenosis had associated disc protrusion or spondylolysis. Less commonly, hypertrophy of the ligamentum flavum and even Paget's disease can produce narrowing. Finally, iatrogenically produced narrowing after laminectomy or fusion can occasionally be seen.

Patients present with back and leg pain. With associated degenerative disease there are also limited motion, mild gelling, and reduction in discomfort with rest. If the narrowing is congenital or if further encroachment occurs, weakness in the lower limbs and achiness of the low back, buttocks, thighs, legs, and calves may occur. There may be associated numbness and tingling. Symptoms are often exacerbated with exertion and in turn relieved with recumbency, which is often initially presumed to be the result of arterial insufficiency rather than neurogenic disease. Neurogenic claudication, however, is not relieved by slowing or standing still.

Patients with lumbar spinal stenosis often have pain simply while standing washing dishes or cooking. In men, bladder dysfunction may be assumed to be secondary to bladder obstruction related to an associated enlarged prostate gland. Ultimately, bowel dysfunction may also develop if no steps are taken to decompress the nerves. Both osteoarthritis of the hips and lumbar disc disease with radiculopathy can occasionally mimic spinal stenosis.

Physical examination is rarely diagnostic, although it can provide further clues to etiology and associated illness. Either the loss of lower limb pulses or abdominal or femoral bruits suggest vascular compromise. Although most patients have a nonfocal neurologic examination, an associated disc protrusion may produce straight-leg-raising pain or restriction as well as loss of reflexes and localized muscular weakness. Associated loss of sphincter control suggests advanced disease with coexistent cauda equina syndrome. Sensory loss should suggest peripheral neuropathy in addition to spinal impingement.

Plain x-rays may show spondylolisthesis with or without spondylolysis. Although EMG/NCVs may be helpful, the most appropriate study is either CT myelogram or MRI of the low back. The normal AP diameter of the canal should be 22 to 25 mm. Narrowing to 15 mm usually produces symptoms. More dramatic narrowing or even a complete block of the flow of dye can be seen in advanced or severe disease.

Conservative treatment with bracing, exercises, or analgesics can sometimes relieve symptoms temporarily. Surgical intervention is directed at increasing the available space for neural contents. This is difficult, however, and often requires multilevel laminectomy. About two-thirds of patients do well with the resulting reduction in pain and freer mobility. Patients with the most severe disease or those in whom restenosis develops may continue to have pain. Additional poor prognosis features include other contributing factors such as peripheral neuropathy, obesity, and generalized debilitated condition. Occasionally, if the surgery is extensive, some instability may occur, also contributing to recurrence of pain.

The source of pain in the neck is quite similar. Patients typically develop spastic pain, hyperreflexia of the lower limbs, and positive Babinski sign. Neck pain and cervical radicular pain are usually present. Weakness and wasting of the small muscles of the hands are common. Again, diagnosis is based on the clinical syndrome and myelogram. EMG and nerve conduction studies can be helpful but are not diagnostic. Surgical treatment often produces less than dramatic results. Such surgeries are complicated and difficult and, because of the risk of instability, often cannot be extensive enough to completely relieve symptoms.

Reference: Epstein NE, et al: Lumbar spinal stenosis. In Camin MB, et al (eds): The Lumbar Spine. New York, Raven Press, 1987, pp 149–162.

SPLENOMEGALY

Causes

Congestive splenomegaly

1. Portal venous hypertension
   a. Cirrhosis: splenomegaly is mild to moderate, not massive
   b. Portal vein thrombosis
   c. Cavernous transformation of portal vein: a rare disorder

    d. Schistosomiasis: intrahepatic presinusoidal portal venous obstruction

    e. Hepatic vein thrombosis: Budd-Chiari syndrome, hepatomegaly, and ascites are prominent

    f. Congestive heart failure: long-standing right ventricular failure with striking hepatic congestion

2. Splenic venous thrombosis

Primary hematologic disorders

1. Hemoglobinopathies
   a. β-Thalassemia major: splenomegaly is often massive
   b. β-Thalassemia minor: mild splenomegaly is frequent
   c. α-Thalassemia
   d. Sickle-cell hemoglobinopathies such as hemoglobin SC disease and S-thalassemia; young children with sickle-cell disease may have splenomegaly, but adults have hyposplenia
2. RBC enzyme deficiencies
   a. Glucose-6-phosphate dehydrogenase (G6PD) deficiency: variants with chronic hemolysis
   b. Pyruvate kinase deficiency
3. Hemolytic anemias with RBC membrane defects
   a. Hereditary spherocytosis
   b. Hereditary elliptocytosis
4. Paroxysmal nocturnal hemoglobinuria: splenomegaly is mild at most
5. Megaloblastic anemia: splenomegaly is mild in degree

Immunologic disorders

1. Systemic lupus erythematosus
2. Felty's syndrome: splenomegaly with rheumatoid-type arthritis and leukopenia
3. Autoimmune hemolytic anemia
4. Idiopathic (immune) thrombocytopenic purpura: splenomegaly is uncommon
5. Immune neutropenic syndrome
6. Angioimmunoblastic lymphadenopathy with dysproteinemia

Infectious disorders

1. Bacterial
   a. Infective endocarditis
   b. Splenic abscess
   c. Brucellosis
2. Granulomatous infections
   a. Disseminated mycobacterial infection
   b. Histoplasmosis
3. Parasitic diseases
   a. Malaria: splenomegaly may be substantial
   b. Leishmaniasis (kala-azar): splenomegaly can be massive
4. Viral disorders
   a. HIV infection and AIDS
   b. Infectious mononucleosis: very common cause of splenomegaly
   c. Cytomegalovirus infection
   d. Viral hepatitis: splenomegaly is uncommon

Malignant infiltrative disorders

1. Chronic myelogenous leukemia: splenomegaly very common and often substantial in degree
2. Myelofibrosis: with agnogenic myeloid metaplasia of the spleen—a major cause of massive splenomegaly
3. Polycythemia vera: splenomegaly usually present; if marked, suspect complicating myeloid metaplasia
4. Essential thrombocythemia: mild splenomegaly is frequent
5. Myelodysplastic syndrome: mild to moderate splenomegaly is common
6. Hodgkin's disease
7. Lymphocytic lymphomas
8. Chronic lymphocytic leukemia: splenomegaly can be substantial
9. Hairy-cell leukemia: a major cause of massive splenomegaly
10. Acute leukemia: mild to moderate, not massive, splenomegaly

Benign infiltrative disorders

1. Hemangiomas, hemangioendotheliomas, lymphangiomas
2. Splenic cysts
3. Sarcoidosis
4. Amyloidosis
5. Histiocytosis X
6. Gaucher's disease: a cause of massive splenomegaly
7. Niemann-Pick disease

STATUS EPILEPTICUS

Status epilepticus is defined as persistent seizures without recovery of consciousness. This may arise in two settings: (1) repeated seizures that recur so close together that there is no recovery of consciousness from the time one ends until the next one begins and (2) a single seizure that persists without cessation. This is a medical emergency, because repeated or persistent seizures will damage neurons and lead to permanent brain damage within approximately 1 hr.

The commonest cause of status epilepticus is anticonvulsant withdrawal—that is, in the case of a known epileptic who has been noncompliant with medications and who thus experiences a breakthrough of seizures. However, virtually any condition that irritates the cerebral cortex can conceivably cause seizures and status epilepticus, including stroke, intracerebral hemorrhage, meningitis, and brain tumor.

Therapy for status epilepticus is not standardized, and numerous algorithms and protocols have been advocated, but the differences between them are generally minor. A useful approach to the patient in status epilepticus would include the following guidelines.

1. *ABC's:* Assess cardiorespiratory function, and be prepared to support the airway. Many neurologists immediately intubate all patients in status epilepticus; others wait until significant respiratory depression actually occurs. In any event, you should always be prepared to immediately intubate the patient.

2. Perform a rapid Hx & PE, and draw blood for anticonvulsant levels, glucose, electrolytes, CBC, and a toxicology screen.

3. Start an IV line, and administer thiamine and glucose.

4. Begin therapy of status epilepticus. Many authorities advocate an initial bolus of diazepam (10 mg) or lorazepam (2 mg) to abruptly terminate seizures. These benzodiazepines effectively stop seizures, but at the cost of respiratory suppression. Their anticonvulsant effects are also brief and may disappear within 20 min. Therefore, other investigators recommend forgoing benzodiazepines unless the patient is having such active seizures that it is essential to terminate them, however briefly, in order to proceed with intubation, start an IV line, or perform a similar stabilizing or therapeutic maneuver.

5. Give IV phenytoin (Dilantin) at a rate no greater than 50 mg/min IV push. Phenytoin can seldom be hung in an IV solution and is best given by IV bolus at the bedside. The total dose is 15 mg/kg, or roughly 1–1.5 gm for the average adult. At a rate of 50 mg/min, this can be accomplished within 20 to 30 min.

6. If seizures persist, many authorities advocate proceeding to treatment with phenobarbital, which can be given as 120 mg ampules IV push over several minutes, repeated every 15 to 20 min, up to approximately 600 mg total. If the patient has not already been intubated, it is highly likely that phenobarbital will produce sufficient respiratory suppression to require support.

7. Over 90% of status epilepticus is terminated by phenytoin infusion and certainly after phenobarbital is given. Should seizures persist, rapid action must be taken because the patient will have been in status epilepticus for over an hour at that point in the protocol. There is little consensus on how to stop seizures that persist after this level of treatment, but many researchers advocate general anesthesia, performed by the anesthesiologist, with inhalation anesthetics, often in the setting of the surgical suite. Other options include an IV drip of diazepam consisting of 100 mg diluted in 500 cc of D5W run in at least 40 ml/hr and titrated as needed to terminate the seizures. IV lidocaine may also be used, at a dose of 100 mg IV push followed by a dilution of 100 mg in 250 cc of D5W dripped in at 1 to 2 mg/min.

References: Aminoff MJ, et al: Status epilepticus: Causes, clinical features and consequences in 98 patients. Am J Med 69:657–666, 1980.

Delgado-Escueta AV, et al: The management of status epilepticus. N Engl J Med 306:1337–1340, 1982.

Brodie MJ. Status epilepticus in adults. Lancet 306:551–553, 1990.

STOMATITIS

Stomatitis is a term describing ulcers or severely denuded superficial oral mucosa. Stomatitis is painful, sometimes to the degree that patients are unable to eat or even to swallow saliva. In patients who have recurrent attacks, the diagnosis includes recurrent aphthous stomatitis, Behçet's syndrome, recurrent herpes simplex infection, recurrent erythema multiforme, and cyclic neutropenia. Stomatitis may also be the result of chemotherapeutic agents used to treat many different cancers.

Recurrent aphthous stomatitis was at one time believed to have a viral etiology, but several studies failed to identify an agent, and it is now generally thought to be an autoimmune phenomenon. Immunoglobulins and complement have been demonstrated in the cytoplasm of the oral mucosal cells of patients afflicted with this problem. Lymphocytes from these patients have also been shown to decrease the survival time of oral epithelial cells. *Streptococcus sanguis* 2A, a normal oral organism, has been implicated in this issue, because delayed hypersensitivity reaction to that organism has been shown in several studies of patients with these lesions. An inherited predisposition to these lesions has also been demonstrated, so it is possible that genetic influences occur. Some researchers found nutritional deficiencies of iron, folate, or vitamin B_{12} in a small number of these patients, and stomatitis is also found in about 5% of patients with celiac disease.

Behçet's syndrome, considered an autoimmune disorder, involves a vasculitis, with presentation of recurrent oral and genital ulcers, as well as uveitis, which can cause blindness. The oral ulcers are painful and range in size from 2 to 10 mm. They may be shallow or deep, with a central necrotic base, and are found on the lips, buccal mucosa, tongue, gingiva, tonsils, and larynx. Such ulcers usually resolve in 1 to 2 weeks without scars.

Herpes simplex stomatitis is usually the primary infection with herpes and is accompanied by fever, malaise, myalgias, and cervical adenopathy lasting from 3 to 14 days. Lesions are found on the tongue, lips, palate, and gingiva. Exudative or ulcerative lesions may be found in the posterior pharynx and tonsils.

Stomatitis may be a toxic effect of chemotherapeutic agents. Bleomycin causes the most striking toxicity, but it is unusual; methotrexate regularly causes mild mucositis. Doxorubicin may also cause a painful stomatitis. However, almost all agents given in sufficiently high doses will cause stomatitis. Stomatitis caused by the drugs required to prevent rejection is often seen in patients receiving organ transplants. Patients with leukemia may also have stomatitis, due to superimposed or opportunistic infections.

STROKE

Stroke refers to brain dysfunction caused by vascular disease and broadly applies to both ischemia and hemorrhage. Most strokes cause abrupt hemiparesis, sometimes accompanied by other neurologic deficits.

There are four main kinds of strokes: thrombotic, embolic, lacunar, and hemorrhagic.

TYPE OF STROKE	% OF ALL STROKES	ONSET	PRECEDING TIAs (%)	SEIZURE AT ONSET (%)	COMA (%)	MRI OR CT SCAN	OTHER FEATURES
Thrombotic	40	Stuttering, gradual	50	1	5	Ischemic infarction	Carotid bruit; stroke during sleep
Embolic	30	Sudden	10	10	1	Superficial (cortical) infarction	Underlying heart disease, peripheral emboli, or strokes in different vascular territories
Lacunar	20	Gradual or sudden	30	0	0	Normal, or small, deep infarction	Pure motor or pure sensory stroke
Hemorrhagic	10	Sudden	5	10	25	Hyperdense mass	Nausea and vomiting; decreased mental status

Strokes in the carotid distribution usually cause contralateral hemiparesis and hemianesthesia, affecting the face, arm, and leg to varying degrees. In the dominant (left) hemisphere, a stroke involving the cortex may also cause aphasia, whereas in the nondominant hemisphere, a cortical stroke may cause neglect and denial of illness. If the ischemia extends deep within the brain, the visual fibers may be affected, resulting in a field cut on the same side as the hemiparesis.

Strokes in the vertebral-basilar distribution, affecting the brain stem, generally also cause hemiparesis but are usually accompanied by cranial nerve deficits such as double vision, dysarthria, dysphagia, or vertigo. Ataxia and cerebellar tremor are also common.

The most important reasons for misdiagnosis of a stroke are:

1. Assuming that any neurologic deficit that occurs abruptly must be vascular in origin.
2. Attributing isolated symptoms to a stroke: The patient who experiences a sudden onset of vertigo alone, or dysarthria alone, or diplopia alone rarely has vascular disease. Except for hemiparesis, a stroke seldom causes isolated neurological deficits.
3. Attributing altered mental status to a stroke: A common mistake is to assign a vascular cause for a decreased level of alertness. Although it is true that intracerebral hemorrhages, either within the substance of the brain or as a subarachnoid hemorrhage, usually cause altered mental status, these represent a very small percentage of all patients with decreased mental status.

Among patients admitted to the hospital with an initial diagnosis of stroke who subsequently prove to have other conditions, the two most common problems mistaken for stroke are seizures and metabolic encephalopathies.

The evaluation of patients with suspected stroke should include early imaging of the brain. Ischemia may not become apparent on CT or MRI for several hours or days, so the major value of brain imaging is not necessarily to confirm a stroke, but rather to rule out tumors, abscesses, subdural hematomas, and other conditions that may mimic stroke. Other diagnostic tests depend on the clinical setting but could include carotid artery evaluation (by angiography, magnetic resonance angiography, or Doppler) or cardiac evaluation (by echocardiogram, transesophageal echo, or Holter monitor).

No therapy has been proven to alter the course of a completed stroke, so treatment focuses on the management of medical problems and complications.

Anticoagulation is generally indicated in two settings:

1. Stroke in evolution: A stuttering, progressive stroke, in which the neurological deficit worsens over a period of minutes or hours. This generally occurs in thrombotic, large-vessel atherosclerotic disease.
2. Embolic strokes from a cardiac source: This generally occurs in a setting of AF or a recent MI with transmural thrombus. Septic emboli from heart, such as bacterial endocarditis, are not anticoagulated.

Commonest Causes of Death among Patients Hospitalized for Stroke

1. Aspiration pneumonia
2. Pulmonary embolus
3. MI or arrhythmia
4. CNS damage or edema from the stroke itself

In these settings, if a CT or MRI shows the stroke to be ischemic, with no bleeding, and the patient has no other contraindications to heparinization, anticoagulation is often initiated.

When a stroke occurs in a young patient, less than 40 years of age, cardiac causes predominate, including congenital valve disease, subacute bacterial endocarditis, patent foramen ovale, mitral valve prolapse, and cardiac arrhythmias. Vasculitis, fibromuscular dysplasia, and other blood vessel anomalies are also common; atherosclerosis is rare. Hematologic problems can include antiphospholipid antibodies, sickle-cell disease, and other hypercoagulable states. Never forget that drugs can cause strokes, especially cocaine.

Reference: Barnett HJM, et al: Stroke, 2nd ed. New York, Churchill Livingstone, 1992.

SUPRAVENTRICULAR TACHYCARDIA

The initial approach to the patient presenting with a tachycardia of supraventricular origin (QRS duration <120 ms) or wide-complex tachycardia of uncertain origin has been outlined by the Emergency Cardiac Care Committee of the American Heart Association. This algorithm helps the clinician to evaluate the severity of a situation and balances the need for immediate treatment with the need for diagnosis of the dysrhythmia.

Adenosine, an endogenous nucleoside that blocks conduction through the AV node, was approved for clinical use in the United States in 1989. It has revolutionized the treatment of certain SVTs and become invaluable in the diagnosis of both narrow-complex tachycardia (helping to determine whether its origin is the atrium or junction) and wide-complex tachycardia of uncertain origin. Adenosine terminates most junctional tachycardias (with or without aberrant conduction), reveals intraatrial arrhythmias by producing AV nodal block, and has no effect on preexcitation atrial arrhythmias or VTs. Distinguishing SVT with aberrant conduction from VT is a challenge, and misdiagnosis can adversely affect outcome. ECG findings suggesting that a wide-complex tachycardia is of ventricular origin include AV dissociation, a QRS duration >140 ms, fusion beats, capture beats, and left axis deviation. Findings suggesting that a wide-complex tachycardia is of supraventricular origin include some slowing of the rate with vagal maneuvers and an RSR′ pattern in V1. Adenosine has been found to be a safe and effective way to distinguish these two entities. Importantly, in contrast to verapamil, adenosine does not cause hemodynamic deterioration in patients with wide-complex tachycardia associated with Wolff-Parkinson-White syndrome.

---

*Unstable condition must be related to the tachycardia. Signs and symptoms may include chest pain, dyspnea, decr. level of consciousness, low BP, shock, pulmonary congestion, CHF, acute MI.

†Carotid sinus pressure is contraindicated in patients with carotid bruits; avoid ice water immersion in patients with ischemic heart disease.

‡If the wide complex tachycardia is known with certainty to be paroxysmal SVT and BP is normal/elevated, sequence can include verapamil.

From Emergency Cardiac Care Committee and Subcommittees of the American Heart Association: The algorithm approach to ECC. JAMA 268:2215–2232, 1992, pp 2223–2234, with permission.

Camm AJ, et al: Adenosine and supraventricular tachycardia. N Engl J Med 325:1621–1629, 1991.

TACHYCARDIA ALGORITHM

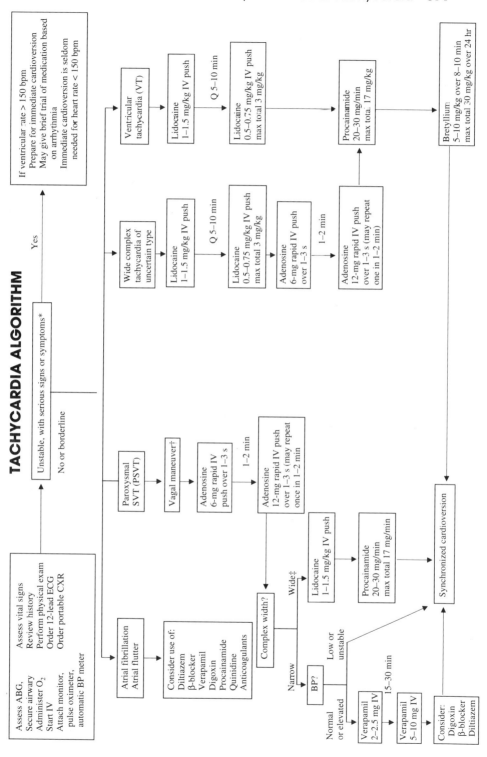

SURGERY

ESTIMATION OF PERIOPERATIVE CARDIAC RISK IN NONCARDIAC SURGERY

The cardiac risk index (CRI) developed by Goldman et al. was a major advance in the systematic evaluation of the risk of cardiac complications faced by patients over age 40 undergoing noncardiac surgery. Even though most now believe the index *overestimates* risk (perhaps because newer anesthetic and surgical techniques are safer), the index retains its usefulness as a way of reminding clinicians to modify risk factors that are modifiable before surgery. The following table summarizes the CRI.

Computation of Cardiac Risk Index

CRITERIA	POINTS
1. History	
a. Age >70 yrs	5
b. MI in previous 6 months	10
2. Physical examination	
a. S_3 gallop or jugulovenous distension	11
b. Important valvular aortic stenosis	3
3. Electrocardiogram	
a. Rhythm other than sinus or PACs on last preoperative ECG	7
b. >5 PVCs/min documented at any time before operation	7
4. General status	3
P_aO_2 <60 or P_aCO_2 >50 mm Hg, K^+ <3.0 or HCO_3^- <20 mEq/liter, BUN >50 or Cr >3.0 mg/dl, abnormal AST, signs of chronic liver disease, or patient bedridden from noncardiac causes	
5. Operation	
a. Intraperitoneal, intrathoracic, or aortic operation	3
b. Emergency operation	4
Total possible	53 points

PAC = premature atrial contraction; PVC = premature ventricular contraction.
From Goldman L, et al: Multifactorial index of cardiac risk in noncardiac surgical procedures. N Engl J Med 297:845–850, 1977, p 848, with permission.

Detsky et al. modified Goldman's original index. Using a somewhat different set of patients (e.g., they included men undergoing TURP, whereas Goldman considered such procedures too minor for concern), they added some variables, simplified the scoring, and tested the index prospectively. They showed how the "average" risk of a patient depends on the actual setting in which the patient undergoes surgery. That is, the patient's actual risk score tally must be modified by the "pretest probability" of a complication, i.e., the cardiac complication rate for that procedure at your hospital. The authors published a nomogram that converts those figures into a "post-test probability" of a cardiac complication.

Incidence of Perioperative Infarction, Cardiac Mortality, and
All-Cause Mortality According to the Preoperative Risk Stratification Scheme

DESCRIPTION	ESTIMATED PREVALENCE OF CAD	OBSERVED MI RATE	CARDIAC DEATH RATE	OVERALL DEATH RATE
High risk for MI: patients with CAD: history of MI or ECG evidence of MI, typical angina pectoris, angiographically documented significant CAD, or history of CABG	Nearly 100%	4.1% (13/319)	2.3% (7/319)	4.1% (13/319)
Intermediate risk: patients without evident CAD but with atherosclerotic disease elsewhere: history of stroke, prior or planned vascular surgery, carotid bruit, TIA, claudication, or atypical chest pain	30–70%	0.8% (2/260)	0.4% (1/260)	3.5% (9/260)
Low risk: patients without evident atherosclerotic disease but who are >age 75 or have a high atherogenic risk factor profile based on age, sex, smoking, BP, glucose tolerance, and cholesterol; patients who have a ≥15% likelihood of a cardiac event within 6 yrs	5–30%	0% (0/256)	0/4% (1/256)	3.1% (8/256)
Negligible risks: patients without evident atherosclerosis and with a low atherogenic risk factor profile	Almost 0%	Not known*	0% (0/652)	1.2% (8/652)

*ECGs, CK = MBs, and daily postoperative surveillance for infarction were not done in this group. Only the occurrence of and cause of death were tabulated.

From Ashton CM, et al: The incidence of perioperative myocardial infarction in men undergoing noncardiac surgery. Ann Intern Med 118:504–510, 1993, with permission.

More recently Ashton et al. took a different approach. In contrast to Goldman and Detsky, who grouped MI, pulmonary edema, and VT into one cardiac complication group, these authors studied only perioperative MI. On the basis of available Hx & PE and ECG data, patients were stratified preoperatively by their likelihood of having CAD, which appears to be the strongest risk factor for perioperative MI. The following table summarizes that risk stratification scheme.

Eagle et al. evaluated risk factors for perioperative cardiac complications and the predictive value of dipyridamole thallium scintigraphy in patients undergoing peripheral vascular surgery. They found that among patients with one or two clinical variables (age >70, DM, angina, Q wave on ECG, ventricular ectopy), those who had thallium redistribution had a perioperative cardiac event rate of 30%, ten times that of patients who did not have thallium redistribution. The cardiac events tabulated were cardiac death, MI, ischemic pulmonary edema, and unstable angina.

References: Detsky AS, et al: Cardiac assessment for patients undergoing noncardiac surgery. A multifactorial clinical risk index. Arch Intern Med 146:2131–2134, 1986.

Eagle KA, et al: Combining clinical and thallium data optimizes preoperative assessment of cardiac risk before major vascular surgery. Ann Intern Med 110:859–866, 1989.

SVC SYNDROME

Superior vena cava syndrome is caused by compression of the SVC, with subsequent obstruction of venous drainage into the right atrium. Any type of lesion in the mediastinum or right upper lung can result in SVC syndrome. In the past, most cases were due to benign etiologies. Today, more than 90% of cases are caused by malignancy.

Causes of SVC Syndrome

NEOPLASTIC CAUSES	BENIGN CAUSES
Lung cancer	Fibrosing mediastinitis
(all types) 76%	Infectious mediastinitis (TB, syphilis, histoplas-
Lymphoma 12%	mosis)
Thymoma	Thrombosis (spontaneous or catheter related)
Metastatic cancer:	Postoperative (Mustard procedure)
Breast cancer	Goiter
Germ cell cancer	Aneurysm
Thyroid cancer	Radiation fibrosis
Others	

Symptoms and Signs of SVC Syndrome

SYMPTOMS	SIGNS
Dyspnea	Jugular venous distention
Facial swelling/head fullness	Dilated veins on chest wall
Cough	Facial/neck edema
Arm swelling	Arm edema
Chest pain	Facial plethora
Dysphagia	Cyanosis
Blurry vision	

The diagnosis may be made clinically if the patient has a right hilar mass with typical signs and symptoms. If not, venograms, CT, or MRI of the chest may be used to demonstrate SVC obstruction.

Treatment

1. Radiation therapy is the treatment of choice for SVC syndrome of malignancy.

2. Chemotherapy can be given for very chemosensitive tumors (e.g., lymphoma). *Chemotherapy and IVs should not be administered into the upper extremities!*

3. Surgical bypass of the SVC may be used for benign disease or for cancer patients with prolonged life expectancy.

Steroids help in reducing inflammation and edema for the first 3 to 7 days of treatment. The use of anticoagulants is controversial, but is generally not recommended because of bleeding complications. Diuretics also must be used with caution, as hemoconcentration may worsen the clotting tendency. Subjective improvement precedes objective signs of improvement by 3 to 7 days.

If the patient has no previous diagnosis of cancer, treatment should be withheld if possible until an etiology for SVC syndrome is established. Indications for emergency treatment are cerebral dysfunction, decreased cardiac output, or upper airway edema.

References: Parish JM, et al: Etiologic considerations in superior vena cava syndrome. Mayo Clin Proc 56:407–413, 1981.

Yellin A., et al: Superior vena cava syndrome: The myth—the facts. Am Rev Respir Dis 141:1114–1118, 1990.

SYNCOPE

Syncope is defined as a sudden loss of consciousness in the absence of obvious trauma or seizure activity. Vasodepressor (also called vasovagal) syncope—the common fainting spell—is seen mostly in young female patients. Syncope is also seen in 2% of persons over age 65 and in 12% of those over age 85. If a cardiovascular cause is found, there is an associated 33% mortality within 1 year. If the syncope is not cardiovascular in etiology, the mortality is 6 to 12%, which is not significantly higher than that of age- and comorbid-condition-matched controls without syncope.

Age Changes Making Older Persons More Likely to Have Syncope

- Decreased beta-adrenergic cardiac chronotropic responsiveness
- Decreased Na^+ and water conservation with higher likelihood of volume depletion
- Decreased thirst drive
- Greater reliance on preload to maintain and augment cardiac output
- Altered cerebrovascular autoregulation

Causes of Syncope (3 Cs: Cerebral, Cardiac, Circulatory)

- Hypotension/hypoxemia/hypoglycemia
- Cardiovascular: ischemia, aortic stenosis, myxoma, arrhythmia, hypertrophic cardiomyopathy
- Medications that exacerbate orthostatic hypotension and arrhythmias, decrease conduction, or decrease heart rate

Evaluation: In older patients with syncope, after an extensive evaluation, one-third are found to have a cardiovascular cause, one-third have a noncardiovascular cause, and in one-third the cause remains unknown. The Hx & PE should pay attention to precipitating factors (exercise, micturition, pressure on carotid, etc.) and to the cardiovascular system on exam. An ECG should be done, looking for bradycardia in sick sinus syndrome or complete heart block. Continuous ECG monitoring can help elicit the diagnosis in both symptomatic tachycardia and bradycardia. Holter monitors give many false positives because dysrhythmias are frequent in healthy older persons. Unless a syncopal episode occurs during monitoring, it may be difficult to implicate any arrhythmia. An echocardiogram with Doppler should be ordered if there is a systolic murmur (or diastolic plop) or if pulmonary HTN is a consideration. The role of cardiac electrophysiological studies is unclear unless the baseline ECG or history is suggestive of arrhythmias.

Treatment: Avoid medications that exacerbate orthostatic hypotension or are cardioactive or proarrhythmic. Treat symptomatic orthostatic hypotension, bradycardia, heart block, or sick sinus syndrome appropriately. Noncardiac cases have a very benign prognosis, and extensive interventions may not be warranted.

Reference: Kapoor WN, et al: A prospective evaluation and follow-up of patients with syncope. N Engl J Med. 309:197–204, 1983.

SYNDROME OF INAPPROPRIATE (SECRETION OF) ANTIDIURETIC HORMONE

Hyponatremia occurring in the presence of euvolemia and in the absence of osmotic or volume stimuli for ADH release denotes SIADH. The diagnosis is made by exclusion and requires the absence of hypovolemia or hypervolemia, renal failure, adrenal failure, hypothyroidism, and drug ingestion known to cause hyponatremia. There are multiple conditions associated with SIADH and they generally fall into three categories as in the following table.

Disorders Associated with SIADH

CARCINOMA	PULMONARY DISORDERS	CNS DISORDERS
Bronchogenic carcinoma	Viral pneumonia	Encephalitis (viral, bacterial)
Carcinoma of the duodenum	Bacterial pneumonia	Meningitis (viral, bacterial,
	Cystic fibrosis	TB, and fungal)
Carcinoma of the pancreas	Pulmonary abscess	Head trauma
Thymoma	Tuberculosis	Brain tumor or abscess
Carcinoma of the ureter	Aspergillosis	Guillain-Barré syndrome
Lymphoma	Positive pressure breathing	Delirium tremens
Ewing's sarcoma	Asthma	CVA
Mesothelioma	Pneumothorax	Acute intermittent porphyria
Carcinoma of the bladder		Subarachnoid or subdural
Prostate cancer		bleeds
		Cerebellar and cerebral
		atrophy
		Cavernous sinus thrombosis
		Neonatal hypoxia
		Hydrocephalus
		Shy-Drager syndrome
		Multiple sclerosis

Diagnosis: As already mentioned, the diagnosis is one of exclusion. Plasma Na$^+$ is often <135 mEq/L, and plasma osmolarity is <280 mOsmol/kg, whereas urinary Na$^+$ is >20 mEq/L (unless the patient is volume depleted or placed on a low-Na$^+$ diet) and urine osmolality is inappropriately high for the plasma osmolality. The plasma K$^+$ and Cl$^-$ concentrations may be normal or low, especially if the patient is not eating adequately. Plasma urea and uric acid are abnormally low due to increased renal clearance of these substances caused by mild, clinically invisible volume expansion. The signs and symptoms are those of hyponatremia as mentioned elsewhere. The main differential diagnosis is from the drugs that cause hyponatremia.

Drug-induced Hyponatremia

POTENTIATE ADH ACTION	CAUSE ADH RELEASE	RELEASE AND POTENTIATE ADH HORMONE
Tolbutamide	Clofibrate	Chlorpropamide
Acetaminophen	Vincristine	Cyclophosphamide
NSAIDs	Carbamazepine	Thiazide diuretics
ADH analogues	Narcotics	
	Barbiturates	

Treatment: There is no specific treatment for SIADH except for management of the underlying disorder. Most often the hyponatremia is asymptomatic and can be managed by water restriction alone, often to 0.5 to 1 L/day. Liberalizing the salt intake in the diet is helpful. If the hyponatremia is severe and/or symptomatic (seizures or coma), prompt and active treatment may be needed. In that setting, the benefits of rapid correction with isotonic or hypertonic saline, preferably in combination with furosemide to promote renal free-water excretion, outweigh the risks. Intramuscular desoxycorticosterone acetate (DOCA) has been employed in some cases because it promotes Na$^+$ reabsorption in the distal tubules.

In chronic situations, water restriction may be difficult to enforce, and in such instances, agents that antagonize the action of ADH have been utilized. Demeclocycline, a tetracycline antibiotic, in doses of 600 to 1,200 mg/day is effective in interfering with the action of ADH on the kidney. It may take several days before its effects are obvious. The drug causes reversible renal failure, especially in patients with cirrhosis and underlying renal disease, and therefore should be avoided. Lithium carbonate in doses of 300 mg three times a day is also effective in interfering with the effect of ADH on the distal nephron. However, it may also interfere with the action of aldosterone and may cause natriuresis. In addition, it is reported to cause nephrogenic DI. Other reported toxicities include vomiting, diarrhea, tremor, and ataxia. On the whole, demeclocycline appears more effective than lithium in the chronic management of these patients. The development of antagonists to the diuretic action of ADH constitutes an exciting step in the management of patients with water excess, and further testing is needed to document antagonist effectiveness in humans.

Reference: Anderson RJ, et al: Hyponatremia: A prospective analysis of its epidemiology and pathogenetic role of vasopressin. Ann Intern Med 102:164–168, 1985.

SYNOVIAL FLUID ANALYSIS

Synovial fluid (SF) analysis is a simple and inexpensive way to acquire otherwise unavailable information and often establish a diagnosis in a patient with arthritis. Joint fluid is produced by synovial lining cells, which secrete hyaluronic acid. The remaining constituents of SF in general are distillates of plasma. Early work in the 1950s suggested that the measuring of various constituents could give clues to the origin of disease. Later, the discovery of monosodium urate as the mediator for gout further confirmed the importance of this bedside procedure. Ultimately, joint fluids were categorized into four groups as in the opposite table.

Evaluation of fluid is warranted in any patient with an undiagnosed arthritis with even a small synovial effusion. One expert follows the motto, "Do not hesitate—aspirate." Patients with known arthritis who develop a new event unexplained by their underlying condition (as a patient with RA who suddenly develops monarticular swelling) should also have arthrocentesis.

Aspiration should be done with sterile technique. Topical anesthesia can be used in the form of ethyl chloride spray. In general, the procedure can be done quickly enough that lidocaine is unnecessary. In addition, local anesthetics can crystallize in SF, confounding interpretation. Bits of synovium can clog the needle and thus make aspiration difficult. Gentler suction, repositioning the needle, or positive pressure before reaspirating can solve the problem.

Certain bedside clues can be helpful in analysis of synovial fluid. Grossly bloody fluid from the start suggests intraarticular hemorrhage. This is contrasted with initially normal-appearing fluid in which a small amount of blood later appears. Free-floating tissue aggregates, called rice bodies, can be clumps of WBCs. Dark particles are often a sign of ochronosis. The more inflammation, the more opaque the fluid appears. If newsprint can be read through the fluid, it is generally normal or noninflammatory. Like clarity, viscosity is decreased with inflammation. These features relate to the number of WBCs and amount of fluid debris. With increased WBCs and proteolytic enzyme release, hyaluronic acid (the principal factor responsible for SF viscosity) is broken down. The string test is the classical bedside test for

Joint Fluid Characteristics

	NORMAL	GROUP I (NONINFLAMMATORY)	GROUP II (INFLAMMATORY)	GROUP III (SEPTIC)
Volume (knee, in ml)	<3.5	>3.5	>3.5	>3.5
Viscosity	Very high	High*	Low	Variable
Color	Clear	Xanthrochromic	Xanthrochromic to opalescent	Variable with organisms
Clarity	Transparent	Transparent	Translucent, opaque at times	Opaque
Mucin clot	Firm	Firm	Friable	Friable
WBC/mm³	200	200–2,000	2,000–100,000	>50,000†, usually >100,000
PMN (%)	<25	<25	>50	>75†
Culture	Negative	Negative	Negative	Usually positive

*Rapid accumulation of fluid will lower viscosity.
†May be lower with partially treated or low-virulence organism.

Differential Diagnoses by Joint Fluid Groups*

GROUP I (NONINFLAMMATORY)	GROUP II (INFLAMMATORY)	GROUP III (SEPTIC)	GROUP IV (HEMORRHAGIC)
Osteoarthritis	Rheumatoid disease	Bacterial	Trauma with or without
Traumatic arthritis	Crystal-induced	infections	fracture
Avascular necrosis	synovitis		Charcot's arthropathy
Internal derangement	Gout		Hemorrhagic diathesis
Osteochondritis disse-	Pseudogout		Anticoagulation
cans	Hydroxyapatite		von Willebrand's
Osteochrondromatosis	Corticosteroid		Hemophilia
Charcot's arthropathy	injection		Scurvy
Subsiding inflamma-	Psoriatic arthritis		Thrombocytopenia
tion	Reactive arthritis		Hemangioma
Villonodular synovitis	Reiter's syndrome		Tumor
Hypertrophic pulmo-	Regional enteritis		Pigmented villonodular
nary osteoarthropa-	Ulcerative colitis		synovitis
thy	Postileal bypass		Synovioma
SLE†	*Yersinia*		
Rheumatic fever†	*Campylobacter*		
Scleroderma†	Whipple's disease		
Amyloidosis†	Connective tissue disease		
Myxedema	SLE		
Acromegaly	Polyarteritis		
Hemochromatosis	Scleroderma		
Gaucher's disease	Polymyositis		
Ochronosis	Vasculitis (nonspecific)		
Paget's disease of bone	Polymyalgia rheumatica		
Sickle-cell disease	Polychondritis		
	Sarcoidosis		
	Behçet's syndrome		
	Ankylosing spondylitis		
	Juvenile rheumatoid arthritis		
	Rheumatic fever		
	Agammaglobulinemia		
	Infectious arthritis (low-viru-		
	lence)		
	Viral		
	Fungal		
	Bacterial		
	Mycobacterial		
	Mycoplasmal		
	Hypersensitivity		
	Serum sickness		
	Erythema multiforme		

*Partial listing.
†May be group I or II.
From Gatter RA: A Practical Handbook of Joint Fluid Analysis. Philadelphia, Lea & Febiger, 1988, with permission.

viscosity. Express a drop of SF from the syringe. Stretching, or stringing, of several inches as it drops to a container suggests normal viscosity. Short drops without a tail occur with inflammatory fluid. Some texts still discuss the mucin clot test. Normal hyaluronic acid forms a tight clot when added to diluted acetic acid, whereas with active inflammation and destruction of hyaluronic acid, the clot forms weakly.

Although clinical/bedside evaluation can suggest an inflammatory or noninflammatory fluid, the most definitive measure of inflammation is the WBC count. This should be ordered on all synovial fluid samples obtained. Evaluation for crystals is another study that should be performed on all synovial fluid samples. Polarized light microscopy is the most efficient way to demonstrate crystals. Urate crystals are needle shaped, often piercing the WBCs. They are negatively birefringent (yellow when a rose compensator filter is aligned parallel to the axis of the crystal). Calcium pyrophosphate crystals, conversely, are usually rectangular, are seen in multiples in WBCs (not to be confused with inflammatory granules), and are positively birefringent (blue when a rose compensator filter is aligned parallel to the axis of the crystal).

Other studies can be ordered but are rarely diagnostic. RF is commonly present in the synovium of patients with RA. In addition, RF has occasionally been documented in the fluid even of seronegative patients. In either case, however, RF adds little definitive diagnostic information to other findings. Synovial fluid glucose ought to parallel plasma glucose, in the fasting state. Synovial fluid glucose lower than plasma suggests inflammation. A synovial fluid level of less than one-half plasma suggests infection, and a profoundly low level suggests tuberculous arthritis. However, culture data remain the diagnostic gold standard in any infectious arthritis. Complement, total protein, and ANA levels can all be measured but in general add little diagnostic information to the simple studies outlined previously.

Sometimes materials can appear in SF that mimic or confound fluid analysis. Cholesterol crystals are not a stimulus to inflammation but appear as thin, rectangular, stacked plates. Talc from gloves can make its way to the wet mount, appearing as Maltese crosses. Glucocorticoids can dissolve quite slowly, and thus one may find crystals if aspirating after intraarticular injection.

In summary, synovial fluid analysis often facilitates better characterization of an arthropathy and may establish a diagnosis, allowing institution of definitive treatment.

SYPHILIS

Syphilis remains a significant disease entity, with some 80,000 cases reported annually. It is caused by the spirochete *Treponema pallidum* and is most often spread by intimate sexual contact, placental transfer, blood transfusion, or direct inoculation. Four stages of the disease are recognized.

Primary: There is an incubation period of 9 to 90 days (average = 21 days). The stage is characterized by a painless chancre most often found on the genitals, lips, or tongue. RPR becomes positive after the chancre has been present at least 7 days. The chancres usually heal spontaneously, within 8 weeks' time, but may persist longer in immunocompromised patients. Spirochetes can be demonstrated in the chancres. Immunocompromised hosts may have multiple chancres.

Secondary: This stage involves dissemination of the spirochete at 4 to 12 weeks after primary inoculation. It is characterized by systemic symptoms such as sore throat, malaise, arthralgias, anemia, lymphadenopathy, rash (macular, papular, annular, or follicular), headaches, anterior uveitis, hepatitis, glomerulonephritis, mucous patches (shallow, painless ulcerations), condyloma lata (grayish, broad, flat-appearing papules that occur in moist areas), and neurologic abnormalities (meningismus, meningitis, cranial nerve palsies, or spinal cord or nerve root involvement).

Latent: Treponemal antibody tests are positive but there are no clinical findings of the disease. During the first 4 years of this period (early latent syphilis), the patient remains potentially infectious due to a relapse, although most relapses actually occur within the first 12 months. After 4 years (late latent syphilis), the patient is considered resistant to reinfection and relapse and is no longer considered infectious (although transfer via the placenta and by contaminated blood may still occur).

Late: This stage consists of a progressive destructive inflammatory process in one-third of untreated patients and has three major manifestations:

A. Neurosyphilis
  1. Asymptomatic (abnormalities of the CSF (↑ WBCs, [+] CSF VDRL, ↑ protein) in absence of symptoms
     a. Early (<5 years)
     b. Late (>5 years)
  2. Meningeal neurosyphilis
     a. Acute syphilitic meningitis
        1. Acute syphilitic hydrocephalus manifested by headache, nausea and vomiting: Physical findings include neck stiffness, Kernig's sign, and papilledema. ↑ intracranial pressure present.
        2. Syphilitic meningitis with cerebral changes characterized by stiff neck, confusion or delirium, papilledema, seizures, aphasia, and hemiplegia: Cranial nerve III and VI palsies may occur.
        3. Syphilitic meningitis with prominent cranial nerve palsies manifested by increased intracranial pressure with prominent cranial nerve palsies
  3. Meningovascular neurosyphilis due to areas of infarction secondary to syphilitic endarteritis in two forms.
     a. Cerebrovascular syphilis manifested by hemiparesis or hemiplegia, aphasia, and seizures
     b. Spinal syphilis characterized by weakness or paresthesias of the legs that progresses to paraparesis or paraplegia and fecal or urinary incontinence
  4. Parenchymatous neurosyphilis
     a. General paresis (tables follow)
     b. Tabes dorsalis (table follows)
     c. Gummas of the nervous system
        1. Cerebral gummas present as subacute development of a space-occupying lesion.
        2. Spinal gummas present similarly to tumors, with root pains, spastic paraplegia, urinary and fecal incontinence, and loss of sensation below the lesion.
B. Cardiovascular syphilis: Aortitis, most commonly of the ascending aorta, aortic aneurysms, CAD, aortic valvular disease
C. Gumma: Granulomatouslike lesions involving the skeleton, skin, liver, or mucocutaneous areas, causing local destruction

Symptoms of General Paresis

EARLY	LATE
Irritability	Defective judgment
Memory loss	Emotional lability (depression, agitation, euphoria)
Personality changes	Lack of insight
Impaired capacity to concentrate and learn	Confusion and disorientation
Carelessness in appearance	Delusions of grandeur
Headache	Paranoia
Insomnia	Seizures

Neurologic Signs of General Paresis

SIGN	%
Common	57
Pupillary abnormalities	
Argyll Robertson pupils	26
Slurred speech	28
Expressionless facies	–
Tremors (tongue, face, hands)	18
Impaired handwriting	–
Reflex abnormalities (↑ or ↓)	52
Uncommon	
Focal signs	1–2
Eye muscle palsies	–
Optic atrophy	2
Extensor plantar responses	–

Symptoms and Signs of Tabes Dorsalis

SYMPTOMS	SIGNS
Lightning pains	Pupillary abnormalities
	Argyll Robertson pupils
Ataxia	Absent ankle jerks
Bladder disturbances	Absent knee jerks
Paresthesias	Romberg's sign
Visceral crises	Impaired vibratory sense
Visual loss (optic atrophy)	Impaired position sense
Rectal incontinence	Impaired touch and pain sense
	Ocular palsies
	Charcot's joints

Foregoing three tables modified from Swartz MN: Neurosyphilis. In Holmes KK, et al (eds): Sexually Transmitted Diseases. New York, McGraw-Hill, 1984, pp 318–334, pp 324–327, with permission.

The diagnosis of syphilis varies depending on the stage of illness. Darkfield examination remains the technique of choice in primary, secondary, and early congenital syphilis. Serologic tests are used for later stages.

Successful treatment of syphilis requires the maintenance of adequate blood antibiotic levels over extended periods of time. Recommended therapy is as in the following table.

Patients should be alerted about the possibility of the Jarisch-Herxheimer reaction, occurring most often in the secondary stage within the first 2 hours following initial therapy. Resulting from the release of pyrogen from spirochetes, this reaction is characterized by headache, myalgias, fever, and tachycardia, which resolve within 24 to 48 hours and are best treated with standard doses of aspirin.

Recommended Therapy for Syphilis

STAGE	REGIMEN
Early syphilis (primary, secondary)	Procaine PCN, 2.4 M units im daily, *plus* probenecid, 1.0 g po qd × 10 days, *or*
	Doxycycline, 200 mg po bid × 21 days, *or*
	Amoxicillin, 3.0 g po bid, *plus* probenecid, 1.0 g po qd × 14 days, *or*
	Ceftriaxone,[c] 250 mg im qd or iv × 5 days or 1 g im qd × 14 days, *or*
	Benzathine PCN G,[d] 2.4 M units im weekly for 2 or 3 doses alone or with any of the above oral regimens
For PCN-allergic patients[a]	Doxycycline, 200 mg po bid × 15 days, *or*
	Tetracycline hydrochloride, 500 mg po qid × 15 days, *or*
	Erythromycin (stearate, ethylsuccinate, or base), 500 mg qid po × 15 days[b]
Late syphilis (tertiary), neurosyphilis, or HIV infection, especially late-stage IV disease	Aqueous crystalline PCN G, 2.0–4.0 M unit iv q4h × 10 days, *or*
	Procaine PCN G, 2.4 M units im, *plus* probenecid, 1 g po daily × 10 days, *or*
	Amoxicillin, 3 g, *plus* 0.5 g probenecid po bid × 15 days, *or*
	Doxycycline, 200 mg po bid × 21 days, *or*
	Ceftriaxone[c] 1 g im or iv × 14 days, *or*
For PCN-allergic patients[a]	Chloramphenicol,[e] 2 g iv or 500 mg q6h po × 30 days
Pregnancy	Same regimen as for nonpregnant; only penicillin therapy reliably treats the infant.
Congenital syphilis	Aqueous crystalline PCN G, 50,000 units/kg iv daily in 2 divided doses for minimum of 10 days, *or*
	Procaine PCN G, 50,000 units/kg im daily for minimum of 10 days

[a]Therapeutic regimens other than penicillin (PCN) have not been well studied, especially in patients with syphilis of > 1 year's duration; therefore, careful follow-up is mandatory.

[b]Erythromycin is effective in immunocompetent hosts only. Not recommended for pregnant patients.

[c]Ceftriaxone should be diluted in 1% lidocaine solution (1 g/3.6 ml) for im injection.

[d]Treatment failures with benzathine PCN have been reported. Therefore, the addition of another drug, e.g., doxycycline, is prudent. Patients treated with benzathine PCN must be reevaluated at 6-month intervals for neurosyphilis.

[e]Chloramphenicol is theoretically beneficial treatment for neurosyphilis.

From Tramont EC: *Treponema pallidum* (syphilis). In Mandell G, et al (eds): Principles and Practice of Infectious Diseases, 3rd ed. New York, Churchill Livingstone, 1990, p 1806, with permission.

Treatment of syphilis in immunocompromised patients, especially those with HIV, may require the use of bactericidal drugs for more prolonged periods. A greater frequency of false-positive tests in these patients complicates the assessment of cure. Last, the chance of contracting syphilis following exposure to an infectious case is 50%, mandating that preventive therapy should be offered to individuals exposed within the preceding 3 months.

Serologic Tests

Serologic tests for syphilis may be either nonspecific or specific. Nontreponemal tests are nonspecific and designed to test serum for the presence of antibody that reacts with a cardiolipin-lecithin antigen and include the VDRL slide test and the RPR card test. Nontreponemal tests can be quantified and therefore are of use to measure serial titers as a measure of response to therapy. With successful therapy, titers should return to zero.

Specific treponemal tests detect antibody that reacts with antigenic components of *Treponema pallidum*. The MHA-TP is the most commonly used test. Specific treponemal tests usually remain positive for life.

Sensitivity of Commonly Used Serologic Tests for Syphilis

	DISEASE STAGE (% POSITIVE)			
	Primary	Secondary	Latent	Late
VDRL slide test	59–87	100	73–91	37–94
FTA-ABS test	86–100	99–100	96–99	96–100
MHA-TP	64–87	96–100	96–100	94–100

FTA-ABS = fluorescent treponemal antibody absorption; MHA-TP = microhemagglutination-*T. pallidum* test.

Modified from Jaffe HW: Management of the reactive syphilis serology. In Holmes KK, et al (eds): Sexually Transmitted Diseases. New York, McGraw-Hill, 1984, p 314.

SYSTEMIC LUPUS ERYTHEMATOSUS

Clinical Manifestations

SLE is a chronic, inflammatory autoimmune condition. Early descriptions of the disease were centered primarily on the cutaneous manifestations. *Lupus* itself means wolf, an analogy used to describe the destructive eating away by the rash. Later, the systemic manifestations of disease were described. SLE has a worldwide distribution, with a predisposition for females as high as 9 to 1. The incidence, morbidity, and mortality of SLE are higher in African-Americans than in white Americans, and African-Americans seem to have an earlier age at onset. There is strong epidemiologic evidence for a hereditary predisposition. There are also data to suggest a polygenic influence involving both HLA- and non-HLA-linked genes. Specifically, HLA DR and DQ are strongly associated with the presence of clinical SLE, as are certain antibody profiles.

Environmental factors also have some influence. UV light is a known external factor, and the development of drug-induced lupus has been described. Hydralazine, diphenylhydantoin, procainamide, and quinidine are best known, although phenothiazines and isoniazid have also been associated. Hormonal medications such as propylthiouracil and oral contraceptives are also commonly used medications that may predispose to the development of a positive ANA or clinically recognizable symptoms.

The diagnosis of SLE is established primarily on clinical features of disease. The American College of Rheumatology has devised criteria for the classification of SLE. Although these criteria were developed for clinical trials and population studies rather than for individual diagnostic purposes, they do highlight common clinical manifestations of SLE.

Symptoms of malaise, fatigue, and even weight loss are common at the onset. Arthralgia and frank arthritis may occur in up to 95% of patients and can be the presenting complaint in up to 50%. Deformity is uncommon but when present is of the Jaccoud type (nondestructive and voluntarily correctable). Subcutaneous nodules are rare but documented. Histologically they appear granulomatous and can be confused with erythema nodosum or lupus panniculitis. Tendinitis and tenosynovitis are other commonly associated problems in lupus. Weight-bearing areas (such as the knee or Achilles tendon) are more commonly affected than non–weight-bearing areas. Myalgia in addition to arthralgia is noted. An inflammatory myopathy is present in up to 10% of patients.

Skin involvement is the second most common presenting manifestation. The classical skin lesion of acute SLE (acute cutaneous lupus) is the well-known malar or butterfly rash. It covers the bridge of the nose but spares the nasolabial folds. Chronic skin involvement most commonly occurs as discoid lupus erythematosus. Patients with discoid lesions have inflammation of the skin with hyperpigmentation and erythema. There is an advancing inflammatory margin of the lesion with central atrophy, depigmentation, and scarring. Subacute cutaneous lupus is recognized as a distinct variant of chronic cutaneous lupus. The lesions are circinate and can appear psoriasiform in about half of patients. They are usually red macules or papules localized primarily over the head, shoulders, and upper back. In contrast to chronic discoid disease, subacute cutaneous lupus usually heals without scarring.

Serositis can present as pleurisy with or without pleural effusion. Although pleural disease is the most common pulmonary manifestation, an interstitial component can develop. Acute pulmonary hemorrhage syndrome has also been described. Pulmonary embolic phenomena are well described, and subsequent pulmonary HTN may develop. Serositis can extend to the heart, and pericarditis is the most common cardiac manifestation of SLE. Myocarditis is also well described and when present is usually associated with pericarditis. Endocarditis of the Libman-Sacks type is a recognized part of SLE.

In the early years of investigation, involvement of the CNS was often the harbinger of death. As testing became more sensitive and treatments improved, however, both a reduced mortality and a broader spectrum of neurologic involvement were noted. Some studies have shown more frequent episodes of CNS involvement in African-Americans and in patients with reduced renal function. The major neurologic manifestations can vary from mild cognitive dysfunction and headache to seizure and altered mental status (increased somnolence or stupor as well as psychosis and depression). Cerebral infarction and myelopathy are well-known complications. Peripheral neuropathy has been documented in 5 to 20% of patients. Mononeuritis multiplex has been seen. Pseudotumor cerebri is also an associated finding.

Psychosis is well-known, with a prevalence of 12 to 71%. Usually patients have some neurologic and psychologic dysfunction. The incidence of frank psychosis has lessened over the years. The contribution of steroid therapy in SLE patients is difficult to assess, and the presence of other evidence of active lupus would make the distinction somewhat simpler. Neuropsychologic testing is important for assessing the impact of neuropsychologic disease.

Pathologic changes were originally felt to be secondary to an active inflammatory vasculopathy. Other pathologic processes such as hemorrhage and infections have been documented to produce CNS dysfunction in lupus patients. Thus, the general rubric of "lupus cerebritis" is not accurate in most patients with CNS symptoms.

Renal disease in SLE has a prevalence of nearly 100%. A renal biopsy even in asymptomatic patients has shown lesions of varying severity. Clinical renal disease is reported in about 50% of patients. Severe renal disease leading to death or renal failure is rarer. Pathologically, the WHO has provided a classification of the morphologic patterns seen in lupus nephritis (see also later discussion). Class I is defined as normal kidneys. Class II lesions are limited to the mesangium. Class III lesions show focal and segmental proliferative glomerulonephritis (GN). By the WHO definition, there is mesangial and endocapillary hypercellularity. There is narrowing of the capillary lumen involving less than 50% of the total surface area of glomerulus. Immune deposits are found in the mesangium and along the peripheral capillary walls in a subendothelial position and may be present in the tubular basement membrane. In class IV lesions, a diffuse proliferative and necrotizing GN is seen. More than 50% of the total area of glomerular turfs is involved. There are more severe and diffuse tubular, interstitial, and vascular changes. Glomerular hypercellularity is global, whereas necrotizing features may be more segmental. Epithelial crescents are more common than in class III. A variant of class IV (membranoproliferative pattern) shows little necrotizing change. Finally, class V lesions are described by membranous glomerulonephropathy. There are global and diffuse glomerular basement membrane thickening and mesangial deposits sometimes associated with hypercellularity, but no necrotizing changes are seen. The generation of these lesions is considered to be secondary to chronic immune complex deposition. Specifically, double-stranded and anti-double-stranded DNA immune complexes can be detected.

Use of renal biopsy has added important adjunctive diagnostic and prognostic information. Mixed forms are sometimes noted and should be treated according to the most active form present on biopsy. Subsequent biopsy may be required. It is noted that up to 30% of patients may actually have a change in their biopsy pathology, although change and progression are less common for patients with only mesangial disease than for patients with evidence of more active disease. The NIH activity and chronicity indices are also important in predicting prognosis and treatment (see later discussion).

Laboratory data can provide important clues to the diagnosis. Lupus is probably the most commonly recognized condition associated with circulating ANA. Anti-DNA and anti-Sm antibodies are more specific for SLE. Low complement values also not only provide a clue to the diagnosis but also tend to be of prognostic significance. Newer data suggest that complement split products (C3a and iC3b) may be predictive of disease activity.

Treatment

Treatment of SLE can be difficult. Careful review of the activity of the disease is important and should be the primary guide to treatment. With a low level of disease activity and no evidence of active tissue destruction (nephritis, etc.), local measures, rest, and symptomatic medication can be quite helpful. Exercise and conditioning remain important management tools. Heat and cold therapy as well as whirlpool baths should be utilized.

Avoidance of stress and trauma should be emphasized, for the onset or flares of disease commonly occur at times of stress. Use of sunscreen and judicious avoidance of UV light are prudent measures for SLE patients. Up to 73% of SLE patients have some degree of photosensitivity, which can flare systemic illness. Lightweight, protective clothing, hats, and sunblocks are effective in this regard.

Although there is some controversy about the use of NSAIDs in SLE, they can be effective in controlling minor clinical manifestations of the disease. Both NSAIDs and aspirin are useful in patients with SLE. Aseptic meningitis has been described in SLE patients taking NSAIDs. With careful monitoring, however, these medications can be safe and effective.

Antimalarial medications have long been effective in treatment of SLE. These preparations are most useful in the treatment of the nondestructive manifestations of disease, specifically, arthralgia, rash, serositis, and alopecia. The mechanism of action is unknown, although UV light absorption, immunologic action, and anti-inflammatory actions have all been hypothesized. Cutaneous changes are common side effects. About 10 to 25% of patients develop cutaneous changes after long-term use of chloroquine or hydroxychloroquine; these can include blue/black discoloration of the skin. Ocular changes, especially corneal and retinal deposits, are the most concerning toxicities. Early changes are often reversible. Ophthalmologic review every 6 months is required.

The cornerstone of treatment remains glucocorticoids, which are useful topically for many of the cutaneous manifestations. Even at low doses, glucocorticoids can provide remarkable symptomatic relief with regard to musculoskeletal symptoms and the more generalized symptom of fatigue. In general, however, they are reserved for treatment of patients with active cardiac, renal, or CNS disease. Once the acute manifestations of the disease are controlled, alternate-day treatment may be less toxic. Cytotoxic medications, because of substantial toxicities, are generally reserved for patients with organ-threatening manifestations of disease.

As noted, treatment regimens in lupus nephritis should be tailored to biopsy data. It is also important to monitor urinary sediment, serum creatinine, 24-hr urine protein excretion, C_{Cr}, BP, albumin, complement, and anti-DNA antibodies. In patients with mesangial disease alone, treatment may not be necessary. Urinary protein excretion over 1.0 gm/day or low serum complement levels may indicate the need for intervention. Hyperphysiologic doses of glucocorticoids are warranted. Patients with class III and IV lesions are treated more aggressively given the risk of renal failure. High doses (1 mg/kg/d) of prednisone or an equivalent should be used for at least 6 weeks. If a suboptimal response occurs, cytotoxic medication should be administered. Cyclophosphamide (750 mg/m2) is given monthly for 6 months and then tapered to bimonthly or even every 3 months depending on the clinical response. Mesna can be given with each infusion to minimize bladder toxicity. A fair number of patients may still be unresponsive or may relapse as the cytotoxic dose administration is reduced. Treatment options include resuming monthly cyclophosphamide or adding oral azathioprine. Some suggest that daily oral cyclophosphamide may be more effective in active vasculitis than monthly IV administration is. Plasmapheresis and monthly IV pulse methylprednisolone are sometimes added, although data suggesting a significant contribution are relatively poor.

Reference: Wallace DJ, et al (eds): Dubois' Lupus Erythematosus, 4th ed. Philadelphia, Lea & Febiger, 1993.

Lupus Nephritis

SLE is an important cause of secondary glomerulopathies. The incidence of renal involvement in SLE is variable depending on the criteria used for the diagnosis. About 70% of patients have either overt clinical symptoms and signs or abnormalities of urinary sediment. If abnormalities in light or electron microscopy are also considered, the renal involvement in lupus is almost universal.

Classification and Clinical Features

The World Health Organization classifications, based on histopathologic criteria, are reviewed in the following table:

Histologic Class, Clinical Presentation, and Prognosis in SLE Nephritis

HISTOLOGIC TYPE	WHO CLASS	FREQUENCY* (%)	PROTEINURIA (%)	NEPHROTIC SYNDROME† (%)	AZOTEMIA‡ %	DEATH (%)	UREMIC DEATH (%)
Normal	I	<5					
Mesangial	II	15	68	0	12	18	0
Focal pro-liferative	III	20	100	15	18	30	11
Diffuse pro-liferative	IV	50	100	87	75	58	36
Membra-nous	V	15	100	88	20	38	6

*Percent of patients with SLE who show this lesion on biopsy.
†Proteinuria exceeding 3.0 gm per 24 hrs.
‡Serum creatinine >1.2 mg/dl or BUN >25 mg/dl.
From Couser WG: Glomerular disorders. In Wyngaarden JB, et al (eds): Cecil Textbook of Medicine, 19th ed. Philadelphia, W. B. Saunders, 1992, p 566, with permission.

Class I is very rare. Class II includes minimal lesion or mesangial lupus nephritis and represents the milder forms of renal involvement in lupus. Minimal lesion is characterized by normal histology on light microscopy and foot process fusion under electron microscopy. Mesangial lupus denotes mesangial hypercellularity and an increase in mesangial matrix with immunoglobulin and C3 deposition in the mesangium. When mesangial lupus is accompanied by focal proliferation, patients are classified as IIB. Proteinuria and hematuria are common, but frank nephrotic syndrome and azotemia are unusual. Progression occurs in 20% of cases, and 5-year survival is >90%.

Focal and segmental proliferative nephritis (class III) demonstrates, as the name indicates, focal changes (<50% of glomeruli involved), and even the involved glomeruli show only segmental changes. Microscopic hematuria with or without proteinuria is common, whereas nephrotic syndrome and renal failure occur in <20% of the cases. The presence of subendothelial deposits is a bad prognostic sign. The 5-year survival rate is 90% unless transformation to class IV disease occurs.

Diffuse proliferative nephritis (class IV) is the most frequent and severest form of renal disease in SLE. It is characterized by generalized diffuse endocapillary proliferation often with fibrinoid necrosis (wire loop nephritis). Nephrotic syndrome and azotemia are seen in over three-fourths of patients. Hypocomplementemia, circulating immune complexes, and high levels of anti-DNA titers are common. The

Ig and C3 deposits in the glomeruli may be large and organized (fingerprinting). Hematoxylin bodies, if present, are pathognomonic of SLE. The proliferation could be of endocapillary, extracapillary, or mesangiocapillary types. With aggressive therapy, the 5-year survival is now about 75%.

Membranous lupus (class V) is indistinguishable from idiopathic membranous nephritis except that electron-dense and Ig deposits are noted in the mesangium in addition to the subepithelial location. The serologic and systemic features are less pronounced than in class IV. The usual presentation is nephrotic syndrome with slowly progressive renal failure. The prognosis is that of class II disease.

Other histologic variants such as diffuse or focal sclerosis (often superimposed on other proliferative lesions), necrotizing vasculitis, and varying degrees of tubulointerstitial nephritis are not uncommon. Transformation from one class to another is not uncommon, especially from class II and III to class IV; class IV and V often change into one another. Extrarenal signs correlate poorly or not at all with renal manifestations.

Prognosis and Treatment

The National Institutes of Health have developed a semiquantitative assessment for therapeutic and prognostic purposes based on activity and chronicity indices. High activity and low chronicity scores indicate a greater chance of reversibility and better prognosis than high chronicity and low activity scores.

Activity and Chronicity Indices

ACTIVITY	CHRONICITY
Proliferation/hypercellularity	Sclerotic glomeruli
Leukocytic infiltration	Fibrous crescents
Necrosis/karyorrhexis	Tubular atrophy
Cellular crescents	Interstitial fibrosis
Hyaline deposits	
Interstitial mononuclear cell infiltration	

Renal biopsy forms a cornerstone in patients with active renal lupus, as it is both a diagnostic and a prognostic indicator. In general, minimal and mesangial lupus requires more specific therapy. Corticosteroids in high doses (1 mg/kg/day) given over 4 to 6 weeks have proven beneficial in class III and IV disease. In patients with formation of crescents and/or nephrosis with azotemia, treatment with steroid pulses followed by oral steroids and/or cyclophosphamide results in better preservation of renal function. Some studies indicate that monthly IV cyclophosphamide pulses are as efficacious as daily oral steroids and have fewer side effects. Treatment of membranous lupus is similar to that of idiopathic membranous nephropathy, involving combinations of steroids and cytotoxic agents. In these patients, if renal function deteriorates rapidly, patients should undergo rebiopsy to detect transformation to other renal lesions. Acute renal vein thrombosis should also be excluded. With the development of ESRD, systemic and serologic activity of SLE fades. Maintenance dialysis and renal transplantation are well tolerated by patients with lupus nephritis.

Reference: Balow JE, et al: Lupus nephritis. Ann Intern Med 106:79–94, 1987.

SYSTEMIC SCLEROSIS

SSc, sometimes called scleroderma, is a connective tissue disorder that causes inflammation and ultimately fibrosis and scarring. The skin, blood vessels, and joint linings are most commonly involved. The disease affects women three to four times more frequently than men. Its incidence increases with age, although onset is usually between ages 30 and 60. Occasional cases in childhood have been reported.

Vascular damage is observed, with small arterioles' manifesting intimal proliferation, medial thinning, deposition of collagen in the adventitia, and chronic inflammation. Anoxic injury after prolonged vasospasm may account for the process, and the intensity of normal fibrosis may be accelerated in SSc.

The first symptom commonly encountered is puffiness of the hands. Over ensuing months, the skin may thicken. As the disease progresses, other areas of the skin become involved, causing limitation of motion. The normal, relative looseness of the skin becomes replaced by a taut, bound-down quality. Patients may notice that exposure to cold or emotional stress causes the fingers to become numb. Raynaud's phenomenon, which may be present for years prior to frank SSc (either the classic triphasic or biphasic response), is one of the most common manifestations. Spasm of the blood vessel is believed to be the cause of the reduced flow.

Arthritis and achiness generally follow. Tendons and synovium become thickened and fibrous, further limiting motion and causing pain. If fibrosis is severe enough, frank contractures develop, and crepitus over the tendon may be audible. In about 30% of SSc patients, muscle pain and weakness occur and can be attributed to the development of an inflammatory myopathy. GI involvement occurs in approximately 50% of patients. Reduced intestinal motility, particularly in the esophagus, may be present, leading to symptoms of dysphagia, constipation, and bloating. Ultimately, bacterial overgrowth may develop, leading to malabsorption (particularly of vitamin B_{12}, folate, and iron). Barium enemas show characteristic widemouthed diverticula.

In years past, the so-called scleroderma renal crisis was a leading cause of death. Patients developed rapidly progressive renal failure usually with malignant HTN and marked increases in circulating renin. Predictive factors for renal involvement include reduction in plasma volume (institution of diuretic), worsening Raynaud's, and rapid progression of skin involvement (particularly over the trunk). Nowadays this syndrome is less common since the advent of ACE inhibitors.

Cardiac involvement is now more commonly recognized. Exposure to cold can lead to spasm of coronary arteries. Myocardial perfusion defects associated with reduced ventricular function in this setting have been well documented.

Pulmonary involvement, including interstitial fibrosis and pleural inflammation, is often present. Ultimately, pulmonary HTN and RV failure can develop. Pulmonary disease is now the most common cause of death in SSc patients. Patients with SCL-70 antibodies and recurrent digital infarction and pitting are more likely to develop pulmonary involvement. Data show that bronchoalveolar lavage (BAL) and pulmonary function testing with reduced diffusion capacity of carbon monoxide (DLCO) can indicate early involvement.

Patients often have laboratory abnormalities including a positive ANA. More specific analysis shows an antibody directed against topoisomerase-1, an enzyme that uncoils DNA. Anti-topoisomerase-1 (also called SCL-70) is quite specific and present in about 70% of patients with scleroderma.

Variants: There are several so-called variants of scleroderma. Occasionally, patients can have more localized disease (*morphea*) appearing in small patches of hidebound skin. Prognostically these patients do much better. The morphea lesions can heal and there are no systemic manifestations in these patients. The *CREST syndrome* is also felt to be a less intense form of the disease causing *C*alcium deposits, *R*aynaud's phenomenon, *E*sophageal motility disorders, *S*clerodactyly (hidebound skin quality confined to the fingers), and *T*elangiectasias (small, dilated blood vessels). Although progression of CREST is slower, serious systemic manifestations such as pulmonary and renal disease can occur. Circulating ANA is present, usually in a centromere pattern. Anti-SCL-70 antibody is absent. *Eosinophilic fasciitis* refers to a condition of intense inflammation of fascia. Systemic features such as Raynaud's are not present. Circulating ANA is also absent, but ESR may be elevated, and peripheral eosinophilia is present. Biopsy shows eosinophilic infiltrate.

Other so-called scleroderma variants can occur after exposure to environmental toxins. In the mid-1970s, contaminated cooking oil caused a sclerodermalike illness in Spain. More recently, contamination of the over-the-counter sleeping medication L-tryptophan produced a sclerodermalike illness called *eosinophilia myalgia syndrome*. Polyvinyl chloride exposure and even certain chemotherapies (bleomycin is the most common) can cause sclerodermalike illnesses. Although much has been written about autoimmune disease after silicone breast implants, scleroderma is probably the most discussed autoimmune condition occurring with increased frequency in these patients. Graft-versus-host disease, particularly as seen in bone marrow transplant patients, has many of the features of scleroderma.

Mixed connective tissue disease (MCTD) refers to a syndrome with features of SSc and SLE. Although apparent overlap occurs commonly in many rheumatic conditions, the designation *MCTD* is quite specific. In addition to its clinical features, high titer of antibody to ribonuclear protein is detected. There remains some controversy over the designation as patients have been reported to develop more distinctly one or the other specific syndrome with time.

Management: Unfortunately, there is no cure for scleroderma, but there are many simple things that can be done to lessen the impact of the disease. Self-contained, chemically activated warmers are now available for shoes and gloves. ACE inhibitors are lifesaving adjuncts for HTN and renal crisis. Antibiotics can keep colonic bacteria overgrowth controlled. D-Penicillamine has some reported usefulness, especially in SSc patients with lung involvement. Cytotoxics are used more as a last resort rather than because of proven efficacy. Experimentally, mast cell inhibitors have been used with good effect. Fish oils show efficacy in Raynaud's when associated with underlying SSc, although there is little evidence that they change the long-term outcome of disease. Prazosin is useful in patients with intractable Raynaud's if hypotension is tolerable. Intra-arterial reserpine is no longer available. Because of the availability of good support, the prognosis for patients with scleroderma has improved remarkably in recent years.

Reference: Smiley DJ. The many faces of scleroderma. Am J Med Sci 34(5):319–333, 1992.

SYSTOLIC HYPERTENSION

Isolated systolic HTN is defined as a systolic BP >160 mm Hg in the presence of a normal diastolic BP (<90 mm Hg). Combined systolic-diastolic HTN requires that both pressures be elevated. In normal people, systolic BP increases with age while diastolic BP does not change. Systolic BP is strongly correlated with the incidence of CVA and MI. Isolated systolic HTN is seen in 10 to 30% of patients over age 70; combined systolic-diastolic HTN is seen in 15 to 25% of those over age 70. Blacks have a higher prevalence of both types of HTN than whites.

The SHEP (Systolic Hypertension in the Elderly Project) trial supports that treatment of systolic HTN decreases the risk of CVA, MI, CHF, and death. However, the study specifically excluded the oldest patients (>85) and those with multiple coexisting illness. SHEP treatment consisted of diuretic first, then atenolol or reserpine, as needed. It is possible that even systolic BP >140 should be considered elevated and therefore treated.

Treatment: Diet (2 gm Na diet), modest weight loss (if the patient is overweight), and walking exercise should normalize BP in over 25% of newly diagnosed elderly persons with mild systolic HTN. Thus, nonpharmacologic therapy should constitute the first step in treatment for both mild systolic HTN and combined systolic-diastolic HTN.

Low-cost, low-dose diuretics have been effective as first-line therapy for systolic HTN in numerous studies. Doses of chlorthalidone or hydrochlorothiazide of more than 25 mg/day are not indicated. Instead, a second-line agent should be added. Specific choice of drug is optimized per patient, but atenolol, calcium channel blockers, and perhaps ACE inhibitors or alpha-blockers may all be considered.

Pseudohypertension: Older patients with stiff (calcified) and noncompressible arteries may give a falsely elevated BP. In these patients, the brachial artery may be palpable even when the BP cuff is inflated to greater than systolic BP (Osler maneuver). Calcified arteries may be demonstrated on radiographs of the upper arm. These patients tolerate antihypertensive therapy very poorly (often with syncope and falls).

Reference: Applegate WB, et al: Advances in management of hypertension in older persons. J Am Geriatr Soc 40:1164–72, 1992.

T

TETANUS

Tetanus is an acute disease resulting from the effects of a neurotoxin produced by the anaerobic gram-positive rod *Clostridium tetani.* Following an incubation period of approximately 14 days, the patient begins to experience generalized muscle rigidity. The diagnosis must be made clinically, as the causative organism often cannot be cultured from the portal of entry, which may include areas of any type of minor injury, operative procedure, or needlestick, including illicit drug use. Trismus, or lockjaw, is a common presenting symptom. Reflex spasms increase in severity over the first 3 days and begin to decline after 10 to 14 days, with the illness resolving within 3 to 4 weeks. Complete recovery can occur but is less common in both the neonatal or geriatric age groups, in which mortality may run as high as 42%.

Treatment should be carried out in a dark, quiet room of an ICU. Benzodiazepines are widely utilized for their sedative, anticonvulsant, and muscle relaxant properties, although more severe cases may require neuromuscular blocking agents such as tubocurarine. Mechanical ventilation is frequently required. Human tetanus immune globulin in a dose of 500 units IM given as soon as possible serves to neutralize any circulating toxin before it enters the nervous system. Wound debridement and penicillin therapy further decrease the toxin load. Autonomic dysfunction related to excessive catecholamine output is best managed by propranolol, morphine, and magnesium sulfate.

Most important, tetanus is a preventable disease through the administration of tetanus toxoid. Recovery from the disease does not confer immunity, as the amount of toxin required to produce the disease state is less than that required to confer immunity.

Schedule of Active Immunization against Tetanus

DOSE	AGE/INTERVAL	VACCINE
Age less than 7 yr		
Primary 1	Age 6 wk or older	DPT
Primary 2	4–8 wk after the first dose	DPT
Primary 3	4–8 wk after the second dose	DPT
Primary 4	About 1 yr after the third dose	DPT
Booster	4–6 yr of age	DPT
Additional boosters	Every 10 yr after the last dose	Td
Age 7 and older		
Primary 1	First visit	Td
Primary 2	4–6 wk after the first dose	Td
Primary 3	6 mo–1 yr after the second dose	Td
Boosters	Every 10 yr after the last dose	Td

Abbreviations: DPT: diphtheria and tetanus toxoids and pertussis vaccine absorbed; Td: tetanus and reduced-dose diphtheria toxoids absorbed (for adult use).

From Cate TR: *Clostridium tetani* (tetanus). In Mandell G, et al (eds): Principles and Practice of Infectious Diseases, 3rd ed. New York, Churchill Livingstone, 1990, pp 1845–1846, with permission.

Guidelines for the Use of Tetanus Toxoid and Human
Tetanus Immune Globulin Following a Wound

PRIOR VACCINATIONS WITH ABSORBED TETANUS TOXOID		CLEAN, MINOR WOUNDS		ALL OTHER WOUNDS	
Total Number	Years Since Last Dose	Td[a]	TIG	Td	TIG
≥3	<5	No	No	No	No
≥3	5–10	No	No	Yes	No
≥3	>10	Yes	No	Yes	No
≤2 or unknown	–	Yes	No	Yes	Yes

[a]Children under 7 years old should receive DPT or absorbed diphtheria and tetanus toxoids (DT) if pertussis vaccine is contraindicated. TIG = tetanus immune globulin.

From Cate TR: *Clostridium tetani* (tetanus). In Mandell G, et al (eds): Principles and Practice of Infectious Diseases, 3rd ed. New York, Churchill Livingstone, 1990, pp 1845–1846, with permission.

THEOPHYLLINE

Dosing Recommendations

Theophylline is a methylxanthine bronchodilator that has been used since the 1930s. Bronchodilatory activity is observed at serum levels as low as 5 µcg/ml, and the degree of bronchodilation increases with the serum level. However, the incidence of side effects increases markedly as serum levels exceed 20 µcg/ml, and so the therapeutic range is ordinarily closed at 20 µcg/ml. That narrow range, together with the significant variation in clearance rates between individuals and even *within* the same individual at various times, means that dosing needs to be individualized and should be guided by determination of serum levels. The most serious side effects of theophylline are seizures and ventricular arrhythmias. Bothersome but not life-threatening side effects include GI problems (anorexia, nausea, vomiting, abdominal pain, diarrhea), tremor, a feeling of nervousness, headaches, insomnia, and palpitations (tachycardia and extrasystoles).

The dosing algorithm that follows was developed in 1990 by the Clinical Pharmacy Section and the Medical Service of the Houston Veterans Affairs Medical Center and is in use there. The algorithm incorporates what is currently known about the volume of distribution of theophylline and factors affecting theophylline clearance. It covers several important situations: calculation of the IV loading dose of aminophylline for a patient not previously taking oral theophylline as well as for a patient who has been using theophylline, calculation of the IV maintenance dose, actions to take when the serum level is supratherapeutic, and how to switch to an oral preparation.

Oral Theophylline-Dosing Algorithm

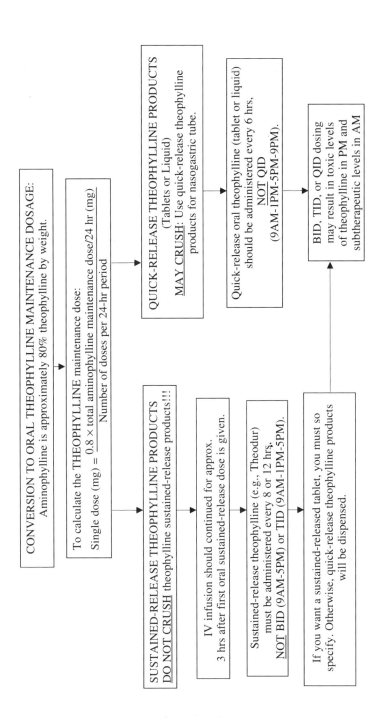

CONVERSION TO ORAL THEOPHYLLINE MAINTENANCE DOSAGE:
Aminophylline is approximately 80% theophylline by weight.

To calculate the THEOPHYLLINE maintenance dose:

$$\text{Single dose (mg)} = \frac{0.8 \times \text{total aminophylline maintenance dose/24 hr (mg)}}{\text{Number of doses per 24-hr period}}$$

QUICK-RELEASE THEOPHYLLINE PRODUCTS
(Tablets or Liquid)
<u>MAY CRUSH</u>: Use quick-release theophylline products for nasogastric tube.

Quick-release oral theophylline (tablet or liquid) should be administered every 6 hrs,
<u>NOT QID</u>
(9AM-1PM-5PM-9PM).

BID, TID, or QID dosing may result in toxic levels of theophylline in PM and subtherapeutic levels in AM

SUSTAINED-RELEASE THEOPHYLLINE PRODUCTS
<u>DO NOT CRUSH</u> theophylline sustained-release products!!!

IV infusion should continued for approx.
3 hrs after first oral sustained-release dose is given.

Sustained-release theophylline (e.g., Theodur) must be administered every 8 or 12 hrs,
<u>NOT BID</u> (9AM-5PM) or TID (9AM-1PM-5PM).

If you want a sustained-released tablet, you must so specify. Otherwise, quick-release theophylline products will be dispensed.

From Hendeles, L, et al: Update on the pharmacodynamics and pharmacokinetics of theophylline. Chest 88(Suppl)103S-111S, 1985, with permission.

THROMBOCYTOPENIA, IMMUNE

Differential Diagnosis

Antibody-related destruction of platelets in the peripheral blood is an important mechanism of thrombocytopenia. Immune thrombocytopenia must be differentiated from other mechanisms. Thrombocytopenia may be due to failure of production of platelets in the bone marrow or to peripheral platelet destruction. Examples of causes of impaired thrombocytopoiesis are aplastic anemia, myelophthisic disorders, and megaloblastic anemias. Examination of the bone marrow ordinarily differentiates failure of production from peripheral destruction. The major mechanisms of excessive peripheral destruction of platelets are as follows:

1. Immune destruction (see following table)
2. Sequestration of platelets in the spleen
3. DIC with consumption of platelets in the formation of microthrombi
4. Microangiopathies such as TTP, hemolytic uremic syndrome (HUS), and preeclampsia
5. Sequestration of platelets in large hemangiomas
6. Paroxysmal nocturnal hemoglobinuria
7. Congenital abnormalities of platelet structure such as Wiskott-Aldrich syndrome

---

Disorders Associated with Immune Thrombocytopenia

---

1. Congenital immunologic thrombocytopenia
   a. Neonatal alloimmune thrombocytopenia: a disorder in which the platelets of the fetus and neonate are destroyed by maternal antibodies, usually directed at platelet-specific antigen Pl^{A1}
   b. Drug sensitivity: in which fetal platelet destruction occurs because of maternal antibodies to a drug taken by the mother
   c. Neonatal thrombocytopenia due to maternal ITP: in which the antibodies cross the placenta to the fetus
2. Posttransfusion purpura: thrombocytopenia, 1 week after transfusions
3. Acute postinfectious thrombocytopenia (acute ITP): acute viral infections, particularly in childhood
4. Idiopathic (immune) thrombocytopenic purpura (chronic ITP): most common immune disorder with thrombocytopenia
5. Drug-induced immunologic thrombocytopenia: most common drugs are heparin, quinine, quinidine, gold, sulfonamides, anticonvulsants, chlorothiazide, furosemide, procainamide, heroin, and antilymphocyte globulin
6. Chronic postinfectious thrombocytopenia (chronic ITP): viral infections (particularly HIV-1, infectious mononucleosis, CMV, and infectious hepatitis), TB, and histoplasmosis
7. Immune disorders: SLE, Evans's syndrome, autoimmune thyroiditis, Sjögren's syndrome, and thyrotoxicosis
8. Malignancies: CLL, lymphoid lymphomas, Hodgkin's disease, and carcinomas
9. Miscellaneous: sarcoidosis, inflammatory bowel disease

THROMBOCYTOSIS

Causes

The normal range for the platelet count is 150,000 to 450,000/mm^3 of blood. An elevation of the platelet count above normal (e.g., thrombocytosis) may be due to primary clonal proliferative disorders of the bone marrow or due secondarily to a wide variety of disorders.

Causes of Thrombocytosis

Primary thrombocytosis (myeloproliferative disorders)
    Primary (essential) thrombocythemia
    Polycythemia vera
    Chronic myelogenous leukemia
    Myelofibrosis (agnogenic myeloid metaplasia)
Secondary thrombocytosis
    Acute hemorrhage
    Chronic infections
    Chronic inflammatory disorders
        Connective tissue disorders
        Inflammatory bowel disease
        Sarcoidosis
    Chronic malignancies
        Hodgkin's disease
        Carcinomas
    Iron deficiency
    Postoperative state
    Splenectomy
    Exercise
    Epinephrine
    Rebound thrombocytosis (after thrombocytopenia)

Thrombocytosis can be responsible for either thrombosis or hemorrhage. However, those complications are uncommon if the platelet count is below 1 million per mm^3. When the thrombocytosis is secondary, the platelet count is usually below 1 million per mm^3 and there are no complications. Thus, thrombocytosis as a mechanism of hemostatic abnormalities is an issue principally in primary thrombocythemia and polycythemia vera and occasionally in chronic myelogenous leukemia and myelofibrosis.

THROMBOTIC THROMBOCYTOPENIC PURPURA

TTP is a syndrome defined by the presence of the characteristic triad of thrombocytopenia, fragmentation hemolysis, and waxing and waning neurologic signs. To this triad may be added two additional criteria to make a pentad: fever and renal involvement. TTP is closely related to the hemolytic uremic syndrome (HUS).

In both disorders there is microangiopathy manifested by intravascular hyaline thrombotic occlusions in small vessels. In HUS this is largely confined to the endothelial cells of the renal vasculature, whereas in TTP the process is focused in the brain, although the kidneys, lungs, pancreas, and heart may also be affected.

The diagnosis of TTP is a good test of clinical judgment and requires a high index of suspicion. The neurologic sequelae include headache, transient strokes, seizures, and coma. TTP is usually recognized when the physician takes the opportunity to look at the peripheral blood film. The dramatic appearance of schistocytes (helmet cells) and spherocytes suggests the diagnosis. Although mild fragmentation hemolysis may be seen in a variety of disorders (particularly those associated with DIC), the picture is one of exuberant hemolysis accompanied by reticulocytosis and sometimes a leukoerythroblastic blood picture. Thrombocytopenia occurs in TTP in the setting of an elevated LDH and without prolongation of the PT or PTT (which more strongly suggests DIC).

TTP occurs during pregnancy or in patients taking birth control pills. In a pregnant woman, TTP must be differentiated from preeclampsia and eclampsia, which are marked by fragmentation hemolysis, thrombocytopenia, proteinuria, and seizures. In eclamptic disorders, fever is seldom present and the degree of fragmentation hemolysis is milder than that seen in TTP. There is also overlap with SLE, and patients may have a positive ANA. TTP has also been associated with HIV infection. In addition, a thrombotic microangiopathy that resembles TTP may be seen in malignancy. Treatment of tumors with the agent mitomycin has been associated with the development of HUS months later.

The pathogenesis of TTP is obscure and the treatment is empiric. Platelet-agglutinating factors, endothelial dysfunction, abnormalities of prostaglandins, and disorders of von Willebrand's factor processing have been proposed. About 10 to 20% of patients follow a relapsing course. In the remission phase of their disease, an unusually large von Willebrand's factor can be identified by electrophoretic gel analysis. These patients tend to relapse during infections, trauma, or surgery.

The most effective form of therapy is usually plasmapheresis-plasma exchange and the administration of prednisone. Some patients have responded to prednisone or plasma infusion alone. Antiplatelet drugs such as aspirin are not routinely used in TTP because they increase the risk of bleeding without demonstrated benefit. Anecdotal cases of dramatic neurologic decompensation have followed platelet transfusions. In refractory patients, pheresis with cryoprecipitate-poor plasma (vWF is removed) may be beneficial. Vincristine has also been utilized. In most patients, neurologic recovery is expected. However, some patients sustain long-term injury, which may be more likely in those who have abnormalities identified on head CT or MRI.

Reference: Lian EC: Thrombotic thrombocytopenic purpura. Annu Rev Med 39:203–212, 1988.

THYROID CANCER

Thyroid cancer accounts for about 1% of all cancers. Although thyroid nodules are common, thyroid cancer is quite rare, and thyroid lumps are usually benign. However, thyroid cancer can be very aggressive, so careful evaluation of nodules is indicated.

There are three types of thyroid cancer: papillary, follicular, and medullary. Papillary cancers occur in a young age group, usually before the fourth decade. The natural history can be very prolonged, metastasizing to local nodes and growing slowly in both areas. The average duration of symptoms before diagnosis of papillary cancer is about 15 months. Differentiating benign and malignant lesions is often a considerable challenge for the pathologist. Pure follicular cancers are even less common and are also a problem for the pathologist. They also have a long duration of symptoms, averaging about 32 months before diagnosis. Unlike papillary cancers, they tend to spread hematogenously, producing lytic bone lesions—often in the spine, pelvis, or skull—and mimicking myeloma; they can also spread to the lungs. In both papillary and follicular cancers, younger patients have a better survival rate. However, pure papillary and pure follicular cancers are rare. Most lesions are mixed-cell types, and the mixture is found in both primary and metastatic lesions, often in dissimilar proportions.

Medullary carcinoma of the thyroid, occurring in only 3% of all thyroid cancers, originates from the parafollicular rather than the follicular cells and produces thyrocalcitonin. One form of this disease is a single nodule, which occurs sporadically in elderly patients; another form is bilateral and may be associated with pheochromocytoma in an autosomal dominant disorder called MEN II. Two subsets of the disease are described: type IIA, which is associated with a defect on chromosome 10 and occurs with parathyroid hyperplasia, and type IIB (also called type III) in which there are a neuroectodermal defect and characteristic facies. Symptoms range from none (with incidental elevation of serum calcitonin) to intractable diarrhea, to Cushing's syndrome, and/or to carcinoid syndrome. Most patients are asymptomatic for an average of 54 months before diagnosis. Study of first-degree relatives has led to early diagnosis and treatment of the disease before clinical manifestations occur.

Symptoms of thyroid cancer include a lump in the neck, hoarseness, and the sensation of pressure or pain in the neck. A history of goiter is found in up to 15% of patients. On physical exam, about a fourth of patients have palpable cervical nodes.

When a thyroid nodule is palpated, patients should have a thyroid scan after testing for hyperthyroidism. If uptake occurs and hyperthyroidism is present, patients may be treated with surgery or radioiodine. If euthyroid, careful observation is indicated, but if the nodule is cold on scan and there is a history of thyroid irradiation, resection should be done. If there is no radiation history and the patient is a female greater than age 30, treatment with thyroxine and careful monitoring are appropriate. However, if the patient is male or is a female less than age 30, a biopsy should be performed, followed by resection if necessary.

For all types of thyroid cancer, however, the 5- and 10-year survival rates are quite good, with more than three-fourths of patients alive at 10 years. This is most probably due to early diagnosis and the generally indolent nature of these cancers.

THYROID DISEASE

Diagnostic Testing for Thyroid Disease

I. **Thyroid function tests**
   A. **Serum total T_4:** measures the total (both free and bound) fractions of T_4.
      1. Total T_4 level is elevated in:
         - Hyperthyroidism (characterized by high T_4 production).
         - Conditions characterized by increased TBG levels: hereditary TBG excess, excess estrogen (pregnancy and oral contraceptives), and acute hepatitis.
         - Other less common conditions (acute psychiatric illness).

2. Total T_4 is reduced in:
   - Hypothyroidism (due to decreased T_4 production).
   - Conditions associated with decreased TBG levels, (e.g., hereditary TBG deficiency, androgens, glucocorticoids, and severe illness).

B. **Serum-free T_4** may be useful because it gives a better assessment of thyroid hormone production. It is low in hypothyroidism and elevated in hyperthyroidism.

C. **T_3 resin uptake (T_3RU):** T_3RU and total T_4 are both decreased in hypothyroidism; both are elevated in hyperthyroidism. With excess TBG, total T_4 is elevated and the T_3RU is decreased. With TBG deficiency, T_3RU is increased. The **free thyroxine index (FTI)** is calculated by multiplying total T_4 level by T_3RU, thus correcting for the changes in thyroid-hormone-binding proteins.

D. **Serum T_3 by radioimmunoassay:** T_3 measurement is important in the diagnosis of hyperthyroidism. However, it is not as useful in diagnosis of hypothyroidism, because it is the last test to become abnormal in this condition.

E. **Radioactive iodine uptake (RAIU):** The uptake of radioiodine 1 to 24 hrs after an oral tracer dose reflects the trapping and organification of iodine and therefore permits direct assessment of glandular activity. Normal values for 24-hr RAIU are 10 to 30% in the United States. RAIU is useful in the differentiation of the causes of hyperthyroidism and hypothyroidism.

F. **TRH stimulation test:** This test amplifies any minimal change in TSH secretion. From 200 to 500 μg of TRH are given as an IV bolus, and the serum is sampled for TSH measurement before and following TRH injection at variable intervals for 1 to 2 hrs. Normal response consists of a rise in TSH level, which peaks at 20 to 30 min. Hyperthyroidism and pituitary hypothyroidism are associated with a blunted TSH response to TRH, whereas mild primary hypothyroidism is associated with an exaggerated response of TSH to TRH.

II. **Imaging techniques**

A. **Thyroid scan:** This scan is valuable in making the diagnosis of a multinodular goiter. It is also very useful in the evaluation of a nodule: cold (hypofunctioning) or hot and warm (hyperfunctioning).

B. **Thyroid ultrasonography and CT:** High-resolution ultrasonography may be helpful both in distinguishing a solid nodule from a cyst and in confirming the presence of a nodule. CT may be useful both in determining whether a neck mass is contiguous with the thyroid and in defining the extension of large nodular goiters in the neck area and substernally.

TFT changes in nonthyroidal illness (euthyroid sick syndrome): Several changes in thyroid hormone levels may occur as the consequence of an acute or chronic medical illness and may give rise to diagnostic difficulties. TFT abnormalities are the consequence of complex responses of thyroid hormone physiology to illness, are not specifically related to the nature of the illness, and occur in as many as 30 to 70% of hospitalized patients.

The most common abnormality is a low T_3 level, which is the result of an impairment in the peripheral conversion of T_4 to T_3. Despite the low T_3, TSH levels usually remain normal or decreased. In individuals with more severe illness, total T_4

is also low. Low T_4 is found in 15 to 20% of hospitalized patients and may cause serious diagnostic difficulties with central hypothyroidism. Hypothyroxinemia seems to be secondary to the presence in serum of factors that inhibit the binding of T_4 to TBG. Free T_4 concentrations are also often reduced in nonthyroidal illnesses. The significance of these changes is unclear.

Euthyroid Sick Syndromes

In elderly patients, this condition is more common than true thyroid disease. These patients are clinically euthyroid and their TFTs will vary depending on which syndrome is present. However, in almost all cases, the TSH is within normal limits.
Three syndromes are identified:

I. Low T_3, normal T_4
  • The most common type
  • Usually seen in acute/reversible illnesses
  • Also seen in caloric restriction and postoperatively
  • Drugs that can produce the syndrome include propranolol, glucocorticoid, amiodarone, and radiocontrast agents.
  • Due to the reduced conversion of T_4 to T_3

II. Low T_4, low T_3
  • Seen in very sick patients
  • May be due to decreased thyroid-binding proteins and increased peripheral thyroid inhibitors of T_4 to T_3 conversion

III. High T_4 (euthyroid hyperthyroxinemia)
  • Increased total T_4, low to normal T_3RU, and normal free T_4
  • Unusual, more common in elderly patients and in acute illness
  • Caused by increased TBG seen with increased estrogen, seen with hepatitis, and produced by drugs (tamoxifen, DES, and methadone)

In general, the role of the TRH stimulation test in euthyroid hyperthyroxinemia is uncertain. Acute illness, true hyperthyroidism, psychiatric illness, and aging will all blunt the normal response. However, a normal response does rule out hyperthyroidism. In ill patients with unclear abnormalities on TFTs, it may be worthwhile to repeat the tests after the acute illness has resolved (6–8 weeks later).

Reference: Surks MI, et al: American Thyroid Association guidelines for use of laboratory tests in thyroid disorders. JAMA 263:1529–1532, 1990.

Goiters

A goiter may or may not be associated with thyroid dysfunction. A goiter may occur in a euthyroid, hyperthyroid, or hypothyroid patient depending on the nature of the underlying thyroid pathology. The causes of a goiter and its clinical characteristics are listed in the following table.

Causes and Clinical Characteristics of Goiters

THYROID CONDITION	GOITER SIZE	FINDINGS ON PALPATION	THYROID FUNCTION
Simple goiter	1.5–4 × normal	Diffuse, spongy, smooth	Normal
Graves' disease	1.5–6 × normal	Diffuse, spongy, smooth	Hyperthyroid, euthyroid
Nodular goiter	1.5–8 × normal	Bilateral multiple nodularities; firm, not painful	Euthyroid, subclinical or overt hyperthyroidism
Hashimoto's thyroiditis	1.5–3 cm	Diffuse, firm, lobulated, granular	Normal or hypothyroid
Silent thyroiditis	2–3 × normal	Diffuse, firm, painless	Increased, decreased, or normal depending on the phase
Subacute thyroiditis	2–3 × normal	Diffuse, firm, painful, tender to palpation	Increased, decreased, or normal
Cancer	<2.5, often focal enlargement	Stony, fixed, irregular contours	Normal
Lymphoma of the thyroid	Variable	Diffuse or focal, firm, nontender	Normal
Reidel's thyroiditis	Small	Diffuse, stony, fixed	Normal or decreased
Suppurative thyroiditis	Small	Often unilateral, fluctuant, painful	Euthyroid

There is frequently a poor correlation between findings of nodularities on palpation and on ultrasound. Ultrasonography of the thyroid is probably the procedure of choice to distinguish diffuse from nodular goiter.

Nontoxic goiter: A diffuse nontoxic goiter may be due to Hashimoto's thyroiditis or other mechanisms (iodine deficiency in endemic areas). Multinodular, nontoxic goiter may be the consequence of progression of a diffuse goiter, and it is more common in the elderly. It is associated with normal thyroid hormone levels, but TSH is often suppressed and the TSH response to TRH is often blunted, suggesting the presence of subclinical hyperthyroidism due to autonomous function of hyperfunctioning nodules. A multinodular nontoxic goiter may enlarge significantly and cause compressive symptoms such as hoarseness, difficulty in breathing, and dysphagia. The occurrence of compressive symptoms is an indication for surgical resection of the goiter.

Nodular toxic goiter (Plummer's disease): This may be due to a single toxic adenoma or to multiple nodularities (multinodular toxic goiter). Such goiters are common causes of hyperthyroidism (mostly in the elderly) and T_3 toxicosis. The treatment is either surgical or radioactive iodine ablation.

Thyroid scan or thyroid ultrasound is helpful in differentiating between Graves' disease and toxic nodular goiter.

Graves' Disease

Graves' disease is an autoimmune disease characterized by the presence of a diffuse goiter, a state of hyperthyroidism, exophthalmos, and, occasionally, pretibial myxedema. The patient may present with one, two, or all of these manifestations.

Pathogenesis: The major pathogenic mechanism of hyperthyroidism is the production of Igs that interact with the TSH receptor to mimic the effects of TSH and activate the biosynthesis of thyroid hormone. The presence of Igs is assessed by ^{125}I-TSH binding inhibitory assay (TBI) and thyroid stimulatory Ig assay (TSI). (Long-acting thyroid stimulating [LATS] assay was the original assay for the same Ig.)

The primary defect in Graves' disease is thought to be a diminution of the ratio of suppressor T cells to helper T cells. Normally, the immune response is modulated by the suppressor function of a subpopulation of T lymphocytes, which inhibit the Ig syntheses by B cells and inhibit helper T cells. When a mutation occurs in a genetically predisposed individual, a population of autoreactive helper T lymphocytes appears, causing the augmented antibody formation and the cell-mediated immune responses characteristic of Graves' disease. Patients with Graves' disease often have a family history of autoimmune disease.

Clinical manifestations: The clinical manifestations of hyperthyroidism reflect the impact of excessive thyroid hormone action on end organs. They are often related to increased metabolism and enhancement of adrenergic activity. The findings are multiple, nonspecific, and of variable severity. The onset may be abrupt or progressive.

Symptoms include nervousness, excessive sweating, heat intolerance, palpitations, increased appetite, weight loss, fatigue, hyperkinetic movements, and insomnia. Other complaints are dyspnea, hair loss, muscle weakness, diarrhea, impotence in the male, oligomenorrhea in the female, and pruritus. Some patients present with symptoms of CHF.

The physical findings may include tachycardia, warm and moist skin, onycholysis, Plummer's sign, and a fine tremor of the outstretched fingers. The heart sounds are often loud, and a mid-systolic ejection murmur may be present. The ankle jerk relaxation time is rapid. Less common findings are AF, CHF, and proximal muscle weakness. Eye findings are very common in hyperthyroid patients. Lid lag, stare, lid retraction, itching, and increased tearing are due to increased adrenergic activity.

In addition to the manifestations of hyperthyroidism, patients with Graves' disease often exhibit a diffuse goiter of variable size with a bruit and no nodularity.

Exophthalmos is present in approximately 50% of patients and is characteristic of Graves' disease. It is the result of periorbital infiltration by mucopolysaccharidelike material and fibrotic and inflammatory changes of the extraocular muscles. Characteristic changes are often seen on CT scan of the orbits, particularly thickening of the eye muscles. Exophthalmos is often accompanied by periorbital edema, congestion, chemosis, conjunctival injection, and, occasionally ocular-muscle-paralysis-causing diplopia. If the exophthalmos is very marked (malignant exophthalmos), it may cause an ulceration of the cornea that predisposes to infection.

Laboratory findings: T_4, T_3, and T_3 RU are usually elevated. In some instances, only T_3 is high (T_3 toxicosis). The most useful diagnostic tests in hyperthyroidism are elevated T_3 and suppressed TSH. RAIU is elevated and differentiates Graves' disease from other causes of hyperthyroidism (e.g., silent thyroiditis, subacute thyroiditis, factitious thyroid hormone intake). Other causes of hyperthyroidism that should be excluded prior to therapy include toxic nodules, hydatidiform mole, choriocarcinoma, TSH-induced hyperthyroidism, and iodine-induced hyperthyroidism.

Treatment: The ultimate objective is achievement of a long-standing remission. The three therapeutic modalities are a long course of antithyroid drugs, radioactive iodine ablation, and subtotal thyroidectomy. The most commonly used form of therapy is radioiodine ablation.

The two major antithyroid medications are propylthiouracil (PTU) and methimazole. Both inhibit thyroid hormone synthesis. In addition, PTU impairs the peripheral conversion of T_4 to T_3. Propranolol may be useful to counteract the peripheral effects of thyroid hormone in symptomatic patients.

Hyperthyroidism

Hyperthyroidism is defined as a clinical state resulting from any one of several causes and is characterized by the following symptoms and signs.

Signs and Symptoms in 247 Patients with Thyrotoxicosis

Symptoms (with % incidence)

Nervousness (99%)	Increased appetite (65%)
Increased sweating (91%)	Eye complaints (54%)
Hypersensitivity to heat (89%)	Swelling of legs (35%)
Palpitation (89%)	Hyperdefecation (without diarrhea) (33%)
Fatigue (88%)	Anorexia (23%)
Weight loss (85%)	Diarrhea (23%)
Tachycardia (82%)	Constipation (4%)
Dyspnea (75%)	Weight gain (2%)
Weakness (70%)	

Signs (with % incidence)

Tachycardia* (100%)	Eye signs (71%)
Goiter (100%)	Atrial fibrillation (10%)
Skin changes (97%)	Splenomegaly (10%)
Tremor (97%)	Liver palms (8%)
Bruit over thyroid (77%)	Gynecomastia (4%)

*In other studies, thyrotoxic patients with normal pulse rate have been observed.

From Larsen PR, et al: The thyroid gland. In Wilson JD, et al (eds): William's Textbook of Endocrinology, 8th ed. Philadelphia, W.B. Saunders, 1992, p 426, with permission.

The various etiologies of thyrotoxicosis may be differentiated by the following findings.

Etiologies of Thyrotoxicosis

CAUSE	THYROID GLAND	TSH	RAIU
Graves' disease	Smooth, firm	Suppressed	↑
Multinodular	Nodular, inconsistent	Suppressed	↑
Toxic adenoma	Nodular (usually ≥3 cm)	Suppressed	↑
Silent thyroiditis	Smooth, firm	Suppressed	↓
Subacute thyroiditis	Exquisitely tender	Suppressed	↓
Thyrotrope pituitary adenoma (rare)	Smooth, firm	Inappropriately detectable	↑
Factitious	Nonpalpable	Suppressed	↓
Hyperfunctioning thyroid carcinoma	Firm	Suppressed	↑

Adapted from Caruso DR, et al: Intervention in Graves' disease. Postgrad Med 92(8):117, 1992, p 122.

Rare causes include HCG-induced hyperthyroidism (from choriocarcinoma or hydatidiform mole) and struma ovarii.

Graves' disease is the most common cause and is characterized by the triad of diffuse goiter, ophthalmopathy, and dermopathy, any one of which may progress or regress independently of the others. It is an autoimmune disorder with familial transmission, is more common in women, and occurs most often during the third or fourth decade. Circulating autoantibodies that stimulate TSH receptors on the thyroid gland induce the thyrotoxic state (thyroid-inhibiting autoantibodies have also been reported). Eye and skin findings result from inflammatory infiltrates of the orbital musculature and dermis, respectively.

Treatment: Three therapeutic options exist: antithyroid medications, radioiodine, and surgery. A recent survey of members of the American Thyroid Association favored radioiodine as the treatment of choice for Graves' disease. Subsequent hypothyroidism must be anticipated, and ophthalmopathy may be aggravated (pretreatment with prednisone is necessary). Antithyroid drugs may be preferable in children and adolescents and are the treatment of choice for pregnant patients and patients who do not wish to take radioiodine. Remission rates of up to 65% have been reported after 2 years of drug therapy, but high relapse rates and potentially lethal side effects (agranulocytosis, exfoliative dermatitis, thrombocytopenia), although admittedly rare, make drug therapy less attractive to many clinicians. Propylthiouracil (PTU) may be started at a dose of 150 mg PO Q 8 hrs, with a maximum of 1,200 mg daily. Methimazole is started at a dose of 10 mg PO Q 8 hrs, with a maximum of 90 mg daily. Dosages are adjusted according to clinical response.

Both a baseline and periodic repeat WBCs should be obtained during the first 3 months of administration, with discontinuation of the medication if the WBC falls below 2,000/mm^3 (most cases of agranulocytosis are reported during this time). Euthyroidism is often established within the first 6 weeks, at which time an attempt to lower the drug dosage by about one-third is warranted. After 12 to 24 months, the thionamide dose is slowly lowered during close observation for possible relapse (usually in the first 3 to 6 months). Successful outcomes with antithyroid medication most often occur in patients with mild hyperthyroidism, small gland size, or gland size that decreases during therapy.

Thyroid storm is an emergency condition treated with PTU (preferred over methimazole because it also inhibits the peripheral conversion of T_4 to T_3) at an initial dose of 300 to 400 mg PO followed by 200 mg PO Q 4 hrs. Dexamethasone is given in a dose of 2 mg IV or PO Q 6 hrs to inhibit conversion of T_4 to T_3. Iodide therapy (e.g., SSKI at a dose of 2 drops PO Q 8 hrs) acts acutely to slow release of thyroid hormone. Beta-adrenergic blockers (40–80 mg PO Q 6–8 hrs or 2 mg IV with monitoring) are administered to reduce symptom severity. With such combined therapy, normalization of serum T_3 values may occur within 24 to 48 hours.

Management of Graves' ophthalmopathy requires close interaction with an ophthalmologist. High-dose corticosteroids and/or external radiation to the orbits is usually tried initially, with decompressive surgery reserved for refractory cases. Graves' dermopathy, if severe, may be treated with topical corticosteroids with or without an occlusive dressing.

Hyperthyroidism associated with toxic multinodular goiter is believed to result from activity of one of the nodules that gradually over many years begins to function autonomously, usually producing symptoms in later life. Because of the need for larger doses of radioactive iodine to treat this condition, as well as the older age of patients, pretreatment with antithyroid drugs is usually recommended, with discontinuation of oral medications 4 to 5 days before treatment with radioiodine. Toxic adenomas may best be managed by surgery in patients less than 20 years of age or in older patients with large, disfiguring tumors. Radioactive iodine remains the treatment of choice in most other cases, usually following pretreatment with antithyroid medications to relieve symptoms.

Atypical Presentations of Hyperthyroidism

Hyperthyroidism is quite common in elderly patients, with a female predominance. Graves' disease is the most common etiology. Also seen is an increase in the proportion due to single or multiple toxic nodules. Less than 50% of older patients present with classic symptoms of weight loss, palpitations, weakness, anxiety and nervousness, and heat intolerance. On physical exam, only 30% of elderly as opposed to 100% of young patients have tachycardia. Exophthalmos, lid lag, and tremor are also infrequent in the elderly. As was seen with President Bush, the new onset of AF, CHF, and exacerbation of angina are common presentations.

Apathetic or Masked Hyperthyroidism

- Apathy, depression, dizziness, syncope, increased tremor, and increased confusion (reversible dementia) are symptoms unique to old persons with hyperthyroidism.
- Constipation is more frequent than diarrhea in the elderly.
- Lab: elevated T_3, decreased TSH
- Often normal or only slightly elevated T_4

Risk factors for hyperthyroidism include a family history for thyroid disease and use of amiodarone and iodine. Propranolol artificially increases T_4, as does acute illness (see Thyroid Disease: Euthyroid Sick Syndromes), and acute illness can decrease TSH. Serum T_3 clarifies diagnosis. The long-term effects of hyperthyroidism include accelerated osteoporosis, A fib, accelerated angina, and chronic delusions or dementia.

Symptomatic patients should be treated initially with beta-blockers and PTU or methimazole. Definitive therapy can proceed with radioactive iodine or surgery. A radioiodine scan will differentiate Graves' disease from nodular goiter.

Reference: Feit H: Thyroid function in the elderly. Clin Geriatr Med 4:151–161, 1988.

Hypothyroidism

Hypothyroidism is the most common thyroid condition. It is defined by a deficiency in circulating and tissue thyroid hormone concentrations. It may be the result of thyroidal failure (primary hypothyroidism, in which the TSH level is high) or deficiency of TSH (central, in which TSH level is low normal). Hypothyroidism may be subclinical, overt (presence of clinical manifestations of thyroid hormone deficiency), or severe (usually associated with myxedema). Myxedema refers to the accumulation of glycosaminoglycans in subcutaneous and interstitial tissue due to profound hypothyroidism.

Common Causes of Hypothyroidism

1. Autoimmune thyroiditis, Hashimoto's thyroiditis (the most common cause of primary hypothyroidism in the adult)
2. Atrophic hypothyroidism (end stage of Hashimoto's thyroiditis or mediated by TSH receptor-blocking antibodies)
3. Postablative therapy for Graves' disease
4. Neck irradiation for lymphoma and other head and neck conditions
5. Postsurgical
6. Infiltrative diseases (scleroderma, amyloidosis)
7. Functional defect in thyroid hormone production or release (iodine deficiency and excess, lithium, antithyroid drugs, numerous inherited enzymatic defects)
8. Transient primary hypothyroidism (silent thyroiditis, subacute thyroiditis, postpartum thyroiditis)
9. Central hypothyroidism (pituitary tumors, other sellar and parasellar processes, particularly hypothalamic disease)

Symptoms and Signs of Hypothyroidism

Symptoms

Fatigue	Cold intolerance
Sleepiness	Decreased appetite
Lethargy	Constipation
Decreased memory	Decreased perspiration
Depression	Dyspnea on exertion
Impaired cognitive functions	Galactorrhea
Slow speech	Hoarseness
Decreased hearing	Slow motion
Lack of interest	Slow speech
Weight gain	Muscle weakness
Menstrual disturbances	Muscle cramps
(menorrhagia)	Hair loss
Arthralgias	Paresthesias
Yellow palms	

Signs

Slow movement	Slow speech
Dry skin	Bradycardia
Hoarseness	Nonpitting edema
Hyporeflexia	Thick tongue
Delayed relaxation of	Puffy face
deep tendon reflexes	Myoedema
Hypercarotenemia (yellow palms)	Ascites (rare)
Hypothyroid heart (cardiomegaly,	Brittle nails
pericardial effusion)	Pleural effusion
Loss of $1/3$ of eyebrows	Pale, waxy skin
Extraocular muscle dysfunction	Goiter
(Hashimoto's thyroiditis)	Bladder atony
Gastric atony and megacolon	(severe hypothyroidism)
(severe hypothyroidism)	

Laboratory Findings in Hypothyroidism

1. Hyponatremia (impaired free-water excretion)
2. Anemia (normochromic, hypochromic, macrocytic, coexistent vitamin B_{12} deficiency)
3. Abnormal LFTs: elevation of transaminases
4. Elevated CPK
5. Decreased FTI and free T_4 level. T_3 is low only in profound hypothyroidism. TSH level is high in primary hypothyroidism (the higher the TSH, the more severe the thyroid hormone deficiency). In central hypothyroidism, TSH is normal or low and the TSH response to TRH is blunted.
6. High serum cholesterol, high LDL cholesterol

Treatment of hypothyroidism consists of the administration of synthetic L-thyroxine. The initial dose should be small in patients with a history of cardiovascular disease (12.5–25 μg daily) with a gradual increase every week or two, up to a maintenance dose necessary to achieve and maintain a euthyroid state.

In younger, healthy individuals, initial starting dose is 50 μg, with a more rapid increase up to the maintenance dose. Other forms of thyroid substitution should be avoided. Follow-up TSH measurement is crucial for titration of the dose.

Subacute Thyroiditis

Subacute thyroiditis (also called de Quervain's thyroiditis or granulomatous or giant-cell thyroiditis) is a common thyroid disorder. Its incidence varies from one region of the world to another. It occurs more frequently between the second and fifth decades. The female-male ratio is approximately 6:1. The etiology is viral in many circumstances (e.g., mumps, influenza, measles, common cold, adenovirus, infectious mononucleosis, coxsackievirus, St. Louis encephalitis, cat scratch fever). Antiviral antibodies are often elevated and the titers correlate with the course of the disease. Although autoimmunity does not seem to play a role in the occurrence of subacute thyroiditis, TSH receptor-blocking antibodies have been documented in some patients with permanent hypothyroidism following subacute thyroiditis. It is believed that the presence of autoimmune markers in subacute thyroiditis constitutes a secondary phenomenon rather than a primary one.

Pathology is characterized by architectural destruction of thyroid follicles, granuloma formation, and giant cells. There is also evidence of inflammatory reaction with histiocytes and lymphocytes in the interstitial tissue. Part of the gland may be replaced by residual fibrosis, and often, as the process resolves, there is regeneration of follicular cells.

Clinical Course and Management

The disease process follows a triphasic course and often resolves completely, with restoration of normal health. However, a few patients will have permanent, postsubacute thyroiditis hypothyroidism. The triphasic course of the disease is often preceded by a prodromal syndrome characterized by fever, malaise, and URI. There may be some neck discomfort and complaint of sore throat. The severity and the duration of the prodromal syndrome are variable. Hyperthyroidism due to subacute thyroiditis should be treated with beta-blockers rather than antithyroid medications. The latter are not effective because the mechanism of hyperthyroidism consists of destruction of follicular cells rather than increased organification. Thyroid ultrasound often shows diffuse hypoechoicity of the gland, which often returns to normal after resolution of the subacute thyroiditis.

Clinical Course, Laboratory Findings, and Management of Subacute Thyroiditis

	PHASE		
	Hyperthyroid	Hypothyroid	Recovery
Thyroid exam	Enlarged, painful, tender	Often enlarged, painless	Normal or slightly enlarged
Systemic manifestations	Variable (fever, neck pain unilateral or bilateral, radiating to ear)	None	None
Duration	1–3 months	1–2 months	Permanent
T_3:T_4	Increased (often T_4 toxicosis)	Decreased	Normal
RAIU	Low (0–5%)	0–27%	Normal
Other lab findings	Leukopenia, high ESR, high thyroglobulin	High TSH	—
Treatment	Aspirin, NSAID (e.g., indomethacin, ibuprofen), steroids, propranolol	Thyroid hormone	None

Subclinical Hypothyroidism

Subclinical hypothyroidism is defined as a slightly elevated basal TSH level or an exaggerated TSH response to TRH stimulation in a patient with normal total T_4 and T_3 levels. Free T_4 is frequently either borderline low or low. It represents the mildest form of primary hypothyroidism. Its prevalence is quite high. It affects approximately 4 to 5% of the general population and is more common in elderly people, particularly postmenopausal women, in whom the prevalence may reach 15 to 17%. Elderly men have a lower prevalence (6–7%). In many patients it is associated with evidence of autoimmune thyroid disease (i.e., positive thyroid antibodies), but many patients do not have an elevated titer of antithyroid antibodies. The rate of progression to overt hypothyroidism in patients with subclinical hypothyroidism and positive thyroid antibody is approximately 4 to 5% a year. A few patients may have symptoms of thyroid hormone deficiency (decreased memory, constipation, menorrhagia).

Causes of TSH elevation other than subclinical hypothyroidism:

1. Nonthyroidal illnesses: TSH is often <20. If the patient is asymptomatic, TSH should be repeated after recovery from the nonthyroidal illness (often thyroid antibody negative).
2. Psychiatric illnesses
3. Chronic renal failure
4. Presence of heterophilic antibodies to TSH
5. Dopamine agonists (used mostly in Europe, e.g., metoclopramide)

6. Addison's disease, isolated ACTH deficiency
7. Generalized and selective pituitary resistance to thyroid hormone
8. Central hypothyroidism

Consequences of subclinical hypothyroidism:

1. Possible association with CAD and peripheral vascular disease
2. Cardiac dysfunction at the subclinical level; clinically not significant
3. Neuropsychological changes, affecting 20% of patients; reversed with thyroid hormone therapy
4. Changes in lipoprotein metabolism; increased LDL cholesterol and apo B
5. Refractory depression, increased severity of bipolar disorder
6. Infertility, possibly mediated by hyperprolactinemia, galactorrhea
7. Menorrhagia

In addition to the elderly, subclinical hypothyroidism is more common in patients with other autoimmune diseases, a history of treated Graves' disease, Down's syndrome, depression, polymyalgia rheumatica, and hyperprolactinemia.

THYROID DYSFUNCTION IN THE ELDERLY

The diagnosis of thyroid dysfunction in the elderly may be difficult both because the clinical expression may be different from that in younger adults and because many features of aging resemble those of thyroid hormone deficiency. In addition, TFTs in the elderly are frequently abnormal because of the effects of aging, illness, use of drugs, and starvation on thyroid hormone metabolism. The most common abnormality is a low T_3 level. Most epidemiologic studies have shown that elevated TSH is quite common in the elderly. Approximately 17% of postmenopausal women and 7% of elderly men have elevated TSH levels consistent with hypothyroidism (subclinical cases are more common than overt cases). The prevalence of positive antithyroid antibody increases with aging. TSH elevation may also be due to a nonthyroidal illness, and normalization of TSH often follows recovery from the illness.

Hypothyroidism: The most common causes of primary hypothyroidism in the elderly are autoimmune thyroiditis and ablative therapy. The typical symptoms and signs of hypothyroidism are observed in only 25 to 70% of all hypothyroid patients. One study showed that only 10% of patients with laboratory confirmation of hypothyroidism were diagnosed on clinical examination. Symptoms and signs of hypothyroidism are often present only in patients with markedly elevated serum TSH. Cold intolerance, depression, decreased cognitive functions, muscle weakness, lethargy, and constipation should be the clinical clues of thyroid hormone deficiency. Other features are muscle cramps, paresthesias, poor balance, deafness, and dementia.

Management includes levothyroxine substitution initiated at a small dose (12.5 μg), which should be gradually increased until normalization of thyroid status is achieved. Cardiovascular function should be monitored very carefully during thyroid hormone replacement.

Hyperthyroidism: Approximately 2% of patients older than 65 years admitted to hospitals may have unsuspected hyperthyroidism. Females are more often affected than males (8:1 ratio). Graves' disease remains the most common cause of hyperthyroidism in the elderly, although there also is increased incidence of toxic nodular goiter in older people. The hyperthyroid condition is often diagnosed during evaluation or management of other conditions such as HTN, DM, and atherosclerotic cardiovascular disease (particularly A fib). In the elderly, catabolic and cardiac symptoms predominate. The diagnosis is established by the findings of elevated free thyroxine index, free T_4, and T_3. T_3 toxicosis may be present in patients with toxic nodular goiter. If thyroid hormone levels are borderline, a TRH stimulation test is indicated and will show a flat response. The treatment of choice for both Graves' disease and nodular toxic goiter is radioiodine ablation. Following treatment, patients should be carefully and frequently monitored so that the physician can recognize and correct thyroid hormone deficiency.

Presenting Features of Hyperthyroidism in the Elderly

SYMPTOMS	SIGNS
Dyspnea	Absence of tachycardia ($\approx$50%)
Weight loss	Exophthalmos rare
Muscle weakness	Goiter absent in 30%
Anorexia	A fib common ($\approx$50%)
Palpitations	CHF (new onset or worsening)
Constipation or diarrhea	Severe muscle weakness
Angina	Depression
Anxiety	Wasting appearance (suggesting malignancy)
Confusion	Apathy (apathetic hyperthyroidism)
Insomnia	

THYROID NODULES

Clinically palpable thyroid nodules are present in 3 to 4% of the population. Autopsy and ultrasound studies have shown an even higher prevalence of thyroid nodularities (exceeding 10%). Most nodules do not exceed 1 cm in diameter and have little clinical implication. Most patients present with an asymptomatic nodule discovered by the patient or the physician during a physical examination. There is no evidence that multinodular goiters carry a higher risk of cancer. Most thyroid cancers are cold on scintiscan, most warm or hot (hyperfunctioning) nodules are benign, and 15% of cold nodules are malignant. In the past, thyroid cysts have been assumed to be usually benign; however, recent studies have suggested a high incidence of malignancy within the walls of cysts (in the range of 10%).

Clinical Features Raising Suspicion of Malignancy in Thyroid Nodules

1. Male patient
2. Presence of compressive symptoms such as dysphonia, dysphagia, or respiratory difficulties
3. History of radiation exposure, particularly treatment with external radiation to the neck and face
4. Irregular contours, hard consistency, and rapid growth over a short period of time
5. Cystic lesion recurring after multiple aspirations

The size of the nodule and the presence or absence of a family history of thyroid disease do not seem to be associated with an increased incidence of malignancy. There is controversy whether autoimmune thyroid disease, particularly Graves' disease, is associated with an increased incidence of malignant lesions. Only medullary thyroid carcinoma is associated with an increased family incidence of such neoplasia.

Evaluation of a nodule: Thyroid scan allows the determination of whether the nodule is cold (hypofunctioning) or warm to hot (hyperfunctioning). Approximately 2 to 6% of thyroid nodules appear hot or warm on scan. Ultrasound is helpful in establishing the diagnosis of a cyst and its simple or complex nature. Ultrasound may also be helpful in determining whether the nodule is single or part of a multinodular goiter. In addition, ultrasound is helpful in differentiating between a distinct nodularity and focal or diffuse thyroiditis. It also provides accurate measurement of the nodule, which may be helpful for subsequent follow-up.

In most centers, fine-needle aspiration (FNA) biopsy has become the gold standard and the initial test in evaluation of thyroid nodules. It has significantly reduced the number of unnecessary surgeries. There has been controversy whether imaging with ultrasound or thyroid scan should precede the FNA. Certainly, using FNA as the initial step is more cost-effective than using imaging techniques in every patient. However, doing a blind aspiration on every single nodule may give rise to false-positive cytological readings due to hyperfunctioning nodules (often associated with high cellularity and nuclear pleomorphism). In addition, cystic lesions can be diagnosed by FNA by the presence of fluid in the aspirate; however, cytology of the fluid aspirate may not be helpful in the diagnosis. Oxyphilic nodules found in Hashimoto's thyroiditis may be confused with Hürthle cell or follicular tumors.

Interpretation of Fine-Needle-Aspiration Biopsy of Thyroid Nodules

1. Benign	60–75%
2. Malignancy	5%
3. Suspicious or undeterminate	20%
Rate of malignancy	20%
False-negative rate	10%

Accuracy depends on the type of tumor and the experience of both the physician performing the procedure and the cytopathologist. Most false-negative results are from inadequate sampling. Adequacy of a sample requires six smears containing 10 to 15 groups of well-preserved clumps of follicular cells. Accuracy in distinguishing between neoplastic and nonneoplastic lesions is approximately 88%, with 7% false-positive and 5% false-negative interpretations.

Management: Patients who have a benign FNA reading should be followed closely because of the high false-negative rate. Repeat aspiration in the follow-up helps in detecting new cases of malignancy. Cystic lesions that reaccumulate fluid or the presence of a residual mass after aspiration should be excised unless ultrasound-guided biopsy of the residual mass has been performed and shows a benign lesion. Undeterminate or suspicious lesions should be subjected to surgery. Repeat FNA should be performed in cases of inadequate sampling.

The use of L-thyroxine suppressive therapy for shrinkage of nodules has become controversial because of the potentially adverse effects of long-term L-thyroxine therapy (i.e., bone loss) and because its effectiveness is not certain.

Warm and hot nodules should be followed conservatively, with repeat thyroid function testing.

THYROID STORM

Thyroid storm is a life-threatening state of severe hyperthyroidism. Its mortality rate ranges from 10 to 75%. The diagnosis is mostly clinical. The clinical features include:

1. Hyperpyrexia: temperature higher than 38.5°C (out of proportion to any underlying infection); may be life threatening.
2. Extreme tachycardia (out of proportion to the fever), arrhythmias, CHF, vascular collapse
3. GI: nausea, vomiting, diarrhea, abdominal pain, hepatomegaly
4. Jaundice, when present, is associated with an ominous prognosis.
5. CNS manifestations: confusion, restlessness, agitation, psychosis, apathy, and even coma

The most common precipitating factor is infection. Other precipitating factors include surgery, trauma, DKA, abrupt withdrawal of antithyroid drug therapy, severe infection, MI, CVA, pulmonary thromboembolism, radioactive iodine therapy, parturition, vigorous palpation of the thyroid, and use of iodinated contrast dyes.

Laboratory Findings

1. Elevated total T_4, T_3, and free T_4 in the same range as uncomplicated thyrotoxicosis; T_4 toxicosis may be present; elevated T_4, normal or slightly elevated T_3 because of coexistent illness.
2. Mild to moderate hyperglycemia
3. Leukocytosis with mild left shift common (even in the absence of infection)
4. Abnormal LFTs (transaminases, bilirubin, alkaline phosphatase)
5. Serum cortisol should be measured to rule out coexistent adrenal insufficiency (association of autoimmune diseases).

Mechanisms of Thyroid Storm

1. Elevation in the free thyroid hormone fraction due to coexistent illness, despite unchanged serum total T_4 and T_3 levels
2. Increased adrenergic activity
3. Exaggerated thyroid hormone action, possibly related to tissue hypoxia, lactic acidosis, and infection

Management

1. Therapy aimed at inhibiting thyroid hormone production and release (antithyroid drugs, oral iodine [SSKI], or IV NaI or lithium carbonate as an alternative to iodine)
2. Inhibition of peripheral thyroid hormone action; corticosteroids (ipodate, propranolol, and PTU); reserpine may be an alternative to propranolol;

removal of excess circulating hormone only in intractable cases (plasmapheresis, dialysis).

3. Supportive measures include correction of hyperthermia (acetaminophen, cooling, fluid and electrolyte balance), oxygen, vasopressors if needed, and treatment of CHF if present.

4. The precipitating or coexistent illness should be identified and treated aggressively.

THYROIDITIS: HASHIMOTO'S THYROIDITIS

General classification of thyroiditis

1. Acute (suppurative, radiation induced)
2. Subacute course
   a. Subacute or granulomatous thyroiditis
   b. Silent thyroiditis (lymphocytic thyroiditis with resolving hyperthyroidism)
   c. Postpartum thyroiditis
3. Chronic course
   a. Hashimoto's thyroiditis (the most common thyroiditis)
   b. Reidel's or fibrous thyroiditis
   c. Miscellaneous: fungal, tuberculosis, parasitic thyroiditis

Hashimoto's thyroiditis is the most common thyroiditis, with a prevalence of 1 to 2%. Female-male ratio is approximately 9:1; it occurs frequently in middle-aged women, but its prevalence increases with age. Histologically, it is characterized by a diffuse lymphocytic infiltration with presence of germinal centers and variable degrees of fibrosis, which is responsible for shrinkage of the gland. The main clinical presentation is a painless, diffuse goiter in a euthyroid patient. The thyroid may be painful in 5% of patients. Occasionally there is a pressurelike sensation in the neck. Hypothyroidism (either mild or overt) may be present in 10 to 20% of patients. Antithyroid antibodies (antithyroglobulin and antimicrosomal antibody) are positive in 80 to 95% of patients. Antiperoxidase antibody is more sensitive in the diagnosis of Hashimoto's. Thyroid function testing (free-thyroxine index, TSH, and free T_4 level) establishes the thyroid status. The presence of slightly elevated TSH indicates a state of subclinical hypothyroidism. Thyroid scan often reveals a patchy uptake, and thyroid ultrasound may show diffuse hypoechoicity.

Almost all autoimmune diseases may coexist with Hashimoto's thyroiditis (e.g., vitiligo, IDDM, pernicious anemia, Addison's disease).

Hashimoto's thyroiditis is treated with levothyroxine therapy. The purpose is to cause shrinkage of the goiter and replacement of the deficit in thyroid hormone. Lymphoma of the thyroid occurs almost exclusively in patients with Hashimoto's thyroiditis. Hashimoto's thyroiditis is often present in patients with Graves' disease. Both diseases may also be present in members of the same family. There is a genetic predisposition (association with certain HLA types).

The pathogenetic factors of Hashimoto's thyroiditis involve the dysfunction of a specific suppressor T lymphocyte, which permits a randomly appearing, forbidden clone of helper T lymphocyte to survive and interact with thyroid antigens in a genetically predisposed individual. Both humoral and cell-mediated autoimmune processes are involved.

Silent thyroiditis or lymphocytic thyroiditis with resolving hyperthyroidism may be linked to autoimmune thyroid disease (i.e., Hashimoto's thyroiditis) in a subset of patients. However, many patients do not have any evidence of underlying autoimmune thyroid disease. The clinical course of silent thyroiditis is identical to that of subacute thyroiditis; it is not due to a viral illness and is not preceded by an upper respiratory tract infection. The goiter is not painful. The mode of presentation is usually a transient hyperthyroidism lasting 2 to 3 months followed by an episode of hypothyroidism and then recovery of thyroid function. The ESR is not high, and there is usually no leukopenia.

Postpartum thyroiditis often follows a similar course to silent thyroiditis and appears to be an exacerbation of autoimmune thyroid disease in the postpartum period in a significant percentage of patients. The most typical presentation of postpartum thyroiditis is also hyperthyroidism followed by hypothyroidism and then recovery. Its occurrence correlates well with the presence of positive thyroid antibody in early pregnancy. Recurrence with subsequent pregnancy is quite common.

TICK-BORNE INFECTIONS

Important Tick-Borne Disorders

A. Bacterial infections
1. **Tularemia:** Caused by the small gram-negative rod *Francisella tularensis*. The disease may be acquired by the bites of vectors such as ticks, deerflies, and mosquitoes; by direct contact with infected animals such as rabbits or muskrats; or by bites of infected animals such as cats or squirrels. The clinical forms of tularemia are glandular (lymphadenitis), oculoglandular, typhoidal, pneumonic, and oropharyngeal.
2. **Lyme disease:** Caused by the spirochete *Borrelia burgdorferi*. The primary vectors of the microorganisms are ticks of the genus *Ixodes*. In the eastern United States, the deer tick *Ixodes dammini* is the vector. Early manifestations of Lyme disease consist of skin lesions (erythema chronicum migrans), malaise, fever, chills, myalgia, and headache. Later manifestations include arthritis, cardiac involvement with conduction abnormalities, and neurologic problems (meningitis, encephalitis, and cranial nerve dysfunction).
3. **Relapsing fever:** Caused by spirochetes of the genus *Borrelia*. Louse-borne relapsing fever is due to *Borrelia recurrentis*. Several *Borrelia* species can be responsible for tick-borne relapsing fever, which is transmitted by ticks of the genus *Ornithodoros*. These ticks acquire the *Borrelia* organisms when they feed on infected rodents. Infected humans experience the abrupt onset of fever, chills, and headache 4 to 18 days after the tick bite. The patient becomes afebrile in a few days, but relapses are likely to occur.

B. Parasitic disorders
1. **Babesiosis:** The protozoan parasite *Babesia microti* is transmitted to humans through the bite of the deer tick *Ixodes dammini*. This parasite infects erythrocytes. The illness is characterized by fever, hemolytic anemia (often severe), jaundice, and splenomegaly. In the United States, the illness is endemic on islands off the coast of Massachusetts and on Long Island in New York State.

C. Rickettsial infections
1. **Rocky Mountain spotted fever** (RMSF): *Rickettsia rickettsii* is the etiologic agent of RMSF. Several ticks may transmit the disease, including *Dermacentor andersoni* in the Rocky Mountain states, *Dermacentor variabilis* in eastern states, and *Amblyomma*

Table continued on next page.

Important Tick-Borne Disorders (Cont.)

americanum and *Rhipicephalus sanguineus* in the southwestern United States. RMSF is a serious illness, with fever, severe headache, malaise, myalgia, and a macular rash.

2. **Q fever:** The etiologic agent of Q fever is *Coxiella burnetii.* Usually the disease is transmitted to humans directly from domestic animals such as cattle, goats, and sheep. However, numerous species of ticks may also serve as vectors of the microorganisms. The illness consists of fever, chills, and headaches, often with pneumonia and hepatitis.

3. **Ehrlichiosis:** The Ehrlichieae are a group of Rickettsiaceae, which parasitize monocytes and macrophages of humans. Ticks serve as vectors of the organisms. Clinical manifestations are fever, myalgia, headache, fleeting rash, abnormal liver function tests, leukopenia, and thrombocytopenia.

4. **Other rickettsial infections:** A number of other rickettsial infections, with symptoms similar to RMSF, are carried by ticks:

Mediterranean spotted fever	Kenya tick-bite fever
North African tick typhus	Indian tick typhus
Queensland tick typhus	Marseilles fever
Siberian tick typhus	Boutonneuse fever

D. Viral infections

1. **Colorado tick fever:** An acute viral infection characterized by fever, headache, back pain, and leukopenia, occurring in the Rocky Mountain area. The causative agent is a reovirus that is transmitted to humans by the bite of the wood tick *Dermacentor andersoni.*

2. **Flavivirus infections:** There are several tick-borne flavivirus infections, characterized by meningoencephalitis or hemorrhagic fever or both.
   a. Omsk hemorrhagic fever occurs in western Siberia and consists of either encephalitis or hemorrhagic fever.
   b. Kyasanur Forest disease—either encephalitis or hemorrhagic fever—is seen in India.
   c. Central European encephalitis
   d. Russian spring-summer encephalitis
   e. Powassan encephalitis of North America
   f. Louping ill, in the British Isles

3. **Bunyavirus infection:** Crimean-Congo hemorrhagic fever is a tick-borne infection of Africa and the Crimean area that is caused by a bunyavirus and is characterized by fever, headache, hemorrhage, leukopenia, and thrombocytopenia.

TOXIC SHOCK SYNDROME

Major Criteria for Diagnosis

- Fever: temperature $\geq$38.9°C (102°F)
- Rash: diffuse macular erythroderma
- Desquamation: 1–2 weeks after onset of illness, particularly of palms and soles
- Hypotension: systolic BP $\leq$90 mm Hg for adults, or below 5th percentile by age for children younger than 16 years; orthostatic drop in diastolic BP $\geq$15 mm Hg from lying to sitting; orthostatic syncope; or orthostatic dizziness

Multisystem Involvement (3 or more of following)

- GI: vomiting or diarrhea at onset of illness
- Muscular: severe myalgia or creatinine phosphokinase level at least twice upper limit of normal

- Mucous membranes: vaginal, oropharyngeal, or conjunctival hyperemia
- Renal: BUN or Cr at least twice upper limit of normal or urinary sediment with pyuria (≥5 WBC per high-power field) in absence of UTI
- Hepatic: total bilirubin, SGOT, SGPT at least twice upper limit of normal
- Hematologic: platelets ≤100,000 mm^3
- CNS: disorientation or alteration in consciousness without focal neurological signs when fever and hypotension are absent

Negative Results on Following Tests (if obtained)

- Blood, throat, or CSF (blood culture may rarely be positive for *Staphylococcus aureus*)
- Rise in titer against Rocky Mountain spotted fever, leptospirosis, or rubeola

Treatment

- Support of BP with IV fluids or pressors, as necessary
- Treatment of underlying infection, if present
- Specific antistaphylococcal therapy with antibiotics is indicated to reduce the chance of subsequent recurrences.

Reference: Wiesenthal AM: Toxic shock syndrome—an update. Drug Ther (Mar):33–39, 1983.

TOXOPLASMOSIS

Toxoplasmosis is caused by the protozoan *Toxoplasma gondii*. This protozoan is an obligate intracellular organism that is distributed worldwide and is ubiquitous in nature. The definitive hosts for *Toxoplasma* are members of the cat family, with other mammals serving only as incidental hosts. Human infection results from ingestion of food containing *Toxoplasma* cysts. Up to 25% of pork specimens suitable for human consumption have demonstrable tissue cysts when tested. The prevalence of prior *Toxoplasma* infection as evidenced by specific anti-*Toxoplasma* antibodies varies across geographical regions, likely due to climatic tolerance or intolerance of *Toxoplasma* oocysts. In France, up to 90% of adults show evidence of infection. In the United States, antibody seropositivity ranges from 5 to 70%, with higher prevalence in warm, moist regions.

Human disease may be due to either acute infection or reactivation of latent infection. Reactivation occurs in the setting of immune dysfunction. Acute infection in immunocompetent individuals is most commonly asymptomatic, with only 10 to 20% of new infections resulting in symptoms. Patients may complain of fever, night sweats, malaise, pharyngitis, or myalgias. Physical exam can reveal adenopathy (usually cervical) or hepatosplenomegaly. EBV- or CMV-related mononucleosis may initially be the suspected diagnosis. The course of illness is self-limited, with resolution of symptoms within 6 to 12 weeks.

Acute infection is also seen in congenitally infected infants. The manifestations are nonspecific and can present a diagnostic dilemma. For congenital infection to occur, the pregnant woman must become infected while pregnant. Therefore, seronegative women with the potential for pregnancy must attempt to avoid sources of high risk for infection. These include cat litter boxes, raw meats, vegetables, eggs, and unpasteurized milk. Hands should be washed immediately after handling any of these, or gloves should be worn. Hand-to-mouth contact should be minimized. Meats should be cooked to sterilize cysts; this requires a temperature of >66°C.

In the era of HIV/AIDS, the most common manifestation of toxoplasmosis is reactivation of infection in immunocompromised patients. This is seen primarily as toxoplasmic encephalitis. Rarely seen is pneumonitis, cardiomyopathy, or myositis. In AIDS patients, toxoplasmosis of the CNS occurs in 5 to 50% of all patients depending on the underlying local seroprevalence. The median CD4+ lymphocyte count of affected patients is 50. Thus, toxoplasmosis is infrequently the initial or presenting complication of HIV infection. The most common presenting symptoms and signs of CNS toxoplasmosis as described in a large retrospective study from San Francisco General Hospital are listed in the table that follows. Duration of symptoms prior to presentation in this study was 5 to 28 days.

Signs and Symptoms at Presentation in 115 Patients with CNS Toxoplasmosis

SYMPTOMS	NO. OF PATIENTS (%)	SIGNS	NO. OF PATIENTS (%)
Headache	63 (55)	Focal signs	79 (69)
Confusion	60 (52)	Hemiparesis	45 (39)
Fever	54 (47)	Ataxia	34 (30)
Lethargy	49 (43)	Cranial-nerve palsies	32 (28)
Seizures	33 (29)	Sensory deficits	14 (12)
Poor coordination/gait	29 (25)	Aphasia	9 (8)
Focal weakness	25 (22)	Hemianopia	8 (7)
Nausea or vomiting	20 (17)	Temperature >38.4°C	54 (47)
Visual disturbance	17 (15)	Abnormal consciousness	48 (42)
Incontinence	8 (7)	Mildly decreased	31 (27)
Neck stiffness	4 (3)	Minimally responsive	13 (11)
		Obtunded	4 (3)
		Psychomotor retardation	44 (38)
		Meningismus	11 (10)
		Behavioral disturbance	5 (4)

From Porter SB, et al: Toxoplasmosis of the central nervous system in the acquired immunodeficiency syndrome. N Engl J Med 327:1643–1648, 1992, p 1644, with permission.

Because the presenting neurologic exam is usually abnormal in these patients, a CNS imaging procedure is often one of the initial diagnostic tests. Either CT scan or MRI is suitable to demonstrate the abnormalities. From the same San Francisco study, the CT findings are listed in the following table.

The differential diagnosis with these findings in an AIDS patient includes other infectious etiologies of mass lesions such as bacterial abscess, tuberculoma, progressive multifocal leukoencephalopathy, cryptococcoma, and lymphoma. Due to the higher prevalence of toxoplasmosis (particularly in a patient seropositive for *Toxoplasma* antibodies) and the difficulties in obtaining tissue specimens, empiric therapy for toxoplasmosis is usually initiated. Clinical and radiographic response is fairly rapid, securing the diagnosis.

Radiographic Findings in 103 Patients Presenting with CNS Toxoplasmosis

CT FINDINGS	NO. OF PATIENTS (%)	CT FINDINGS	NO. OF PATIENTS (%)
Normal	3 (3)	Location	
Nonenhancing lesions	6 (6)	Frontal	49 (48)
Enhancing lesions	94 (91)	Basal ganglia	49 (48)
Ring enhancement	85 (82)	Parietal	38 (37)
Diffuse enhancement	9 (9)	Occipital	20 (19)
No. of lesions		Temporal	18 (18)
1	28 (27)	Cerebellum	15 (15)
2	23 (22)	Centrum semiovale	10 (10)
3	22 (21)	Thalamus	10 (10)
≥4	27 (26)	Edema	80 (78)
		Mild	23 (22)
		Mass effect	57 (55)

From Porter SB, et al: Toxoplasmosis of the central nervous system in the acquired immunodeficiency syndrome. N Engl J Med 327:1643–1648, 1992, p 1645, with permission.

Therapy in the immunocompromised patient with acute toxoplasmosis is necessary because spontaneous regression will not occur. A combination of pyrimethamine and sulfadiazine has been the most frequently reported therapy. Pyrimethamine is given as a 200-mg loading dose on day 1 followed by a daily dose of 50 to 75 mg per day. Sulfadiazine is given at 4 to 6 gm per day in divided doses every 6 hrs. Because of the hematologic toxicity of pyrimethamine, folinic acid should also be routinely prescribed. In patients with sulfa intolerance, clindamycin is an alternative medication prescribed at doses of 1,200 to 4,800 mg per day in divided doses every 6 hrs.

Therapy in the immunocompetent patient is not necessary unless some unusual degree of visceral involvement is present or if the constitutional symptoms are severe and disabling.

Duration of therapy in both groups is prolonged because the medications are effective only against the tachyzoite and not the cyst. In the immunocompetent patient, therapy is given for 2 to 4 months and then discontinued. In the immunocompromised patient, initial therapy is similarly prolonged, but then chronic suppressive therapy is administered for the duration of immunosuppression—lifelong in AIDS.

TRANSFUSIONS

Risks and Associated Problems

The most feared complication of blood transfusions is a major cross-match error resulting in a hemolytic transfusion reaction. This is an infrequent event (see following table) and is usually due to clerical errors in identification of the unit of blood, the cross-match tube sent for the patient, or administration of the blood to the wrong patient. It is important to realize that such errors often affect *two* patients. Occasionally, hemolytic transfusion reactions are delayed 3 to 21 days. These delayed reactions result from the inability of the cross-match to detect very low levels of antibody in the previously transfused patient or in women who have been pregnant. The anamnestic response occurring a few days later results in hemolysis with jaundice, arthralgias, myalgias, fever, and anemia. Immediate hemolytic transfusion reactions are marked by back pain, chest tightness, dyspnea, fever, chills, passage of dark urine, jaundice, and bleeding due to DIC. When any of these occur, the transfusion should be discontinued, as morbidity is roughly proportional to the amount of blood transfused. IV saline should be administered and an investigation begun. Tests for hemolysis should be ordered. Treatment should be aimed at the major complications: shock, DIC, and acute tubular necrosis. Urine output should be maintained with 20 to 80 mg of furosemide, if necessary. Corticosteroids and antihistamines may be of benefit.

Major Risks of RBC Transfusion

RISK	FREQUENCY PER TRANSFUSION
Infectious	
Cytomegalovirus	Common
Non-A, non-B hepatitis	1:100*
Hepatitis B	1:200–300
HIV	1:40,000–1,000,000
Immunologic	
Fever, chills, urticaria	1:50–100
Hemolytic transfusion reactions	1:6000
Fatal hemolytic transfusion reactions	1:100,000
Graft-versus-host reaction	Unknown

*Before implementation of the screening test for hepatitis C.
From Welch HG, et al: Prudent strategies for elective red blood cell transfusion. Ann Intern Med 116:394, 1992, Table 1, with permission.

Urticarial reactions accompany 1 to 2% of transfusions. Transfusions need not be interrupted. Symptoms are improved by antihistamines. A small percentage of individuals (1 in 800) are IgA deficient and may experience anaphylaxis when transfused with components that contain small amounts of IgA. Fever is uncommon in these reactions, but nausea, abdominal pain, hypotension, and dyspnea signal the need for immediate discontinuation of the infusion and administration of epinephrine (0.4 ml of 1:1,000 dilution).

Febrile reactions are caused by antileukocyte antibodies and are effectively treated with antipyretics or by using leukocyte-poor RBCs. The febrile reaction needs to be differentiated from fever caused by a hemolytic transfusion reaction or bacterial contaminant.

Infectious complications include the following.

1. **Hepatitis:** Studies of transfusion recipients have shown that 5 to 15% of patients had increments in serial ALT (SGPT) by 8 weeks. Hepatitis B accounts for a small proportion of these. Hepatitis C is probably the most important viral etiology of posttransfusion hepatitis and can be serologically detected in blood donors. Screening of blood donors for hepatitis C has reduced the risks for transfusion of this

form of hepatitis from 1:100 units to 1:300–900 units of blood. Patients who do develop hepatitis C often do poorly, with some developing a chronic active hepatitis and cirrhosis. Now that most centers are screening donor bloods, this disorder will probably decrease in frequency but will not disappear.

2. **AIDS:** The development of HIV infection and AIDS after transfusion remains a serious threat in the public's perception, although the risk is very low. The risk of infection is now related to the number of donors recently infected who do not yet have detectable anti-HIV antibodies.

3. **Other infections:** A rare complication is gram-negative septicemia or endotoxemia. Because platelets are stored at room temperature for as long as 4 or 5 days, bacterial contamination is more frequent with these products. Some patients, after receiving blood from CMV or EBV$^+$ donors, develop a mono-like illness a few weeks after transfusion. Neonates and immunocompromised individuals are at great risk for fatal CMV infections. Rare cases of transmission of syphilis, malaria, Chagas' disease, *Yersinia,* and babesiosis have also occurred as a result of transfusion.

Volume overload is a common and potentially dangerous, unfavorable outcome of transfusion. It can be prevented by close attention to the patient's volume status and physical exam during administration of blood. The indications and goals for blood transfusion have to be clearly determined.

Noncardiogenic pulmonary edema occurs uncommonly after transfusion of 2 to 6 units of RBCs and is thought to be caused by leukoagglutinins in the plasma of some donors. Bilateral, fluffy infiltrates on CXR accompanied by cough, fever, urticarial rash, dyspnea, and hypotension occur within 4 hrs of transfusion. Many patients require ventilatory support, but the outcome is usually favorable. In some instances, massively transfused patients develop ARDS that may in fact be due to the underlying condition requiring transfusion, although some authorities suggest that microaggregates in the transfused components contribute to pulmonary injury.

Coagulation abnormalities occur when patients receive components adding up to 1 or 1.5 blood volumes over 24 hrs or less. The laboratory evaluation shows prolonged PT and PTT, as well as thrombocytopenia caused by dilution of labile clotting factors (V and VIII) and platelets. Other complications of massive transfusions include citrate toxicity, hypocalcemia, and alkalosis. Hypokalemia may also occur in the alkalotic patient. RBCs stored for long periods may leak K$^+$, and thus hyperkalemia may result when these cells are infused. If a blood warmer is not used, hypothermia may result from massive transfusion.

Some patients demonstrate alloimmunization (positive indirect Coombs). This makes identification of the antigenic specificity important and selection of compatible units difficult. Iron overload requiring chelation therapy also occurs as the result of many RBC transfusions.

In patients who have undergone conditioning for a bone marrow transplant, or in children with severe combined immunodeficiency disease, graft-versus-host disease has resulted from lymphocytes in donor blood products. These patients should receive only irradiated blood products. Graft-versus-host disease after transfusion has been recognized in adults with Hodgkin's disease and in immunocompetent recipients of blood from related donors. In the latter circumstance, the recipient is heterozygous for an HLA haplotype shared by a homozygous relative. The recipient does not reject the donor cells, but the donor's homozygous lymphocytes recognize the unshared haplotype and spark a fulminant graft-versus-host disease in the recipient. These patients have a skin rash and die of pancytopenia. Thus it is the practice in some centers to irradiate directed donor units coming from family members and to irradiate blood given to patients receiving blood during chemotherapy, particularly those with Hodgkin's disease.

Reference: Welch HG, et al: Prudent strategies for elective red blood cell transfusion. Ann Intern Med 116:393–402, 1992.

TRANSIENT ISCHEMIC ATTACK

A TIA is defined as a focal decrease of blood flow in the brain, producing ischemic symptoms that resolve completely in 24 hours or less. In fact, the vast majority of TIAs last less than 30 minutes, and virtually every ischemic episode that persists more than 4 hours causes actual cell death, i.e., a stroke.

TIAs arise from the same mechanism as completed strokes, namely, thrombosis of a large vessel, emboli from the heart or a proximal artery, or small-vessel disease such as lacunae. Most often, however, TIAs imply atherosclerotic thrombotic narrowing of a large vessel. Approximately 50% of all thrombotic strokes are preceded by TIAs, whereas 30% of lacunar strokes and only 10% of embolic strokes have such prior warnings.

The differential diagnosis of a transient CNS deficit is extensive, but most TIAs prove to be, in fact, atherosclerotic cerebrovascular disease. Conditions that may mimic a TIA include:

1. Focal seizures
2. Metabolic encephalopathies
3. Mass lesions such as tumors and subdural hematomas
4. Demyelinating disease
5. Psychogenic symptoms

TIAs, because they resolve completely, are important primarily as warnings of impending or future stroke. Figures differ, but patients with a TIA suffer subsequent strokes at a rate of approximately 5% per year. Statistically, a patient with a TIA will survive 7 more years before succumbing to CAD, which is by far the commonest cause of death in such patients.

Management for the patient with TIA includes admission to the hospital and MRI of the brain to exclude other processes. If there is a history of cardiac disease, such as AF, prosthetic valve, or recent MI, the heart should be studied as a source of emboli causing a TIA, using echocardiography, transesophageal echocardiogram, or Holter monitoring. Such cardiac evaluation is not mandatory unless indicated by the Hx & PE.

Imaging of the carotid arteries is essential, because carotid endarterectomy is proven to be beneficial for TIAs. Magnetic resonance angiography may soon be the procedure of choice for studying carotid artery morphology and flow, but a battery of noninvasive tests may also include ultrasound and Dopplers. Conventional cerebral angiography is the gold standard, and most surgeons demand such imaging prior to operation.

Carotid endarterectomy effectively reduces subsequent occurrence of stroke in patients who have a 70% or greater stenosis of the ipsilateral carotid artery. In the absence of contraindications, endarterectomy should be performed on all such patients. However, for those with significant lesions who are not surgical candidates or for those whose carotid artery is not diseased, medical management can also lower the risk of subsequent stroke as follows.

1. Treat risk factors, especially BP.
2. Aspirin: Data regarding the effectiveness of this antiplatelet agent are controversial, but many experts believe that aspirin does reduce the risk of subsequent stroke in patients who have suffered a TIA, at least in men.
3. Ticlopidine: Controlled trials of this antiplatelet agent, in doses of 200 mg BID, confirm its effectiveness for preventing stroke and suggest that it is superior to aspirin and other agents for that indication. It has not yet become the first-line drug, however, because of side effects, including diarrhea, GI upset, and a 1% incidence of reversible bone marrow suppression necessitating CBC checks every 2 weeks for the first 6 months of use.

Other agents that inhibit platelets have not shown any ability to reduce subsequent stroke, including sulfinpyrazone (Anturane) and dipyridamole (Persantine).

References: North American Symptomatic Carotid Endarterectomy Trial Collaborators: Beneficial effect of carotid endarterectomy in symptomatic patients with high-grade carotid stenosis. N Engl J Med 325:445–453, 1991.

Sze PC, et al: Antiplatelet agents in the secondary prevention of stroke: Meta-analysis of the randomized control trials. Stroke 19:436–442, 1988.

Hass WK, et al, and the Ticlopidine Aspirin Stroke Study Group: A randomized trial comparing ticlopidine hydrochloride with aspirin for the prevention of stroke in high risk patients. N Engl J Med 321:501–507, 1989.

TREMOR

A tremor is a rhythmic, to-and-fro movement, with symmetric contraction of agonist and antagonist muscles. Tremors are the most common of all abnormal movement disorders.

There are four major types of tremor:

1. Physiologic tremor
2. Parkinsonian tremor
3. Essential tremor
4. Cerebellar tremor

Differential Diagnosis of Tremor

CHARACTERISTICS	PHYSIOLOGIC	PARKINSONIAN	ESSENTIAL	CEREBELLAR
Present at rest	1+	4+	1+	1+
Present with action	4+	2+	3+	4+
Goal directed	2+	2+	2+	4+
Location	Distal	Distal as well as head	Distal as well as head	Proximal and distal
Frequency	6–12 Hz	3–7 Hz	6–12 Hz	2–5 Hz

A certain degree of fine physiologic tremor is normal, but this can be accentuated by anxiety, fatigue, and some metabolic derangements such as thyrotoxicosis. Drugs that accentuate a physiologic tremor include caffeine, amphetamines, lithium, and tricyclic antidepressants.

A parkinsonian tremor, seen in idiopathic Parkinson's disease, is the commonest resting tremor and has a coarse, high-amplitude, slow, pill-rolling movement. It is aggravated by stress and improved with relaxation. (See also Parkinson's Disease.)

Essential tremor often appears as an autosomal dominant condition, with symptoms beginning in the fourth or fifth decade of life. It is a postural tremor, which often interferes with writing, drinking liquids, and other daily activities. A striking feature of essential tremor is its alleviation by alcohol. Despite folklore to the contrary, the incidence of alcoholism is not increased in patients with essential tremor, although alcohol undeniably mitigates the abnormal movements. Propranolol and primidone are also useful therapies. (The famous film and stage actress Katharine Hepburn is perhaps the best-known example of a person with essential tremor.)

Cerebellar tremor, arising from damage to the cerebellum or its inflow and outflow pathways, produces a tremor that is most prominent by its goal-directed, targeted activity. It is best seen during routine physical examination when the patient attempts to touch the examiner's finger, or slide the heel down the shin. Activities of daily living that are usually impaired include inserting a key into a lock or reaching for an object, all of which are goal-directed activities. Cerebellar tremor is difficult to treat, but it may be improved by clonazepam (Klonopin), which potentiates the cerebellar neurotransmitter gamma-aminobutyric acid (GABA). Another effective drug is isoniazid, which prevents the breakdown of GABA and so also enhances its activity, but the doses of isoniazid required are from 900 to 1,200 mg/day, which often produces hepatotoxicity and peripheral neuropathy.

Reference: Jankovic J: Tremors: Pathophysiology, differential diagnosis and pharmacology. Neurol Consult 2(3):1–8, 1984.

TUBERCULOSIS

In the United States, transmission of TB declined annually from 1953 through 1984. Beginning in 1986, the annual number of new cases began to increase. Much of that increase can be attributed to the occurrence of TB in patients infected with HIV and, to a lesser extent, new immigrants. In order to control the spread of TB, effective screening programs are necessary, especially in high-risk populations.

Host factors associated with increased risk of TB

1. Persons with previously untreated TB, including persons with a positive PPD and stable, fibrotic pulmonary lesions
2. Silicosis
3. Malignancy
4. Chronic renal failure
5. Alcoholism
6. Diabetes mellitus
7. Postgastrectomy
8. HIV infection

9. Immunosuppression
10. Malnutrition

Classification of TB

TB 0	No TB exposure: not infected
TB 1	TB exposure, no evidence of infection: (+) history of exposure, (−) PPD
TB 2	TB infection, no evidence of active disease: (+) PPD, (−) clinical presentation, (−) CXR, (−) bacteriology

Candidates for preventive therapy

TB 3	TB, current disease: (+) culture or (+) PPD and evidence of active disease (clinical or CXR)
TB 4	TB, no current disease: past history of TB or stable abnormal CXR, (+) PPD, no clinical disease
TB 5	TB suspect: Diagnosis pending

PPD Screening

Populations to be screened by PPD testing
1. Persons infected with the HIV
2. Close contacts of persons known or suspected of having TB or sharing the same household or other enclosed environments
3. Persons with medical risk factors known to increase the risk of disease if infection has occurred, which include:
   a. Silicosis
   b. Postgastrectomy
   c. Postjejunoileal bypass
   d. Weight of 10% or more below ideal body weight
   e. Chronic renal failure
   f. Diabetes mellitus
   g. Conditions requiring prolonged high-dose corticosteroid therapy and other immunosuppressive therapy
   h. Some hematologic disorders (e.g., leukemia and lymphoma)
   i. Other malignancies
   j. Persons with abnormal CXRs demonstrating fibrotic lesions suggestive of healed TB
4. Foreign-born persons from countries with high TB prevalence
5. Medically underserved low-income populations, including high-risk racial or ethnic minority populations (e.g., African-Americans, Hispanics, and Native Americans)
6. Alcoholics and IV drug abusers
7. Residents of long-term-care facilities, correctional institutions, mental institutions, nursing homes/facilities, other long-term-residential facilities

Recommendations for preventive therapy

The main goals of preventive therapy are to prevent latent (asymptomatic) infection from progressing to clinical disease and to prevent initial infection after significant exposure. The usual preventive therapy regimen consists of isoniazid 300 mg daily for adults. The recommended duration in patients with HIV infection and CXR evidence of past infection is 12 months. Other groups should receive treatment for a minimum of 6 months. The following table outlines the recommendations for preventive therapy.

Criteria for Determining Need for Preventive Therapy
for Persons with Positive Tuberculin Reactions

	AGE GROUP (YRS)	
CATEGORY	<35	≥35
With risk factor*	Treat at all ages if reaction to 5TU purified protein derivative (PPD) ≥10 mm (or ≥5 mm and patient is recent contact, is HIV infected, or has radiographic evidence of old TB).	
No risk factor, high-incidence group[†]	Treat if PPD ≥10 mm	Do not treat
No risk factor, low-incidence group	Treat if PPD ≥15 mm[§]	Do not treat

*Risk factors include HIV infection, recent contact with infectious person, recent skin test conversion (<2 years), abnormal CXR, IV drug abuse, and medical risk factors described in foregoing text.

[†]High-incidence groups include foreign-born persons, medically underserved low-income populations, and residents of long-term-care facilities.

[§]Lower or higher cut points may be used for identifying positive reactions depending on the relative prevalence of *Mycobacterium tuberculosis* infection and nonspecific cross-reactivity in the population.

Modified from CDC: The use of preventive therapy for tuberculous infection in the United States. MMWR 39:11, 1990.

Indications for isoniazid prophylaxis (300 mg/day for 1 year)

1. Persons of any age should receive isoniazid if they:
   a. Are positive for antibody to HIV or are suspected to be HIV positive and have a tuberculin skin test (TST) of ≥5 mm of induration.
   b. Are close contacts of newly diagnosed TB cases and have a TST of ≥5 mm of induration.
   c. Have an abnormal CXR with fibrotic lesions suggesting old TB and have a TST of ≥5 mm of induration.
   d. Are IV drug abusers, negative for HIV, and have a TST of ≥10 mm of induration.
   e. Have a medical condition that increases their risk of TB and have a TST of ≥10 mm of induration.
2. Persons <35 years of age should receive isoniazid if they have a TST of ≥10 mm of induration and they:
   a. Are born in a high-prevalence country.
   b. Are in a medically underserved population.
3. Recent converters (within the past 2 years):
   a. With a TST of ≥10 mm of induration and age <35 years.
   b. With a TST of ≥15 mm of induration and age >35 years.

Commonly Used Drugs for TB Treatment

DRUG	DOSAGE FORMS	DAILY DOSE**		MAXIMUM DAILY DOSE IN CHILDREN AND ADULTS	TWICE WEEKLY DOSE		MONTHLY COST*		MAJOR ADVERSE REACTIONS
		Children	Adults		Children	Adults	Daily	Twice Weekly	
Isoniazid	Tablets: 100 mg ††‡ 300 mg; Syrup: 50 mg/5 ml; Vials: 1 gm	10–20 mg/kg PO or IM	5 mg/kg PO or IM	300 mg	20–40 mg/kg Max. 900 mg	15 mg/kg Max. 900 mg	Less than $1	Less than $1	Hepatic enzyme elevation, peripheral neuropathy, hepatitis, hypersensitivity
Rifampin	Capsules: 150 mg ††‡ 300 mg; Syrup: formulated from capsules 10 mg/ml	10–20 mg/kg PO	10 mg/kg PO	600 mg	10–20 mg/kg Max. 600 mg	10 mg/kg Max. 600 mg	$13–$21	$4–$6	Orange discoloration of secretions and urine, nausea, vomiting, hepatitis, febrile reaction, purpura (rare)
Pyrazinamide	Tablets: 500 mg ‡	15–30 mg/kg PO	15–30 mg/kg PO	2 mg	50–70 mg/kg	50–70 mg/kg	$19–$48	$17–$32	Hepatotoxicity, hyperuricemia, arthralgias, skin rash, GI upset
Streptomycin	Vials: 1 gm, 4 gm	20–40 mg/kg IM	15 mg/kg ††† IM	1 gm †††	25–30 mg/kg IM	25–30 mg/kg IM	$23–$27	$16–$20	Ototoxicity, nephrotoxicity
Ethambutol	Tablets: 100 mg 400 mg	15–25 mg/kg PO	15–25 mg/kg PO	2.5 gm	50 mg/kg	50 mg/kg	$27–$72	$23–$36	Optic neuritis, decreased red-green color discrimination, decreased visual acuity, skin rash

*Approximate cost to health departments for drugs purchased in quantities based on a 70-kg adult (1984–86).

†Isoniazid and rifampin are available as a combination capsule containing 150 mg of isoniazid and 300 mg of rifampin.

‡A combination of isoniazid, rifampin, and pyrazinamide in a single capsule is being introduced

†††In persons above age 60 the daily dose of streptomycin should be limited to 10 mg/kg, with a maximum dose of 750 mg.

**Doses based on weight should be adjusted as weight changes

From Farer LS: Tuberculosis: What the Physician Should Know. American Lung Association, New York, NY, 1986, with permission.

Second-Line Antituberculosis Drugs*

DRUG	DOSAGE FORMS	DAILY DOSE** IN CHILDREN AND ADULTS	MAXIMUM DAILY DOSE IN CHILDREN AND ADULTS	MAJOR ADVERSE REACTIONS	RECOMMENDED REGULAR MONITORING
Capreomycin	Vials: 1 gm	15–30 mg/kg IM	1 gm	Auditory, vestibular, and renal toxicity	Vestibular function, audiometry, BUN and creatinine
Kanamycin	Vials: 75 mg 500 mg 1 gm	15–30 mg/kg IM	1 gm	Auditory and renal toxicity, rare vestibular toxicity	Vestibular function, audiometry, BUN and creatinine
Ethionamide	Tablets: 250 mg	15–20 mg/kg PO	1 gm	GI disturbance, hepatotoxicity, hypersensitivity	Hepatic enzymes
Para-aminosalicylic acid (PAS)	Tablets: 500 mg 1 gm Bulk powder	150 mg/kg PO	12 gm	GI disturbance, hypersensitivity, hepatotoxicity, sodium load	
Cycloserine	Capsules: 250 mg	15–20 mg/kg PO	1 gm	Psychosis, personality changes, convulsions, rash	Assessment of mental status

*These drugs are more difficult to use than drugs listed in the foregoing table. They should be used only when necessary and should be given and monitored by health providers experienced in their use.

**Doses based on weight should be adjusted as weight changes.

From Farer LS: Tuberculosis: What the Physician Should Know. American Lung Association, New York, NY, 1986, with permission.

4. All persons <35 years of age who are likely to have a low incidence of TB but have a TST of ≥15 mm of induration.

Centers for Disease Control: Screening for tuberculosis infections in high-risk populations, and the use of preventive therapy for tuberculosis infection in the United States: Recommendations of the Advisory Council for the Elimination of Tuberculosis. MMWR 39(RR-8).1–12, 1990.

Regimen Options for the Preferred Initial Treatment of Children and Adults with TB

Option 1	Administer daily isoniazid, rifampin, and pyrazinamide for 8 wk followed by 16 wk of isoniazid and rifampin daily or 2–3 times/wk.* In areas where the isoniazid resistance rate is not documented to < 4%, ethambutol or streptomycin should be added to the initial regimen until susceptibility to sioniazid and rifampin is demonstrated. Consult a TB medical expert if the patient is symptomatic or smear or culture positive after 3 mo.
Option 2	Administer daily isoniazid, rifampin, pyrazinamide, and streptomycin or ethambutol for 2 wk followed by 2 times/wk* administration of the same drugs for 6 wk (by DOT), and subsequently, with 2 times/wk administration of isoniazid and rifampin for 16 wk (by DOT). Consult a TB medical expert if the patient is symptomatic or smear or culture positive after 3 mo.
Option 3	Treat by DOT, 3 times/wk* with isoniazid, rifampin, pyrazinamide, and ethambutol or streptomycin for 6 mo. Consult a TB medical expert if the patient is symptomatic or smear or culture positive after 3 mo.

*All regimens administered 2 times/wk should be monitored by directly observed therapy (DOT) for the duration of therapy.

Adapted from Joint Statement of the American Thoracic Society and the Centers for Disease Control: Treatment of tuberculosis and tuberculosis infection in adults and children. Am J Respir Crit Care Med 149:1359–1374, 1994.

TUMOR LYSIS SYNDROME

We owe the recognition of tumor lysis syndrome to the late Sir Denis Burkitt, an intrepid British surgeon, who described it as a consequence of the treatment of the aggressive B-cell lymphoma that bears his name. Burkitt was alarmed by the rapid development of renal failure after cyclophosphamide therapy in his patients. Although Burkitt's lymphoma offers the most spectacular opportunity for tumor lysis, the syndrome has been observed in acute leukemia, non-Hodgkin's lymphoma, and, occasionally, in solid neoplasms.

It is now apparent that rapidly proliferating tumors are also very sensitive to chemotherapy, resulting in a huge population of dead and dying cells, which release their contents into the blood. Thus there are hyperkalemia, hyperuricemia, and hyperphosphatemia followed by urate nephropathy and hypocalcemia. Persistent hypocalcemia in some patients may be due to a lowered level of calcitriol. The syndrome may be blunted or avoided by reducing the level of chemotherapy used in the first course of therapy. Administration of both fluids (to keep the patient well hydrated) and allopurinol is helpful. Alkalinization of the urine by the addition of bicarbonate to the IV fluids may be of use prior to chemotherapy. However, this maneuver is seldom required for more than 2 days. Dialysis is indicated when there is severe hyperkalemia, volume overload, or symptomatic hypocalcemia.

Reference: Cohen LF, et al: Acute tumor lysis syndrome. A review of 37 patients with Burkitt's lymphoma. Am J Med 69:486–491, 1990.

U

ULCERS, LOWER EXTREMITY

Etiology of Lower Extremity Ulcers

TYPE OF ULCER	USUAL LOCATION	EDEMA	PIGMENTATION	EVIDENCE OF ARTERIAL INSUFFICIENCY
Varicose	Medial leg	0 to +	0 to +	0
Stasis	Medial leg	+ + to + + + +	+ + +	0 to +
Arterial	Lateral leg, foot	0 to +	0	+ + + +
Dystrophic	Sole, tip of foot	+ +	0	0
Traumatic	Midleg, toe	0	0	0 to + + + +
Diabetic	Toes, dorsum of foot	+ +	0	+ to + + +
Factitious	Anywhere	+	0	0

From Munster AM, et al: Lower extremity ulcers and varicose veins. In Barker LR, et al (eds): Principles of Ambulatory Medicine, 3rd ed. Baltimore, Williams & Wilkins, 1991, p 1225, with permission.

The therapy for leg ulcers depends on their etiology. The above table lists diagnostic clues for different types of ulcers.

Varicose ulcers are treated with bed rest, leg elevation, and compression stockings. The ulcer itself should be treated either with an Unna's boot (gauze covered with a zinc-gelatin dressing) that is changed weekly or with wet-to-wet dressings—covered with an Ace wrap—that are changed twice a day. A wet-to-wet dressing is made by moistening a gauze pad with normal saline, applying it over the ulcer, and covering with a dry gauze. The gauze is moistened again before removal.

Stasis ulcer treatment is similar to that of varicose ulcers, but stasis ulcers are usually harder to heal. Their occurrence suggests impairment of the deep venous system and venous HTN. When such ulcers are covered with debris and exudate, wet-to-dry dressings should be used twice a day. These dressings are made the same way as wet-to-wet dressings, except they are not re-moistened before removing. In removal of a "dry" dressing, some of the debris from the ulcer is removed. Bed rest, elevation, and compression are essential to heal these ulcers. For both varicose and stasis ulcers, graduated-pressure stockings are the preferred means to provide compression. These stockings are made to fit each individual patient and are available from hospital supply stores through prescription.

Patients with ulcers due to **arterial** insufficiency should be referred to a vascular surgeon for management because restoration of blood flow through surgery is frequently needed before healing will occur. Also, a nonhealing ulcer due to vascular disease may portend limb-threatening ischemia.

Dystrophic ulcers (due to neuropathy and insensitivity) require meticulous wound care with wet-to-wet dressing changes, debridement, and appropriate antibiotic therapy. **Traumatic** and **factitious** ulcers are treated in a similar manner.

All patients with foot ulcers should also be counseled to avoid future injury by means of preventive measures as follows.

1. Wear comfortable, closed-toe shoes with adequate room for the toes.
2. Wear cotton or wool socks to avoid moisture retention.
3. Cleanse feet daily, using tepid, not hot, water.
4. Trim nails carefully with nail clippers (not scissors).
5. Place lamb's wool between toes.
6. Apply lubricating lotion to the soles of the feet (*not between the toes*) to avoid cracking.
7. Inspect feet daily and call physician if any sign of injury is found.

UNIVERSAL PRECAUTIONS

In 1985, the CDC developed the strategy of universal blood and body fluid precautions to deter the transmission of HIV and other blood-borne pathogens to health care workers. Now generally referred to as Universal Precautions, the approach is based on the fact that it is difficult, on the basis of Hx & PE alone, to determine whether a patient has a blood-borne infection. Thus *all* patients are assumed to be infected, and health care workers are to take precautions with all patients.

Universal precautions comprise four broad categories.

1. **Protective equipment** should be used so as to eliminate or minimize exposure. Gloves should be worn anytime there is the possibility the worker will come in contact with blood, body fluids containing blood, other body fluid to which universal precautions apply (see later), mucus membranes, or broken skin. In almost all settings, gloves are recommended during phlebotomy, although even gloves cannot guard against penetrating injury. Masks and protective eyeware should be worn during procedures likely to generate droplets of blood or body fluids. Gowns or aprons should be added whenever blood or body fluids may be splashed during a procedure.

2. **Hands or other skin surfaces should be washed** immediately after coming in contact with blood or body fluids.

3. **Extreme caution around sharp objects** (needles, scalpels, broken lab glass, etc.) should be exercised to limit the risk of penetrating injury. No attempt should be made to recap needles after use. All sharps should be disposed of in appropriately identified puncture-resistant containers.

4. **Health care workers with exudative skin lesions** should avoid direct patient contact.

Universal precautions apply to blood, any body fluid with visible blood in it, semen, vaginal secretions, and CSF, synovial, pleural, peritoneal, pericardial, and amniotic fluids. Universal precautions do not apply to feces, breast milk, nasal secretions, saliva, sputum, sweat, tears, urine, and vomitus unless visible blood is present.

Universal Precautions to Prevent Transmission of HIV

Universal Precautions

Because a medical history and physical examination cannot reliably identify all patients infected with HIV or other blood-borne pathogens, blood and body-fluid precautions should be consistently used for all patients, especially those in emergency care settings in which the risk of blood exposure is increased and the infection status of the patient is usually not known.

1. Use appropriate barrier precautions to prevent skin and mucous membrane exposure when exposure to blood, body fluids containing blood, or other body fluids to which universal precautions apply (see below) is anticipated. Wear gloves when touching blood or body fluids, mucous membranes, or nonintact skin of all patients; when handling items or surfaces soiled with blood or body fluids; and when performing venipuncture and other vascular access procedures. Change gloves after contact with each patient; do not wash or disinfect gloves for reuse. Wear masks and protective eye wear or face shields during procedures that are likely to generate droplets of blood or other body fluids to prevent exposure of mucous membranes of the mouth, nose, and eyes. Wear gowns or aprons during procedures that are likely to generate splashes of blood or other body fluids.

2. Wash hands and other skin surfaces immediately and thoroughly afer contaminations with blood, body fluids containing blood, or other body fluids to which universal precautions apply. Wash hands immediately after gloves are removed.

3. Take care to prevent injuries when using needles, scalpels, and other sharp instruments or devices; when handling sharp instruments after procedures; and when cleaning used instruments; and when disposing of used needles. Do not recap used needles by hand; do not remove used needles from disposable syringes by hand; and do not bend, break, or otherwise manipulate used needles by hand. Place used disposable syringes and needles, scalpel blades, and other sharp items in puncture-resistant disposal containers, which should be located as close to the use area as is practical.

4. Although saliva has not been implicated in HIV transmission, the need for emergency mouth-to-mouth resuscitation should be minimized by making mouthpieces, resuscitation bags, or other ventilation devices available for use in areas in which the need for resuscitation is predictable.

5. Health care workers with exudative lesions or weeping dermatitis should refrain from all direct patient care and from handling patient-care equipment until the condition resolves.

Universal precautions are intended to supplement rather than replace recommendations for routine infection control, such as hand washing and use of gloves to prevent gross microbial contamination of hands. In addition, implementation of universal precautions does not eliminate the need for other category- or disease-specific isolation precautions, such an enteric precautions for infectious diarrhea or isolation for pulmonary tuberculosis. Universal precautions are not intended to change waste management programs undertaken in accordance with state and local regulations.

Body Fluids to Which Universal Precautions Apply

Universal precautions apply to blood and other body fluids containing visible blood. Blood is the single most important source of HIV, hepatitis B virus, and other blood-borne pathogens in the occupational setting. Universal precautions also apply to tissues, semen, vaginal secretions, and the following fluids: cerebrospinal, synovial, pleural, peritoneal, pericardial, and amniotic.

Universal precautions do not apply to feces, nasal secretions, sputum, sweat, tears, urine, and vomitus unless they contain visible blood. Universal precautions also do not apply to human breast milk, although gloves may be worn by health care workers in situations in which exposure to breast milk might be frequent. In addition, universal precautions do not apply to saliva. Gloves need not be worn when feeding patients or wiping saliva from skin, although special precautions are recommended for dentistry, in which contamination of saliva with blood is predictable. The risk of transmission of HIV, as well as HBV, from these fluids and materials is extremely low or nonexistent.

Table continued on next page.

Universal Precautions to Prevent Transmission of HIV (Cont.)

Use of Gloves for Phlebotomy

Gloves should be effective in reducing the incidence of blood contamination of hands during phlebotomy (drawing of blood samples), but they cannot prevent penetrating injuries caused by needles or other sharp instruments. In universal precautions, all blood is assumed to be potentially infectious for blood-borne pathogens. Some institutions have relaxed recommendations for the use of gloves for phlebotomy by skilled health care workers in settings in which the prevalence of blood-borne pathogens is known to be very low (e.g., volunteer blood-donation centers). Institutions that judge that routine use of gloves for all phlebotomies is not necessary should periodically re-evaluate their policy. Gloves should always be available for those who wish to use them for phlebotomy. In addition, the following general guidelines apply:

1. Use gloves for performing phlebotomy if cuts, scratches, or other breaks in the skin are present.
2. Use gloves in situations in which contamination with blood may occur—e.g., when performing phlebotomy on an uncooperative patient.
3. Use gloves for performing finger or heel sticks on infants and children.
4. Use gloves when training persons to do phlebotomies.

Precautions for Laboratories

Blood and other body fluids from all patients should be considered infective. To supplement the universal precautions listed above, the following precautions are recommended for workers in clinical laboratories:

1. Put all specimens of blood and body fluids in a well-constructed container with a secure lid to prevent leakage during transport. Take care when collecting each specimen to avoid contaminating the outside of the container or the laboratory form accompanying the specimen.
2. Wear gloves when processing blood and body-fluid specimens (e.g., when removing tops from vacuum tubes). Wear masks and protective eye wear if it is anticipated that mucous membranes will come in contact with blood or body fluids. Change gloves and wash hands after completion of specimen processing.
3. For routine procedures, such as histologic and pathologic studies or microbiological culturing, a biologic safety cabinet is not necessary. However, use a biologic safety cabinet (class I or II) when procedures are conducted that have a high potential for generating droplets, such as blending, sonicating, and vigorous mixing.
4. Use a mechanical pipetting device for manipulating all liquids in the laboratory. Do not pipette by mouth.
5. Limit use of needles and syringes to situations in which there is no alternative.
6. Decontaminate laboratory work surfaces with an appropriate chemical germicide after a spill of blood or other body fluids and after work is completed.
7. Decontaminate materials contaminated during laboratory tests before reprocessing them. Place contaminated materials for disposal in bags and discard in accordance with institutional policies for disposal of infective waste.
8. Decontaminate and clean scientific equipment that has been contaminated by blood or body fluids if repair in the laboratory or transport to the manufacturer is necessary.
9. Wash hands after completing laboratory work and remove protective clothing before leaving the laboratory.

Implementation of universal precautions eliminates the need for warning labels on specimens because blood and body fluids from all patients should be considered infective.

From Rubin R: Acquired immunodeficiency syndrome. In Rubenstein E, Federman DD (eds): Scientific American Medicine. New York: Scientific American, 1993, p 7(XI):17, with permission.

UPPER RESPIRATORY TRACT INFECTIONS

Upper respiratory tract infections in adults are caused by a number of viruses. The most common etiologic agents for the common cold are the 100 strains of rhinoviruses, several strains of coronaviruses, and some parainfluenza and respiratory syncytial viruses, coxsackieviruses, echoviruses, and polioviruses. Symptoms include coryza, slight fever alternating with chills, and general malaise. Most adults have two or three colds per year. Diagnosis of a specific agent is difficult because these agents can produce more than one symptom complex, and many are identical in their presentation. If diagnosis of a specific agent were essential, the age of the patient, the time of year, and epidemiologic clues could help to make the determination. Respiratory tract viruses are more common in children than adults, but adults who are frequently in contact with children will become infected. Travel to new areas often exposes patients to new pathogens to which they are susceptible. There is no specific treatment, and symptomatic therapy is recommended.

Bacterial superinfection can occur 3 to 4 days after the onset of these viral infections, which most often involves *Staphylococcus aureus* or *Streptococcus pneumoniae,* although *Haemophilus influenzae* is also seen. In patients who are immunocompromised or who have chronic diseases, superinfection is more likely. These patients should be monitored closely for symptoms and signs of bacterial infection, which can then be treated with antibiotics. Acute sinusitis may present with fever and nasal discharge, but the discharge is purulent rather than thin and watery. There is tenderness over the sinuses, often in the frontal sinuses. Treatment should include epinephrine or ephedrine, which may be applied topically to the middle meatus so that the passage may be opened enough for drainage. Antibiotics are indicated, and penicillin or an analogue remains the treatment of choice in nonallergic patients. Heat over the sinuses provides comfort, and steam inhalations are also helpful.

Treatment of uncomplicated upper respiratory infections is symptomatic, with the usual advice of intake of fluids, control of fever with antipyretics, rest, antihistamines, decongestants, analgesics, and cough medications as needed.

Conditions that may superficially present as upper respiratory tract infections include CSF leaks through the ethmoid plate, foreign bodies in the nasal passages, deviated nasal septum, cocaine use, chronic allergies, vasomotor rhinitis, nasal polyps, and carcinomas of the sinuses causing obstruction.

URINARY INCONTINENCE

The prevalence of urinary incontinence increases with a patient's age and is seen in 10 to 20% of the community-dwelling elderly. This frequency increases to 50% among nursing home residents. The frequency is higher in women than in men.

Acute Causes of Incontinence (very likely to be reversible)

Delirium	Restricted or impaired mobility
Infections (symptomatic UTI)	Fecal impaction
Polyuria from diuretics	Diabetes mellitus
Sedation	Diabetes insipidus
Depression	

Resnick has identified four mechanisms, but combinations of mechanisms are quite common as well.

1. *Detrusor overactivity:* local irritation or decreased inhibitory control from cortex as in dementia (probably the most common mechanism)
2. *Detrusor underactivity:* decreased neurogenic, parasympathetic influence (also sometimes seen after an obstruction is removed)
3. *Excessive bladder outlet resistance (obstruction):* seen in BPH, urethral stricture, fecal impaction, or other pelvic mass
4. *Insufficient bladder outlet resistance (stress incontinence):* seen following childbirth, functional incontinence, impairment of mobility or cognition that prevents toileting, accidental trauma to sphincter during prostate surgery

Evaluation of urinary incontinence:

History
Amount of urine lost per episode	Incontinence diary
Precipitated by cough or laugh	Tumors
Diabetes, pelvic surgery	Constipation
Medications	High parity

Physical
Fecal impaction	Large prostate
Mental status, depression	Absent anal wink
Impaired perineal sensation	

Lab exam
Large residual volume	Pyuria, bacteriuria
Elevated blood glucose	

Treatment (guided by mechanism):

1. *Obstruction:* prostatectomy, urethral dilation for strictures, prazosin or terazosin (1–2 mg BID or TID) to decrease tonic obstruction
2. *Detrusor underactivity:* decompression of bladder with catheter for 10 to 14 days, urologic evaluation to rule out obstruction, bethanechol or urecholine to increase contractility
3. *Detrusor overactivity:* ditropan 2.5 to 5 mg BID to QID, antidepressants (anticholinergic), calcium channel blockers
4. *Stress incontinence:* pelvic floor exercise, topical or oral estrogens in postmenopausal females, urologic referral for corrective surgery

The absolute last resort in management of incontinence should be indwelling catheterization. The frequency of urosepsis with a chronic urethral catheter is very high and generally unacceptable. Intermittent self-catheterization for obstructive or stress incontinence is very successful for young spinal cord injury patients but has not been translated to older persons.

Note: New-onset incontinence plus back pain in a person with cancer may be a medical emergency (it may indicate spinal cord compression).

Reference: Resnick MN, et al: Management of urinary incontinence in the elderly. N Engl J Med 313:800–808, 1985.

URINARY TRACT INFECTIONS

UTIs constitute a major source of morbidity in any medical practice. Most UTIs occurring in people up to age 50 are found in females. After age 50 the incidence in men increases due to the development of prostatic hyperplasia. The classic symptoms of a lower UTI are urinary frequency, dysuria, and suprapubic pain. Fever and flank pain usually signal upper tract involvement. The diagnosis is made with a midstream urine specimen containing more than 5 WBCs per high-power field, although 2 to 5 WBCs per high-power field or more than 15 organisms per high power field may be considered diagnostic in symptomatic patients. The leukocyte esterase test may be considered diagnostic if positive, but false-negative results have been reported with very dilute urine, glycosuria, or the presence of vitamin C or cranberry juice. Cultures may be reserved for all children and men with UTI, as well as women with an immunocompromised state or renal abnormalities and/or a history of three or more UTIs in the preceding 12 months, pregnancy, or suspected pyelonephritis.

Treatment for men usually involves 10 to 14 days of an appropriate antibiotic, frequently trimethoprim-sulfamethoxazole (TMP-SMX), tetracycline, doxycycline, or amoxicillin. In women, single-dose or short-course (3-day) therapy may be effective, TMP-SMX having been studied the most in this setting. However, a high relapse rate of between 20 and 60% may dictate a more traditional 10- to 14-day course. Furthermore, short-course therapy is ineffective for eradication of *Chlamydia* and may therefore be inappropriate for the management of sexually active young women, in whom a 10- to 14-day course of doxycycline 100 mg BID or TMP-SMX (one double-strength tablet BID) would be effective. Resistant infections in any patient may require the use of the newer quinolones or amoxicillin with clavulanic acid. All men should be referred for thorough urologic evaluation, but the decision to proceed with such evaluation in women may be individualized. Pregnant women are best treated with ampicillin or cephalexin 500 mg or nalidixic acid 1 gm QID.

Pyelonephritis may be managed in the outpatient setting unless dehydration, inability to take oral fluids and medications, or severe toxic symptoms including unremitting fever and hypotension develop. Treatment with TMP-SMX (one double-strength tablet BID) is usually effective, or, in patients allergic to sulfa, norfloxacin or ciprofloxacin (250–500 mg BID). Inpatient therapy may be initiated with parenteral TMP-SMX, a third-generation cephalosporin, or an aminoglycoside pending the results of blood and urine cultures. An extended-spectrum penicillin in combination with an aminoglycoside is recommended for immunocompromised or elderly or diabetic patients or in patients with a history of recent urinary tract instrumentation.

Prophylaxis for recurrent UTIs has been demonstrated to be a cost-effective means of reducing morbidity. Intermittent prophylaxis, either postcoital or at the onset of symptoms, with a single dose of antibiotic is usually effective. In other cases, low-dose continuous prophylaxis may be indicated (e.g., TMP-SMX, one single-strength tablet every night or every other night) for a 6-month course, with trimethoprim, nitrofurantoin, or cephalexin as alternatives in patients allergic to sulfa. Women should also be advised to void after intercourse and to avoid the use of diaphragms for contraception. Before initiation of prophylaxis, a urine culture must be performed to ensure that the urine is sterile. If infection is present, a 6- to 8-week course of therapeutic full-dose antibiotics may be required prior to the initiation of prophylaxis. Prophylactic doses are continued for approximately 6 months, with longer-term therapy being reserved for cases that recur when prophylaxis is discontinued.

Asymptomatic bacteriuria in geriatric patients occurs frequently. However, it is usually transient and should not be treated routinely. UTIs in the geriatric population may present with findings such as a change in mental status, loss of appetite, weakness, urinary incontinence, or low-grade fever. Short-course regimens are associated with a high failure rate in the elderly.

Patients with an indwelling bladder catheter should be treated only if symptomatic. As in the elderly, many of these patients have neurologic conditions that make diagnosis by conventional symptoms difficult, and therefore a high level of suspicion based on more generalized systemic symptoms may be necessary.

References: Fihn SD: Urinary tract infection: Diagnosis and treatment differences in women and men. Consultant 32(10):43–58, 1992.

Howes, DS: UTI: Advances and controversies. Emerg Med 24:218–227, 1992.

Considerations in the Elderly

Asymptomatic bacteriuria: This is defined as finding 10^5 bacteria/ml of the same organism on two consecutive urine samples in a patient with no signs or symptoms of UTI. The condition is associated with decreased survival in institutionalized populations (seen in 50–70% of females in nursing homes). Antibiotics are ineffective, and treatment is needed only when symptoms occur. It is probably a marker for associated diseases, impaired immune function, increased debility, or all three. About 25% of female patients with asymptomatic bacteriuria have sterile urine without treatment 1 year later.

Infections: UTI implies invasion by pathogens, not just colonization, and it parallels the presence of symptoms of urgency, frequency, dysuria, and incontinence. *Escherichia coli* is the most frequent organism, but its predominance decreases with increasing debility, and enterococci and other gram-negatives make up the difference. In elderly men, up to 50% of UTIs are due to gram-positive organisms. There is a female predominance of UTI in young adults (20–30:1); in the elderly the ratio decreases to 2–3:1.

UTIs in an elderly patient often present in a nonspecific fashion with confusion, anorexia, lethargy, abdominal pain, and falls. Age-related changes that predispose the elderly to UTIs include alterations in the vaginal and urinary mucosa leading to improved adherence by enterobacteria, decreased bactericidal activity by prostate secretions, impaired bladder emptying, and thinning of bladder epithelium.

If the bacterial count is 100,000 (10^5) colony-forming units/ml in a clean-catch midstream urine, then there is a high likelihood the urine is infected. False positives can be minimized with catheter-obtained specimens. If urine is collected in first-morning void, it has been incubating in the bladder for 6 or more hours, which elevates colony counts. Similarly, urine that sat in the lab at room temperature for a number hours before plating will have artificially elevated colony counts.

Symptomatic UTI in a man should increase one's index of suspicion of anatomic abnormality, including BPH or obstructive uropathy. In patients with an indwelling catheter who have a temperature elevation, lower abdominal pain, or other reason to consider UTI, a new, sterile catheter should be inserted to obtain a good specimen. As long as the indwelling catheter is present, it will be impossible to keep the urine sterile. The catheters must be changed as part of treatment.

Treatment: Single-dose or very short courses of antibiotics for symptomatic cystitis may be unsatisfactory in the elderly: 1 to 2 weeks of TMP/SMX (one DS tablet BID) is our first-choice regimen. Quinolones may be used as secondary agents after the culture results are available or in sulfa-allergic cases; however, treatment should be guided by the antibiotic sensitivity of cultured organisms.

Reference: Baldassarre JS, et al: Special problems of urinary tract infection in the elderly. Med Clin North Am 75:375–390, 1991.

URINE

Red Urine

Although it is common to assume that "red urine" means RBCs in the urine, there are a number of other important causes of red urine. The main ones are:

1. **Hematuria:** This term means RBCs in the urine. Gross hematuria exists if the urine is red to reddish-brown. Microscopic hematuria is the circumstance in which RBCs are present in the urine but not in a sufficient number to change the color of the urine. RBC casts in the urine indicate glomerular disease. If the gross hematuria is noted only in the initial portion of the urine sample, a distal urethral lesion is suspected as the cause of the hematuria. Terminal hematuria, with the initial portion grossly clear, suggests the source is the posterior urethra, trigone, or base of the bladder. Total hematuria, that is, red coloration that is equal throughout voiding, occurs when the source of blood is the kidneys, ureters, or bladder.

2. **Hemoglobinuria:** The urine is red or reddish-brown in color due to free hemoglobin in the urine. There are no RBCs or RBC casts present in relationship to the hemoglobinuria. Intravascular hemolysis is the cause of hemoglobinuria. Free hemoglobin in the plasma is filtered at the glomerulus and excreted in the urine, or iron may be extracted from the hemoglobin by renal tubular cells and incorporated into ferritin and/or hemosiderin. Thus, with intravascular hemolysis there are ferritinuria and hemosiderinuria. These compounds do not impart color to urine.

3. **Myoglobinuria:** Myoglobin imparts a red to reddish-brown color to the urine. Myoglobinuria occurs because of necrosis of muscle cells (i.e., rhabdomyolysis).

4. **Uroporphyrinuria:** Patients with porphyria cutanea tarda pass red to reddish-brown urine because of large amounts of uroporphyrins in the urine. Uroporphyrins are also increased in the urine in congenital erythropoietic porphyria, yielding red urine. In acute intermittent porphyria (AIP), the urine is usually of normal color. However, nonenzymatic conversion of porphobilinogen (excreted in large amounts in the urine in AIP) to porphobilin in the urinary bladder or after the urine is excreted gives it a dark reddish-brown appearance.

5. **Drugs:** Red or orange urine is observed with the use of drugs such as rifampin, phenazopyridine (Pyridium), anthracycline compounds, and phenolphthalein.

6. **Foods:** Beets and a few food additives color the urine red.

V

VALVULAR PROSTHESES

Major breakthroughs were witnessed in the development of prosthetic heart valves since the first prosthetic valve was successfully implanted by Starr in March 1960. Except for patients with a pliable, noncalcified, stenotic, nonregurgitant mitral valve, the surgical procedure of choice is replacement of a native valve with a prosthetic heart valve.

There are two main types of prosthetic heart valves: mechanical heart valves and bioprosthetic heart valves. The era of mechanical heart valves began with the first implantation of a caged-ball mechanical prosthetic heart valve in 1960. Use of bioprosthetic heart valves was stimulated by Carpentier's invention of the process of glutaraldehyde preservation of tissue valves. The most commonly used bioprosthetic heart valve is the porcine xenograft prepared from porcine pericardium.

Mechanical Heart Valves: In the years since their introduction, many new and promising mechanical heart valve devices were developed in an attempt to address certain limitations of the original caged-ball mechanical valve design. Another mechanical prosthetic heart valve design is the tilting disc valve, as exemplified by the Bjork-Shiley and Lillihei-Kaster valves.

The major complications of both types of mechanical prosthetic heart valves are:

1. **Thromboembolism:** With in situ thrombosis or embolism in the arterial circulation. Thromboembolism is the most common and potentially most devastating complication of mechanical heart valve implantation. Changes in the design of heart valves such as cloth covering of exposed metal components to encourage endothelial tissue growth may decrease the risk of thromboembolism. However, even the newest and least hemodynamically obstructive prosthetic valve—the St. Jude Medical heart valve—is still associated with substantial risk of thromboembolism.

2. **Intravascular hemolysis:** Due to red cell trauma resulting in elevations in serum LDH, indirect bilirubin, and urinary iron excretion. A mild degree of hemolysis is expected in patients with a normally functioning heart valve. Mild intravascular hemolysis results in elevations of LDH to levels not exceeding 500 IU/L and occurs more commonly in patients with a small prosthetic valve or a cloth-covered prosthetic valve. A greater degree of intravascular hemolysis often indicates the presence of a perivalvular leak due to valve dehiscence. Prosthetic valve endocarditis and resultant perivalvular leak should be considered in patients with excessive intravascular hemolysis with serum LDH levels in excess of 1,000 IU/L.

3. **Mechanical valve dysfunction:** This can be in the form of a fracture of the ball, strut, or valve diaphragm; ball variance (a change in the shape of the valve ball due to a change in the physical properties of the ball); or embolization either of a valve or of valve components.

4. **Trauma to periprosthetic tissues:** Results in coronary ostial narrowing and LV outflow obstruction.

5. **Transvalvular pressure gradients:** Such gradients are present in all prosthetic valves, regardless of valve design. The major reason for the presence of a

significant pressure gradient across mechanical prosthetic heart valves is the centrifugal flow of blood around the ball or disc of the mechanical valve. The lowest transvalvular gradients can be obtained using the all-pyrolytic carbon St. Jude Medical valve with the unique bileaflet valve design.

Bioprosthetic Heart Valves: The first successful clinical implantation of an aortic valve allograft was reported by Ross in 1962. The procedure rapidly gained widespread use in the ensuing years. Compared to mechanical heart valves, bioprosthetic heart valves are less durable but are associated with both a significantly lower rate of thromboembolic events and much lower transvalvular pressure gradients. Thus, patients with a bioprosthetic heart valve do not require oral anticoagulation. However, because of those valves' lesser durability, bioprosthetic heart valves are recommended only for patients who cannot receive oral anticoagulation because of either a bleeding tendency, active peptic ulcer disease, or contraindication for the use of warfarin compounds, such as pregnancy. Warfarin compounds are absolutely contraindicated in pregnant women because of their potential teratogenic effects.

VASCULITIS

Vasculitis is one of the most confusing areas of rheumatic disease. Multiple classification schemes exist, etiologies remain mysterious, prognosis is difficult to judge, and intensity of disease is variable. Nonetheless, certain unifying features are recognizable.

In the simplest terms, vasculitis represents inflammation of blood vessels leading to damage to the vessel wall, occlusion of the vessel lumen, and, ultimately, tissue destruction. Thrombosis, aneurysm formation, or rupture also may occur. Many theories about the pathogenesis of vessel destruction have been proposed. Immunologic mechanisms are generally believed to be responsible. Immune complex deposition, although difficult to document, remains the prevailing theory for the pathogenesis of vessel injury. Complement activation then accentuates the immune attack, contributing to ongoing damage. Cell-mediated injury to vessels has been proposed to mechanistically explain the presence of granulomatous destruction. In addition, antibodies can also add to active vasculopathy and inflammation. Neutrophil- and eosinophil-induced vasculopathies have been documented. Finally, the contribution of cytokines in driving vessel injury remains under active investigation. The impact of the pathologic process depends on the vessels affected and the extent of involvement.

The clinical signs and symptoms of inflammatory vasculopathy are recognizable: Constitutional symptoms such as fevers, malaise, and arthralgias are perhaps the most common. Rash in the form of nonpalpable purpura or livedo reticularis is commonly present. Other features such as abdominal pain and renal and neurologic involvement may also suggest systemic inflammatory vasculopathy. Conditions such as atrial myxoma, multiple cholesterol emboli, and ergotism can mimic the clinical presentation of vasculitides and must be ruled out.

Some clearly identifiable clinical syndromes are recognized. Idiopathic or primary vasculitis such as polyarteritis nodosa (PAN), Wegener's granulomatosis, and Churg-Strauss vasculitis, among others, are of unknown cause and arise de novo. Conversely, vasculitis can be present as part of an existing condition (secondary vasculitis) such as RA or SLE. In some cases, these can be pathologically identical to an idiopathic counterpart. Infections with spirochetes, rickettsial organisms, and even pyogenic bacteria can be associated with vasculitis as well. In addition to the grouping of these conditions by potential etiologies, they are subcategorized by vessel size and type of inflammation present, as shown in the following table.

Classification of Vasculitides by Etiology

Infectious angiitis
1. Spirochetal (syphilis; Lyme disease)
2. Mycobacterial
3. Pyogenic bacterial or fungal

4 Rickettsial
5. Viral
6. Protozoal

Noninfectious angiitis

Involving large, medium-sized, and small blood vessels
1. Takayasu arteritis (primary or nonspecific aortitis and arteritis)
2. Granulomatous (giant cell) arteritis
   —Cranial (temporal) arteritis and extracranial giant cell arteritis
   —Disseminated visceral granulomatous angiitis
   —Primary angiitis of the central nervous system
3. Arteritis of rheumatic diseases and spondyloarthropathies

Involving predominantly medium-sized and small blood vessels
1. Thromboangiitis obliterans (Buerger's disease)
2. Polyarteritis (periarteritis)
   —Polyarteritis nodosa
   —Microscopic polyarteritis
   —Infantile polyarteritis
   —Kawasaki disease
3. Pathergic-allergic granulomatosis and angiitis
   —Wegener's granulomatosis
   —Churg-Strauss syndrome
   —Necrotizing sarcoid granulomatosis
4. Vasculitis of collagen-vascular disease
   —Rheumatic fever
   —Rheumatoid arthritis
   —Spondyloarthropathies
   —Systemic lupus erythematosus
   —Dermatomyositis/polymyositis
   —Relapsing polychondritis
   —Systemic sclerosis
   —Sjögren's syndrome
   —Behçet's syndrome
   —Cogan's syndrome

Involving predominantly small blood vessels (hypersensitivity angiitis; syn. allergic vasculitis; leukocytoclastic vasculitis)
1. Serum sickness
2. Schönlein-Henoch purpura
3. Drug-induced angiitis
4. Mixed cryoglobulinemia
5. Hypocomplementemia
6. Lymphocytic vasculitis

7. Malignancy-associated vasculitis
8. Retroperitoneal fibrosis
9. Inflammatory bowel disease
10. Primary biliary cirrhosis
11. Goodpasture syndrome
12. Organ transplant vasculitis

Vasculitis look-alikes or simulators
1. Arterial coarctation/hypoplasia or dysplasia
2. Idiopathic arterial calcification of infancy
3. Vasculopathy of antiphospholipid syndromes
4. Ehlers-Danlos syndrome
5. Pseudoxanthoma elasticum

6. Ergotism
7. Atheroembolism
8. Myxoma embolism
9. Neurofibromatosis
10. Köhlmeier-Degos disease

From Lie JT: Diagnostic histopathology of major systemic and pulmonary vasculitis syndromes. Rheum Dis Clin North Am 16(2):269–292, 1990, p 271, with permission.

Classification by Pathologic Process

General recognition of the clinical aspects associated with blood vessel inflammation will guide the clinician to further diagnostic evaluations as needed. Thus if one takes a broader approach to the problem, much of the mystery falls away.

A. **Vasculitis of arterioles and venules**

The skin is the organ most commonly involved. The main clinical findings are palpable purpura and chronic urticaria. The histologic picture is leukocytoclastic vasculitis, particularly involving the postcapillary venules. There is infiltration of the vessel wall with segmented neutrophils, fibrinoid necrosis of the vessel wall, and nuclear debris (leukocytoclasis). In most instances, deposition of immune complexes is responsible for the vascular damage. Causes (or associations) of leukocytoclastic vasculitis are:

Henoch-Schönlein purpura: mediated by IgA immune complexes

Essential mixed cryoglobulinemia: usually an IgM RF against IgG

Connective tissue disorders: SLE, RA, Sjögren's syndrome, or mixed connective tissue disease

Serum-sickness-like reactions

Drug reactions

Infective endocarditis

Gonococcemia

Viral infections

Chronic active hepatitis

Primary biliary cirrhosis

Lymphoproliferative disorders: chronic lymphocytic leukemia, lymphocytic lymphoma, hairy-cell leukemia, multiple myeloma, or Waldenström's macroglobulinemia

Hodgkin's disease

Acute leukemia

B. **Vasculitis of small arteries and veins**

This type of vasculitis involves particularly the blood vessels of the panniculus. Disorders with this type of vasculitis are as follows.

Erythema nodosum: May be either idiopathic (most common) or associated with sarcoidosis, TB, coccidioidomycosis, other fungal infections, leprosy, streptococcal infections, inflammatory bowel disease, Behçet's disease, and drugs (esp. sulfonamides, oral contraceptives).

Erythema induratum (rare disorder): idiopathic or seen in TB

Weber Christian disease: e.g., relapsing febrile nodular nonsuppurative panniculitis; idiopathic or associated with pancreatic fat necrosis, pancreatic cancer, or SLE

C. **Cutaneous vasculitis of medium-sized vessels**

Syndrome of ulcerative skin lesions, livedo reticularis, subcutaneous nodules, and occasional digital gangrene; associations are SLE, RA, and PAN

Sweet's syndrome: acute febrile neutrophilic dermatosis; manifested by fever, sustained neutrophilia of blood, painful red skin plaques, and neutrophilic infiltration of the skin

D. **Systemic vasculitis of medium-sized arteries**

Polyarteritis nodosa (PAN): with clinical manifestations of fever, weight loss, hypertension, renal disease, mononeuropathy multiplex, abdominal pain, and aneurysms by angiography; PAN may be associated with hepatitis B antigenemia (in 30% of cases) or amphetamine abuse.

Allergic angiitis and granulomatosis (Churg-Strauss syndrome): with clinical picture of pulmonary vascular involvement, eosinophilia, systemic vasculitis, and history of asthma and eczema

Polyangiitis overlap syndrome: showing features of PAN, allergic angiitis, and leukocytoclastic vasculitis

Cogan's syndrome: characterized by fever, abrupt loss of hearing, interstitial keratitis, and systemic vasculitis

Kawasaki disease: an illness of children manifested by fever, red and dry buccal mucosa, conjunctivitis, cervical lymphadenopathy, rash of skin leading to desquamation, and coronary arteritis

E. Granulomatous vasculitis

Wegener's granulomatosis: a systemic granulomatous vasculitis with necrotizing granulomas in the upper respiratory tract and lungs, renal arteritis and glomerulitis

Giant-cell arteritis (temporal arteritis): a granulomatous arteritis affecting the temporal arteries and other branches of the carotid arteries

Takayasu's arteritis: a granulomatous process involving large arteries such as the aorta and the carotid, subclavian, innominate, renal, celiac, and pulmonary arteries

Lymphomatoid granulomatosis (LG): Previously classified as a vasculitis, LG is probably a lymphoproliferative disorder rather than a primary disease of blood vessels. In this disorder, lymphocytes surround large pulmonary vessels (angiocentric distribution). The disease shows pulmonary, renal, dermatologic, and CNS involvement

References: Fan PT, et al: A clinical approach to systemic vasculitis. Semin Arthritis Rheum 9:248–304, 1980.

Fauci AS, et al: The spectrum of vasculitis: Clinical pathologic, immunologic, and therapeutic considerations. Ann Intern Med 89:660–675, 1978.

Haynes BF, et al: Diagnostic and therapeutic approach to the patient with vasculitis. Med Clin North Am 70:355–369, 1986.

VENOUS VALVULAR INSUFFICIENCY

Venous insufficiency produces two important problems: venous stasis ulcers and varicose veins. Symptoms include aching and swelling of lower legs and night cramps. Both problems are due to increased venous pressure caused by valvular incompetence in the perforating, or central veins or by a deep venous thrombosis. In the United States, approximately 500,000 people have stasis ulcers.

Differentiation of Venous from Arterial Ulcers in Lower Extremities

VENOUS	ARTERIAL
Varicosities, fibrosis present	No varicosities or fibrosis
Edema present	Usually no edema unless 2nd process present
Pulses usually present	Decreased peripheral pulses
Ulcers on medial malleolar area	Ulcers on distal forefoot, heels, toes, or anterior tibia
Stasis dermatitis	Not present
Proliferation of capillaries	Not present
Rusty/brownish discoloration of local skin	Surrounding skin pale or mottled
Pain minimal, decreases with elevation	Pain moderate to severe; pain increases with elevation and decreases with dependency.

Treatment of Venous Stasis Ulcer

- Compression (elastic) stockings, Unna's boots, elastic bandages: Unna's boots are uncomfortable, changed only weekly, and must not be removed overnight, but they are superior to elastic stockings and they prevent patients from disturbing the healing process (a big problem with demented patients).

- Initial debridement of ulcer because necrotic debris inhibits epithelial growth
- Systemic antibiotics for cellulitis, but not for colonization
- Topical antibiotics of little efficacy
- Surgery, occlusive dressings, valvelike prosthesis may be helpful in difficult-to-control cases.
- Leg elevation (venous HTN is present only when sitting, or standing)
- Topical corticosteroids for dermatitis and pruritus (emollients for mild cases)
- After successful treatment of an ulcer, *lifelong* preventative measures are needed.

VENTILATION, MECHANICAL

Indications for Use

Causes of Acute Respiratory Failure

1. Decompensation of chronic lung disease
2. Acute airway obstruction
   a. Epiglottitis   d. Asthma
   b. Croup   e. Bronchiolitis
   c. Aspiration of a foreign body
3. Pneumonia
4. Pulmonary emboli
5. Pneumothorax
6. Chest trauma (fractured ribs, flail chest)
7. Cardiogenic pulmonary edema
8. ARDS (noncardiogenic pulmonary edema)
9. Alveolar hypoventilation
   a. Neuromuscular disorders
        Spinal cord injuries
        Polyneuritis (Guillain-Barré)
        Poliomyelitis
        Myasthenic crisis
   b. CNS suppression: sedatives, analgesics, alcohol
   c. Severe hypothyroidism
   d. Severe metabolic alkalosis
   e. Apnea

General Guidelines for Mechanical Ventilation

1. Absolute indications (all patients)
      Apnea
      Administration of paralyzing agents
2. Clinical examination alone
      Ineffectual respiratory muscle
      Inspiratory muscle fatigue
3. Blood gas values plus clinical evaluation
      Hypoxemia not corrected by other means
      Progressive hypercarbia with acidosis

From Johanson WG, et al: Critical care. In Murray JF, et al (eds): Textbook of Respiratory Medicine. Philadelphia, W.B. Saunders, 1988, Table 95–5 on p 1994, with permission.

Physiologic Guidelines for Ventilatory Support in Respiratory Failure

PARAMETER	READING
Respiratory rate	>35/min
Vital capacity	<15 ml/kg
FEV_1	<10 ml/kg
Inspiratory force	<25 cm H_2O
P_aO_2	<70 mm Hg with O_2
$P_{(A-a)}O_2$	>450 mm Hg
P_aCO_2	>55 mm Hg
V_D/V_T	>60%

From Johanson WG, et al: Critical care. In Murray JF, et al (eds): Textbook of Respiratory Medicine. Philadelphia, W. B. Saunders, 1988, Table 95–6 on p 1994, with permission.

Modes and Complications

There are two basic types of positive-pressure mechanical ventilators that are used to support ventilation, and these are classified according to the basic mechanism limiting the inspiratory cycle.

1. **Pressure-cycled ventilators:** These devices deliver a variable volume of gas, and inspiration is terminated when a preselected airway pressure is reached. The amount of gas delivered is dependent on the elastic properties of the lung and chest wall, as well as the resistance of the tubing and airways.
2. **Volume-cycled ventilators:** These devices deliver a preset volume of gas, and inspiration is terminated when this volume is delivered. Most ventilators are equipped with pressure-limiting valves to prevent excessive pressure from developing within the airways. This is the most commonly used ventilator in adults.

Techniques of Mechanical Ventilation

1. **Assist-control ventilation:** A spontaneous effort triggers the ventilator to deliver a preset volume of gas. Controlled ventilation is determined by a preset respiratory rate and tidal volume. The controlled breath is automatic and does not require inspiratory effort. Ideally, this allows the patient to set the pattern of respiration while ensuring a minimum number of predetermined breaths if inspiratory effort fails. Patients who are paralyzed, sedated, or extremely weak must be followed carefully in order to avoid underestimating needed minute ventilation.

2. **Intermittent mandatory ventilation (IMV) or synchronized intermittent mandatory ventilation (SIMV):** This allows spontaneously breathing patients to breathe on their own, with mechanical breaths delivered at a preset rate and tidal volume regardless of patient effort. In SIMV, the mechanical breath is synchronized to begin with an inspiratory effort. These modes are often used in the weaning process.

3. **Positive end-expiratory pressure (PEEP):** PEEP is the application of end-expiratory pressure to increase functional residual capacity, which may enhance alveolar recruitment, reduce shunt, and improve oxygenation.

4. **Continuous positive airway pressure (CPAP):** CPAP consists of continuous flow at an elevated pressure during both inspiration and expiration and is used in spontaneously breathing patients. CPAP maintains a pressure above atmospheric throughout the breathing cycle.

5. **Pressure-support ventilation:** Accelerated inspiratory flow at a predetermined level is achieved, is maintained, and then slowly decelerates. This inspiratory support decreases the inspiratory work of breathing.

Complications of Endotracheal Intubation

Immediate
  Difficult intubation
  Local trauma
  Malposition of the tube
Delayed
  Self-extubation
  Infections: sinus/otitis media, tracheobronchitis/pneumonia
  Mucosal edema, denudation
Late
  Tracheomalacia
  Tracheal perforation
  Laryngeal dysfunction
  Subglottic/tracheal stenosis

From Johanson WG, et al: Critical care. In Murray JF, et al (eds): Textbook of Respiratory Medicine. Philadelphia, W. B. Saunders, 1988, Table 95–1 on p 1979, with permission.

Extubation

Various parameters are evaluated to determine if a patient can tolerate extubation (i.e., the ventilatory capability can meet ventilatory demands). The ventilatory demand is determined by the amount of CO_2 produced, the amount of wasted ventilation, and the ventilatory drive. The ventilatory capability is determined by the central respiratory drive and the strength of the respiratory muscles. The following table lists factors that influence ventilation and weaning from mechanical ventilation.

Guidelines for Assessing Withdrawal of Mechanical Ventilation

Mental	Awake and alert
F_IO_2 requirement	Adequate P_aO_2 (>60 mmHg) with F_IO_2 <0.5 PEEP <5
Ventilatory capacity	Capable of self-support for >30 min on T-tube with acceptable gases, heart rate, and respiratory rate
	P_aCO_2 acceptable, pH within normal range
	Vital capacity >10–15 ml/kg
	Minute ventilation <10 L/min
	Respiratory rate <25
	Max voluntary ventilation 2× minute ventilation
	Peak inspiratory pressure more negative than −25 cm H_2O
Secretions	Clearance adequate

Adapted from Marcy TW, et al: Modes of mechanical ventilation. In Simmons DH, et al (eds): Current Pulmonology. St. Louis, Mosby Year Book, 1992, p 76.

VERTIGO

The best evaluation of a dizzy patient is by means of a Hx & PE, directed at determining whether the symptoms arise from the vestibular system (vertigo) or from another localization. The clinical examination can accurately localize the site of the dizziness.

1. Disease anywhere in the vestibular system, whether peripherally in the ear or centrally in the brain stem, causes true vertigo, which is a spinning or other perception of movement.
2. Disease in the cerebellum causes a staggering, drunken sensation.
3. Disease in the cardiovascular system causes light-headedness and near-syncope.
4. Disease of a psychiatric nature causes chronic, continuous, vague dizziness, usually accompanied by other signs of depression or anxiety.
5. Disease that impairs sensory input, such as vision, hearing, and touch, causes most complaints of dizziness.

It is often useful to say to patients, "Describe what you feel without using the word *dizzy*."

Vertigo is almost a hallucination—that is, it is the sensation or perception of motion when none is truly present. Such patients may feel they themselves are spinning, or the room is spinning, or the floor is tilting, or there is some other motion present. This abnormal sensation of movement, called vertigo, is diagnostic of disease in the vestibular system. Determining whether the problem is central—in the brain stem—or peripheral—in the ear—is best done by analyzing the symptoms accompanying the vertigo.

1. **Central vertigo** is accompanied by other CNS signs and symptoms. The brain stem is a small, compact structure, and damage to even an isolated area, such as the vestibular nuclei at the top of the medulla, is likely to cause deficits in the adjacent structures. Therefore, vertigo from a central cause is almost always accompanied by diplopia, ataxia, hemiparesis, hemianesthesia, dysarthria, or other CNS signs.

2. **Peripheral vertigo,** affecting the eighth cranial nerve or the labyrinthine structures themselves, generally is also accompanied by other signs and symptoms referable to the auditory apparatus, such as tinnitus or hearing loss.

Most causes of true vertigo arise from the ear, not the brain. Benign positional vertigo is by far the most frequent etiology. This condition produces vertigo when the head is placed in certain positions and is a self-limited problem.

The best treatment for the symptom of vertigo, regardless of the etiology, is to suppress the vestibular input. This can be accomplished most effectively with scopolamine, which is by far the most useful drug for vertigo. It is administered as a transdermal patch with a sustained, continuous action. (See also Dizziness.)

References: Baloh RW, et al: Clinical Neurophysiology of the Vestibular System, 2nd ed. Philadelphia, F.A. Davis, 1990.

Stronger SP, et al: Diagnosis, causes and management of vertigo. Compr Ther 16:34–41, 1990.

VITAMIN DEFICIENCIES

Manifestations of Vitamin Deficiencies

VITAMIN	MANIFESTATIONS OF DEFICIENCY
Vitamin A (retinol)	Loss of night vision, xerophthalmia, Bitôt's spots Keratomalacia: ulceration of cornea leading to perforation, prolapse of the iris, panophthalmitis, and blindness; dryness of the skin and hyperkeratinization
Vitamin B_1 (thiamine)	Beriberi: paresthesias, diminished reflexes, weakness, muscle fatigue, cramps, myalgias, foot and wrist drop Peripheral vasodilation: high-output CHF, tachycardia, circulatory collapse, edema Wernicke-Korsakoff syndrome: ophthalmoplegia, nystagmus, ataxia, amnesia, confusion, confabulation
Vitamin B_2 (riboflavin)	Soreness and burning of mouth and tongue, cheilosis, seborrheic dermatitis, photophobia, conjunctivitis, sore throat, anemia
Niacin (nicotinic acid)	Pellagra: dermatitis, dementia, diarrhea (and death) —Symmetrical bilateral dermatitis due to photosensitivity —Fatigue, apathy, disorientation, memory loss, organic psychosis —Diarrhea
Vitamin B_6 (pyridoxine)	Nausea, vomiting, dizziness, cheilosis, glossitis, convulsions, peripheral neuropathy
Vitamin B_{12} (methylcobalamine)	Pernicious anemia: megaloblastic anemia plus any of the following: anorexia, irritability, confusion, glossitis, fever, orthostatic hypotension Subacute combined degeneration: stocking-glove paresthesias, clumsiness, ataxia, weakness, spasticity
Vitamin C (ascorbic acid)	Scurvy: perifollicular hemorrhages, purpura, bleeding in muscles and joints, poor wound healing. Gum disease: swelling, bleeding, and loosening of teeth
Vitamin D (D_2 and D_3)	Osteomalacia due to failure of bone mineralization Hypocalcemia: muscle cramps, decreased muscle tone and strength, seizures
Vitamin E (α-tocopherol)	Edema, anemia, areflexia, reduced proprioception and vibratory sense, gait disturbance, ophthalmoplegia
Vitamin K	Bleeding disorders
Folic acid	Megaloblastic anemia, glossitis

Adapted from Margolis S, et al: Nutritional disorders. In Harvey AM, et al (eds): The Principles and Practice of Medicine, 22nd ed. Norwald, CT, Appleton & Lange, 1988, pp 988–989, with permission.

Vitamin B_{12} Deficiency

Deficiency of vitamin B_{12} results in a macrocytic anemia, commonly with pancytopenia, megaloblastic hematopoiesis, glossitis, and the neurologic abnormalities of subacute combined-system disease with degeneration of the posterior and lateral columns of the spinal cord. In addition, affected patients may have peripheral neuropathy and cerebral dysfunction manifested by dementia and neuropsychiatric abnormalities, including psychosis. Serum B_{12} levels are low in 80 to 90% of patients with B_{12} deficiency.

In consideration of the causes of a megaloblastic anemia, B_{12} deficiency must be discriminated from folic acid deficiency and from a diverse group of disorders with megaloblastic changes such as erythroleukemia, myelodysplastic syndrome, congenital dyserythropoietic anemia, hereditary orotic aciduria, long-term exposure to nitrous oxide, and use of chemotherapeutic agents that interfere with nucleic acid metabolism. Values of the serum B_{12}, serum and RBC folate levels, when analyzed together, usually permit differentiation of deficiencies of B_{12} and folic acid.

Classification of Vitamin B_{12} Deficiency

Dietary deficiency
Gastric disorders
    Pernicious anemia
    Gastrectomy
Intestinal disorders
    Mucosal disorders
    Blind loop syndrome
    Diphyllobothrium latum infestation
Pancreatic insufficiency
Congenital disorders

Vitamin B_{12} deficiency by reason of deficient dietary intake is very rare, being limited to strict vegetarians of long duration. In pernicious anemia, atrophic gastritis results in achlorhydria and diminished secretion of intrinsic factor, which is required for absorption of B_{12} in the ileum. The presence of antiparietal cell antibodies in 90 % of patients with pernicious anemia supports the concept of autoimmune causation of the disease by reason of immunologic destruction of gastric mucosal cells. Pernicious anemia is one of a number of disorders (autoimmune thyroiditis, Addison's disease, DM, and vitiligo) composing the autoimmune endocrine deficiency syndromes. There is a hereditary predisposition in patients with pernicious anemia. Vitamin B_{12} deficiency inevitably occurs within 5 to 6 years after total gastrectomy and may be observed eventually in about 5% of patients after partial gastrectomy.

Failure to absorb B_{12} in the ileum is the cause of B_{12} deficiency in disorders such as Crohn's disease, sprue, and intestinal lymphoma and after ileal resection. In blind loop syndrome, microorganisms within the blind small bowel loops utilize the B_{12}, preventing absorption. The fish tapeworm *Diphyllobothrium latum* competes effectively with its human host for B_{12} in the intestinal lumen.

In patients with pancreatic insufficiency, B_{12} deficiency occurs because of the lack of normally secreted pancreatic proteases that destroy R binder, a compound that binds to B_{12} and prevents its absorption.

An abnormal stage I of the Schilling test with a normal stage II indicates a gastric cause of B_{12} deficiency, whereas the cause is intestinal or pancreatic if both stages show impaired absorption of the radiolabeled vitamin.

A rare congenital disorder of infancy is Imerslund-Gräsbeck disease, in which there are both selective ileal malabsorption of B_{12} and albuminuria. Congenital intrinsic factor deficiency—transmitted as an autosomal recessive trait—leads to B_{12} deficiency in infancy or childhood. Deficiency of the transport protein transcobalamin II results in severe megaloblastic anemia in infancy. In such infant patients, serum B_{12} levels are normal (carried by transcobalamin I), but tissue levels are very low.

VOMITING IN CANCER

Vomiting associated with cancer and cancer chemotherapy is debilitating and distressing. Any physician caring for cancer patients must address this problem and pay special attention to its amelioration. Besides negatively affecting the quality of life, it may limit sufficient food intake and further compromise ability to tolerate treatment.

The mechanism of vomiting occurs through multiple routes. The vomiting center in the CNS is located in the lateral reticular formation of the medulla and receives signals from (1) the midbrain receptors of intracranial press; (2) the GI tract via vagal and sympathetic afferents; (3) the labyrinthine apparatus; (4) the chemoreceptor trigger zone, a medullary center located in the floor of the fourth ventricle; and (5) higher CNS structures such as the limbic system reacting to psychic stimuli. The **chemoreceptor trigger zone** (CTZ) is stimulated by toxic substances and is rich in neuroreceptors responding to histamine, dopamine, and acetylcholine. Efferent pathways include the phrenic nerves to the diaphragm, spinal nerves to the abdominal muscles, and visceral nerves to the stomach and esophagus. Autonomic nervous system output such as salivation, tachycardia, diaphoresis, and pallor accompany vomiting. Somatic efferent nerves coordinate the musculature of respiration, causing retching and then expulsion of gastric contents.

Antiemetic Agents

1. *Metoclopramide* is a substituted benzamide that blocks dopamine receptors at the CTZ, increases lower esophageal sphincter tone, promotes gastric emptying, and accelerates small bowel transit. It is particularly useful in cisplatin-induced vomiting.

2. *Phenothiazines* are dopamine antagonists that block dopamine receptors at the CTZ. They are useful for vomiting caused by chemotherapy with low emetogenic potential such as methotrexate, cyclophosphamide, and melphalan. Piperazine phenothiazines such as prochlorperazine and triethylperazine maleate have higher antiemetic potency with less sedation, hypotension, and extrapyramidal symptoms.

3. *Butyrophenones* such as haloperidol and droperidol are useful for cisplatin-induced vomiting.

4. *Antihistamines* similar to diphenhydramine may be used in conjunction with other dopamine blockers such as phenothiazine or metoclopramide.

5. *Corticosteroids* work by blocking prostaglandin synthesis.

6. *Benzodiazepines* such as diazepam and lorazepam are usually used in combination with other antiemetics and are most useful in treatment of anticipatory vomiting due to their anamnestic properties.

7. *Cannabinoids* are believed to decrease vomiting by inhibiting efferent pathways from the vomiting center, and they may inhibit prostaglandin synthesis. However delta-9-THC, nabilone, and levonantradol have frequent side effects of euphoria, sedation, and confusion.

8. *Ondansetron* is a potent and highly selective 5-hydroxytryptamine antagonist. It prevents emesis induced by both cisplatin and noncisplatin chemotherapy as well as by radiation. There is no antagonism of dopamine D2 receptors, so extrapyramidal side effects that are seen with other agents are not observed.

VON WILLEBRAND'S DISEASE

VWD is an autosomal disorder associated with abnormalities of the von Willebrand factor (vWF)—a high-molecular-weight, multimeric protein that is an important mediator of platelet adhesion to injured endothelial surfaces. Von Willebrand factor is also important as a carrier for Factor VIII:C (the Factor VIII coagulant activity missing in the sex-linked disorder hemophilia A). VWD results in prolongation of the bleeding time and has a variable impact on the PTT or Factor VIII coagulant activity when it is specifically assayed. Patients with vWD are clinically heterogenous—many types have been identified. The four most important types of vWD are summarized in the following table.

Laboratory Values in Principal vWD Subtypes

	I	IIa	IIb	III
Bleeding time	Prolonged	Prolonged	Prolonged	Markedly prolonged
VWF antigen	↓	→ or ↓	→ or ↓	Markedly ↓
Ristocetin cofactor	↓Proportionatly to vWF Ag	Less than vWF Ag	Variable	Absent
Ristocetin aggregation in platelet-rich plasma	↓	↓	↑	Absent
Gel electrophoretic pattern	→	↓ high molecular weight	↓ high molecular weight	Absent

From Triplett, DA: Laboratory diagnosis of von Willebrand disease. Mayo Clin Proc 66:839, 1991, with permission.

Patients are troubled by purpura, epistaxis, GI bleeding, hematuria, and menorrhagia. Because vWD affects platelet function, some of these manifestations are exacerbated by aspirin. Postdental extraction and trauma may be complicated by excessive bleeding.

The vWF gene has been localized to chromosome 2 and cloned. It is likely that defects leading to vWD reside in this gene or in the regulation of its expression. In type I vWD there is a quantitative reduction in the vWF in the plasma and in platelets. The pattern of vWF multimer size is not affected, although the plasma level may be significantly decreased. VWD is sometimes observed in patients with hemorrhagic telangiectasia, so it is also possible that a gene regulating the excretion of vWF by endothelial cells is disordered. In type II disease there is a qualitative dysfunction of vWF, which results in functional abnormalities or changes in the pattern of electrophoretic mobility of the vWF multimers. In type IIa disease, the qualitative defect results in impaired interaction with platelets. In contrast, type IIb vWD is associated with increased avidity of platelets for vWF, especially in the presence of ristocetin. These patients sometimes have mild thrombocytopenia. Type III vWD patients are homozygous or double heterozygous for dominant and recessive defects, are severely affected, and have very low levels of vWF in the plasma.

The clinical features of vWD are variable even among families. Some of this variability within families may be due to the presence of two different abnormal genes. Affected members possess one abnormal but mild gene, one gene with modest effects, or both genes and therefore more serious hemostatic impairment. The blood type, for unknown reasons, also affects the level of vWF, with type O individuals having lower vWF levels. Acquired vWD also occurs, but its pathogenesis remains obscure. Disorders associated with acquired vWD include lymphoma, multiple myeloma, autoimmune disorders, myeloproliferative diseases, and Wilms' tumor.

Management in the past was based solely on the use of plasma and cryoprecipitate that was enriched in vWF and Factor VIII:C. Today several alternatives are available. A significant number of patients with type I vWD respond to desmopressin by increase in their vWF levels and normalization of bleeding time. If successful in a trial, desmopressin may be used prior to elective, usually minor, procedures or for bleeding—without the need for reestablishing its effect on hemostasis. Desmopressin is usually given IV once daily and often in conjunction with an antifibrinolytic agent—either epsilon-aminocaproic acid or transexemic acid. It is generally a safe drug, although hyponatremia has occurred. This complication can be avoided by following the patient's Na$^+$ and limiting hypotonic fluids. One of the newer Factor VIII:C preparations contains a significant amount of native vWF. As these products undergo steps to inactivate viruses, they may be safer to use than multiple single-donor cryoprecipitate units. Because of the decreased Factor VIII:C level in many vWD patients, the aim of therapy is to increase the Factor VIII:C level to 50% and to shorten the bleeding time.

W

WARTS

Warts, also known as verrucae, are seen throughout the world in every ethnic group. They affect 7 to 10% of the population and can be associated with various age groups and occupations. Caused by infection with any one of many human papillomaviruses (HPV), warts are benign tumors of the epithelial and mucosal surfaces, although infection with certain HPV may be associated with increased risk of certain genital tract malignancies. As a viral infection, warts are transmissible through inoculation.

Papillomaviruses infect many species of mammals but are species specific, with no transmission between species. Over 60 HPVs have been identified by DNA homology studies. Distinct viruses are associated with distinct types of warts. Cell-mediated immunity appears to play an important role in the response to HPV infection and the extent and duration of warts. In most cases the lesions are self-limited and regress spontaneously, but in individuals with impaired immunity there may be indefinitely continued extension of lesions. In immunocompetent individuals some HPVs induce neutralizing antibody, and recurrence is prevented.

Three types of cutaneous warts are most common: common warts (verruca vulgaris), deep plantar warts (myrmecia), and plane or flat warts (verruca plana).

Types of Cutaneous Warts

	COMMON	PLANTAR	PLANE
Age group	<20	10–25	Any
Distribution	Dorsa hand, palms/ soles, mucosal (rare)	Soles, palms	Face, neck, hands
Size	2–10 mm	2–10 mm	1–5 mm
Pain	No	Yes	No
HPV types	2 (more), 1 (less)	1	3, 10

Anogenital warts (condylomata acuminata) are increasing rapidly in incidence and now represent approximately 10% of all STDs. They are cauliflowerlike clusters of white-gray or pink-red papules that may be on the skin or pedunculated. The size can range from 1 mm for an isolated lesion to more than several centimeters for a confluent group lesion. Normal-appearing skin may have HPV DNA present and is potentially infectious. In circumcised men, the penile shaft is most commonly involved; in those uncircumcised, the preputial cavity is most common. Involvement of the perianal area is based on sexual practices and potential contact. The scrotum is rarely affected. In women, the posterior introitus and the labia majora and minora are most frequently involved. Again, the perianal area is involved only with prior exposure. As with cutaneous warts, the extent and duration of lesions depend on immune status. With the profound defects in cell-mediated immunity seen in HIV/AIDS, the extent of perianal warts can progress to interfere with evacuation of anal contents.

661

Therapy against warts is usually minimal because the lesions will regress spontaneously in the vast majority of cases. Often, the release of antigens with the destruction of one lesion prompts an immune response that clears other lesions. For those lesions requiring therapy due to location, cosmetic concerns, or pain, cryotherapy with liquid nitrogen is the most common therapeutic modality. Often, a single treatment is sufficient to eliminate the lesion. Podophyllin is still commonly used for genital warts because there can be less inflammation and irritation if used properly. Surgical excision may be required for some of the larger, confluent lesions seen in the perianal areas.

WEGENER'S GRANULOMATOSIS

Wegener's granulomatosis is an example of a systemic vasculopathy involving medium-sized vessels that is recognizable by its clinical presentation. By definition, the respiratory tract is always involved. Sinusitis is common (most often maxillary), and superimposed bacterial infections can make the diagnosis difficult. Nasal involvement also occurs and leads to actual destruction of the cartilaginous nasal septum, leading to a saddle-nose deformity. The granulomatous inflammation and destruction can occur anywhere in the respiratory tract, from the mouth through the lungs. The eyes can be involved, with conjunctivitis, episcleritis, scleritis, or optic nerve vasculopathy. Pancarditis can also occur. Mononeuritis multiplex due to vasculopathy of the vaso nervorum is perhaps the most common neurologic manifestation. Renal disease is present in the majority of patients, manifested primarily by glomerulonephritis. Constitutionally, symptoms such as joint pain, fever, and weight loss are common presenting symptoms.

Laboratory features include anemia and elevated ESR. ANCA is a cytoplasmic staining pattern present in over 90% of patients. Plain x-rays of the sinus may show severe pansinusitis and even bony destruction. Elevated BUN and creatinine as well as active urinary sediment are present. As many as 50% of patients may have a positive RF. Circulating immune complexes have also been found.

Pathologic features include a focal, segmental, necrotizing glomerulonephritis often associated with crescent formation. Classic leukocytoclastic vasculopathy can occur in small skin vessels. Larger vessels can be involved and are usually associated with granulomatous change, although a fibrinoid necrosis similar to that seen in polyarteritis nodosa can also occur. Granulomas can sometimes occur in extravascular foci, causing destruction. Other destructive granulomatous diseases that commonly occur in the differential include lymphomatoid granulomatosis (also called midline granuloma) and sarcoidosis.

Treatment should include glucocorticoids and cytotoxic agents. Although originally pulse cyclophosphamide was thought to be of equal efficacy, it now appears that daily oral doses of cyclophosphamide are more likely to lead to steady improvement. There is little added improvement if plasma exchange is added to this regimen.

WEIGHT LOSS IN CANCER

Weight loss in cancer is one of the most common symptoms of widespread disease. The tumor types most frequently associated with weight loss—gastric and pancreatic—also have the greatest degree of weight loss. It is a well-described phenomenon that weight loss is a prognostic factor in cancer. For sarcoma, some lymphomas, colon cancer, and prostate cancer, the median survival is approximately twice as long in patients who have not lost weight as in the patients who do. The prognosis is poorer the greater the weight loss. Response to treatment is also correlated with weight loss, and overall response rates for patients who do not lose weight are longer.

The reasons for weight loss in cancer are not completely understood but are thought to be related to energy balance, altered carbohydrate metabolism, and altered protein metabolism. Energy balance in the cancer patient may be negative because of decreased caloric intake and/or increased caloric expenditure. When measured, caloric intake in those who lose weight is usually insufficient. Alterations in taste and smell occur. An elevated threshold for sweet taste is described in one-quarter of patients who were tested in one study. Increased sensitivity to bitter taste and elevated thresholds for salty taste have also been described. These abnormalities increase with tumor burden but not tumor type. Early satiety is also reported frequently, possibly related to alterations in GI sensing or delays in gastric emptying. Energy expenditure in cancer patients shows modest increases: about 20 to 50% higher than expected based on age, sex, body size, and activity level. It is believed this is due to the energy requirements of the growing cancer cells. It has also been found that intake of carbohydrate in cancer patients leads to increased plasma lactate, which causes anorexia, nausea, and anxiety leading to a learned aversion to carbohydrate foods. Decreased glucose tolerance has also been seen, with decreased insulin output and insulin resistance. Continued elevations of blood glucose decrease the appetite stimulus and also lead to delayed gastric emptying. Experiments with TPN have found that this expensive and somewhat risky therapy made no contribution to overall response rate or survival. Furthermore, increased nutritional intake may accelerate tumor metabolism, leading to a hypermetabolic state, with fever, tachycardia, and mild tachypnea. In animal model studies, mild reductions in caloric intake decreased tumor growth and increased survival. (See also Anorexia in Cancer.)

WHEEZING

Wheezing is a high-pitched sound produced when airway size is narrowed such that the turbulence of air produces oscillation of the airway walls. The pitch of the wheeze depends on the velocity of airflow and the degree of airway narrowing. Therefore, any disease that causes airway narrowing can be included in the differential diagnosis. In its intensity and predominance during *inspiration,* stridor heard with laryngeal or tracheal obstruction differs from wheezing.

Characteristics of wheezing that may help to identify a specific etiology include whether the wheezing is chronic or intermittent, localized or diffuse, inspiratory or expiratory, and associated with passive or associated with forced respiration.

Differential Diagnosis of Wheezing

Laryngeal obstruction
  Foreign body
  Edema
  Anaphylaxis
  Vocal cord dysfunction
  Epiglottitis and abscess
  Trauma, hemorrhage
  Tumors

Table continued on next page.

Differential Diagnosis of Wheezing (Cont.)

Central airway obstruction
  Foreign body
  Trauma
  Enlarged thyroid
  Tumors
  Anomalous arteries, aneurysm
Peripheral airway obstruction
  Asthma and other diseases associated with reactive airways disease
  Nonasthmatic causes of peripheral airway obstruction
    Acute
      Pulmonary embolism
      Pulmonary edema (cardiac asthma)
      Aspiration of gastric contents or toxic liquids
      Inhalation injury (thermal or irritant)
      Carcinoid tumors
      Eosinophilic pneumonia
    Chronic
      Cystic fibrosis
      Bronchiectasis
      Bronchiolitis
      Sarcoid

From Hunter RS: Sudden onset of wheezing and dyspnea. In Schwarz MI (ed): Pulmonary Grand Rounds. Toronto, B. C. Decker, 1990, Table 1, p 265, with permission.

WOLFF-PARKINSON-WHITE SYNDROME

Recognition

Preexcitation syndrome is a syndrome characterized by earlier activation of part or the whole ventricle by an atrial impulse than expected if the impulse traveled through the normal specialized conduction system. WPW, the most common type of preexcitation, is characterized by muscular connections composed of working myocardial fibers connecting the atrium and ventricle. The term *WPW* is applied when a patient has symptoms, generally due to tachycardias, in addition to the following classic ECG triad:

1. Short P-R interval: <120 msec during sinus rhythm
2. Prolonged QRS duration: >120 msec
3. Delta wave: causing a slurred, slowly rising onset of the QRS in some leads with a normal terminal QRS portion

To facilitate anatomic delineation of the site of the accessory pathway in preexcitation syndromes, an algorithm based on a 12-lead ECG has been developed and is illustrated in the figure that follows. Although the algorithm can be conveniently used in most patients, the exact anatomic delineation of the accessory pathway in patients with preexcitation syndromes requires electrophysiologic testing. That anatomic delineation is necessary in order to plan the definitive surgical resection of the accessory pathway.

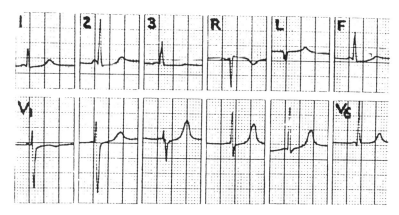

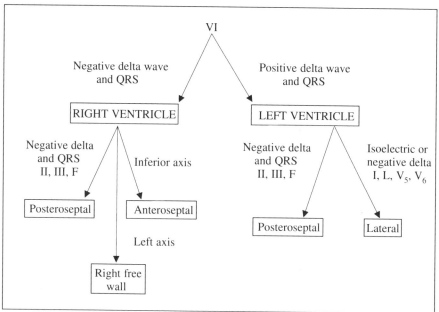

Localization of accessory pathways. Begin with analysis of V_1 to determine whether the delta wave and the QRS complex are negative or positive. That establishes the ventricle in which the accessory pathway is located. Next, determine whether the delta wave and QRS complex are negative in leads II, III, and AVF. If so, then the accessory pathway is located in a posteroseptal position. If the accessory pathway is located in the RV, an inferior axis indicates an anteroseptal location, whereas left axis indicates a right free wall location. If the accessory pathway is located in the LV, an isoelectric or negative delta wave and QRS complex in leads I, aVI, V_5, and V_6 indicate a left lateral (free wall) location. (From Zipes DP: Specific arrhythmias: Diagnosis and treatment. In Braunwald E (ed): Heart Disease, 4th ed. Philadelphia, W. B. Saunders, 1992, p 695, with permission.)

Associated Cardiac Anomalies

WPW syndrome is associated with a variety of congenital and acquired cardiac defects.

1. Ebstein's anomaly: Patients with Ebstein's anomaly often have multiple accessory pathways, right-sided accessory pathways either in the posterior septum or in the posterolateral wall, and preexcitation localized in the atrialized portion of the right ventricle.
2. Mitral valve prolapse
3. Cardiomyopathies

A careful physical examination and a two-dimensional echocardiogram are essential in the diagnostic workup of patients with WPW syndrome to exclude various associated congenital anomalies.

Z

ZOLLINGER-ELLISON SYNDROME

Zollinger-Ellison syndrome is the result of a non-beta cell endocrine neoplasm secreting excessive amounts of gastrin into the serum. Increased levels of circulating gastrin result in extreme gastric acid hypersecretion leading to severe PUD and its complications. More than 80% of gastrinomas can be localized to an anatomic area known as the gastrinoma triangle. The boundaries of that triangle are the confluence of the cystic duct and common bile duct superiorly, junction of the second and third portion of the duodenum inferiorly, and junction of the neck and body of the pancreas medially. Although the pancreas itself is the most common site of tumor, the duodenum is the most common extrapancreatic site. Tumors have also been found within the stomach, bones, ovaries, liver, and lymph nodes. Tumors are generally considered to be malignant and have metastatic potential.

Diagnosis: Clinically, patients typically present with symptoms related to gastric acid hypersecretion. Most patients develop PUD at some point during the course of their disease but frequently are unresponsive to traditional medical therapy, which should raise the suspicion of a hypersecretory state. Ulcers may be found in unusual locations, including the second, third, and fourth portions of the duodenum and the jejunum. Other symptoms include diarrhea related to excessive acid secretion as well as complicated ulcer disease presenting initially with obstruction, perforation, or bleeding.

The diagnosis of gastrinoma rests with an initial high index of suspicion. Elevation of fasting serum gastrin, particularly greater than 1,000 pg/ml, is highly suggestive of gastrinoma. In conjunction with elevation of serum gastrin, acid production must be present (achlorhydria may result in elevation of serum gastrin as well). At this point, to differentiate between the many possible additional causes of hypergastrinemia, a provocative test must be performed: a secretin stimulation test has proven to be the easiest and most reliable study to perform. Here, IV secretin is injected, and, in the normal host, serum gastrin either remains constant or is reduced. In the presence of a gastrinoma, a paradoxical rise in serum gastrin occurs, usually >200 pg/ml. Less commonly utilized gastrin provocative tests include calcium infusion (results in an increased gastrin ≥400 pg/ml over baseline).

Treatment: Curative therapy may be undertaken by way of surgical resection of the primary tumor. However, gastrinomas are notoriously difficult to localize, and in 50% of cases no tumor can be found. Preoperative attempts to localize tumors should include abdominal CT scan with contrast. If evidence of extensive tumor with metastases is present, then no further evaluation is necessary, and medical therapy should be undertaken. If no tumor is seen by CT scan or if a single tumor site is identified without metastases, then selective mesenteric angiography should be performed to help with localization of the primary tumor site and identification of metastases. If angiography is negative, then portal venous sampling for gastrin levels may be useful in localizing a primary site. More recently, endoscopic ultrasound has been used successfully to localize pancreatic endocrine tumors that have not been identified by CT or angiography in the preoperative state.

If a single tumor site is identified, surgical resection may be undertaken. If the tumor cannot be resected, medical therapy to control gastric acid hypersecretion is necessary. High-dose H_2 receptor antagonists or, more recently, H^+–K^+ ATPase inhibition with omeprazole has resulted in excellent ulcer healing and symptom resolution. In addition, highly selective vagotomy or total gastrectomy may be used to control acid secretion in conjunction with medical treatment. Effective therapy for metastatic tumor has not been forthcoming. The most useful combination chemotherapy regimen has been streptozocin, 5-fluorouracil, and doxorubicin.

ZOONOSES

A zoonosis is a disease communicable from lower animals to humans under natural conditions.

Zoonoses

ORGANISM	DISEASE IN HUMANS	RESPONSIBLE ANIMAL
Parasitic infections		
Toxocara canis	Visceral larva migrans	Dog
Ancyclostoma caninum	Cutaneous larva migrans	Cats and dogs
A. braziliense	Cutaneous larva migrans	Cats and dogs
Dirofilaria immitis	Solitary pulmonary nodule	Dog
Echinoccus granulosus	Cysts in many different organs	Dogs and other carnivores
E. multilocularis	Cysts in many different organs	Dogs, cats, foxes, and other carnivores
Dipylidium caninum	Diarrhea, pruritus ani	Dogs and cats
Toxoplasma gondii	Acute: mononucleosis syndrome Late: myocarditis, encephalitis; congenital infection	Cats
Cryptosporidium	Diarrheal disease	Cows
Bacterial infections		
Brucella canis	Systemic or focal illness	Dogs
B. abortus	Systemic or focal illness	Cows
B. suis	Systemic or focal illness	Pigs
B. melitensis	Systemic or focal illness	Sheep, goats
Leptospira canicola, and *L. icterohaemorrhagiae*	Septicemic illness with headache, myalgias, fever, and renal and hepatic impairment; immune phase with fever, rash, and meningitis	Dogs Dogs, rats, cows, pigs, mice
Campylobacter jejuni	Enteritis	Poultry, dogs, cows, horses, sheep, pigs
Salmonella sp.	Enteritis, typhoidal illness	Poultry, dogs, cows
Pasteurella multocida	Bite wound infection, pneumonia, endocarditis	Cats, dogs
Borrelia recurrentis	Endemic or tick-borne relapsing fever	Rodents, rabbits, and foxes
B. burgdorferi	Lyme disease (arthritis, rash, encephalitis, myocarditis)	White-footed mice, white-tailed deer
Listeria monocytogenes	Meningitis, bacteremia	Many animals and birds

Table continued on next page.

Zoonoses (Cont.)

ORGANISM	DISEASE IN HUMANS	RESPONSIBLE ANIMAL
Bacterial infections (cont.)		
Erysipelothrix rhusiopathiae	Cutaneous lesions (erysipe-loid), bacteremia	Marine mammals, fish, crus-taceans, birds, pigs
Capnocytophaga canimorsus (DF-2)	Wound infections, bactere-mia, endocarditis	Dogs
Streptobacillus moniliformis	Rat-bite fever	Wild and laboratory rodents
Spirillum minus	Rat-bite fever	Wild and laboratory rodents
Chlamydia psittaci	Psittacosis, pneumonia	Psittacine birds, fowl
Yersinia enterocolitica and *Y. pseudotuberculosis*	Enteritis, typhoidal syn-drome, arthritis, adenitis	Rodents, birds, dogs, cats, pigs, sheep
Rochalimaea henselae	Cat-scratch disease	Cats
Coxiella burnetii	Pneumonia	Cats, cows, sheep, goats, fowl
Ectoparasite-borne infections		
Rickettsia rickettsii	Rocky Mountain spotted fe-ver	Wild rodents, rabbits, dogs
Bacillus anthracis	Cutaneous lesions, pneumo-nia	Cows, goats, sheep
Francisella tularensis	Tularemia (pneumonic, ulcer-oglandular, oropharyngeal)	Rabbits, dogs, cats
Yersinia pestis	Plague (pneumonic, bubonic, septicemic)	Rodents, cats
Ehrlichia canis	Systemic illness	Dogs
R. prowazekii	Epidemic typhus	Eastern flying squirrel
R. akari	Rickettsialpox	Mice
R. tsutsugamushi	Scrub typhus	Mice
Dermatophytes		
Microsporum canis	Tinea or ringworm	Dogs, cats
Viral infections		
Rabies virus	Rabies	Wild carnivores, bats, dogs, cats, horses, cows, raccoons
Lymphocytic chorio-meningitis virus	Aseptic meningitis	Rodents
Herpesvirus simiae	Encephalitis	Primates of the genus *Macaca*

References: Elliot DL, et al: Pet-associated illness. N Engl J Med 313:985–995, 1985.
Weinberg AN, et al (eds): Animal-associated human infections. Infect Dis Clin North Am 5:1–181, 1991.

ABBREVIATIONS

AAA	abdominal aortic aneurysm
ABGs	arterial blood gases
ACD	anemia of chronic disease
ACE	angiotensin converting enzyme
ACLS	advanced cardiac life support
ACTH	adrenocorticotropic hormone (corticotropin)
ADH	antidiuretic hormone
AF/A fib	atrial fibrillation
AFB	acid-fast bacillus (smear test)
αFP	alpha fetoprotein
Ag	antigen
AIDS	acquired immunodeficiency syndrome
AIHA	autoimmune hemolytic anemia
ALL	acute lymphoblastic leukemia
ALS	amyotrophic lateral sclerosis
ALT	alanine transaminase (SGPT)
AMA	antimitochondrial antibody
AML	acute myelogenous (or myeloblastic) leukemia
ANA	antinuclear antibodies
ANCA	antineutrophilic cytoplasmic antibodies
AP	anteroposterior
aPL	antiphospholipid antibodies
APTT	activated partial thromboplastin time
APUD	amine precursor uptake and decarboxylation
ARDS	adult respiratory distress syndrome
ARF	acute renal failure
ASD	atrial septal defect
AST	aspartate transaminase (SGOT)
ATG	antithymocyte globulin
ATN	acute tubular necrosis
AV	arteriovenous, atrioventricular
BBB	bundle branch block
ß-HCG	beta subunit of human chorionic gonadotropin
BID	twice daily
BP	blood pressure
BPH	benign prostatic hypertrophy
bpm	beats per minute
BUN	blood urea nitrogen
CABG	coronary artery bypass graft surgery
CAD	coronary artery disease

cAMP	cyclic adenosine monophosphate
CAPD	continuous ambulatory peritoneal dialysis
CBC	complete blood count
CDC	Centers for Disease Control and Prevention
CEA	carcinoembryonic antigen
CFS	chronic fatigue syndrome
CHF	congestive heart failure
CLL	chronic lymphocytic leukemia
CML	chronic myelogenous leukemia
CMML	chronic myelomonocytic leukemia
CMV	cytomegalovirus
CNS	central nervous system
COPD	chronic obstructive pulmonary disease
CPAP	continuous positive airway pressure
CPDD	calcium pyrophosphate deposition disease
CPK	creatine phosphokinase
CPR	cardiopulmonary resuscitation
Cr	creatinine
CREST	calcinosis, Raynaud's, esophageal disorders, sclerodactyly, telangiectasia
CRH	corticotropin-releasing hormone
CRF	chronic renal failure
CRP	C-reactive protein
CSF	cerebrospinal fluid
CT	computed tomographic (scan)
CUP	carcinoma of unknown primary (syndrome)
CVA	cerebrovascular accident
CVP	central venous pressure
CXR	chest x-ray, chest radiograph

D5W	5% dextrose in water
DES	diethylstilbestrol
DHEA	dehydroepiandrosterone
DI	diabetes insipidus
DIC	disseminated intravascular coagulation
DKA	diabetic ketoacidosis
DL_{co}	diffusion capacity for carbon monoxide
DM	diabetes mellitus
DTR	deep tendon reflex
DTs	delirium tremens
DVT	deep venous thrombosis

EBV	Epstein-Barr virus
ECF	extracellular fluid
ECG	electrocardiogram, electrocardiographic
ECM	erythema chronicum migrans
ED	emergency department
EEG	electroencephalogram
EF	ejection fraction

EGD	esophagogastroduodenoscopy (gastroscopy)
ELISA	enzyme-linked immunosorbent assay
EMG	electromyogram
ENG	electronystagmogram
EPO	erythropoietin
ERCP	endoscopic retrograde cholangiopancreatography
ESR	erythrocyte sedimentation rate
ESRD	end-stage renal disease
FAB	French-American-British (classification)
FE_x	fractional excretion of substance ''x''
$FEF_{25-75\%}$	forced expiratory flow from 25 to 75% of FVC
FEV_1	forced expiratory volume in 1 sec
F_IO_2	fraction of inspired oxygen
FM	fibromyalgia
FSH	follicle-stimulating hormone
FTA/ABS	fluorescent treponemal antibody absorption (test)
FTI	free thyroxine index
FUO	fever of unknown origin
FVC	forced vital capacity
GERD	gastroesophageal reflux disease
GFR	glomerular filtration rate
GGT	gamma-glutyltransferase
GH	growth hormone
GHRH	growth hormone–releasing hormone
GI	gastrointestinal
GNRH	gonadotropin-releasing hormone
GN	glomerulonephritis
GU	genitourinary
HAV	hepatitis A virus
Hb	hemoglobin (e.g., Hb S, Hb F, Hb A)
HBcAg	hepatitis B core antigen
HBeAg	hepatatis B e antigen
HBsAg	hepatitis B surface antigen
HBV	hepatitis B virus
HCG	human chorionic gonadotropin
HCL	hairy-cell leukemia
HCO_3	bicarbonate ion
Hct	hematocrit
HDL	high-density lipoprotein
HEENT	head, eyes, ears, nose, and throat
HELLP	hemolysis, elevated liver enzymes, and low platelet (count)
HIV	human immunodeficiency virus
HLA	human leukocyte antigen
HPF	high-power field (on microscopy)
HPV	human papillomavirus

HSV	herpes simplex virus
HTLV I	human T-lymphotrophic virus type I
HTN	hypertension
HUS	hemolytic uremic syndrome
Hx & PE	history and physical examination

IBD	inflammatory bowel disease
ICF	intracellular fluid
ICP	intracranial pressure
ICU	intensive care unit
IDA	iron deficiency anemia
IDDM	insulin-dependent diabetes mellitus
IFN	interferon
Ig	immunoglobulin (eg., IgE, IgG, IgH)
IHSS	idiopathic hypertrophic subaortic stenosis
IL	interleukin (e.g., IL-1, IL-6)
IM	intramuscular, intramuscularly
INR	international normalized ratio
ISI	International Sensitivity Index
ITP	idiopathic thrombocytopenic purpura
IUD	intrauterine device
IV	intravenous, intravenously
IVC	inferior vena cava
IVDU	intravenous drug use
IVP	intravenous pyelogram
IVSS	intravenous soluset

JRA	juvenile rheumatoid arthritis

KS	Kaposi's sarcoma

LAC	lupus anticoagulant
LAE	left atrial enlargement
LAK	lymphokine-activated killer (cells)
LBBB	left bundle branch block
LBP	low back pain
LBW	lean body weight
LDH	lactic dehydrogenase
LDL	low-density lipoproteins
LEMS	Lambert-Eaton myasthenic syndrome
LES	lower esophageal sphincter
LFTs	liver function tests
LGV	lymphogranuloma venereum
LH	luteinizing hormone
LHRH	luteinizing hormone–releasing hormone
LMWH	low-molecular-weight heparins
LUQ	left upper quadrant
LV	left ventricle, left ventricular

LVEDP	left ventricular end-diastolic pressure
LVEF	left ventricular ejection fraction
LVH	left ventricular hypertrophy
MAC	*Mycobacterium avium-intracellulare* complex
MCV	mean cell (or corpuscular) volume
MEN	multiple endocrine neoplasia (syndrome)
MG	myasthenia gravis
MGUS	monoclonal gammapathy of uncertain significance
MI	myocardial infarction
MM	multiple myeloma
MMR	measles, mumps, rubella
MMSE	Mini Mental Status Exam
MRI	magnetic resonance imaging
MS	multiple sclerosis
MSH	melanocyte-stimulating hormone
MVP	mitral valve prolapse
MVV	maximal voluntary ventilation
MW	molecular weight
NCV	nerve conduction velocity
Nd/YAG	neodymium-yttrium aluminum garnet (surgical laser)
NG	nasogastric
NIDDM	non-insulin-dependent diabetes mellitus
NIH	National Institutes of Health
NPH	normal-pressure hydrocephalus
NS	normal saline
NSAID	nonsteroidal anti-inflammatory drug
NSGCT	nonseminomatous germ cell tumors
OA	osteoarthritis
OI	opportunistic infection
OTC	over-the-counter (medications)
PA	pernicious anemia
PAC	premature atrial contraction
PAN	polyarteritis nodosa
PAS	para-aminosalicylic acid
PBC	primary biliary cirrhosis
PCA	patient-controlled analgesia
PCO_2	partial pressure of carbon dioxide
P_aCO_2	partial pressure of carbon dioxide in arterial blood
P_vCO_2	partial pressure carbon dioxide in venous blood
PCP	*Pneumocystis carinii* pneumonia
PCR	polymerase chain reaction
PCWP	pulmonary capillary wedge pressure
PD	peritoneal dialysis
PDA	patent ductus arteriosus

PE	pulmonary embolus
PEEP	positive end-expiratory pressure
PEFR	peak expiratory flow rate
PFTs	pulmonary function tests
PID	pelvic inflammatory disease
PMNs	polymorphonuclear leukocytes
PMR	polymyalgia rheumatica
PO	oral (route)
PO_2	partial pressure of oxygen
P_aO_2	partial pressure of oxygen in arterial blood
P_vO_2	partial pressure of oxygen in venous blood
$P_{(A-a)}O_2$	alveolar-arterial oxygen gradient
PPD	purified protein derivative
PSA	prostate-specific antigen
PSC	primary sclerosing cholangitis
PT	prothrombin time
PTCA	percutaneous transluminal coronary angioplasty
PTH	parathyroid hormone
PTT	partial thromboplastin time
PTU	propylthiouracil
PUD	peptic ulcer disease
PVC	premature ventricular contractions

Q	quaque (Latin for every, each)
QID	four times daily

RA	rheumatoid arthritis
RAE	right atrial enlargement
RAEB	refractory anemia with excess blasts
RAIU	radioactive iodine uptake
RBBB	right bundle branch block
RBC	red blood cell
RES	reticuloendothelial system
RF	rheumatoid factor
RPGN	rapidly progressive glomerulonephritis
RPR	rapid plasma reagin
RTA	renal tubular acidosis
RUQ	right upper quadrant
RV	right ventricle, right ventricular

SBE	subacute bacterial endocarditis
SBP	spontaneous bacterial peritonitis
SC	subcutaneous, subcutaneously
SCC	squamous cell carcinoma
SD	standard deviation
SF	synovial fluid
SIADH	syndrome of inappropriate (secretion of) antidiuretic hormone
SIDS	sudden infant death syndrome

SLE	systemic lupus erythematosus
SSc	systemic sclerosis
STD	sexually transmitted disease
SVC	superior vena cava
SVT	supraventricular tachycardia
T_3	triiodothyronine
T_4	thyroxine
TB	tuberculosis
TBG	throxin-binding globulin
TENS	transcutaneous electrical nerve stimulation
TFT	thyroid function test
TG	triglycerides
THC	tetrahydrocannabinol
TIA	transient ischemic attack
TIBC	total iron-binding capacity
TID	three times daily
TMP/SMX	trimethoprim/sulfamethoxazole
TNF	tumor necrosis factor
TPN	total parenteral nutrition
TRH	thyrotropin-releasing hormone
TSH	thyroid-stimulating hormone (thyrotropin)
TTP	thrombotic thrombocytopenic purpura
TURP	transurethral resection of the prostate
UA	urinalysis
URI	upper respiratory tract infection
UTI	urinary tract infection
UV	ultraviolet
VC	vital capacity
V_D/V_T	ratio of dead space ventilation to total pulmonary ventilation
VDRL	Venereal Disease Research Laboratory
VF	ventricular fibrillation
VIP	vasoactive intestinal polypeptide
VLDL	very low density lipoproteins
V/Q	ventilation perfusion ratio
VSD	ventricular septal defect
VT/V tach	ventricular tachycardia
vWD	von Willebrand's disease
vWF	von Willebrand's factor
WBC	white blood cell
WHO	World Health Organization
WPW	Wolff-Parkinson-White syndrome
ZDV	zidovudine

INDEX